T0190046

Lecture Notes in Computer Science 3765

Commenced Publication in 1973
Founding and Former Series Editors:
Gerhard Goos, Juris Hartmanis, and Jan van Leeuwen

Yanxi Liu   Tianzi Jiang
Changshui Zhang (Eds.)

Computer Vision for Biomedical Image Applications

First International Workshop, CVBIA 2005
Beijing, China, October 21, 2005
Proceedings

 Springer

Volume Editors

Yanxi Liu
Carnegie Mellon University
School of Computer Science
The Robotics Institute
4109 Newell-Simon Hall, 5000 Forbes Ave., Pittsburgh, PA 15213
E-mail: yanxi@cs.cmu.edu

Tianzi Jiang
Chinese Academy of Sciences
National Laboratory of Pattern Recognition
Institute of Automation
100080, Beijing, China
E-mail: jiangtz@nlpr.ia.ac.cn

Changshui Zhang
Tsinghua University
Department of Automation
Beijing,100084, China
E-mail: zcs@mail.tsinghua.edu.cn

Library of Congress Control Number: 2005934416

CR Subject Classification (1998): I.4, I.5, I.3.5-8, I.2.10, J.3, J.6

ISSN   0302-9743
ISBN-10   3-540-29411-2 Springer Berlin Heidelberg New York
ISBN-13   978-3-540-29411-5 Springer Berlin Heidelberg New York

Springer is a part of Springer Science+Business Media

springeronline.com

© Springer-Verlag Berlin Heidelberg 2005
Printed in Germany

Typesetting: Camera-ready by author, data conversion by Scientific Publishing Services, Chennai, India
Printed on acid-free paper   SPIN: 11569541   06/3142   5 4 3 2 1 0

Preface

With the rapid increase in the variety and quantity of biomedical images in recent years, we see a steadily growing number of computer vision technologies applied to biomedical applications. The time is ripe for us to take a closer look at the accomplishments and experiences gained in this research subdomain, and to strategically plan the directions of our future research. The scientific goal of our workshop, "Computer Vision for Biomedical Image Applications: Current Techniques and Future Trends" (CVBIA), is to examine the diverse applications of computer vision to biomedical image applications, considering both current methods and promising new trends. An additional goal is to provide the opportunity for direct interactions between (1) prominent senior researchers and young scientists, including students, postdoctoral associates and junior faculty; (2) local researchers and international leaders in biomedical image analysis; and (3) computer scientists and medical practitioners. Our CVBIA workshop had two novel characteristics: each contributed paper was authored primarily by a young scientist, and the workshop attracted an unusually large number of well-respected invited speakers (and their papers). We had the good fortune of having Dr. Ayache of INRIA, France to talk about "Computational Anatomy and Computational Physiology," Prof. Grimson of MIT to discuss "Analyzing Anatomical Structures: Leveraging Multiple Sources of Knowledge," Dr. Jiang of the Chinese Academy of Sciences to present their work on "Computational Neuroanatomy and Brain Connectivity," Prof. Kanade of CMU to reveal their recent work on "Tracking of Migrating and Proliferating Cells in Phase-Contrast Microscopy Imagery for Tissue Engineering," Prof. Noble of Oxford to answer the question: "Cardiology Meets Image Analysis: Just an Application or Can Image Analysis Usefully Impact Cardiology Practice?," and Prof. Stewart of RPI to summarize "Computer Vision Algorithms for Retina Images."

We received an overwhelming response from the computer vision community to our call for papers. A total of 82 full papers were received from 12 countries. Through careful reviews of each paper by at least three members of our Program Committee, 50 contributed papers were accepted for this volume of the LNCS book series. This large number of paper acceptances reflects the high quality of the submissions.

We received generous support from our sponsors: National Science Foundation of China, Chinese Association for Artificial Intelligence, Siemens Research, Intel Research, and Dr. Enming Song.

A workshop of this size would not be possible without the hard work of many people. In particular, we would like to thank each member of the Program Committee for their prompt and critical reviews, which ensured high standards for this workshop. We would like to express our sincere gratitude to our administrative coordinator, Ms. Janice Brochetti of Carnegie Mellon University, for her dedicated, tireless effort; to Dr. Zhongbao Kou of Tsinghua University for his effective plans; and to Ms. Fang Qian of the National Lab of Pattern Recognition for her care and attention to detail.

Last, but not least, we would like to thank the Advisory Committee and Prof. Stewart. Without their insightful guidance, we would not have made.

We hope our readers will benefit from this timely collection of excellent papers in CVBIA research as much as we enjoyed putting the volume together.

August 2005

Yanxi Liu
Tianzi Jiang
Changshui Zhang

Organization

Chair

Yanxi Liu, Carnegie Mellon University, USA

Local Chairs

Changshui Zhang, Tsinghua University, China
Tianzi Jiang, LNPR, Chinese Academy of Sciences, China

Advisory Board

Nicholas Ayache, INRIA, France
James Duncan, Yale University, USA
Takeo Kanade, Carnegie Mellon University, USA
Stephen M. Pizer, University of North Carolina at Chapel Hill, USA
Ron Kikinis, Harvard Medical School, USA

Program Committee

Howard Aizenstein, University of Pittsburgh Medical Center, USA
Jonas August, Carnegie Mellon University, USA
James Becker, University of Pittsburgh Medical Center, USA
Margrit Betke, Boston University, USA
Owen Carmichael, University of Pittsburgh and CMU, USA
Albert Chung, University of Science and Technology
Christos Davatzikos, University of Pennsylvania, USA
Yong Fan, University of Pennsylvania, USA
Fernando De La Torre Frade, Carnegie Mellon University, USA
Polina Golland, Massachusetts Institute of Technology, USA
Eric Grimson, Massachusetts Institute of Technology, USA
David Hawkes, King's College London, UK
William Higgins, Pennsylvania State University, USA
Tianzi Jiang, NLPR, LNPR, Chinese Academy of Sciences, China
Nicole Lazar, University of Georgia, USA
Shuqian Luo, Capital University of Medical Science, China
Carolyn Meltzer, University of Pittsburgh Medical Center, USA
Alison Noble, Oxford University, UK
Linda Shapiro, University of Washington, USA
Dinggang Shen, University of Pennsylvania, USA

Peng Cheng Shi, University of Science and Technology, Hong Kong, China
Larry Staib, Yale University, USA
George Stetten, University of Pittsburgh and CMU, USA
Charles Stewart, Rensselaer Polytechnic Institute, USA
Rahul Sukthankar, Intel and Carnegie Mellon University, USA
Paul Thompson, University of California, Los Angeles, USA
Max Viergever, Utrecht, Netherlands
Baba Vemuri, University of Florida, USA
Yonmei M. Wang, University of Illinois at Urbana-Champaign, USA
Simon Warfield, Harvard University, USA
William (Sandy) Wells III, Harvard University, USA
James Williams, Siemens Research, USA
Guang-Zhong Yang, Imperial College, London, UK
Faguo Yang, University of Pennsylvania, USA
Xiaolan Zeng, EDDA Technology, Inc., USA
Changshui Zhang, Tsinghua University, China
Tu Zhuowen, Siemens Research, USA

Sponsors

Chinese Association for Artificial Intelligence
Intel Research
National Science Foundation of China
Siemens Research
Dr. Enmin Song

Table of Contents

Computational Anatomy and Computational Physiology for Medical
Image Analysis
  Nicholas Ayache 1

Analyzing Anatomical Structures: Leveraging Multiple Sources
of Knowledge
  Eric Grimson, Polina Golland 3

Advances on Medical Imaging and Computing
  Tianzi Jiang, Xiaobo Li, Gaolong Gong, Meng Liang, Lixia Tian,
  Fuchun Li, Yong He, Yufeng Zang, Chaozhe Zhu, Shuyu Li,
  Songyuan Tang 13

Tracking of Migrating and Proliferating Cells in Phase-Contrast
Microscopy Imagery for Tissue Engineering
  Takeo Kanade, Kang Li 24

Cardiology Meets Image Analysis: Just an Application or Can Image
Analysis Usefully Impact Cardiology Practice?
  J. Alison Noble 25

Computer Vision Algorithms for Retinal Image Analysis: Current
Results and Future Directions
  Charles V. Stewart 31

3D Statistical Shape Models to Embed Spatial Relationship Information
  Jurgen Fripp, Pierrick Bourgeat, Andrea J.U. Mewes,
  Simon K. Warfield, Stuart Crozier, Sébastien Ourselin 51

A Generalized Level Set Formulation of the Mumford-Shah Functional
with Shape Prior for Medical Image Segmentation
  Lishui Cheng, Xian Fan, Jie Yang, Yun Zhu 61

A Hybrid Eulerian-Lagrangian Approach for Thickness,
Correspondence, and Gridding of Annular Tissues
  Kelvin R. Rocha, Anthony J. Yezzi, Jerry L. Prince 72

A Hybrid Framework for Image Segmentation Using Probabilistic
Integration of Heterogeneous Constraints
  Rui Huang, Vladimir Pavlovic, Dimitris N. Metaxas 82

A Learning Framework for the Automatic and Accurate Segmentation
of Cardiac Tagged MRI Images
    Zhen Qian, Dimitris N. Metaxas, Leon Axel 93

A Local Adaptive Algorithm for Microaneurysms Detection in Digital
Fundus Images
    Ke Huang, Michelle Yan 103

A New Coarse-to-Fine Framework for 3D Brain MR Image Registration
    Terrence Chen, Thomas S. Huang, Wotao Yin, Xiang Sean Zhou 114

A New Vision Approach for Local Spectrum Features in Cervical
Images Via 2D Method of Geometric Restriction in Frequency Domain
    Viara Van Raad 125

Active Contours Under Topology Control – Genus Preserving Level Sets
    Florent Ségonne, Jean-Philippe Pons, Eric Grimson,
    Bruce Fischl 135

A Novel Multifaceted Virtual Craniofacial Surgery Scheme Using
Computer Vision
    A.S. Chowdhury, S.M. Bhandarkar, E.W. Tollner, G. Zhang,
    J.C. Yu, E. Ritter 146

A Novel Unsupervised Segmentation Method for MR Brain Images
Based on Fuzzy Methods
    Xian Fan, Jie Yang, Yuanjie Zheng, Lishui Cheng, Yun Zhu 160

A Pattern Classification Approach to Aorta Calcium Scoring
in Radiographs
    Marleen de Bruijne 170

A Topologically Faithful, Tissue-Guided, Spatially Varying Meshing
Strategy for Computing Patient-Specific Head Models for Endoscopic
Pituitary Surgery Simulation
    M.A. Audette, H. Delingette, A. Fuchs, O. Astley, K. Chinzei 178

Applying Prior Knowledge in the Segmentation of 3D Complex
Anatomic Structures
    Hong Shen, Yonggang Shi, Zhigang Peng 189

Automatic Extraction of Femur Contours from Hip X-Ray Images
    Ying Chen, Xianhe Ee, Wee Kheng Leow, Tet Sen Howe 200

Automatic Landmarking of 2d Medical Shapes Using the Growing
Neural Gas Network
 Anastassia Angelopoulou, Alexandra Psarrou,
 José García Rodríguez, Kenneth Revett 210

Biomedical Image Classification with Random Subwindows and
Decision Trees
 Raphaël Marée, Pierre Geurts, Justus Piater, Louis Wehenkel 220

Combining Binary Classifiers for Automatic Cartilage Segmentation
in Knee MRI
 Jenny Folkesson, Ole Fogh Olsen, Paola Pettersen, Erik Dam,
 Claus Christiansen 230

Computer-Aided Diagnosis (CAD) for Cervical Cancer Screening
and Diagnosis: A New System Design in Medical Image Processing
 Wenjing Li, Viara Van Raad, Jia Gu, Ulf Hansson,
 Johan Hakansson, Holger Lange, Daron Ferris 240

Constrained Surface Evolutions for Prostate and Bladder Segmentation
in CT Images
 Mikael Rousson, Ali Khamene, Mamadou Diallo, Juan Carlos Celi,
 Frank Sauer 251

Curvilinear Structure Based Mammographic Registration
 Lionel C.C. Wai, Michael Brady 261

Deformable Registration for Generating Dissection Image of an
Intestine from Annular Image Sequence
 Suchit Pongnumkul, Ryusuke Sagawa, Tomio Echigo, Yasushi Yagi ... 271

Distance-Intensity for Image Registration
 Rui Gan, Albert C. S. Chung 281

Efficient Population Registration of 3D Data
 Lilla Zöllei, Erik Learned-Miller, Eric Grimson, William Wells 291

Efficient Symbolic Signatures for Classifying Craniosynostosis Skull
Deformities
 H. Jill Lin, Salvador Ruiz-Correa, Raymond W. Sze,
 Michael L. Cunningham, Matthew L. Speltz, Anne V. Hing,
 Linda G. Shapiro 302

Elastic Interaction Models for Active Contours and Surfaces
 Albert C.S. Chung, Yang Xiang, Jian Ye, W.K. Law 314

Estimating Diameters of Pulmonary Nodules with
Competition-Diffusion and Robust Ellipsoid Fit
  Toshiro Kubota, Kazunori Okada 324

Fast 3D Brain Segmentation Using Dual-Front Active Contours with
Optional User-Interaction
  Hua Li, Anthony Yezzi, Laurent D. Cohen 335

Improved Motion Correction of fMRI Time-Series Corrupted with
Major Head Movement Using Extended Motion-Corrected Independent
Component Analysis
  Rui Liao, Martin McKeown, Jeffrey Krolik 346

Local or Global Minima: Flexible Dual-Front Active Contours
  Hua Li, Anthony Yezzi 356

Locally Switching Between Cost Functions in Iterative Non-rigid
Registration
  *William Mullally, Margrit Betke, Carissa Bellardine,
  Kenneth Lutchen* 367

Multi-modal Image Registration by Quantitative-Qualitative Measure
of Mutual Information (Q-MI)
  Hongxia Luan, Feihu Qi, Dinggang Shen 378

Multi-scale Vessel Boundary Detection
  Hüseyin Tek, Alper Ayvacı, Dorin Comaniciu 388

Non-rigid Registration for Colorectal Cancer MR Images
  Sarah L. Bond, J. Michael Brady 399

Quantizing Calcification in the Lumbar Aorta on 2-D Lateral X-Ray
Images
  *Lars A. Conrad-Hansen, Marleen de Bruijne, François Lauze,
  Laszlo B. Tanko, Mads Nielsen* 409

Real-Time Simulation of Deformable Soft Tissue Based on Mass-Spring
and Medial Representation
  Shaoting Zhang, Lixu Gu, Pengfei Huang, Jianfeng Xu 419

Registration of 3D Angiographic and X-Ray Images Using Sequential
Monte Carlo Sampling
  Charles Florin, James Williams, Ali Khamene, Nikos Paragios 427

Registration of PET and MR Hand Volumes Using Bayesian Networks
Derek Magee, Steven Tanner, Michael Waller, Dennis McGonagle,
Alan P. Jeavons 437

Segmentation and Volume Representation Based on Spheres for
Non-rigid Registration
Jorge Rivera-Rovelo, Eduardo Bayro-Corrochano 449

Segmentation of 3D CT Volume Images Using a Single 2D Atlas
Feng Ding, Wee Kheng Leow, Shih-Chang Wang 459

Segmenting Brain Tumors with Conditional Random Fields and
Support Vector Machines
Chi-Hoon Lee, Mark Schmidt, Albert Murtha, Aalo Bistritz,
Jöerg Sander, Russell Greiner 469

Segmenting Cardiopulmonary Images Using Manifold Learning with
Level Sets
Qilong Zhang, Robert Pless 479

Shape Based Segmentation of Anatomical Structures in Magnetic
Resonance Images
Kilian M. Pohl, John Fisher, Ron Kikinis, W. Eric L. Grimson,
William M. Wells 489

Simultaneous Segmentation and Motion Recovery in 3D Cardiac Image
Analysis
Ling Zhuang, Huafeng Liu, Wei Chen, Hujun Bao, Pengcheng Shi ... 499

Spatial and Temporal Analysis for Optical Imaging Data Using CWT
and tICA
Yadong Liu, Guohua Zang, Fayi Liu, Lirong Yan, Ming Li,
Zongtan Zhou, Dewen Hu 508

Stereo Matching and 3-D Reconstruction for Optic Disk Images
Zhang Kai, Xu Xi, Zhang Li, Wang Guoping 517

Total Variation Based Iterative Image Reconstruction
Guoqiang Yu, Liang Li, Jianwei Gu, Li Zhang 526

Voronoi-Based Segmentation of Cells on Image Manifolds
Thouis R. Jones, Anne Carpenter, Polina Golland 535

Parcellating the Intra-splenium Based on the Traced Fiber from
Tractography
Gaolang Gong, Tianzi Jiang, Sheng Xie, Fuchun Lin 544

Motion Compensation and Plane Tracking for Kinematic MR-Imaging
  Daniel Bystrov, Vladimir Pekar, Kirsten Meetz, Heinrich Schulz,
  Thomas Netsch 551

Author Index 561

Computational Anatomy and Computational Physiology for Medical Image Analysis

Nicholas Ayache

Research Director,
Epidaure/Asclepios Laboratory,
INRIA, 2004 Route des Lucioles, 06902, Sophia-Antipolis, France

Medical image analysis brings about a revolution to the medicine of the 21st century, introducing a collection of powerful new tools designed to better assist the clinical diagnosis and to model, simulate, and guide more efficiently the patient's therapy. A new discipline has emerged in computer science, closely related to others like computer vision, computer graphics, artificial intelligence and robotics.

In this talk, I will describe the increasing role of computational models of anatomy and physiology to guide the interpretation of complex series of medical images, and illustrate my presentation with three applications: the modeling and analysis of 1) brain variability from a large database of cerebral images, 2) tumor growth in the brain and 3) heart function from a combined exploitation of cardiac images and electrophysiology.

I will conclude with a presentation of some promising trends, including the analysis of *in vivo* microscopic images.

References (also available at http://www-sop.inria.fr/epidaure/BIBLIO/)

- N. Ayache, editor. *Computational Models for the Human Body*, Handbook of Numerical Analysis (Ph. Ciarlet series editor). Elsevier, 2004. 670 pages.
- V Arsigny, P Fillard, X Pennec, and N Ayache. *Fast and Simple Calculus on Tensors in the Log-Euclidean Framework*. In J. Duncan and G. Gerig, editors, Proceedings of MICCAI'05, LNCS, October 2005. Springer Verlag.
- O. Clatz, P.Y. Bondiau, H. Delingette, G. Malandain, M. Sermesant, S. K. Warfield, and N. Ayache. *In Silico Tumor Growth: Application to Glioblastomas;* MICCAI, LNCS 3217, pp 337-345,Springer Verlag, 2004. Longer version accepted by IEEE Trans. on Medical Imaging, in press 2005.
- H. Delingette, X. Pennec, L. Soler, J. Marescaux, N. Ayache, *Computational Models for Image Guided, Robot-Assisted and Simulated Medical Interventions,* Proc. of the IEEE, 2006, submitted.
- J. Duncan and N. Ayache. *Medical Image Analysis: Progress over two decades and the challenges ahead*. IEEE Transactions on Pattern Analysis and Machine Intelligence, 22(1):85-106, 2000.
- P. Fillard, V. Arsigny, X. Pennec, P.Thompson, and N. Ayache. *Extrapolation of Sparse Tensor Fields: Application to the Modeling of Brain Variability*. IPMI, LNCS, Springer, 2005.
- G Le Goualher, A Perchant, M Genet, C Cave, B Viellerobe, F Berier, B Abrat, and N Ayache. *Towards Optical Biopsies with an Integrated Fibered Confocal Fluorescence Microscope*. In Proc. of MICCAI'04, volume 3217 of LNCS, pages 761-768, 2004. Springer Verlag.

Y. Liu, T. Jiang, and C. Zhang (Eds.): CVBIA 2005, LNCS 3765, pp 1-2, 2005

- V. Moreau-Villéger, H. Delingette, M. Sermesant, H. Ashikaga, O. Faris, E. McVeigh, N. Ayache, *Estimating Local Apparent Conductivity with a 2-D Electrophysiological Model of the Heart*; Proc. of Functional Imaging and Modeling of the Heart, Springer, LNCS, June 2005.
- X. Pennec, P. Fillard, and N. Ayache. *A Riemannian Framework for Tensor Computing.* International Journal of Computer Vision, 65(1), October 2005. Also INRIA Research Report 5255.
- M. Sermesant, H. Delingette, and N. Ayache. *An Electromechanical Model of the Myocardium for Cardiac Image Analysis and Medical Simulation.* Res. Rep. 5395, INRIA, 2004. sub.to IEEE-TMI.
- M. Sermesant, K. Rhode, G. Sanchez-Ortiz, O. Camara, R. Andriantsimiavona, S. Hegde, D. Rueckert, P. Lambiase, C. Bucknall, E. Rosenthal, H. Delingette, D. Hill, N. Ayache, R. Razavi. *Simulation of cardiac pathologies using an electromechanical biventricular model and XMR interventional imaging.* Medical Image Analysis. 2005, In Press.

Analyzing Anatomical Structures: Leveraging Multiple Sources of Knowledge

Eric Grimson and Polina Golland

Computer Science and Artificial Intelligence Laboratory,
Massachusetts Institute of Technology,
Cambridge MA 02139

Abstract. Analysis of medical images, especially the extraction of anatomical structures, is a critical component of many medical applications: surgical planning and navigation, and population studies of anatomical shapes for tracking disease progression are two primary examples. We summarize recent trends in segmentation and analysis of shapes, highlighting how different sources of information have been factored into current approaches.

1 Background and Motivation

The application of computer vision techniques to detailed anatomical information from volumetric medical imaging is changing medical practice, in areas ranging from surgery to clinical assessment. Automated reconstruction of precise patient-specific models of anatomic structures from medical images is becoming *de rigeur* for many surgical procedures, disease studies, and clinical evaluation of therapy effectiveness.

For example, neurosurgeons often use navigational aids linked to labeled imagery in order to localize targets. Even the registration to the patient of unprocessed volumetric imagery, such as MRI, is of value to the surgeon. It allows her to see beneath exposed surfaces to localize nearby structures, and to track instruments during minimally invasive procedures, providing faster navigation through narrow openings. But raw imagery is often insufficient, since it is often cluttered and filled with subtle boundaries. By segmenting out distinct anatomical structures, by co-registering functional, biomechanical, or other information to those segmented structures, and by relating all that information to the patient's position, the surgeon's ability to visualize the entire surgical space is greatly enhanced, as is her ability to avoid critical structures while ensuring that targeted tissue is fully excised. This allows surgeons to execute surgeries more quickly, and with less impact on neighboring tissues. Hence, extracting anatomical models from imagery is a key element of emerging surgical techniques. An example is shown in Figure 1.

Understanding healthy development and disease progression also can benefit from computational methods that extract precise models of anatomical substructures from volumetric imagery. For example, in studies of schizophrenia accurately measuring shapes of cortical and subcortical structures and identifying significant differences in shape between diseased and normal populations provides an invaluable tool for

Y. Liu, T. Jiang, and C. Zhang (Eds.): CVBIA 2005, LNCS 3765, pp. 3–12, 2005.

understanding the disease's progression. This is particularly true when shapes of structures also can be tracked over time. In Alzheimer's disease, understanding the relationship between changes in shape and volume of neural structures in correlation with other factors, such as genetic markers or distributions of functional information during specific mental tasks, may provide neuroscientists with computational tools for deepening the understanding of the disease, and its progression. Hence, extracting anatomical models from imagery, especially group statistical properties of those models, is an essential component of emerging neuroscience techniques.

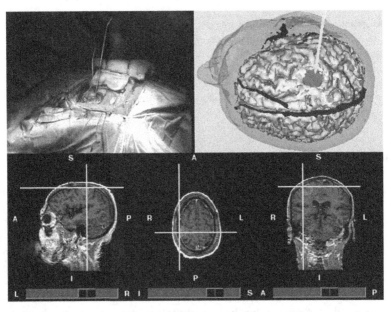

Fig. 1. Example of segmented images in surgical navigation. Segmented structures are overlaid on cross-sectional views of an MRI scan (bottom). The position of a surgical probe is tracked relative to the patient and the segmented scans.

To enhance surgical practice, and to extend neuroscientific understanding of diseases, we need models of shapes, and thus we need segmentation algorithms to extract structures from multi-modal images. These methods have evolved in capability, as increasingly sophisticated models of anatomy and of the image formation process have been embedded within them. Early methods simply relied intensity thresholds to separate structures. These methods fail when confronted with bias fields in the imagery, so approaches were developed that either model the field as a smooth function (e.g., a polynomial) or employ non-parametric techniques, (e.g., Expectation Maximization (EM)), to account for image acquisition artifacts and to create statistical models of tissue response. Because individual voxel responses can be consistent with several tissue types, especially in the presence of noise, Markov Random Field (MRF) methods have been added to impose local continuity. They capture the notion that nearby labels for tissue type should influence the labeling of a particular voxel, since tissue is generally locally continuous. Atlas-based methods capture more global constraints, especially the expected position and spatial extent of structures, by providing spatial templates in which to interpret voxel intensities, either by defining prior probabilities on tissue type as a function of position, or by defining initial positions for boundaries of structures, which are then warped to best match the intensity data.

Structural measurements in morphological studies have seen a parallel refinement. Early methods simply recorded volumes of structures, measurements that have improved in specificity as segmentation methods enabled increasingly detailed and accurate delineation of the structures of interest. However, volume alone is often insufficient to detect changes in a structure or to differentiate different populations. Often a difference in structure between two distinct populations is localized in specific components of that structure; or the progression of a disease will result in variations in a particular component of a structure.

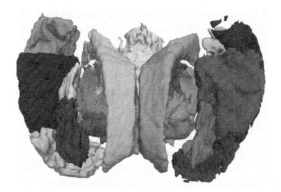

Fig. 2. An example segmentation from a neurosurgical case. Thirty-one different brain structures have been segmented using MRF-based voxel classification methods. The goals of the proposed project include improving on such segmentation by adding shape constraints. While these segmentations are a good start, there are residual errors near subtle boundaries that would be improved by adding shape information.

Thus, we believe that a natural next stage in the evolution of segmentation methods and associated measurements of structures is the incorporation of shape information into the process. To do this, we need to learn the typical shapes of structures and their statistical variation across normal populations. We believe that this information can be extracted from sets of training images, and that the resulting statistical distributions on shape can be used to guide segmentation of new images. Moreover, if we can capture shape distributions, we can use them as a comparative too: to identify differences in shape between populations or to track changes in shape with time.

We have suggested that capturing statistics of shape can aid in segmenting new scans. One clear application of this tool is in surgical planning and guidance. By providing the surgeon with a detailed reconstruction of the anatomy, she can plan access to the operative site, and by registering the model to the actual position of the patient, she can track the position of surgical instruments relative to structures in the

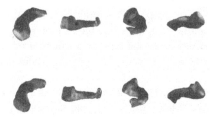

Fig. 3. Visualization of the shape differences in the right hippocampus between the schizophrenia group and the normal controls captured by a discriminative model learned from example images. Using the learned classifier based on the two groups, one can examine the amount of deformation, from blue (moving inwards) to red (moving outwards) needed to shift a normal example towards the schizophrenia group, and vice versa.

reconstructed model. Figure 2 shows an example segmentation of a neuroimage into 31 structures derived using atlas-based segmentation, followed by a MRF label regularization.

Shape based methods can provide more than just better segmentation, however. The shape analysis methods also may improve the quantitative assessment of anatomical development during disease progression. In particular, we can create shape-based classifiers, using machine learning tools applied to our shape distributions, to distinguish between different populations. Such classifiers not only provide a mechanism for assigning new instances to the appropriate class, they can be used to determine what parts of the shape change in significant ways between the two classes, as illustrated in Figure 3 for a study of hippocampal shape in schizophrenia. The colormap indicates the amount of deformation required to make the normal hippocampus shown here be likely to come from the schizophrenia group with respect to the trained classifier function. Such visualization techniques allow one to isolate shape changes to key elements of a structure.

2   Classes of Segmentation Methods

Segmentation is a central component in many medical image analysis applications. It provides a fundamental basis for surgical planning, surgical navigation, analysis of disease progression, and therapy evaluation in essence by extracting geometrically accurate, patient-specific reconstructions of anatomical structures, segmentation provides a foundation for understanding structural correlates with disease and for visualizing and planning interventions. Unfortunately, segmentation is inherently under-constrained: the image intensity alone is often insufficient to delineate anatomical structures. Human operators employ their knowledge of anatomy when they perform segmentation; thus incorporating such knowledge into the automatic methods has improved the quality of segmentation results. However, the problem of accurate automatic segmentation of neuroimages is not yet fully solved, and we believe that building computational mechanisms for modeling anatomical shape and its variability will significantly improve segmentation accuracy.

To understand the role of shape in segmentation, we find it useful to group image segmentation methods into three broad classes: voxel classification, atlas-based segmentation, and boundary localization. The output of the first class of algorithms is a volume in which each voxel is labeled with an associated tissue class. The second group infers segmentation through registering a previously segmented image (atlas) to a new input image. Algorithms in the third class are based on deformable contours that are evolved to explain the novel image.

2.1 Voxel Classification

The original methods in this class used intensity information at a specific voxel to decide on the tissue type enclosed by that voxel [1,2,3,4]. These methods measured intensity responses for different tissue classes from training data (such as voxels selected by a user based on uniqueness of tissue type) and derived a set of optimal thresholds for assigning a tissue class to each voxel. This approach has been refined by our group and other researchers to deal with non-linear gain (bias) artifacts by simultaneously solving for a smooth spatially variant gain field and the identification of tissues at voxels [5,6,7]. To handle noise and uncertainty in the intensity information, the next group of algorithms in this class incorporated local geometric information by employing Markov Random Field (MRF) models [8,9]. The idea is to use information about tissue likelihoods at neighboring voxels to influence the assignment of a tissue label at a specific voxel. The original formulation has been refined by several groups, including ours, to include local estimation of individual and pairwise priors from a set of scans previously segmented by an expert and registered together to form an atlas. This probabilistic atlas is then registered to a new scan to transform the likelihoods into appropriate locations [10,11].

Algorithms in this class provide excellent quality segmentation for gross voxel assignment into three large classes: white matter, gray matter, and cerebrospinal fluid (CSF). The results can be used for analysis of overall (total volume) tissue changes in an individual or a population, but since the methods operate on an implicit representation of the anatomy as a discrete map of tissue labels, they do not produce an explicit representation of the structure boundaries. Instead, an additional step of extracting the boundary surfaces is required if we are to utilize the results of voxel classification in visualization for surgical planning and navigation, or population studies focusing on anatomical shape. Moreover, explicit shape models that involve global descriptors do not easily fit within this intrinsically local framework. Recent work focuses on more detailed segmentation into individual subcortical structures and cortical parcelation by constructing location-specific Markov priors for every structure [10,12] effectively reducing the representation of the anatomy to the level of individual voxels and voxel neighborhoods.

2.2 Atlas-Based Segmentation

The methods in this class seek to induce a segmentation of a new scan by deforming a given segmented atlas image to the novel grayscale image and by applying the estimated transformation, or warp, to the label map of the atlas. The atlas generally includes at least one scan that has been carefully annotated, perhaps along with likelihoods used to describe the variance seen across a population. If the atlas can be successfully matched to a novel scan, then all information present in the atlas, such as the tissue labels, is known with respect to the new image. The registration process is often reduced to an optimization of a weighted sum of two terms: the quality of the image fit, i.e., how well the atlas grayscale image matches the novel scan, and a penalty term on the amount of deformation between the atlas and the image. The deformations required to adequately match the atlas to novel scans are typically sufficiently high-dimensional, requiring a substantial amount of regularization. Examples of regularization methods include representing the deformation field as a sum of basis vectors, which allows for a coarse to fine solution [13,14], or representing the large deformation as a concatenation of a set of small deformations that more efficiently fit into the optimization framework [15] or employing a cascade of similarity groups beginning with rigid transformations, and subsequently allowing more flexible warps, such as piece-wise affine [16,17] or elastic [18,19]. Tissue deformation models can also assist in regularizing the deformation field when dealing with anatomy containing very different structures such as bone, muscle, and CSF [20,21]. Depending on the image properties, the quality of the fit is evaluated using image intensity, its gradient, texture measures, or discrete landmark points. A comprehensive survey of relevant registration techniques can be found in [22].

The algorithms in this class have also been used to map tissue class priors onto a new scan as an initialization step in voxel classification methods that further refine the initial segmentation by evoking MRF-based segmentation [10,11]. Like the voxel classification algorithms, these methods operate on the implicit voxel-based representation of anatomy and thus take little advantage of information on anatomical shape variability. They typically rely on the intensity information and the inherent geometric properties of the mapping (continuity, smoothness, etc.) to guide registration. Active Appearance Models [23,24] are a notable exception, as they achieve registration of a template to a novel image based on the shape variability model. However, we group this particular method with the boundary detection algorithms, as it manipulates an explicit boundary representation both for shape modeling and for registration.

2.3 Boundary Detection

Rather than label each voxel by tissue type, the methods in this group search for boundaries between different tissue types. Standard methods use deformable contours, or ``snakes'' [25]: they evolve a contour (or a surface in 3D), typically by shrinking or expanding it in proportion to its local curvature, until it reaches a strong intensity boundary. Robust variants that use regularization to reduce the sensitivity to noise include balloons [26], t-snakes [27], and pedal snakes [28].

Boundary evolution techniques explicitly manipulate the object boundary surface and therefore lend themselves naturally to shape-based extensions. The Active Shape Models method [29,30] extracts a set of corresponding points on the outline of every training example and employs Principal Component Analysis (PCA) to build a linear model of variation, typically keeping only a few principal components. The resulting probabilistic model is then used to constrain the space of deformations of the ``representative'' example (mean shape) when matching it to a new image. In addition to the variance of point positions, Active Appearance Models [23,24] include the intensity distributions over the object. The model fitting stage searches over the eigen-coefficients with the goal of matching the grayscale values of the model and the image. This framework has also been extended to multi-shape segmentation, where the statistical model captures shape of several structures, as well as their relative position and orientation, helping to overcome poor local intensity contrast [31]. Variants of this approach have been demonstrated that manipulate parametric representations of the boundary -- the Fourier descriptors in 2D [32, 33] and the spherical harmonics in 3D [34] -- by transferring the problem of modeling and template matching into the space of the representation coefficients instead of the boundary points.

The level-set implementation of curve evolution [35,36] overcomes several shortcomings of the traditional snakes. It is more robust to initialization, allows topology changes, and is more stable numerically as it operates on the volumetric grid, thus eliminating the need for re-parameterization of the snake. Similarly to the original snakes, the level-set implementation can be augmented to include prior shape information in steering the evolving boundary towards the ``typical" shape. Examples of application-specific shape constraints include coupled evolution of two surfaces for cortical segmentation [37], or topology preservation of the resulting surface through local constraints [38,39]. We demonstrated a level-set counterpart of the Active Shape Models by applying PCA to the signed distance transforms of the training examples and by introducing a term into the evolution dynamics that ``pulls" the evolving distance transform towards the most likely shape under the probability distribution obtained through PCA [40,41,42]. A multi-shape segmentation based on this principle has recently been demonstrated by our and other groups [43,44].

3 Next Steps in Segmentation

To summarize, segmentation methods have seen a series of developments, each stage incorporating additional information. Thus, early methods simply relied on intensity thresholds to separate structures. These methods fail when confronted with bias fields in the imagery, so approaches were developed that either model the field as a smooth function or employ non-parametric techniques to account for image acquisition artifacts and to create statistical models of tissue response. Because individual voxel responses can be consistent with several tissue types, especially in the presence of noise, Markov Random Field (MRF) methods have been added to impose local continuity. They capture the notion that nearby labels for tissue type should influence the labeling of a particular voxel, since tissue is generally locally continuous. Atlas-based methods capture more global constraints, especially the expected position and spatial extent of structures, by providing spatial templates in which to interpret voxel intensities, either by defining prior probabilities on tissue type as a function of position, or by defining initial positions for boundaries of structures, which are then warped to best match the intensity data. Finally, template-based segmentation has served as a basis for most methods that incorporate prior shape information into segmentation. Both the original deformable contour methods and the more recent level-set implementations have been augmented with probabilistic shape models that modify the evolution of the boundary.

Although considerable progress has been made in creating sophisticated segmentation algorithms and in analyzing populations of segmented structures to capture statistical models of variation, important challenges remain. Key among these are as follows:

- methods that robustly leverage shape information to enhance segmentation;
- a demonstration that shape information significantly improves the quality of segmentation;
- a demonstration that such improved segmentation provides an added value in surgical planning and navigation;
- methods that capture statistical variations in distributions of shape information;
- a demonstration that these statistical models can be used to create classifiers that distinguish between diseased and normal populations;
- a demonstration that classifiers based on shape differences are more accurate than simple volumetric measures;
- methods that use these classifiers to visualize differences in shapes of populations; and
- using the results of the statistical analysis to find correlations between disease states and changes in shapes of structures.

References

1. Cline, H., Lorensen, W., Kikinis, R., Jolesz, F., Three-dimensional segmentation of MR images of the head using probability and connectivity. Journal of Computer Assisted Tomography, 14(6):1037-1045, 1990.
2. Kohn, M.I., Tanna, N.K, Hermann, G.T., Resnick, S.M., Mozley, P.D., Gur, R.E., Alavi, A., Zimmerman, R.A., Gur, R.C., Analysis of brain and cerebrospinal fluid volumes with MR imaging. Part I. Methods, reliability, and validation. Radiology, 178:115-122, 1991.
3. Lim, L.O., Pfefferbaum, A., Segmentation of MR brain images into cerebrospinal fluid spaces, white and gray matter. J. Comput. Assisted Tomography. 13:588 1989.
4. Vannier, M.W., Pilgram, T.K., Speidal, C.M., Neumann, L.R., Rickman, D.L., Schertz, L.D., Validation of magnetic resonance imaging (MRI) multispectral tissue classification. Computer Medical Imaging and Graphics, 15:217- 223, 1991.
5. Brechbuhler, C., Gerig, G., Szekely, G., Compensation of spatial inhomogeneity in MRI based on a multi-valued image model and a parametric bias estimate. In: Proc. VBC'96, LNCS 1131:141-146, Springer, 1996.
6. Wells, W., Grimson, W.E.L., Kikinis, R., Jolesz, F., Statistical intensity correlation and segmentation of MRI Data. Visualization in Biomedical Computing, 1994
7. Van Leemput, K., Maes, F., Vanermeulen, D., Suetens, P., Automated model-based bias field correction of MR images of the brain, IEEE TMI, 18(10): 885–895, 1999.
8. Kapur, T., Grimson, W.E.L., Wells, W.M., Kikinis, R., Enhanced spatial priors for segmentation of magnetic resonance imagery. Proceedings MICCAI 457-468, 1998.
9. Leahy, R., Hebert, T., Lee, R., Applications of Markov random field models in medical imaging. In Proceedings of IMPI'89, 1-14, 1989.

10. Fischl, B., Salat, D.H., Busa, E., Albert, M., Dieterich, M., Haselgrove, C., van der Kouwe, A., Killiany, R., Kennedy, D., Klaveness, S., Montillo, A., Makris, N., Rosen, B., Dale, A.M., Whole brain segmentation: Automated labeling of neuroanatomical structures in the human brain, Neuron, 33, 2002.

11. Pohl, K.M., Wells, W.M., Guimond, A., Kasai, K., Shenton, M.E., Kikinis, R., Grimson, W.E.L., Warfield, S.K., Incorporating non-rigid registration into expectation maximization algorithm to segment MR images, Fifth MICCAI, Tokyo, Japan, pp. 564-572, 2002.

12. Pohl, K.M., Bouix, S., Kikinis, R., Grimson, W.E.L., Anatomical guided segmentation with non-stationary tissue class distributions in an Expectation-Maximization Framework, 2004 IEEE International Symposium on Biomedical Imaging, Arlington, VA, 2004, 81-84.

13. Christensen, G., Rabbitt, R., Miller, M., Deformable templates using large deformation kinematics. IEEE Trans. on Image Processing 5(10):1435-1447, 1996.

14. Christensen, G., Consistent linear-elastic transformations for image matching. IPMI 1999.

15. Christensen, G.E., He, J., Consistent nonlinear elastic image registration, IEEE MMBIA, Kauai, Hawaii, Dec. 2001, pp. 37-43.

16. Collins, D.L., Holmes, C.J., Peters, T.M., Evans, A.C., Automatic 3D model-based neuroanatomical segmentation, Human Brain Mapping, 3(3):190-208, 1995.

17. Grenander, G., Miller, M., Representations of knowledge in complex systems. Journal of the Royal Statistical Society B, 56:249-603, 1993.

18. Bajcsy, R., Kovacic, S., Multiresolution elastic matching. Computer Vision, Graphics, and Image Processing, 46:1-21, 1989.

19. Warfield, S., Robatino, A., Dengler, J., Jolesz, F., Kikinis, R. Nonlinear registration and template driven segmentation. in brain warping. Ed. Arthur W. Toga, (Progressive Publishing Alternatives) Ch.4:67-84, 1998.

20. Edwards, P., Hill, D., Little, J., Hawkes, D., Deformation for image-guided interventions using a three component tissue model. Medical Image Analysis, 2(4): 355-367, 1998.

21. Little, J., Hill, D., Hawkes, D., Deformations Incorporating Rigid Structures. Mathematical Methods in Biomedical Image Analysis, 1996.

22. Maintz, J., Viergever, M., A survey of medical image registration. Medical Image Analysis, 2(1):1-36, 1998.

23. Cootes, T.F., Edwards, G.J., Taylor, C.J., Active appearance models. In Proceedings of the European Conference on Computer Vision. 2:484-498, 1998.

24. Cootes, T.F., Edwards, G.J., Taylor, C.J., Active appearance models. IEEE Transactions on Pattern Analysis and Machine Intelligence. 23(6):681 685, 2001.

25. Kass, M., Witkin, A., Terzopoulos, D., Snakes: Active contour models. IJCV 1:321-331, 1988.

26. Cohen, L., On active contour models and balloons. CVGIP: IU, 53(2):211-218, 1991.

27. McInerney, T., Terzopoulos, D., Medical image segmentation using topologically adaptable surfaces.   Conf. Computer Vision, Virtual Reality, and Robotics in Medicine and Medical Robotics and Computer-Assisted Surgery (CVRMed-MRCAS), 23-32, 1997.

28. Guo, Y., Vemuri, B., Hybrid geometric active models for shape recovery in medical images. Int'l Conf. Inf. Proc. in Med. Imaging, pages 112-125, Springer-Verlag, 1999.

29. Cootes, T., Taylor, C., Cooper, D., Graham, J., Training models of shape from sets of examples. Proceedings British Machine Vision Conference, 9-18, Springer-Verlag, 1992.

30. Cootes, T., Taylor, C.., Cooper, D., Graham, J., Active shape models - their training and application. Computer Vision and Image Understanding, 1995.

31. Cootes, T., Beeston, C., Edwards, G., Taylor, C., Unified framework for atlas matching using active appearance models. Information Processing in Medical Imaging 1999.

32. Wang, Y., Staib, L., Boundary finding with correspondence using statistical shape models. CVPR 1998.
33. Szekely, G., Kelemen, A., Brechbuler, C., Gerig, G., Segmentation of 2D and 3D objects from MRI volume data using constrained elastic deformations of flexible fourier contour and surface models. Medical Image Analysis, 1(1):19-34, 1996.
34. Kelemen, A., Szekely, G., Gerig, G., Three-dimensional model-based segmentation. In Proceedings of IEEE International Workshop on Model Based 3D Image Analysis, Bombay, India, 87-96, 1998.
35. Caselles, V., Kimmel, R., Sapiro, G., Geodesic active contours. IJCV, 22(1):61-79, 1997.
36. Kichenassamy, A., Kumar, A., Olver, P., Tannenbaum, A., Yezzi, A., Gradient flows and geometric active contour models. In Proc. IEEE ICCV, 810-815, 1995.
37. Zeng, X., Staib, L.H., Schultz, R.T., Duncan, J.S., Segmentation and measurement of the cortex from 3D MR images using coupled surfaces propagation. IEEE TMI, 18(10), 1999.
38. Han, X., Xu, C., Prince, J.L., A topology preserving level set method for geometric deformable models, IEEE Trans. PAMI, 25(6):755-768, 2003.
39. Ségonne, F., Grimson, E., Fischl, B., A Genetic algorithm for the topology correction of cortical surfaces, IPMI 2005
40. Leventon, M., Grimson, W.E.L., Faugeras, O., Statistical shape influence in geodesic active contours. CVPR, 2000.
41. Leventon, M., Faugeras, O., Grimson, W.E.L., Wells, W.M., Level set based segmentation with intensity and curvature priors. MMBIA, 2000.
42. Tsai, A., Yezzi, A., Willsky, A.S., A curve evolution approach to smoothing and segmentation using the Mumford-Shah functional. CVPR 2000: 1119-1124
43. Tsai, A., Wells, W., Tempany, C., Grimson, E., Willsky, A., Coupled Multi-shape model and mutual information for medical image segmentation, In Proceedings IPMI, LNCS 2732:185-197, 2003.
44. Yang, J., Staib, L.H., Duncan, J.S., Neighbor-constrained segmentation with 3d deformable models. In Proceedings of Information Processing in Medical Imaging (IPMI'03), LNCS 2732:198-209, 2003.
45. Pohl, K.M., Warfield, S.K., Kikinis, R., Grimson, W.E.L., Wells, W.M., Coupling statistical segmentation and PCA shape modeling, MICCAI, LNCS 3216, Springer 2004, 151-159.

Advances on Medical Imaging and Computing

Tianzi Jiang, Xiaobo Li, Gaolong Gong, Meng Liang, Lixia Tian, Fuchun Li,
Yong He, Yufeng Zang, Chaozhe Zhu, Shuyu Li, and Songyuan Tang

National Laboratory of Pattern Recognition, Institute of Automation,
Chinese Academy of Sciences, Beijing 100080, P. R. China
jiangtz@nlpr.ia.ac.cn

Abstract. In this article, we present some advances on medical imaging and
computing at the National Laboratory of Pattern Recognition (NLPR) in the
Chinese Academy of Sciences. The first part is computational neuroanatomy.
Several novel methods on segmentations of brain tissue and anatomical
substructures, brain image registration, and shape analysis are presented. The
second part consists of brain connectivity, which includes anatomical
connectivity based on diffusion tensor imaging (DTI), functional and effective
connectivity with functional magnetic resonance imaging (fMRI). It focuses on
abnormal patterns of brain connectivity of patients with various brain disorders
compared with matched normal controls. Finally, some prospects and future
research directions in this field are also given.

1 Introduction

It is well known that information technology and biomedical technology are two of
the hottest sciences in twenty-first century. Medical imaging is the convergence of
them. Under such a trend, the Division of Medical Imaging and Computing (MIC) at
the National Laboratory of Pattern Recognition (NLPR) in the Chinese Academy of
Sciences was established in 2001. It is a new group that brings together
multidisciplinary expertise in computer science, mathematics, physics, medical
imaging, medicine, and neuroscience. It pursues a scientifically coherent program of
internationally competitive research in Quantitative Imaging, Image and Signal
Computing, and Medical Computer Vision - building on established strengths in these
areas. Three major fields have been involved. One is Computational Neuroanatomy
(especially on relationships between anatomical abnormalities and mental diseases)
including brain tissue segmentation of MR images, intra- and inter-modality image
registration, automatic lesion detection and segmentation, brain structure
segmentation, registration and shape analysis. The second one is Brain Connectivity,
which includes detection of brain activation regions and functional connectivity
analysis with functional Magnetic Resonance Imaging (fMRI), Diffusion Tensor
Imaging (DTI) based white matter bundle tracking and analysis, and studies on brain
connectivity abnormalities of patients with mental diseases with fMRI and DTI. The
third one is the imaging genome. The motivation is to understand genetic bases for
various anatomical and functional abnormalities of patients with brain diseases and

Y. Liu, T. Jiang, and C. Zhang (Eds.): CVBIA 2005, LNCS 3765, pp. 13–23, 2005.

disorders based on neuroimages. We will introduce the historical achievements, current progress, and future plans of these research fields in the follow on sections respectively.

2 Computational Neuroanatomy

In this part, we focus on human brain morphemetry with Magnetic Resonance Imaging (MRI), especially on brain image and lesion segmentation, registration, and shape analysis.

2.1 Image Segmentation

Brain Tissue Segmentation: Brain tissue segmentation is an important preprocessing step in many medical research and clinical applications. However, intensity inhomogeneities in MR images, which can change the absolute intensity for a given tissue class in different locations, are a major obstacle to any automatic methods for MR image segmentation and make it difficult to obtain accurate segmentation results. In order to address this issue, we proposed a novel method called Multi-context fuzzy clustering (MCFC) based on a local image model for classifying 2D and 3D MR data into tissues of white matter, gray matter, and cerebral spinal fluid automatically [1]. Experimental results on both real MR images and simulated volumetric MR data show that the MCFC outperforms the classic fuzzy c-means (FCM) as well as other segmentation methods that deal with intensity inhomogeneities, as shown in Fig. 1.

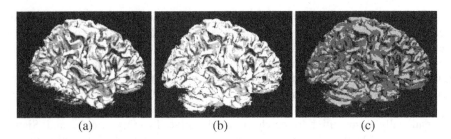

(a)   (b)   (c)

Fig. 1. 3-D renderings of the segmentation results of WM   (a) FCM segmentation (b) MCFC segmentation (c) true model

Another related work done in the MIC is Pixon based image segmentation. Markov random fields (MRF)-based methods are of great importance in image segmentation, for their ability to model a prior belief about the continuity of image features such as region labels, textures, edges. However, the main disadvantage of MRF-based methods is that the objective function associated with most nontrivial MRF problems is extremely nonconvex, which makes the corresponding minimization problem very time consuming. We combined a pixon-based image model with a Markov random field (MRF) model under a Bayesian framework [2]. The anisotropic diffusion equation was successfully used to form the pixons in our new pixon scheme. Experimental results demonstrate that the proposed method performs fairly well and computational costs decrease dramatically compared with the pixel-based MRF algorithm.

Brain Sub-Structure Segmentation: Accurate volumetric segmentation of brain structures, such as the brain ventricles, is needed for some clinic applications. In recent years, the active-models-based segmentation methods have been extensively studied and widely employed in medical image segmentation and have achieved considerable success. Unfortunately, the current techniques are going to be trapped in undesired minimum due to the image noise and pseudoedges. We proposed a parallel genetic algorithm-based active model method and applied it to segment the lateral ventricles from magnetic resonance brain images [3]. First, an objective function was defined. Then one instance surface was extracted using the finite-difference method-based active model and used to initialize the first generation of a parallel genetic algorithm. Finally, the parallel genetic algorithm was employed to refine the result. We demonstrate that the method successfully overcomes numerical instability and is capable of generating an accurate and robust anatomic descriptor for complex objects in the human brain, such as the lateral ventricles. This is first time in literature to introduce clustering distributed computing in medical image analysis. It is very promising and cheap to increase the speed, which is especially needed for some real time clinic applications.

Active shape models (ASM) was proposed by Cootes [4] as shape and appearance models. The method makes full use of priori shape and appearance knowledge of object and has the ability to deform within some constraints. Rather than representing the image structure using intensity gradients, we extracted local edge features for each landmark using steerable filters in [5], which provided richer edge information than intensity. We proposed a machine learning algorithm based on AdaBoost, which selected a small number of critical features from a larger set and can yield extremely efficient classifiers. These non-linear classifiers were used, instead of the linear Mahalanobis distance, to find optimal displacements for landmarks by searching along the direction perpendicular to each landmark. These features give more accurate and reliable matching between models and new images than modeling image intensity alone. Experimental results demonstrated the ability of this improved method to accurately align and locate edge features.

2.2 Image Registration

Image registration is a key component of computational neuroanatomy. In terms of satisfying the technical requirements of robustness and accuracy with minimal user interaction, rigid registration has been considered by many works in the field to be a solved problem. Now the research focus of medical image registration has been shifted to the non-rigid registration. Neuroscientists and clinicians are in dire need of the automatically medical image registration tools to process intra-subject, inter-subject and atlas registration. The method of non-rigid medical image registration usually include physics-based and geometry-based. We have made our effort on both of them.

Physics-Based Method: We developed a fast fluid registration method in [6], which was based on the physics rule of fluid mechanics, and developed another non-rigid medical image registration algorithm, by assuming that the displacement fields were constrained by Maxwell model of viscoelasticity. In Fig. 3, applications of the proposed method to synthetic images and inter-subject registration of brain anatomical structure images illustrate the high efficiency and accuracy.

A non-rigid Medical Image Registration by Viscoelastic Model was presented in [7], by assuming the local shape variations were satisfied the property of Maxwell model of viscoelasticity, the deformable fields were constrained by the corresponding partial differential equations. Experimental results showed that the performance of proposed method were satisfactory in accuracy and speed.

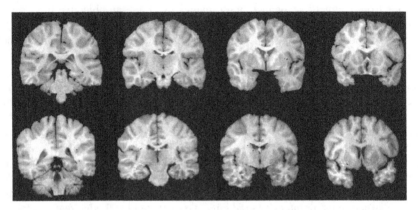

Fig. 2. Top: the template slices; and Bottom: the corresponding slices of reference

Geometry-Based Method: Non-rigid registration of medical image by linear singular blending techniques was proposed by Tang and Jiang [8]. A free-form deformation was based on a LSB B-Spline, which can enhance the shape-control capability of B-Spline. The experiment results indicate that the method is much better to describe the deformation than the affine algorithm and B-Spline techniques.

2.3 Shape Analysis

Statistical Shape Analysis (SSA) is a powerful tool for noninvasive studies of pathophysiology and diagnosis of brain diseases. It is another key component of computational neuroanatomy. The population-based shape analysis not only reveals the difference between the healthy and diseased subjects, but also provides the dynamic variations of the patients' brain structures over time. We proposed a new method which incorporated shape-based landmarks into parameterization of banana-like 3D brain structures to address this problem [9]. First, the triangulated surface of the object was obtained and two landmarks were extracted from the mesh, i.e. the ends of the banana-like object. Then the surface was parameterized by creating a continuous and bijective mapping from the surface to a spherical surface based on a heat conduction model. The correspondence of shapes was achieved by mapping the two landmarks to the north and south poles of the sphere. The approach was applied to the parameterization of lateral ventricle and a multiresolution shape representation was obtained by using the Discrete Fourier Transform, as shown in Fig.3.

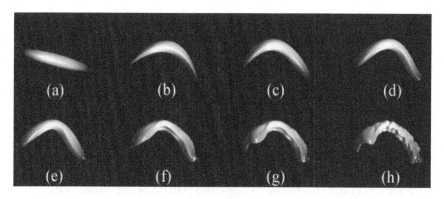

Fig. 3. Parameterization of lateral ventricle and a multiresolution shape representation obtained by using the Discrete Fourier Transform, with Fourier coefficient 9, 13, 29, 49, 81, 1257, and 7845, respectively

3 Diffusion Tensor Imaging

Diffusion tensor imaging, as a relatively new MRI technique, provides information about the random displacement of water molecules in the brain tissue. Using this information, ones could investigate the white matter characteristic and the anatomical connections between different regions non-invasively. Our research efforts cover a wide range from developing new approaches to fiber tracking and the white matter analysis using DTI.

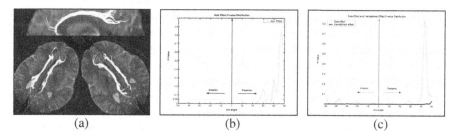

Fig. 4. (a) The reconstructed cingulum tract. (b) The statistical results for asymmetry of right-handers. (c) The statistical results for the effects of handerness and side in cinulum.

Analysis of white matter from DTI is mostly based on region of interesting (ROI) in image data set, which is specified by user. However, this method is not always reliable because of the uncertainty of manual specification. In [10], we developed an improved fiber-based scheme rather than ROI-based analysis to study the cingulum, the most prominent white matter fiber tract of the limbic system. In this work, cingulum bundles were first reconstructed by fiber-tracking algorithm and then were parameterized by arc-angle, which was scale-invariant. All fibers centered at a common origin, and anatomic correspondence across subjects in cingulum was established. This method was used to explore the asymmetry of cingulum in DTI datasets of right-hander normal subjects. As in Fig. 4, statistical results show a significant left-greater-than-right asymmetry pattern in most segments of cingulum bundle, except the most posterior portion.

4 Functional Brain Connectivity

fMRI is an important functional brain imaging technique. Since its advent in the early 1990's, a variety of analytic methods have been developed. This is one important research field in the MIC. Recently, what we have been mostly concerning about are methods for steady-state (including resting-state) fMRI data and connectivity.

4.1 fMRI Activation Detection

Both the spatial and temporal information of fMRI data have been considered in our research on fMRI activation detection. The temporal information is typically the time variant characteristics of the hemodynamic responses, and the spatial information is the fMRI activated regions typically occur in clusters of several spatially contiguous voxels [11, 12]. Another research direction was how to model the trial to trial variability of the hemodynamic responses in human brain. Since the typical model-based methods for fMRI data analysis, for instance, the General Linear Model (GLM) and the deconvolution method, are based on the following assumption: the hemodynamic responses are same across trials, i.e., the trial-to-trial variability is considered as noise. When hemodynamic responses vary from trial to trail [13], an alternative approach is needed to include the trial-to-trial variability.

A region-growing and a split-merge based method have been proposed for fMRI activation detection [14, 15]. Main feature of the region-growing and split-merge based methods was that they can utilize the neighboring information of each time series. As for the second aim, an optimization based framework for single trial variability was proposed in [16]. The main features of this proposed method were as follows: (1) The trial-to-trial variability was modeled as meaningful signal rather than assuming that same HR was evoked in each trial; (2) Since the proposed method was a constrained optimization based general framework, it could be extended by utilizing of prior knowledge of HR; (3) The traditional deconvolution method could be included into our method as a special case.

4.2 Regional Homogeneity (ReHo)

As a result that no specific stimulus was given for resting-state, we proposed a data-driven method call regional homogeneity (ReHo) in [17]. ReHo assumed that voxels within a functional cluster should share similar characteristics and such similarity could vary from state to state. By this method, we found significant higher ReHo in bilateral primary motor cortex (M1) during unilateral finger tapping. Higher ReHo was also detected in posterior cingulate cortex (PCC) during resting-state.

4.3 Functional Connectivity

A large quantity of fMRI studies traditionally focused on identifying activated regions of the brain during an experimental task. However, brain function may be as a result of information integration among brain regions, described in terms of functional connectivity [18] or effective connectivity [19]. Recently, increasing attention has been focused on detecting interregional connectivity, especially in a resting state. Our research efforts cover a wide range from developing new methodology to using established methods for the understanding of the resting brain mechanism and clinical validation. Some representative contributions were as follows.

All-To-All Functional Connectivity [20]: We developed a new approach based on graph theory taking into account n-to-1 connectivity using 1-to-1 connectivity measures instead of conventional pairwise connectivity. It can better reflect the joint interactions among multiple brain regions. With it, a large organized functional connectivity network related to motor function in the resting brain with fMRI was shown. More importantly, we found that such a network can be modulated from a conscious resting state to a voluntary movement state by the measure.

ReHo and Functional Connectivity [21]: So far, the resting state functional connectivity (RSFC) has been performed mainly by seed correlation analysis (SCA) on fMRI studies. On the basis of our previous work based on the ReHo [17], functional network in the resting brain was detected by using the model-free method. Our method identified a parietal-frontal network of brain regions utilizing only resting state data. We proposed the ReHo to serve as the selection of the seed before functional connectivity based on the SCA is performed [21]. It provides a novel way to select the desired seeds by taking the natures of resting state data into account, compared with the previous studies about the selection of the seed utilizing prior anatomical information [22] or previously performed activation maps [20]. Using this technique, the bilateral anterior inferior cerebellum (AICb) showing higher ReHo were identified and used as the seeds for resting state functional connectivity patterns studies. The results show that the bilateral AICb has significant functional connectivity with the bilateral thalamus, the bilateral hippocampus, the precuneus, the temporal lobe, and the prefrontal lobe.

5 Current Activities

Much of our current work on computational neuroanatomy is concerned with structural abnormalities in human brain. This is essential for the research of mental diseases. Under the consideration of the limited resolution of the existing imaging sensors and the low contrast of brain structures to their peri-structures, robust tools for the identification of such structures are highly expected, so that the structures can be quantitatively and statistically analyzed. The research on geometrical fairing mapping using Mean Curvature Flows is now undergoing. It is applicable for arbitrary genus surfaces and avoids shape shrinkage in discrete space. The global geometry of the original object and its area are theoretically preserved. This mapping method has the potential applicability in skeleton regularization and brain surface matching.

Our previous study on DTI was confined to right-handers without considering the role of handedness. It should be interesting to ascertain the relationship of the cingulum microstructure with the handedness and side. We therefore recruited another group of left-handed healthy subjects to examine this issue with the same method mentioned above. The statistical results also showed a remarkable left-greater-than-right asymmetry pattern of anisotropy in most segments of cingulum bundles except the most posterior segment. Higher anisotropy of the right-hander than the left-hander was found in the bilateral cingulum bundles. However, no significant handedness-by-side interaction was observed. Besides the applications to brain research based on DTI, a lot of computational issues are also under our consideration. The tensor model is explicit, however is too simple to characterize the property in some complicated regions such as fiber crossing regions and boundary regions between different brain tissues. More suitable models are under construction in our group.

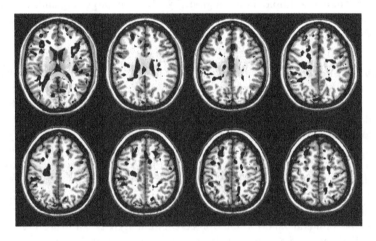

Fig. 5. Highly discriminative regions identified by Fisher brain

Discriminative analysis on fMRI has also been concerned. A discriminative model of attention deficit hyperactivity disorder (ADHD) was newly presented on the basis of multivariate pattern classification and fMRI [23]. This model consists of two parts, a classifier and an intuitive representation of discriminative pattern of brain function between patients and normal controls. Regional homogeneity (ReHo), a measure of brain function at resting-state, is used here as a feature of classification. Fisher discriminative analysis (FDA) is performed on the features of training samples and a linear classifier is generated. The classifier is also compared with linear support vector machine (SVM) and Batch Perceptron. Our classifier outperforms its counterparts significantly. Fisher brain, the optimal projective-direction vector in FDA, is used to represent the discriminative pattern. As shown in Fig. 5, some abnormal brain regions identified by Fisher brain, like prefrontal cortex and anterior cingulate cortex, are well consistent with that reported in neuroimaging studies on ADHD. Moreover, some less reported but highly discriminative regions are also identified. The discriminative model has potential ability to improve current diagnosis and treatment evaluation of ADHD.

We also apply discriminative analysis on DTI. We use two-dimensional histogram of ADC and FA to discriminate Neuromyelitis optica (NMO) from healthy subjects. The correct recognition rate reaches 85%, which is much higher than that of based on the traditional FA histogram (50%) and ADC histogram (73%). The results indicate that our method based on combined feature from two-dimensional histogram is more effective for classification than that of based on one type of feature. Furthermore, some discriminative regions that contribute most to separating the patients with NMO and normal controls can be obtained based on our method. It implies that NMO has diffuse damages of brain tissue on such a small scale that conventional MRI cannot detect it. This challenges the classic notion of a sparing of the brain tissue in the course of NMO. In addition, our method based on two-dimensional histogram can also be used in other brain tissue, especially the diffuse damage of brain tissue, such as multiple sclerosis.

The application of functional connectivity analysis in ADHD is undergoing. We investigate the difference of functional connectivity between the Attention-Deficit/Hyperactivity Disorder (ADHD) children and the normal controls in Flanker task and resting state, respectively. In Flanker task, we found that ADHD children show enhanced functional connectivity between dACC and several other brain areas as shown in Fig. 6. Such an enhanced functional connectivity pattern may suggest that children with ADHD need greater effort, and accordingly a wider network of brain areas to complete the same task as the normal controls do. In a resting state, we found that the ADHD patients exhibited more significant functional connectivity of the dACC with the dACC, as well as with the left medial frontal cortex/ventral anterior cingulate cortex, bilateral thalamus, bilateral cerebellum, bilateral insula, right superior frontal cortex, and brainstem (pons), and only within the brainstem (medulla) did the controls exhibit more significant connectivity than the patients. More information is available at http://www.nlpr.ia.ac.cn/jiangtz.

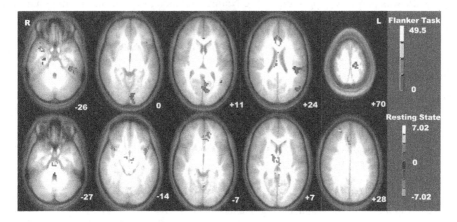

Fig. 6. The brain regions showing significant between-group differences in the Flanker task (p<0.05 corrected, upper row) and in the resting state (p<0.05 & cluster size >600mm^3, lower row)

The application of ReHo in AD is being evaluated. We used resting-state fMRI to examine LFFs activity in terms of regional homogeneity (ReHo) to explore the pathophysiology of dementia of the Alzheimer type (DAT). Compared with healthy controls, DAT subjects showed decreased ReHo in the posterior cingulate cortex (PCC) and increased ReHo in the right inferior temporal cortex and bilateral occipital lobe. In addition, examination of the behavioral correlates revealed significant positive correlation of PCC ReHo versus Mini-Mental State Examination score. Our finding, together with a recent fMRI result that DAT subjects showed decreased resting-state activity in the PCC and hippocampus explored by using a non-pure resting-state paradigm, suggests that PCC LFFs activity measured using resting-state fMRI may be a promising marker for characterization and detection of early DAT.

6 Conclusions and Future Directions

We have developed various techniques to detect the anatomical and functional abnormalities of human brain with neurological and psychiatric diseases. We have been applying various modern neuroimaging techniques to combat the neurological and psychiatric diseases, especially Alzheimer's Diseases and Schizophrenia. A long-term goal of the MIC is to find the early markers based on neuroimages and genome datasets for the neurological and psychiatric diseases. It would be very interesting to identify the genetic basis of the anatomical and functional abnormalities of human brain with neurological and psychiatric diseases. In fact, several publications have been available and a new field - imaging genomics, named by Hariri and Weinberger, has emerged [24]. It is at its infant stage and we expect a lot of important progress can be made in the future.

Acknowledgements

This work was partially supported by the Natural Science Foundation of China, Grant Nos. 30425004 and 60121302, and the National Key Basic Research and Development Program (973), Grant No. 2004CB318107.

References

1. Zhu CZ, Jiang TZ: Multi-context Fuzzy Clustering for Separation of Brain Tissues in MR Images. NeuroImage 18 (2003) 685–696
2. Yang FG, Jiang TZ: Pixon-Based Image Segmentation With Markov Random Fields. IEEE Trans Imag Proc 12 (2003) 1552–1559
3. Fan Y, Jiang TZ, Evans DJ: Volumetric Segmentation of Brain Images Using Parallel Genetic Algorithm. IEEE Trans Med Imaging 21(2002) 904–909
4. Cootes TF, Taylor, CJ, Cooper, DH, Graham, J: Active shape models- their training and application. Computer vision and image understanding 61(1995) 38–59
5. Li SY, Zhu LT, Jiang TZ (2004): Active Shape Model Segmentation Using Local Edge Structures and AdaBoost. In proceedings of MIAR 2004, 121–128, Beijing, China

6. Tang SY, Jiang TZ: Fast Nonrigid Medical Inage Registration by Fluid Model. In proceedings of ACCV'04, vol. II, (2004a) 914-919, Jeju, Korea
7. Tang SY, Jiang TZ: Nonrigid Registration of Medical image By Maxwell Model of Viscoelasticity. In proceedings of ISBI'04, (2004b) 1443–1446, Arlington, USA
8. Tang SY, Jiang TZ: Non-rigid Registration of Medical Image by Linear Singular Blending Techniques. Pattern Recogn Lett 25(2004c) 399–405
9. Zhu LT, Jiang TZ: Parameterization of 3D Brain Structures for Statistical Shape Analysis. In proceedings of SPIE Medical Imaging'04, (2004) 14-17, California, USA
10. Gong GL, Jiang TZ, Zhu CZ, Zang YF, Wang F, Xie S, Xiao JX, Guo XM: Asymmetry Analysis of Cingulum Based on Scale-Invariant Parameterization by Diffusion Tensor. Hum Brain Mapp 24(2005) 92-98
11. Tononi G, McIntosh AR, Russell DP, Edelman GM: Functional clustering: identifying strongly interactive brain regions in neuroimaging data. Neuroimage 7(1998) 133–149
12. Katanoda K, Matsuda Y, Sugishita M: A spatial-temporal regression model for the analysis of functional MRI data. Neuroimage 17(2002) 1415–1428
13. Duann JR, Jung TP, Kuo WJ, Yeh TC, Makeig S, Hsieh JC, Sejnowski JT: Single-Trial Variability in Event-Related BOLD Signals. NeuroImage 15(2002) 823-835
14. Lu YL, Jiang TZ, Zang YF: A Split-merge Based Region Growing Method for the Analysis of fMRI Data. Hum Brain Mapp 22(2004) 271–279
15. Lu YL, Jiang TZ, Zang YF: Region Growing Method for the Analysis of fMRI Data. NeuroImage 20(2003) 455–465
16. Lu YL, Jiang TZ, Zang YF: Single-Trial Variable Model for Event-Related fMRI Data Analysis, IEEE Transactions on Medical Imaging 24(2005) 236-245
17. Zang YF, Jiang TZ, Lu YL, He Y, Lixia Tian: Regional Honogeneity Based Approach to fMRI Data Analysis. NeuroImage 22 (2004) 394–400
18. Friston KJ, Frith CD, Liddle PF, Frackowiak RS: Functional connectivity: the principal component analysis of large (PET) data sets. J Cereb Blood Flow Metab 13(1993a) 5–14
19. Friston KJ, Frith CD, Frackowiak RS: Time-dependent changes in effective connectivity measured with PET. Hum Brain Mapp 1(1993b) 69–80
20. Jiang TZ, He Y, Zang YF, Weng XC: Modulation of Functional Connectivity During the Rest State and the Task State. Hum Brain Mapp 22 (2004) 63–71
21. He Y, Zang YF, Jiang TZ, Liang M, Gong GL: Detecting Functional Connectivity of the Cerebellum Using Low Frequency Fluctuations (LFFs). In proceedings of MICCAI'04, vol. II, (2004) 907-915, St Malo, France
22. Stein T, Moritz C, Quigley M, Cordes D, Haughton V, Meyerand E: Functional connectivity in the thalamus and hippocampus studied with fMRI. Am J Neuroradiol 21(2000) 1397–1401
23. Zhu C, Zang Y, Liang M, Tian L, He Y, Li X, Sui M, Wang Y, Jiang T: Discriminative Analysis of Brain Function at Resting-state for Attention-Deficit/Hyperactivity Disorder. In proceedings of MICCAI'05, USA, (2005) in press.
24. Hariri AR, Weinberger DR: Imaging genomics. Br Med Bull. 65(2003) 259-70.

Tracking of Migrating and Proliferating Cells in Phase-Contrast Microscopy Imagery for Tissue Engineering

Takeo Kanade and Kang Li

Robotics Institute,
Carnegie Mellon University,
Pittsburgh PA, 15213

Abstract. Tissue Engineering is an interdisciplinary field that applies the principles of biology and engineering to develop tissue substitutes to restore, maintain, or improve the function of diseased or damaged human tissues. One approach for engineering tissue involves seeding biodegradable scaffolds with hormones, then culturing and implanting the scaffolds by means of a printing technology to induce and direct the growth of new, healthy tissue cells. Precise and quantitative tracking of the migrating and proliferating cells by non-invasive phase-contrast video microscopy is a vital component to studying and understanding how the concentration-modulated patterns of hormones direct the migration and proliferation of tissue cells. The varying density of the cell culture and the complexity of the cell behavior (shape deformation, division/mitosis, close contact and partial occlusion) pose many challenges to existing tracking techniques. We propose a multi-target tracking algorithm that simultaneously tracks a very large number of cells based on a topology-constrained level-set method and Markov-chain Monte Carlo particle filtering. We apply our methodology to *in vitro* tissue cell tracking under phase-contrast microscopy and demonstrate that the cells proliferate and migrate in alignment with the printed hormone patterns.

Y. Liu, T. Jiang, and C. Zhang (Eds.): CVBIA 2005, LNCS 3765, p. 24, 2005.
© Springer-Verlag Berlin Heidelberg 2005

Cardiology Meets Image Analysis: Just an Application or Can Image Analysis Usefully Impact Cardiology Practice?

J. Alison Noble

Wolfson Medical Vision Laboratory, Department of Engineering Science,
University of Oxford, Parks Road, Oxford OX1 3PJ, UK
noble@robots.ox.ac.uk

Abstract. A decade ago, cardiovascular image analysis very much meant the application of image analysis methods to a cardiac image sequence obtained from a friendly cardiologist. 10 years on, have things changed? In this short paper, I overview research conducted in Oxford in the area of cardiovascular image analysis over this period, aimed at developing clinically useful methods for diagnosing heart disease. This has mainly concerned echocardiography (ultrasound imaging of the heart). I also consider how this area may develop in the future and the influence that computer vision may have on this development.

1 Introduction

More people in the Western World, both women and men[1], are killed by cardiovascular disease (CVD) than any other disease; according to recent figures, it annually accounts for almost 1 million deaths in the USA and over 4.3 million deaths in Europe [1,2]. Coronary heart disease (CHD) accounts for around half of these deaths in both Europe and the USA.

Echocardiography (ultrasound of the heart), PET/SPECT (nuclear medicine), cardiac magnetic resonance imaging (MRI) and X-ray-based cardiac imaging are now widely employed in cardiology departments. However, it is only in the last decade, with advances in spatial and temporal resolution, and the increased availability of digital imagery in hospitals that automated image analysis has become viable. It is even more recently that we have started to see a strong *clinical pull* for image analysis technology as cardiology departments have become flooded with digital data when what is needed is useful digital information. The earliest image analysis technology, developed to track heart chamber walls, and mostly derived based on original ideas from computer vision, is now moving from research laboratories into commercial products. Cardiologists are now questioning how we can provide more advanced quantitative image-based tools for measuring the thickness of the heart walls and how this changes over the cardiac cycle (myocardial thickening), tissue health (or perfusion), and integrating imaging modalities such as PET-MRI and ultrasound-

---

[1] With, in Europe, according to [2], the exception of France and San Marino for men.

Y. Liu, T. Jiang, and C. Zhang (Eds.): CVBIA 2005, LNCS 3765, pp. 25–30, 2005.

MRI, ideally from truly 3D acquisitions; all to provide integrated cardiac function models that in turn provide more useful clinical measurements for early diagnosis and treatment monitoring.

The cardiac image analysis research area is relatively small. To place this is perspective, at a leading international meeting on medical image analysis this year (MICCAI 2005, www.miccai20005.org), by clinical application area only 2% of the papers concern cardiology, compared to 34% on computer aided detection (CAD) and 22% on the brain and neurology. Increasingly, in medical image analysis, we are seeing specialized meetings established; in the case of the heart, there is an established meeting on functional imaging and modeling of the heart (FIMH) which covers both modeling and analysis for understanding physiological function and clinical disease management. However, today, given the clinical (and economic) need for cardiac image analysis methods, the level of effort in image analysis is remarkably out of proportion to its potential impact.

A large amount of our own research at Oxford has concerned analysis of echocardiography. Echocardiography is the most widely used imaging method in cardiology, but has high patient-to-patient variability in quality – indeed it has been estimated that only approximately 40% of patient data is "good" quality. The key to successful image analysis in this case is to make use of as many constraints on interpretation as possible, for instance, models of imaging physics, knowledge of expected shape change, and temporal models. In the following sections I briefly overview both the work we have done and general trends in different aspects of echocardiographic image analysis. I conclude by outlining some general areas in which perhaps computer vision research and researchers might help advance this field.

2   2D Echocardiographic Image Sequence Motion Analysis

Motion analysis, specifically tracking the endocardial (inner) border of the left ventricle is the most widely investigated problem in cardiac image analysis. In the literature, most research validated on a reasonable number of datasets (more than 20 subjects) has been 2D image sequence analysis.

The idea in cardiac motion analysis is to develop (semi)-automatic methods to track the boundaries and then either measure the ejection fraction of the heart as a global measure of heart function or quantify the motion of heart wall segments. This is challenging as the motion is non-rigid. In addition, for ultrasound-based analysis the bloodpool-tissue border has poor definition in routine echocardiography data which makes detection of the border difficult. Along with other groups we have focused on spatio-temporal model-based methods which use a shape-space and a temporal model to constrain the possible deformation of the tracking algorithm [3, 4]. We have also looked at spatio-temporal border detection using phase-based methods in an attempt to overcome the limitation of using intensity gradients to find boundaries [5]. For routine clinical use, in collaboration with Mirada Solutions Ltd, the Gregario Maranon Hospital, Madrid, and the Oxford John Radcliffe Hospital, we have developed a prototype clinical system which works on ultrasound data enhanced by a contrast agent. Results from a large study (under review for a clinical journal) evaluating this approach will be presented at the workshop. Early results were reported in [6]. A conclusion from this work is that 2D echocardiographic image tracking technology is now sufficiently well-developed for application on good-to-medium quality routine clinical data. The technical challenges remain how to analyze low quality data, and hence make analysis truly applicable for all routine use. Our own research effort is now turning to look at automatic quantification of myocardial thickening (strain) and analysis of stress echocardiography. In the former case, an unknown today is how to best model the biomechanics of the heart for this application; in the latter case, the quality of images is lower than for a rest sequence.

3 Assessment of Tissue Health or "Perfusion"

A new and largely un-developed area of automated cardiac image analysis relates to assessing the health of the heart tissue (myocardium) by the rate of uptake of a contrast agent. The rate of uptake or "perfusion" rate is normally observed earlier than a motion change so this is advocated as a way to perform earlier detection of coronary heart disease. When ultrasound imaging is used to measure tissue "perfusion" the technique is known as myocardial contrast echocardiography (MCE) [7]. In MCE, a microbubble contrast agent is injected into the bloodstream. Special ultrasound imaging protocols are used to acquire images as the contrast agent is taken up into the walls of the heart (the myocardium). Typically, image sequences are assessed "by-eye" which is both tedious and subjective. The image sequence in this case is a sampled acquisition of a spatio-temporal functional model of contrast agent uptake which is often assumed to take on the form of a parameterized exponential model. In [8,9] we developed a novel way to estimate both the parameters of the tissue perfusion model and segment the myocardium using a combined Bayesian Factor Analysis and Markov Random Field (BFA-MRF) approach. This fully spatio-temporal method has been evaluated in a 22 patient study showing that automated image analysis gives a better diagnosis than an experienced MCE reader and rather than just detect the presence of an abnormality localizes the extent of disease. The method is now undergoing a larger clinical evaluation. To improve clinical MCE quantification further, we need new protocols to compensate for acquisition artefacts such as signal attenuation and perform quantification on the ultrasound signal rather than image; i.e. work towards a new generation of *combined* ultrasound signal acquisition and image analysis methods. This trend to consider acquisition and analysis together rather than treat them as separate processing stages is one that we are increasingly seeing in medical image analysis as the limitations of physics-free medical image analysis are being reached.

4 3D Analysis – The Way Forward

2D cardiac image analysis makes the assumption that the important components of motion (or perfusion) are restricted to in-plane. In practice, although often a good approximation for acquisitions gated to the cardiac cycle, this is a strong assumption as the heart undergoes a complex 3D motion. Thus in the future 3D+T (here 'T' means times) cardiac imaging and image analysis is likely to predominate. In the case of echocardiography, until a couple of years ago state-of-art 3D echocardiography machines involved mechanically rotating a conventional linear array transducer around an axis. Rotational 3D echocardiography has relatively poor image quality and respiration artifacts were a problem. Sanchez-Ortiz et al (2002) [10] describes the evaluation of a heart tracking method we developed using a 'feature detection then surface-tracking' approach which is representative of the state-of-art that could be achieved using this technology.

Real-time 3D or RT3D (such as the Philips Medical Systems system) is the newest generation of 3D echocardiography and indeed 3D cardiac imaging modality[2]. It is based on matrix-array (rather than linear-array technology) and offers advantages over conventional 2D ultrasound imaging in that 3D volumes can be acquired very quickly ("real-time") minimizing acquisition artifacts due to respiration and transducer movement. Compared with other 3D cardiac imaging techniques, RT3D systems are portable, and acquire 3D data quickly. There are a few early papers reporting on analysis using RT3D but its full utility as a 3D imaging modality is still being evaluated both from the clinical and image analysis perspectives. At Oxford we have recently being extending our previous work on multiple-acquisition (or "acoustic window") analysis applied to rotational 3D echocardiography [11] to fuse RT3D acquisitions from different transducer positions [12]. In this approach we take a probabilistic view, and fuse features from different acquisitions based on their magnitude and orientation with respect to the transducer. This produces an output "saliency" image volume with enhanced structures relative to any individual acquisition. We are currently investigating the advantages of using a 3D saliency representation as the basis for segmentation and tracking. We are also looking at alignment of cardiac MR and RT3D data for multi-modality cardiac disease diagnosis and treatment monitoring [13].

5 Conclusion

In this overview, I have used examples from research in my own laboratory in Oxford to highlight the state-of-art in the field of echocardiographic image analysis.

In general, there has been significant technical progress in this field over the last decade, aided by improvements in acquisition technology, but particularly due to the success of using spatio-temporal models to guide image interpretation and segmentation. However, the literature shows that only a limited number of methods have been well-validated on routine clinical images. It is clear that more attention needs to be given to working with cardiologists on validation to better establish the strengths and weaknesses of different approaches. This is important for the field as a whole, not only to gain credibility with practicing cardiologists, but also this acceptance will open up new opportunities to look at more advanced modeling and analysis problems.

---

[2] There is an earlier version of RT3D, developed at Duke University and commercialized by Volumetrics. However, Volumetrics has ceased trading, and the newer Philips Medical Systems system has superior image quality.

I have not touched on the related area of analysis of clinical cardiac magnetic resonance (MR) imaging (1.5T or 3T). Cardiac MR offers superior tissue differentiation to echocardiography, temporal resolution has significantly improved, and acquisition times are reducing. This is making cardiac MR increasingly a viable alternative to echocardiography in clinical diagnosis. Segmentation issues are different in this case, and non-trivial for automated analysis, but spatial-temporal modeling issues are the same (motion) or similar (perfusion). Nor, have I discussed how one might adapt methods developed for diagnosis, to assess heart recovery after treatment/surgery. This is one of the exciting new opportunities for the application of cardiac image analysis research area in the future.

I have focused on describing methods aimed at clinical diagnosis which employ relatively simple models of the heart. At the other extreme, there is a very active research area developing detailed computational electro-mechanical models of the heart [14, 15]. Unfortunately, such models can not be derived from routine clinical data today. It will be interesting to see how the computational models used in these two fields converge in the future.

Turning to methodology development, computer vision played a role in early work on cardiac motion analysis, although most approaches today are not only governed by the choice of motion model but also knowledge of cardiology and imaging physics. However, there are a number of ways in which ideas from computer vision might be applied in cardiovascular image analysis in the future; particularly relating to spatio-temporal modeling and spatio-temporal segmentation. Multi-modality fusion also offers interesting challenges in terms of how to fuse images/information of time-varying entities with different spatial and temporal resolutions.

Acknowledgments

I wish to acknowledge members, past and present, of the Wolfson Medical Vision Laboratory who have contributed to the development of the WMVL cardiac image analysis research programme. I also wish to acknowledge the strong support we have received from Dr Harald Becher at the Cardiology Department, Oxford John Radcliffe Hospital, Professor Stefan Neubauer at the Oxford Centre for Clinical Magnetic Resonance Research and their respective research teams. Funding for this research has principally come from project grants from the UK Engineering and Physical Sciences Research Council and Medical Research Council.

References

1. American Heart Association, Heart disease and stroke statistics – 2005 update, 2005.
2. British Heart Foundation and European Heart Network, European cardiovascular disease statistics, 2005 ed., 2005.
3. Jacob, G, Noble, J.A. and Blake, A., Robust contour tracking in echocardiographic sequences, 1998 International Conference on Computer Vision, Bombay, India, January 1998, p. 408-413.

4. Jacob, G, Noble, J.A., Behrenbruch, C., Kelion, A.D. and Banning, A.P., A shape-space based approach to tracking myocardial thickening and quantifying regional left ventricular function, IEEE Trans. Medical Imaging, 21(3), p. 226-238, 2002.
5. Mulet-Parada, M. and Noble, J.A., 2D+T boundary detection in echocardiography, Med.Image Anal., 4(1):21-30, 2000.
6. Bermejo J, Mulet-Parada M, Moreyra C, Feldmar J, Noble JA, et al. Endocardial tracking of acoustic quantification and contrast power-Doppler echocardiographic images: clinical validation against cine-MRI and manual segmentation. *Circulation.* 1999;100 (Suppl I):I-445 - I-446.
7. Becher, H. and Burns, PN, A handbook of contrast echocardiography, Springer, Heidelberg, 2000.
8. Williams, Q and Noble, J.A., A spatio-temporal analysis of contrast ultrasound image sequences for assessment of tissue perfusion, Proceedings of MICCAI 2004.
9. Williams, Q, Noble, JA, Ehlgen, A. and Becher, H., Tissue perfusion diagnostic classification using a spatio-temporal analysis of contrast ultrasound image sequences, 19th Int. Conf. IPMI, 2005, p. 222-233.
10. Sanchez-Ortiz, GI, Wright, GJT, Clarke, N, Declerck, J, Banning A and Noble, JA, Automated 3D echocardiography compared to manual delineations and MUGA, IEEE Trans Med. Imag. 21(9):1069-1076, 2002.
11. Ye, X, Atkinson D, and Noble, JA 3D freehand echocardiography for automatic LV reconstruction and analysis based on multiple acoustic windows, IEEE Trans Medical Imaging, 21(9):1051-1058, 2002.
12. Grau, V, and Noble, J.A., Multiscale ultrasound compounding using phase information, Proceedings of MICCAI, to appear 2005.
13. Zhang, W. and Noble, J.A., 2005 (submitted for publication 2005).
14. Hunter, PJ, Pullan, AJ and Smaill, BH, Modelling total heart function, Annual Review of Biomedical Engineering, 5:147-177, 2003.
15. Sermesant, M., Coudiere Y, Delingette H, Ayache N, et al., Progress towards an electro-mechanical model of the heart for cardiac image analysis, IEEE International Symposium on Biomedical Imaging, p. 10-14, 2002.

Computer Vision Algorithms for Retinal Image Analysis: Current Results and Future Directions

Charles V. Stewart

Department of Computer Science,
Rensselaer Polytechnic Institute,
Troy, NY 12180, USA
stewart@cs.rpi.edu

Abstract. Automated image analysis tools have the potential to play an important role in assisting in the diagnosis and treatment of retinal diseases.[1] Problems that must be addressed in developing these tools include extraction of vascular and non-vascular features, segmentation of pathologies, unimodal and multimodal image registration, mosaic construction, and real-time systems. Research at Rensselaer Polytechnic Institute since the late 1990's has focused on several of these problems. Most significantly, we have developed a series of registration and mosaic formation algorithms which have been validated on thousands of retinal images and have been extended beyond the retina application. While the core fundus image registration problem is essentially solved, important problems remain in many aspects of retinal image analysis.

1 Introduction

Diabetic retinopathy, age-related macular degeneration (AMD) and glaucoma, the three leading blindness-causing retinal diseases, currently affect approximately 8 million individuals over age 40 in the United States [45, 44, 46]. These numbers are projected to increase to over 13 million individuals in the next 15 years as the population ages. World-wide the incidence of these diseases is dramatically higher. Much of this blindness can be prevented through periodic screening, early detection, and treatment [40]. Unfortunately, many of the most at-risk individuals do not have regular eye exams.

The first step in diagnosing retinal diseases is a dilated-eye examination. This visual diagnosis may be confirmed through more detailed studies, including color or red-free photography to record the appearance of various parts of the retina,

---

[1] The author would like to thank the entire Retina Project team at Rensselaer, especially Badri Roysam for his project leadership, Drs Howard Tanenbaum and Anna Majerovics for their inspiration and encouragement, and Michal Sofka, Chia-Ling Tsai and Gehua Yange for their help with the figures. This work was supported by National Science Foundation Experimental Partnerships grant EIA-0000417 and the National Institutes for Health grant RR14038.

Y. Liu, T. Jiang, and C. Zhang (Eds.): CVBIA 2005, LNCS 3765, pp. 31–50, 2005.

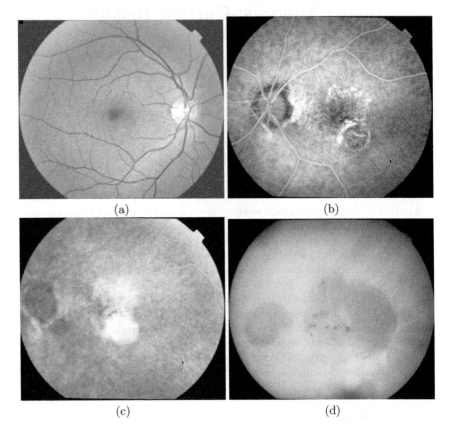

Fig. 1. Three different types of images of the retina: (a) shows a red-free fundus photograph, (b) and (c) show fluorescein angiograms (FA) early and late in the profusion of the fluorescein dye, (d) shows an idocyanine green (ICG) angiogram

fluorescein angiography (FA) to analyze blood flow in the retinal vasculature, or indocyanine-green (ICG) angiography to study blood flow in the choroid (see Figure 1). More specialized imaging sensors, including retinal tomography, optical coherence tomography and scanning laser ophthalmoscopes may be used as well to obtain 3D and subsurface measurements. This expensive equipment is used in larger clinics.

The combination of the large number of at-risk patients, the incidence of disease, and the ease of acquiring images makes the development of automatic retinal image analysis techniques a fertile and critical area of research. Moreover, since the primary acquisition devices are cameras, the image analysis problems are closely related to problems in pattern recognition and computer vision. Image analysis algorithms can potentially be used in a number of ways. Automatic screening tools may be used to label and count the pathologies such as drusen [37, 33, 6], microaneurysms [15, 30], cotton-wool spots [55], and exudates [50, 31,

24, 55] that are early indicators of disease. Registration techniques [9, 29, 34, 43, 47, 53] may be used to combine multiple images to provide a more complete view of the retina, to align and combine multimodal imagery, and to visualize and measure change. Stereo algorithms may be applied to measure three-dimensional structures, especially near the optic disk [12]. Tracking and real-time systems [25, 39] may be used as tools to guide treatment devices such as lasers.

Since the late 1990's, a team at Rensselaer Polytechnic Institute, led by Professors Badrinath Roysam and Charles Stewart, the current author, has been working toward the development of image analysis tools to aid in the diagnosis and treatment of retinal diseases. Our initial goal was tools to aid in the control of lasers during surgery – especially the treatment of macular degeneration. Early in the project we decided to focus first on the core image analysis algorithms, treating them as generally as possible. This turned out to be critically important, since treatment protocols for specific diseases change frequently. In particular, photo-dynamic therapy, which requires significantly less precise control of the laser, is now the recommended treatment for the wet form of macular degeneration [38]. Since we developed the core algorithms first, however, we have been able to move far beyond the original application and now have algorithms that can be used in many different ways.

This paper summarizes current research in algorithms for retinal image analysis, focusing on our own work at Rensselaer and emphasizing our work in image registration in particular. Registration is where we have made the most important algorithmic breakthroughs, and we have extended our algorithms well-beyond retinal images. Registration is also a fundamental underlying technology for many prospective applications of retinal image analysis. The paper emphasizes problems, motivating insights, and inter-relationship between algorithms rather than specific details.

The main body of the paper starts with background on retinal image analysis and its associated challenges. It then proceeds to discuss the main problem areas and algorithms. The paper concludes with an outline of both lessons learned in this work and a set of important open problems.

2   Challenges of Retinal Imaging

The characteristic appearance of the retina is illustrated by the red-free photograph in Figure 1(a). The optic disk is the bright region on the right — on the nasal side of the retina — and the central, bright region of the disk is the optic cup. Emerging from the top and bottom of the optic disk are two relatively large arterial and venous trees. Nerve ganglion fibers, not usually visible in fundus images, cross the retinal surface and meet at the optic disk to form the optic nerve. The macula — where the fovea lies — is to the left of the optic disk and slightly below it. The macula is darker than its surroundings, and is not vascularized: unlike other parts of the retina which are fed by the surface vasculature, the macula is fed from underneath by the choroidal vessels. Overall, the retina appears to have a relatively simple structure — the bright disk, upper and lower branching vessels, relatively dark macula, and a fairly uniform background.

This apparent simplicity is deceiving. It only characterizes what is seen in images of healthy eyes showing both the optic disk and the macular regions. Retinal images taken in routine clinical settings often vary significantly in structure and appearance, with variations arising from both the imaging process and disease conditions. Some of these are illustrated by the images shown in Figure 2. The issues include the following.

- Since the illumination is introduced through the dilated pupil of the eye, it tends to be non-uniform and sometimes has sharp glare artifacts.
- The retina is seen through the lens and the vitreous humor, both of which may be clouded by the effects of disease.
- The retina is imaged using a fundus camera whose optics are designed to minimize distortion of the retina when seen through the lens of the eye.
- The retina is a smoothly curved surface, with a slight depression in the macular region, and a much deeper depression at the optic disk.
- Hemorrhages and other artifacts of disease may obscure part or all of the retina. Diseases such as diabetic retinopathy may cause some vessels to die and new vessels to grow (angiogenessis).
- Images may be acquired of many different parts of the retina as the eye rotates. Aligning these images and building a mosaic must therefore handle potentially low overlap between images. Moreover, images taken of the far periphery of the retina tend to have much less structure because there are far fewer blood vessels.
- For diseased retinas, the characteristic and dark bright appearances of the optic disk and macula, respectively, are often lost.
- The retina may become transparent so that the choroid, with its larger and more complicated vascular structure, dominates fundus images.

Certainly it is not necessary to address all of these issues in any particular application of retinal image analysis. Ignoring them, however, will lead to algorithms that work only on hand-selected images or in controlled circumstances. Moreover, facing the issues is not merely a matter of tuning algorithms developed for a small set of images. Instead, addressing the issues directly can lead to fundamental insights and to algorithms that work well in many different circumstances. This is illustrated here in the context of retinal image registration.

3   Feature Extraction

Most approaches to retinal image analysis, regardless of the application, start with some form of feature extraction. Feature extraction includes the vascular structure [7,21,32], the optic disk location and boundary [20,27], the macula [32], and regions of pathologies [6, 15, 22, 30, 31, 37, 50, 55]. Even when the primary feature extraction goal is detection of pathologies, the location of the optic disk, the macula and the vessels are still important, both as an aid in detection and

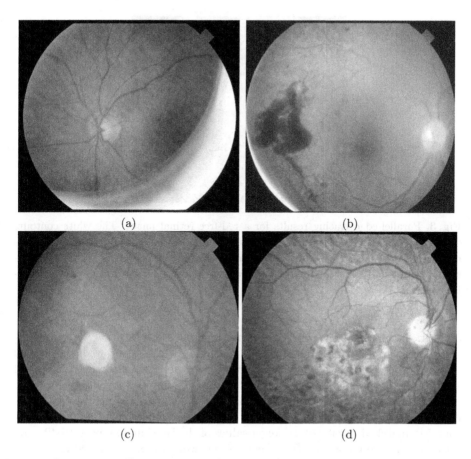

Fig. 2. These images illustrate some of the challenges of retinal image analysis: (a) shows non-uniform illumination caused by glare as well as a partially-effaced retina where the choroidal vessels are starting to appear; in (b) substantial sections of the retina are obscured by a hemorrhage (on the left) and a slight clouding of the vitreous; in (c) the optic disk is not the brightest region of the image, the macula is not clearly visible, and as in (a) the choroidal vasculature is starting to appear; in (d) vasculitis has caused the appearance of pathological regions, the narrowing of vessels, and the neovascularization appearing below and to the left of the optic disk

in interpretation — pathologies such as drusen appearing near the macula are of much greater concern in the progression of macular degeneration than drusen appearing elsewhere on the retina.

3.1 Vascular Structure

The first question in vessel extraction is whether the goal should be segmentation of pixels corresponding to vascular structure or extraction of more geometric

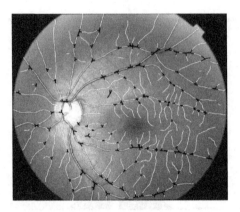

Fig. 3. Parallel-edge tracing results for a red-free retinal image. The white contours show the extracted vessel centerline points. Landmarks detected where these contours meet are show as dark segments. Landmarks are used in our first retinal image registration algorithm, while landmarks and traces are both used in the subsequent Dual-Bootstrap ICP.

quantities such as the location of the centerlines of vessels together with the associated vessel orientations and widths. In our work at Rensselaer, we have stressed geometric descriptions because they are more closely matched to the needs of algorithms that follow. See [21] and [42] for results on pixel-level segmentation.

The next issue is to determine the primary image measurement used to indicate the presence of a vessel. Common techniques include morphological operators [54], matched-filters [10,21], eigenvalues of the Hessian matrix [1,16,42], and a two-sided edge model [7,17]. In most of our work we have stressed the latter. Centerline points of the vessels are placed halfway between anti-parallel edge elements [7], each located to subpixel accuracy [17]. The primary thresholds are determined adaptively based on robustly-computed statistics of intensity gradients in relatively small, overlapping image regions. In very recent work [41], we have built a hybrid vessel measurement model, combining multiscale matched filter responses, Hessian measures, two-sided edge models, and associated confidence measures into a 6-component feature vector at each pixel, which is then mapped into a likelihood ratio. This gives better response to low-contrast vessels and narrow vessels, while avoiding false responses due to the appearance of pathologies.

Our vessel extraction algorithms, like many others [1], use a recursive tracing framework. Seed points on vessels are detected using 1-D searches along vertical and horizontal lines. Tracing starts from these seed points, one at a time, and steps along the vessel centerlines. At each step, the vessel model is applied and the centerline position, the vessel orientation, and the vessel width are all estimated. Tracing for a given seed point ends when the strength of the response is too low, or when a vessel is reached that has already been traced. The two-sided edge algorithm runs in less than a second on megapixel images, whereas the new

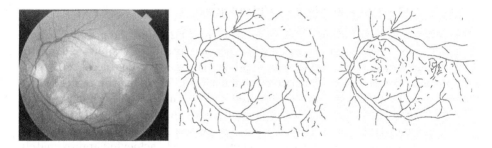

Fig. 4. An example image with parallel-edge (center) and likelihood-ratio (right) tracing results. The new likelihood-ratio results are more complete, especially for narrow and low-contrast vessels.

and more expensive likelihood ratio technique runs in about 10 seconds. The final step of vessel extraction is location of vascular landmarks, which are placed at the branching and cross-over points of the centerline tracings. These are subsequently refined to subpixel accuracy [48]. Thus the final output of tracing is a set of centerline points with their widths and orientations and a set of landmarks with their locations and the orientations of the vessels that meet to form them. Figure 3 shows an example of detecting traces and landmarks, while Figure 4 shows a side-by-side comparison between the results of parallel-edge tracing and likelihood-ratio tracing.

While these results appear nearly complete, several challenges remain:

- On larger vessels there is sometimes a bright strip running along the center of a vessel called the "central reflex". Locally such vessels can easily be misinterpreted as two smaller vessels running side-by-side.
- The most subtle vessels are difficult to detect in small image regions — they disappear into the noise. This might not seem to be a significant problem except that the presence of small vessels above and below an image region, but not running through it, is a good cue for the location of the macula.
- Vessels are particularly difficult to detect in the later stages of a fluorescein angiography sequence.
- Neovascularization (Figure 2(d)), a sign of proliferative diabetic retinopathy, is not easily detected using standard techniques for extracting retinal vasculature. Specialized algorithms are needed to handle their short, thin, tortuous appearance.
- Finally, an important issue in mapping out the structure of the retina is the higher-level organization of the vasculature, including complete trees of veins and arteries.

One key to addressing many of these questions appears to be application of higher-level information over larger image domains. Some important preliminary steps in this direction are reported in [42].

3.2   Optic Disk, Macula and Pathologies

Detection and localization of the optic disk [14, 20, 28] and the macular region, as well as segmentation of pathologies such as cotton-wool spots and micro-aneurysms (for diabetic retinopathy) and drusen (macular degeneration) are all important. Because optic disk detection must work for unhealthy retinas where the typical bright appearance is obscured and because pathologies may appear brighter than the disk, the most important cue is the convergence of the large-scale vascular structure. In Hoover's work [20], vessel endpoints are used together with brightness and shape measures to detect the disk, achieving approximately 90% detection on a challenging data set.

In unhealthy retinas, the characteristic dark shape of the macula is often lost. Additional cues must be used including the position of the optic disk and the position of the vessels, as discussed above. To the best of our knowledge, this remains an open problem.

Techniques for detecting pathologies typically use a suite of methods, including illumination correction [33, 55], morphological shape operations [15, 37, 50], vessel detection [22], and classifier systems [30, 31, 6, 55]. A detailed discussion of these methods is beyond the scope of this paper.

4   Registration

Retinal image registration is challenging for all the reasons outlined in Section 2. Examples of the application of registration, including multisensor fusion and mosaic construction to obtain broader views of the retina, are illustrated in Figure 5.

4.1   Transformation Model

In developing a registration algorithm, one of the first considerations is determining an appropriate transformation model for mapping the pixels from one image into the coordinate system of the other. Earlier retinal image registration algorithms used affine transformations or planar projective transformations [4, 29, 53]. These models are accurate for lower resolution images (e.g. 512x512 or below), especially when images are taken from roughly the same viewpoint. For higher resolution images and images taken from differing viewpoints, a higher-order transformation is needed. In [8, 9] we derived a quadratic transformation using three assumptions: rigid motion of the retina between views, a quadratic retinal surface, and a weak-perspective camera. From these we obtained a 12-parameter quadratic model of the form

$$\mathbf{T}(\mathbf{p}; \boldsymbol{\theta}) = \begin{pmatrix} \theta_{11} & \theta_{12} & \theta_{13} & \theta_{14} & \theta_{15} & \theta_{16} \\ \theta_{21} & \theta_{22} & \theta_{23} & \theta_{24} & \theta_{25} & \theta_{26} \end{pmatrix} \begin{pmatrix} 1 & x & y & x^2 & xy & y^2 \end{pmatrix}^T , \qquad (1)$$

where $\mathbf{p} = (x, y)^T$ is an image location and $\boldsymbol{\theta}$ is formed from the entries in the 2x6 parameter matrix. Estimating the values of $\boldsymbol{\theta}$ is the algorithmic goal

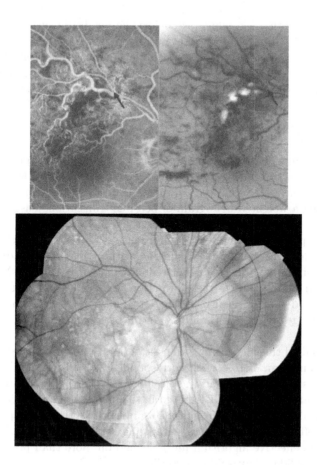

Fig. 5. Example applications of retinal image registration. The top shows a chip from a fluorescein angiogram (left) mapped into the same coordinate system as a fundus image (right). The arrow points to a vein occlusion, seen clearly in the fluorescein angiogram and automatically mapped onto the visible surface of the fundus image. The bottom image shows a mosaic of retinal images constructed using the results of registration.

of registration. The derived quadratic model is accurate to less than 1 pixel on 1024x1024 images, whereas the affine transformation can be off by as many as 5 pixels, depending on the movement of the retina [9]. It is perhaps surprising that the quadratic model is so accurate even though the combined optic system of the fundus camera and the lens of the eye appear to be so complicated. The fundus camera, however, is designed to compensate for the average optics of the human eye, allowing for the effectiveness of the simple model used.

   Applying the quadratic transformation to a retinal image assumes, in effect, that the points on the retina corresponding to the pixels are sitting on a quadratic surface. To the level of precision available in current fundus images, this is true almost everywhere on the retina. However, in the macula and especially in the optic disk, which are below the quadratic surface, application of the transformation can lead to slight misalignments. The amount of misalignment depends on a number of factors, including the effective focal length of the camera, the amount of motion, and the depth of the optic disk and cup. No registration algorithm has yet been developed that compensates for these local misalignments.

4.2   Landmark-Based Algorithm

Our first algorithm is based on landmarks (Figure 3) [8,9]. The quadratic transformation between two images is estimated using a hierarchy of transformation models and estimation techniques. An initial translation between the images is estimated using a weighted histogram of possible translations based on all possible landmark matches. The match set is then culled based on proximity to the histogram peak. An affine transformation is estimated from the resulting matches using a robust random sampling algorithm. The final quadratic transformation is estimated using a further-reduced match set and an M-estimator initialized from the best affine transformation. Experimental evaluation of this algorithm showed that on healthy retinas it almost never fails when the overlap between images is greater than 67% and it often succeeds for lower-overlap images.

The downfall of this algorithm is the restriction to only matching landmarks. It requires a minimum of 10 correct correspondences — 6 to fully constrain the quadratic transformation and at least 4 more to confirm the estimate. Landmark features are not densely distributed in the images, and are quite sparse far from the optic disk. Moreover, in images of unhealthy retinas the appearance of landmarks is often obscured, and repeatable detection of landmarks is difficult. Clearly, a more effective algorithm must depend on more than just landmarks. The obvious candidate is vascular centerlines.

4.3   Dual-Bootstrap

Our second algorithm, the Dual-Bootstrap ICP [43], is neither a revision nor an extension of the first algorithm. It is radically different and novel. The motivation behind the algorithm is the desire to work with as few initial landmark matches as possible. We began to explore this idea in work on real-time indexing and registration in [39], where constellations of two or three matches are used to initialize an affine transformation and matching of vessel centerline points is used to refine it. However, our biggest breakthrough came with the insight that we could get started with just one landmark match. This match gives a limited initial estimate of the mapping between two images. The locations of the matching landmarks in the two images provide an initial indication of the inter-image translation, while comparing the widths and orientations of the vessels meeting to form the landmarks provide the remaining parameters of a similarity transformation. As illustrated in Figure 6 (upper left), this transformation is accurate in a small image region surrounding the matching landmark, but much less accurate farther away.

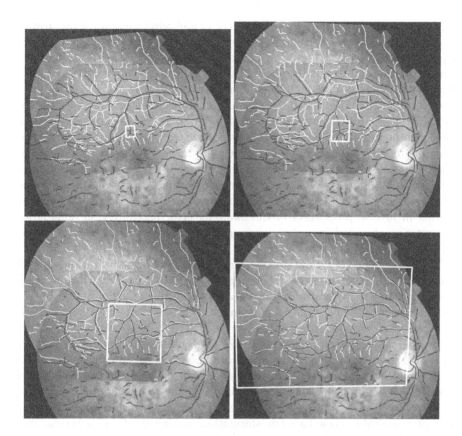

Fig. 6. The Dual-Bootstrap ICP algorithm. The upper left shows the initial similarity-transformation alignment of two retinal images based on a single landmark correspondence. (The black contours are vessel centerline points extracted from one image and the white contours are vessel centerline points extracted from the other.) The transformation is only well-aligned within the bootstrap region, shown as a white rectangle. The other three panels show the progress of the Dual-Bootstrap algorithm, with the alignment becoming better and better as the iterations proceed and the region grows.

This insight raised two questions: (1) how to generate the initial landmark match, and (2) how to generate a quadratic transformation that is accurate throughout the images from the initial similarity transformation. To address the first issue we compute a signature vector of similarity invariants at each landmark, and then match these signature vectors between images. Matches are rank-ordered by signature vector distance, and then tested one-by-one starting with the match that has the lowest distance. Each match is used to generate a similarity transformation as described in the previous paragraph and then each is tested using the following algorithm, which addresses the second question.

Starting from the initial similarity transformation and using the vessel centerline points extracted by tracing, the Dual-Bootstrap ICP algorithm iterates three steps until convergence: re-estimation, model selection and region growing (Figure 6). (1) The transformation parameters are re-estimated by applying one step of a robust form of the iterative closest points (ICP) algorithm [5, 11, 35] using **only** the centerline points within the small region (the "bootstrap region") surrounding the initial match in the moving image. (2) The alignment error and covariance matrix of the transformation parameters are used in model selection, automatically choosing between the initial similarity transformation, an affine transformation, a simplified form of the quadratic transformation (called the "reduced quadratic" [43]), and the full quadratic model for the current bootstrap region. As the region grows, more vessel centerline points are included and more matching constraints are generated, allowing the model to switch from lower-order to higher-order models. (3) The bootstrap region is expanded outward, growing in inverse proportion to the mapping error on the region boundaries. This error is computed from the covariance matrix of the transformation parameters using error propagation techniques [19, Ch. 4].

The Dual-Bootstrap iterations converge when the bootstrap region expands to cover the overlap between images, model selection reaches the quadratic model, and the ICP iterations converge. The resulting transformation is then tested for accuracy (centerlines alignment error is less than 1.5 pixels) and stability (full-rank parameter estimate covariance matrix). If it passes these tests it is excepted as correct and the whole algorithm terminates. Otherwise the next initial estimate is evaluated. The algorithm ends and indicates that it can not align two images when a user-defined number of initial transformations has been tried. Interestingly, in more than half the cases the first match is correct and the Dual-Bootstrap converts this into a correct overall transformation. Figure 6 illustrates several intermediate transformations during the Dual-Bootstrap iterations, and the final mapping between the two images.

Experimental evaluation of the Dual-Bootstrap has produced impressive results. Tests on over 10,000 image pairs have shown that it always succeeds in producing an accurate transformation when (a) the images overlap by at least 30%, (b) at least one common landmark has been detected in the two images and (c) there are enough trace centerline points detected in the overlap between the images to obtain a stable transformation estimate. We have also applied this algorithm to aligning color or red-free fundus images with the images of a FA sequence. The algorithm succeeds quite well in doing so, failing only in extreme cases where the fluorescein dye leaks immediately into the retina or late in the sequence ("late recirculation") where the dye is heavily diluted [47]. Figure 5 shows an example of the alignment of a red-free image and fluorescein angiogram.

4.4   Generalized Dual-Bootstrap

Our next innovation in registration came by moving the Dual-Bootstrap approach beyond the retinal application [52]. Doing so requires addressing two primary issues: an initialization method is needed that does not depend on extracting vascular landmarks, and image information other than the location of vascular centerlines is needed to drive the Dual-Bootstrap growth and refinement

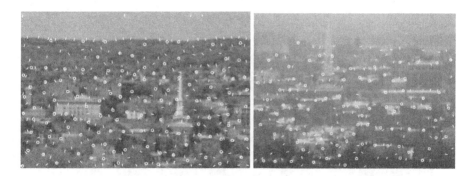

Fig. 7. Two images taken during the winter and sumer, with some the generic features needed to drive the Generalized Dual-Bootstrap algorithm. Face points are shown with line segments and corners are shown with small circles. Features are shown only at a single coarse scale, even though features at all scales are used simultaneously.

process. Solving the first issue simply requires applying recent keypoint matching algorithms from the computer vision literature, Lowe's in particular [26]. Multiscale keypoints are detected by finding peaks in the Laplacian-of-Gaussian response in both spatial and scale dimensions. These keypoints are matched according to a locally-computed signature vector and the matches are rank-ordered according to their distinctiveness. These matches play the same role as landmark correspondences in generating initial matches for the Dual-Bootstrap growth and refinement process.

In order to address the second issue we developed a new generic, multiscale feature extraction technique. The idea is to evaluate the gradient distribution in neighborhoods surrounding each pixel, characterizing each according to whether there are one or two dimensions of signifiant spatial variation in the intensity near the pixel. Features of the first type are "face points", while features of the second type are "corners". Thresholds on the required strengths of these features are determined from robustly-computed local image statistics. The features used in registration are chosen to ensure wide-spread distribution throughout an image. The result, as shown in Figure 7, is not necessarily a perceptually-pleasing set of features. Instead it is a set of features sufficient to drive Dual-Bootstrap registration in place of the original vessel centerlines.

Several other innovations are used to make the Dual-Bootstrap work on a diverse set of images. First, matching is applied symmetrically from the fixed image to the moving image and vice-versa. The transformation parameters are estimated in both directions. This produces a denser and more reliable set of matches, especially in handling small bootstrap regions and scale changes between images. Second, features at all scales are used simultaneously during registration. Third, two different types of distance constraints are used during estimation, one for corners and one for face points. These are combined during parameter estimation using both a standard (though robust) linear least-squares estimation and using Levenberg-Marquardt. Finally, a much more sophisticated

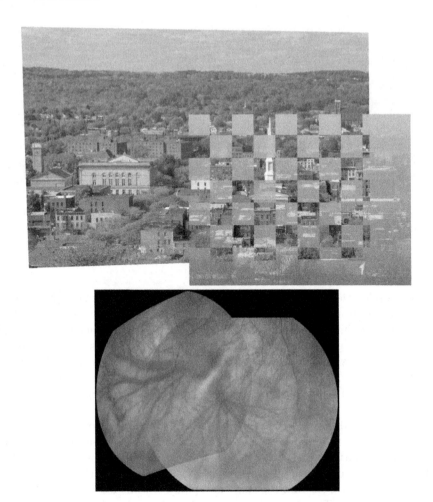

Fig. 8. Two registration results using the Generalized Dual-Bootstrap. The top shows a checkerboard of the alignment of the winter-summer pair from Figure 7, while the bottom shows a mosaic of two retinal images that the original Dual-Bootstrap did not successfully align because of the appearance of the choroidal vessels.

decision criteria is needed, one that requires images to be well-aligned, the mapping to be stable on the boundaries of the bootstrap region, and the resulting face-point matches to have closely-aligned orientations.

This "Generalized Dual-Bootstrap" algorithm has proven to be effective in tests on an extremely challenging database of images, including successful alignments of overlapping images taken day and night and winter and summer. Examples are shown in Figure 8. Interestingly, and importantly, one of the two pairs shown is a retinal image pair that the original Dual-Bootstrap could not align: The images are dominated by the appearance of the choroidal vasculature, which is much larger than the retinal vasculature. The tracing-based vessel and landmark extraction algorithm could not produce enough constraints to drive the Dual-Bootstrap, but the more generic technique, which does not rely on the appearance of particular structures, was successful.

4.5 Multi-image Registration and Mosaics

In combination with our algorithms for aligning pairs of retinal images ("pairwise registration"), we have developed algorithms for simultaneously aligning multiple images. These can be used to play aligned images of a FA sequence as a movie loop, to visualize changes over multiple visits, and to build a mosaic of images, providing a broader view than available from a single image alone.

Each of the N images to be aligned may be thought of as nodes in a graph. Each of the $N(N-1)/2$ possible pairs of the images may be tested individually using the Dual-Bootstrap or Generalized Dual-Bootstrap, and when a pair is successfully aligned the associated nodes are linked to form an edge in the graph. The final ICP feature correspondences are saved with this edge. (Simple heuristics may be used to avoid testing pairs that obviously do not overlap once the graph is partially constructed.) If the final graph is connected, all images may be jointly aligned; otherwise only the images in each connected-component may be aligned separately. In computing the final set of transformations, one image is chosen as the anchor to determine the final coordinate frame, and the quadratic transformation parameters mapping each image onto this anchor are estimated jointly using the final correspondence sets. Unlike other multi-image registration techniques [36], no bundle adjustment is necessary because the final positions of the mapped feature points are not explicitly constructed.

This overall procedure is capable of consistent alignments even for images that do not overlap the anchor or for image pairs that overlap but the Dual-Bootstrap could not align. (In more recent work, we've introduced the capability of adding new constraints between such images [51], improving the results for datasets with extremely low overlaps.) An example mosaic is shown in Figure 5. In extensive tests on the retrospective data set described in Section 4.3, we found that the overall procedure left only 2 of the 855 images unaligned with other images from the same retina (recall that there are images from 46 retinas in this set) [47]. Both these images are completely featureless and can not be aligned manually. Multi-image registration also works extremely well in aligning fluorescein angiogram sequences, except occasionally for images taken in the "late recirculation" stage, after the dye has pooled and been diluted by recirculation through the body (see Figure 1(c)). These results show that our pairwise and multi-image registration algorithms are sufficiently accurate and reliable for many routine clinical applications.

5 Other Problems and Algorithms

Research on retinal image analysis has focused on other problems as well. This includes work at Rensselaer. Here are three important problem areas:

- We have developed real-time versions of some of our earlier registration algorithms [39, 25], together with underlying supporting systems implementations [49]. The goal is accurate knowledge of the position of a surgical tool, such as a laser, with respect to a map of the retina (built off-line), within a guaranteed response time. Related work is reported in [2, 3].
- Researchers have begun to address the problem of using stereo images of the optic disk to construct a depth map of the optic cup [12]. One problem in doing so is that true stereo fundus cameras are not widely available, so that stereo images must be created through movement of the head and eye. Since this movement must be small, is uncontrolled, and involves rotations that do not add significant information about depth, accurate 3d reconstructions are difficult to obtain in many circumstances. If true stereo fundus cameras become available, stereo reconstruction of the disk will become an important problem.
- While the wide-spread availability and predominant clinical use of fundus cameras has led most research on retinal image analysis to concentrate on fundus (color and red-free) images and fluorescein angiography, image analysis algorithms have been developed for other modalities as well. Of particular interest are the use of edge detection, boundary models and active contour techniques in delineating fluid-filled regions [13] and measuring retinal thickness [23] in optical coherence tomography.

6   Discussion

A number of lessons may be gleaned from the success of our retinal image registration algorithms. First, it is important to work with a wide range of data sets indicative of what might be seen in practice. It is not sufficient to work from a small sampling and assume the algorithms will generalize with minor modification. Instead, building the algorithm needed to work on a diverse set of data and on the most challenging cases requires fundamental innovations. Second, extensive testing of algorithms, including careful analysis of the causes of failure, is important not only to validate particular techniques but to lay the ground work for future innovations. Finally, even though algorithm development may be motivated by particular applications, it is important to push toward generality. By trying to minimize the assumptions on which an algorithm depends, the probability that the algorithm will be useful beyond the original application and development data set will be substantially increased.

There are a number of open issues in retinal image analysis. Many of these have already been mentioned in the paper, but they are gathered here for completeness.

- Within the context of registration there are two major issues. One is handling especially challenging imagery from late in the recirculation phases of fluorescein angiography and from indocyanine green angiography which is dominated by the appearance of choroidal vasculature. The second is handling the elevations and depressions of the retinal surface caused by the macula, the optic disk and macular edema. These can cause distracting misalignments of image regions after registration.

- Within the context of feature extraction, a major problem remains building a complete map of the retina that includes labeling the arteries and veins and their branching structure and identifying the optic disk and macula. Significant progress has been made in some of these areas, but a fully-reliable system has not yet been developed.
- Feature extraction also includes automatic pathology detection as an aid to large-scale, rapid screening for diabetic retinopathy and macular degeneration. Challenges include handling the small size of the features, accommodating variations in illumination, and employing knowledge of the map of the retina to interpret the significance of the results.
- Further work in feature detection is needed to detect and characterize neovascularization both near the optic disk and on the periphery of the retina. These small, narrow and tortuous vessels are not captured by standard feature extraction methods.
- Finally, the success of registration has opened the door to automatic change detection, both in the vascular structure [18] and to signal the presence of pathologies. While pathologies appear and disappear frequently during the progress of disease, the ability to align longitudinal images and detect changes provides additional information for the detection and characterization of disease.

In conclusion, the success of current algorithms for retinal image analysis, the challenge of remaining problems, and the societal importance of building tools to aid in the diagnosis and treatment retinal diseases ensure that retinal image analysis will remain an important area of research in medical imaging and computer vision for the foreseeable future.

References

[1] S. Aylward and E. Bullitt. Initialization, noise, singularities, and scale in height-ridge traversal for tubular object centerline extraction. *IEEE Trans. Med. Imaging.*, 21:61–75, 2002.

[2] S. F. Barrett, W. C. H. G., and M. R. Jerath. Computer-aided retinal photocoagulation system. *J. Biomed. Optics*, 1:83–91, 1996.

[3] S. F. Barrett, C. H. G. Wright, H. Zwick, M. Wilcox, B. A. Rockwell, and E. Naess. Efficiently tracking a moving object in two-dimensional image space. *J. Electronic Imaging*, 10(3):785–793, 2001.

[4] J. W. Berger, M. E. Leventon, N. Hata, W. Wells, and R. Kikinis. Design considerations for a computer-vision-enabled ophthalmic augmented reality environment. In *Lecture Notes in Computer Science: 1205*, pages 399–408, 1997.

[5] P. Besl and N. McKay. A method for registration of 3-d shapes. *IEEE T. Pattern Anal.*, 14(2):239–256, 1992.

[6] L. Brandon and A. Hoover. Drusen detection in a retinal image using multi-level analysis. In *Proc. 6th MICCAI*, pages 618–625, 2003.

[7] A. Can, H. Shen, J. N. Turner, H. L. Tanenbaum, and B. Roysam. Rapid
     automated tracing and feature extraction from live high-resolution retinal fun-
     dus images using direct exploratory algorithms. *IEEE Trans. on Inf. Tech. in
     Biomedicine*, 3(2):125–138, 1999.
[8] A. Can, C. Stewart, and B. Roysam. Robust hierarchical algorithm for construct-
     ing a mosaic from images of the curved human retina. In *Proc. CVPR*, pages
     286–292, 1999.
[9] A. Can, C. Stewart, B. Roysam, and H. Tanenbaum. A feature-based, robust,
     hierarchical algorithm for registering pairs of images of the curved human retina.
     IEEE T. Pattern Anal., 24(3):347–364, 2002.
[10] S. Chaudhuri, S. Chatterjee, N. Katz, M. Nelson, and M. Goldbaum. Detection
     of blood vessels in retinal images using two-dimensional matched filters. *IEEE
     Trans. Med. Imaging.*, 8(3):263–269, September 1989.
[11] Y. Chen and G. Medioni. Object modeling by registration of multiple range
     images. *IVC*, 10(3):145–155, 1992.
[12] E. Corona, S. Mitra, M. Wilson, T. Krile, Y. H. Kwon, and P. Soliz. Digital stereo
     image analyzer for generating automated 3-d measures of optic disc deformation
     in glaucoma. *IEEE Trans. Med. Imaging.*, 21(10):1244–1253, 2002.
[13] D. C. Fernández. Delineating fluid-filled region boundaries in optical coherence
     tomography images of the retina. *IEEE Trans. Med. Imaging.*, 24(8):929–945,
     2005.
[14] M. Foracchia, E. Grisan, and A. Ruggeri. Detection of optic disc in retinal images
     by means of a geometrical model of vessel structure. *IEEE Trans. Med. Imaging.*,
     23(10):1189–1195, Oct. 2004.
[15] A. Frame, P. Undrill, M. Cree, J. Olson, K. McHardy, P. Sharp, and J. Forrester.
     A comparison of computer based classification methods applied to the detection
     of microaneurysms in ophthalmic fluorescein angiograms. *Comp. Bio. and Med.*,
     pages 225–38, MAY 1998.
[16] A. Frangi, W. J. Niessen, K. L. Vincken, and M. A. Viergever. Multiscale vessel
     enhancement filtering. In *Proc. 1st MICCAI*, pages 130–137, 1998.
[17] K. Fritzsche, A. Can, H. Shen, C. Tsai, J. Turner, H. Tanenbuam, C. Stewart, and
     B. Roysam. Automated model based segmentation, tracing and analysis of retinal
     vasculature from digital fundus images. In J. S. Suri and S. Laxminarayan, editors,
     *State-of-The-Art Angiography, Applications and Plaque Imaging Using MR, CT,
     Ultrasound and X-rays*, pages 225–298. Academic Press, 2003.
[18] K. H. Fritzsche. *Computer Vision Algorithms for Retinal Vessel Detection and
     Width Change Detection.* PhD thesis, Rensselaer Polytechnic Institute, Troy, New
     York, Dec 2004.
[19] R. Hartley and A. Zisserman. *Multiple View Geometry.* Cambridge University
     Press, 2000.
[20] A. Hoover and M. Goldbaum. Locating the optic nerve in a retinal image using the
     fuzzy convergence of the blood vessels. *IEEE Trans. Med. Imaging.*, 22(8):951–
     958, 2003. http://www.parl.clemson.edu/stare/nerve/.
[21] A. Hoover, V. Kouznetsova, and M. Goldbaum. Locating blood vessels in retinal
     images by piecewise threshold probing of a matched filter response. *IEEE Trans.
     Med. Imaging.*, 19(3):203–210, 2000.
[22] J. Jomier, D. K. Wallace, and S. R. Aylward. Quantification of retinopathy of
     prematurity via vessel segmentation. In *Proc. 6th MICCAI*, pages 620–626, 2003.
[23] D. Koozekanani, K. Boyer, and C. Roberts. Retinal thickness measurements from
     optical coherence tomography using a markov boundary model. *IEEE Trans. Med.
     Imaging.*, 20:900–916, Sept. 2001.

[24] H. Li and O. Chutatape. A model-based approach for automated feature extraction in fundus images. In *Proc. ICCV*, pages 394–399, 2003.

[25] G. Lin, C. V. Stewart, B. Roysam, K. Fritzsche, and G. Yang. Predictive scheduling algorithms for real-time feature extraction and spatial referencing: Application to retinal image sequences. *IEEE Trans. on Biomed. Eng.*, 51:115–124, 2004.

[26] D. G. Lowe. Distinctive image features from scale-invariant keypoints. *IJCV*, 60(2):91–110, November 2004.

[27] J. Lowell, A. Hunter, D. Steel, A. Basu, R. Ryder, and E. Fletcher. Optic nerve head segmentation. *IEEE Trans. Med. Imaging.*, 23(2):256–264, 2004.

[28] J. Lowell, A. Hunter, D. Steel, A. Basu, R. Ryder, and R. Kennedy. Measurement of retinal vessel widths from fundus images based on 2-D modeling. *IEEE Trans. Med. Imaging.*, 23(10):1196–1204, Oct. 2004.

[29] G. K. Matsopoulos, N. A. Mouravliansky, K. K. Delibasis, and K. S. Nikita. Automatic retinal image registration scheme using global optimization techniques. *IEEE Trans. on Inf. Tech. in Biomedicine*, 3(1):47–60, 1999.

[30] M. Niemeijer, B. van Ginneken, J. Staal, M. Suttorp-Schulten, and M. Abramoff. Automatic detection of red lesions in digital color fundus photographs. *IEEE Trans. Med. Imaging.*, 24(5):584–592, May 2005.

[31] A. Osareh, M. Mirmehdi, B. Thomas, and R. Markham. Comparative exudate classification using support vector machines and neural networks. In *Proc. 5th MICCAI*, pages 413–420, 2002.

[32] A. Pinz, S. Bernogger, P. Datlinger, and A. Kruger. Mapping the human retina. *IEEE Trans. Med. Imaging.*, 17(4):606–620, Aug 1998.

[33] K. Rapantzikos, M. Zervakis, and K. Balas. Detection and segmentation of drusen deposits on human retina: Potential in the diagnosis of age-related macular degeneration. *Med. Image Anal.*, 7(1):95–108, Mar. 2003.

[34] N. Ritter, R. Owens, J. Cooper, R. Eikelboom, and P. van Saarloos. Registration of stereo and temporal images of the retina. *IEEE Trans. Med. Imaging.*, 18(5):404–418, 1999.

[35] S. Rusinkiewicz and M. Levoy. Efficient variants of the ICP algorithm. In *Proc. Third Int. Conf. on 3DIM*, pages 224–231, 2001.

[36] H. Sawhney, S. Hsu, and R. Kumar. Robust video mosaicing through topology inference and local to global alignment. In *Proc. 5th ECCV*, volume II, pages 103–119, 1998.

[37] Z. B. Sbeh, L. D. Cohen, G. Mimoun, and G. Coscas. A new approach for geodesic reconstruction in mathematical morphology and application to image segmentation and tracking in ophtalmology. *IEEE Trans. Med. Imaging.*, 20(12):1321–1333, Dec. 2001.

[38] U. Schmidt-Erfurth et al. Photodynamic therapy with verteporfin for choroidal neovascularization caused by age-related macular degeneration: results of retreatments in a phase 1 and 2 study. *Arch. Ophth.*, 117(9):1177–87, 1999.

[39] H. Shen, C. Stewart, B. Roysam, G. Lin, and H. Tanenbaum. Frame-rate spatial referencing based on invariant indexing and alignment with application to laser retinal surgery. *IEEE T. Pattern Anal.*, 25(3):379–384, March 2003.

[40] J. A. Shoemaker. Vision problems in the U.S. Technical report, U.S. National Institute of Health, 2002.

[41] M. Sofka and C. V. Stewart. Retinal vessel extraction using multiscale matched filters, confidence and edge measures. Technical Report 05-20, Department of Computer Science, Rensselaer Polytechnic Institute, 2005.

[42] J. Staal, M. Abramoff, M. Niemeijer, M. Viergever, and B. van Ginneken. Ridge based vessel segmentation in color images of the retina. *IEEE Trans. Med. Imaging.*, 23(4):501–509, Apr 2004.

[43] C. Stewart, C.-L. Tsai, and B. Roysam. The dual-bootstrap iterative closest point algorithm with application to retinal image registration. *IEEE Trans. Med. Imaging.*, 22(11):1379–1394, 2003.

[44] The Eye Diseases Prevalence Research Group. Prevalence of age-related macular degeneration in the united states. *Arch. Ophth.*, 122(4):564–572, 2004.

[45] The Eye Diseases Prevalence Research Group. The prevalence of diabetic retinopathy among adults in the united states. *Arch. Ophth.*, 122(4):552–563, 2004.

[46] The Eye Diseases Prevalence Research Group. Prevalence of open-angle glaucoma among adults in the united states. *Arch. Ophth.*, 122(4):532–538, 2004.

[47] C.-L. Tsai, A. Majerovics, C. V. Stewart, and B. Roysam. Disease-oriented evaluation of dual-bootstrap retinal image registration. In *Proc. 6th MICCAI*, volume II, pages 754–761, 2003.

[48] C.-L. Tsai, C. Stewart, B. Roysam, and H. Tanenbaum. Repeatable vascular landmark extraction from retinal fundus images using local vascular traces. *IEEE Trans. on Inf. Tech. in Biomedicine*, to appear 2003.

[49] J. A. Tyrrell, J. M. LaPre, C. D. Carothers, B. Roysam, and C. V. Stewart. Efficient migration of complex off-line computer vision software to real-time system implementation on generic computer hardware. *IEEE Trans. on Inf. Tech. in Biomedicine*, 8(2):142–153, 2004.

[50] T. Walter, J.-C. Klein, P. Massin, and A. Erginay. A contribution of image processing to the diagnosis of diabetic retinopathy - detection of exudates in color fundus images of the human retina. *IEEE Trans. Med. Imaging.*, 21(10), Oct. 2002.

[51] G. Yang and C. V. Stewart. Covariance-driven mosaic formation from sparsely-overlapping image sets with application to retinal image mosaicing. In *Proc. CVPR*, pages 804– 810, 2004.

[52] G. Yang, C. V. Stewart, M. Sofka, and C.-L. Tsai. The Generalized Dual-Bootstrap ICP algorithm with application to registering challenging image pairs. Technical Report 05-19, Department of Computer Science, Rensselaer Polytechnic Institute, 2005.

[53] F. Zana and J. C. Klein. A multimodal registration algorithm of eye fundus images using vessels detection and Hough transform. *IEEE Trans. Med. Imaging.*, 18(5):419–428, 1999.

[54] F. Zana and J.-C. Klein. Segmentation of vessel-like patterns using mathematical morphology and curvature evaluation. *IEEE Trans. Image Process.*, 10(7):1010–1019, 2001.

[55] X. Zhang and A. Chutatape. Top-down and bottom-up strategies in lesion detection of background diabetic retinopathy. In *Proc. CVPR*, pages 422–428, 2005.

3D Statistical Shape Models to Embed Spatial Relationship Information

Jurgen Fripp[1,2], Pierrick Bourgeat[1], Andrea J.U. Mewes[3], Simon K. Warfield[3], Stuart Crozier[2], and Sébastien Ourselin[1]

[1] BioMedIALab,
CSIRO ICT Centre, Australia
{jurgen.fripp, pierrick.bourgeat, sebastien.ourselin}@csiro.au
[2] School of ITEE,
University of Queensland, Australia
stuart@itee.uq.edu.au
[3] Computational Radiology Laboratory,
Harvard Medical School,
Departments of Radiology, Brigham and Women's Hospital
and Children's Hospital, 75 Francis St, Boston MA 02115
{mewes, warfield}@bwh.harvard.edu

Abstract. This paper presents the creation of 3D statistical shape models of the knee bones and their use to embed information into a segmentation system for MRIs of the knee. We propose utilising the strong spatial relationship between the cartilages and the bones in the knee by embedding this information into the created models. This information can then be used to automate the initialisation of segmentation algorithms for the cartilages. The approach used to automatically generate the 3D statistical shape models of the bones is based on the point distribution model optimisation framework of Davies. Our implementation of this scheme uses a parameterized surface extraction algorithm, which is used as the basis for the optimisation scheme that automatically creates the 3D statistical shape models. The current approach is illustrated by generating 3D statistical shape models of the patella, tibia and femoral bones from a segmented database of the knee. The use of these models to embed spatial relationship information to aid in the automation of segmentation algorithms for the cartilages is then illustrated.

1   Introduction

Osteoarthritis (OA) of the knee is usually characterized by the degeneration of the articular cartilage. However, the progression of OA is much more complicated, usually consisting of changes in all the cartilages, bones and other tissues in the knee. Nevertheless, the loss of the few millimeters of thickness in the articular cartilage is still regarded as the most important feature to monitor OA progression. As OA develops, the changes undergone by the articular cartilage are not simply degenerative, rather it usually consists of localised thinning or thickening that develops slowly over time. The ability to accurately measure this

Y. Liu, T. Jiang, and C. Zhang (Eds.): CVBIA 2005, LNCS 3765, pp. 51–60, 2005.

degeneration is essential to the development of pharmaceuticals and therapies for OA.

Several MR sequences now exist that provide a non-invasive way to obtain high contrast accurate images of the knee cartilage morphology [1]. The potential of MRI to more accurately diagnose and monitor OA compared to other imaging modalities has now been shown in numerous studies. These studies usually monitored the progression of OA using measurements like thickness [2][3], volume [4] and surface area [5].

To obtain these measures from 3D MR images requires the articular cartilage to be segmented, preferably in an accurate and repeatable way. Unfortunately due to the low contrast in several areas particularly in the joint contact areas, tendons and ligaments, fully automated segmentation of the cartilage has not been achieved. Current clinical studies have favored the use of supervised semi-automated 2D algorithms like region growing [6], active shape models [7], active contours [8] and live wire [9]. These algorithms all require various degrees of user interaction, verification and correction of the segmentations results on a slice by slice basis. These approaches have significantly reduced the time taken to segment a dataset and provide provide higher intra- and inter-observer consistency than fully manual methods. However, for routine clinical use they are still too time consuming, so a fully automated approach is desirable.

To fully automate the segmentation of the cartilages requires the segmentation to be performed directly in 3D. There have only been a few attempts to do this, including a model based approach [10], immersion based watershed [11] and statistical classification [12]. The most promising work uses a modified watershed metric that utilises prior information to perform the segmentation of the cartilages [13]. This algorithm can be combined with an atlas registration to fully automate the segmentations, however this has yet to be performed with the cartilages.

1.1   Segmentation System for the Knee

The philosophy behind our segmentation system for the knee is similar to the thoughts of both Kapur [10] and Hamarneh [14] and is focused on the effective but flexible incorporation of *a priori* knowledge, which is utilised intelligently to obtain automated, accurate and robust segmentations of the knee. Different types of knowledge needs to be used in order to attain the required automation, accuracy and the robustness.

Shape information is the most important piece of knowledge for the knee as it allows us to compensate for the missing or poor delineation seen in the cartilages. This primarily is used to improve the robustness of the segmentation algorithm, which is essential if full automation is desired. In 2D, active shape models (ASMs) have been shown to produce accurate and robust results for the articular cartilage [7]. The primary problem with ASM type approaches is that they are sensitive to initialisation, and for many providing a good automatic initialisation is difficult. Spatial relationship information is one of the primary piece of knowledge that can be used to aid in automating the initialisation of segmentation algorithms.

The core of the segmentation system will be a statistical map of the knee based around 3D statistical shape models (SSMs). Besides the use of the SSM to incorporate shape information we propose to use it as a framework to include *a priori* knowledge by utilising the corresponding landmarks to extract information from the set of training images. This type of approach is used in grey level modeling of ASMs; however, our segmentation system incorporates various other types of information including texture and spatial relationship information. This information is used either by embedding it inside the SSM or modeling the associated information separately. The incorporation of image derived information will aid the accuracy and robustness of the segmentations, while spatial relationship information will aid in automating and self correcting the segmentation system.

The first part of this paper presents the automatic creation of 3D SSMs of the patella, tibia and femoral bones using an implementation based on the Point Distribution Model optimisation scheme of Davies [15]. The second part of the paper presents how these models are then extended to include associated or embedded spatial relationship information. The strong spatial relationship between the bones and the cartilages is used to illustrate how this information could be used to automatically initialise segmentation algorithms of the cartilages.

2 Methodology

2.1 Subjects and Imaging

This work used a knee database provided by Brigham and Women's Hospital that consisted of 15 normal adults scanned using 1.5 and 3 T G.E. MR scanners with a fat suppressed 3D SPGR MR sequence. The sequence parameters were $t_e = 5$ or 7 msec, $t_r = 60$ msec and a flip angle of 40°. The FOV was 120×120 and the acquisition matrix was either 512×512 or 256×256. These were reconstructed to images with dimension of 0.23×0.23 or 0.46×0.46 and slice thickness of 1.5mm. The bones and cartilages in the images were then interactively segmented by experts. To retain the variability of the shaft lengths in the SSM, the femoral and tibia shafts were not concatenated to be proportional to the head widths.

This database is sufficient to evaluate the feasibility and effectiveness of 3D SSM for the knee segmentation system. However, the final knee segmentation system will either require the use of a much larger database or the use of a more sensitive modeling technique than principal component analysis (ie wavelets).

2.2 Statistical Shape Models for the Bones

SSMs provide a compact representation of the shape variability from a training set [16]. A SSM is built from a set of N training shapes s_i ($i = 1, \ldots, N$). Each shape s_i has M points sampled on its surface. These shapes are aligned using generalised Procrustes alignment. Principal Component Analysis (PCA) allows each shape to be written as

$$s_i = \tilde{s} + Pb_i = \tilde{s} + \sum_k p^k b_i^k \qquad (1)$$

where $\tilde{s}$ is the mean shape and $P = p^k$ contains the k eigenvectors of the co-variance matrix. The corresponding eigenvalues (λ^k) describe the amount of variation expressed by each eigenvector. The shape parameters $b = b^k$ are used to control the modes of variation.

To obtain a valid SSM it is necessary that the coordinates are in a common frame of reference and all the points on each surface correspond in an anatomically meaningful way. Several approaches can be used to obtain point correspondence including non-rigid registration [17], deformable models [18] and Point Distribution Model optimisation [15].

The primary problem with using non-rigid registration is that the correspondence obtained is not unique and dependent on the accuracy of the registration, which for objects like cartilage can be highly inaccurate. Deformable models do not generate any true correspondence and Davies Point Distribution Model framework is restricted to genus 0 surfaces and requires already segmented training sets.

For the knee segmentation system we have implemented an automated scheme to generate 3D SSMs based on the Point Distribution Model optimisation framework of Davies et al [15]. The primary reason for this is the flexibility the optimisation scheme allows, where the target results obtained can be altered simply by changing the objective function or the type of model we are optimising[1] This flexibility as well as the known improvement in the correspondence obtained compared to other techniques are the reason we chose this approach.

3   Implementation

The implementation we used for the Point Distribution Model optimisation framework of Davies can be broken down into 3 stages: pre-processing, generation of initial landmarking and the optimisation of the landmarking.

3.1   Pre-processing and Initial Landmarking

The 15 manually segmented knee datasets are pre-processed as outlined in Figure 1. In the literature the surfaces are usually extracted before being decimated (or remeshed) and then smoothed before being parameterized onto a unit sphere. In this work we have used a subdivision based parameterized surface extraction algorithm to guarantee we obtain genus 0 surfaces and parameterization. The full algorithm is similar to shrink wrap algorithms [19] however it is still under development and beyond the scope of this paper.

---

[1] Eg. inclusion of curvature, thickness and other derived measures into the model or objective function.

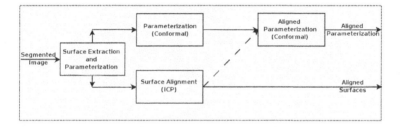

Fig. 1. Overview of Pre-processing

The bone surfaces and parameterization that is used consisted of 4098 vertices for the patella and 16,386 vertices for the tibia and femoral bones. These surfaces are then rigidly ICP aligned, centroid matching and RMS normalisation. The resulting surfaces are then used to align the set of parameterizations.

3.2   Initial Landmarking

The initial SSM is created by quasi-uniformly sampling[2] the parameter space of each ICP aligned surface as outlined and illustrated in Figure 2. The set of re-parameterized surfaces are then used to generate a 3D SSM (see Section 2.2).

To inverse map each vertex in parameter space to the surface, an efficient intersection algorithm using a partitioned parameter space and barycentric coordinates has been utilised.

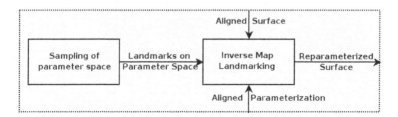

Fig. 2. A surface is re-parameterized by sampling its parameter space and inverse mapping the sampled landmarks onto the surface

3.3   Optimisation of Landmarking

Although the parameter spaces are rotationally aligned there is no true correspondence from the parameterization; the correspondence is obtained by using an implementation of the Point Distribution Model optimisation scheme of Davies [15] (See Figure 3). The Nelder Mead simplex algorithm was used to optimise an eigenspace objective function, $F = \sum_i \log(\lambda_i + \epsilon)$ with $\epsilon = 0.01$.

---

[2] The patella consisted of 1026 vertices and the tibia and femur 4,098 vertices.

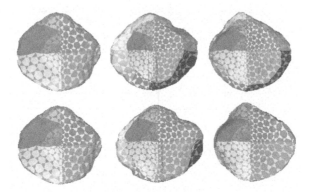

Fig. 3. 3 Patella bones pairs where the left pair is held fixed during the optimisation process. **Top** Initial landmarking **Bottom** Optimised landmarking **Note:** Colouring of surface based on corresponding triangles.

3.4   Associating or Embedding Information into 3D SSM

The creation of corresponding point distribution models allows the extraction of accurate information from the training datasets. The simplest approach is to associate with each point in the model the set of extracted or derived information. An example of this is the expected thickness of the cartilage above a point on the tibia, or the variance of the thickness across the training set (see Figure 4 and 5).

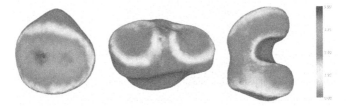

Fig. 4. The mean thickness of the cartilage above each landmark in the SSM

Ideally, rather than having a static representation of the information at each point in the model, it is often preferable that the information varies based on the parameters of the model. One approach to this is to embed the information extracted from the training sets directly into the model by simply extending the dimensionality from R^3 to R^{3+m}, where m is the number of different types of information to be included in the model. This type of approach has been previously used to incorporate thickness variability into the optimisation of a model for the Levator Ani [20]. However, spatial relationship information between the cartilages and bone is disassociated from the whole shape, because the thickness is only defined for a subset of the model. As a result, by directly incorporating the information into the model, the expected thickness values obtained as

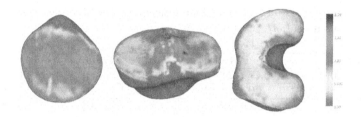

Fig. 5. The standard deviation of the thickness of the cartilage above each landmark in the SSM

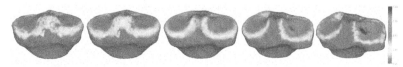

Fig. 6. The primary mode of the combined tibia shape and thickness (of the meniscus) model varied by $\pm\sqrt{3}$ standard deviations **Note:** The cartilage thickness extending beyond 5mm

the model is varied extend beyond the range that is expected anatomically (see Figure 6).

As we are still examining how best to combine several types of disassociated information into one model, the current models are optimised in the standard way and from the corresponding points the information of interest is extracted. The information is associated with each point and kept constant, rather than being modeled in a way that would allow its value to vary based on the parameters of the shape model. Several examples of the type of spatial relation information that we are interested in are illustrated in Figure 4, 5 and 8.

4   Results and Discussion

The initial landmarking obtained for the patella, tibia and femur provide a satisfactory initial approximation for correspondence landmarks. The optimisation scheme improves this correspondence significantly as can be seen in Figure 3 and by the improvement in compactness shown in Table 1. The primary mode of variation of the optimised models can be seen in Figure 7.

Associating or embedding information into the SSM will aid the automation of the initialisation of the cartilage models. After segmenting the bones using these models, the information embedded in these models (like cartilage thickness) will be used to determine the placement and parameters used to initialise them. The type of information includes the probability that the cartilage exists above a point, its expected thickness and the variation of the thickness (see Figures 4, 5 and 8).

Table 1. Compactness and the first four primary modes of variation of the bone models: Optimised (Initial)

Mode	Patella	Tibia	Femur
0	5.77 (12.98)	13.32 (14.01)	13.37 (22.17)
1	1.92 (2.62)	9.34 (9.44)	10.60 (12.53)
2	1.71 (2.16)	2.31 (2.93)	4.06 (4.87)
3	1.27 (1.72)	1.68 (2.38)	2.20 (2.80)
Compactness	14.78 (25.00)	33.11 (36.51)	37.03 (51.86)

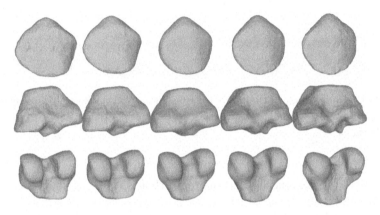

Fig. 7. The primary mode of the bone models varied by $\pm\sqrt{3}$ standard deviations

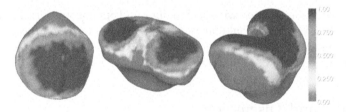

Fig. 8. The probability that cartilage is above each landmark in the SSM

5   Conclusion

The optimisation process presented has allowed the automatic creation of 3D SSMs of the knee bones. We propose the use of these models as a basis to associate or embed *a priori* knowledge like spatial relationship information. The initial use of this information is to aid in the automatic initialisation of 3D segmentation models of the cartilages using the probability and expected thickness. This information can also be utilised by each model to improve their segmentation process and allow for the development of cooperative or competitive segmentations of difficult regions like the meniscus/articular cartilage boundary.

The incorporation of information such as thickness into the models will become even more important with models created from a database of osteoarthritis sufferers. This approach extends naturally to the embedding of other *a priori* knowledge and is an ideal way to aid in the development of 3D *intelligent* deformable models [14] for use in an automated segmentation system.

Acknowledgements

The authors wish to thank Johannes Pauser for help in acquiring and interactively segmenting the scans.

This investigation was supported in part by a research grant from the National Multiple Sclerosis Society and by NIH grants R21 MH67054, R01 LM007861, P41 RR13218 and P01 CA67165 and NSF grant 0426558.

References

1. Hargreaves, B.A., Gold, G.E., Beaulieu, C.F., Vasanawala, S.S., Nishimura, D.G., Pauly, J.M.: Comparison of new sequences for high resolution cartilage imaging. Magnetic Resonance in Medicine **49** (2003) 700–709
2. Cohen, Z.A., McCarthy, D.M., Kwak, S.D., Legrand, P., Fogarasi, F., Ciaccio, E.J., Ateshian, G.A.: Knee cartilage topology, thickness and contact areas from MRI: in-vitro calibration and in-vivo measurements. Osteoarthritis Cartilage **7** (1999) 95–109
3. Williams, T.G., Taylor, C.J., Gao, Z., Waterton, J.C.: Corresponding articular cartilage thickness measurements in the knee joint by modelling the underlying bone. In: MICCAI'03. Volume 2879. (2003) 480–487
4. Wluka, A.E., Stuckey, A., Snaddon, J., Cicuttini, F.: The determinants of change in tibial cartilage volume in osteoarthritic knees. Arthritis and Rheumatism **46** (2002) 2065–2072
5. Hohe, J., Ateshian, G., Reiser, M., Englmeier, K.H., Eckson, F.: Surface size, curvature analysis and assessment of knee joint incongruity with MRI in vivo. Magnetic Resonance in Medicine **47** (2002) 554–561
6. Eckstein, F., Schnier, M., Haubner, M., Priebsch, J., Glaser, C., Englmeier, K.H., Reiser, M.: Accuracy of cartilage volume and thickness measurements with magnetic resonance imaging. Clinical Orthopaedics and related research **352** (1998) 137–148
7. Solloway, S., Hutchinson, C., Waterton, J., Taylor, C.: The use of active shape models for making thickness measurements of articular cartilage from MR images. Magnetic Resonance in Medicine **37** (1997) 943–952
8. Lynch, J., Zaim, S., Zhao, J., Stork, A., Peterfly, C.G., Genant, H.: Cartilage segmentation of 3D MRI scans of the osteoarthritic knee combining user knowledge and active contours. SPIE **3979** (2000) 925–935
9. Gougoutas, A., Wheaton, A., Borthakur, A., Shapiro, E., Kneeland, J., Udupa, J., Reddy, R.: Cartilage volume quantification via live wire segmentation. Academic Radiology **11** (2004) 1389–1395
10. Kapur, T., Beardsley, P., Gibson, S., Grimson, W., Wells, W.: Model-based segmentation of clinical knee MRI. In Proc. IEEE Int'l Workshop on Model-Based 3D Image Analysis (1998) 97–106

11. Ghosh, S., Beuf, O., Ries, M., Lane, N., Steinbach, L.S., Majumdar, S.: Watershed segmentation of high resolution magnetic resonance images of articular cartilage of the knee. Engineering in Medicine and Biology Society **4** (2000) 3174–3176
12. Warfield, S.K., Kaus, M., Jolesz, F.A., Kikinis, R.: Adaptive, template moderated, spatially varying statistical classification. Medical Image Analysis **4** (2000) 43–55
13. Grau, V., Mewes, A., Alcaniz, M., Kikinis, R., Warfield, S.: Improved watershed transform for medical image segmentation using prior information. IEEE Transactions on Medical Imaging **23** (2004) 447–458
14. Hamarneh, G., McInerney, T., Terzpopoulos, D.: Intelligent deformable organisms: An artificial life approach to medical image analysis. Technical report CSRG-432 (2001)
15. Davies, R., Twining, C., Cootes, T., Waterton, J., Taylor, C.: 3D statistical shape models using direct optimisation of description length. In: 7th European Conference on Computer Vision. Volume 3. (2002) 3–21
16. Cootes, T., Taylor, C., Cooper, D., Graham, J.: Active shape models - their training and application. Computer Vision and Image Undertanding **61** (1995) 38–59
17. Rueckert, D., Frangi, A.F., Schnabel, J.A.: Automatic construction of 3d statistical shape models using non-rigid registration. IEEE Transactions on Medical Imaging **22** (2003) 1014–1025
18. Siers, M., Frangi, A., Kaus, M., Niessen, W.: Comparison of two 3D automatic landmarking methods for a large training set of cardiac MR images. (citeseer) citeseer.ist.psu.edu/529161.html.
19. Kobbeltm, L., Vorsatz, J., Labsik, U., Seidel, H.: A Shrink Wrapping Approach to Remeshing Polygonal Surfaces. In: Proceedings of the 20th Annual Conference ot the European Association of Computer Graphics (Eurographics-99). (1999)
20. Lee, S.L., Horkaew, P., Darzi, A., Yang, G.Z.: Statistical Shape Modelling of the Levator Ani with Thickness Variation. In: MICCAI'04. Volume 3216. (2004) 258–265

A Generalized Level Set Formulation of the Mumford-Shah Functional with Shape Prior for Medical Image Segmentation

Lishui Cheng[1], Xian Fan[1], Jie Yang[1], and Yun Zhu[2]

[1] Institute of Image Processing and Pattern Recognition, Shanghai Jiao Tong
University (SJTU),Shanghai, 200030,P.R. China
[2] Department of biomedical engineering, Yale University, New Haven, CT, USA

Abstract. Image segmentation is an important research topic in medical image analysis area. In this paper, we firstly propose a generalized level set formulation of the Mumford-Shah functional by a sound mathematical definition of line integral. The variational flow is implemented in level set framework and thus implicit and intrinsic. By embedding a weighted length term to the original Mumford-Shah functional, the paper presents a generic framework that integrates region, gradient and shape information of an image into the segmentation process naturally. The region force provides a global criterion and increases the speed of convergence, the gradient information allows for a better spatial localization while the shape prior makes the model especially useful to recover objects of interest whose shape can be learned through statistical analysis. The shape prior is represented by the zero-level set of signed distance maps of images and is well consistent with level set based variational framework. Experiments on 2-D synthetic and real images validate this novel method.

1   Introduction

Medical applications, visualization and quantification methods for computer-aided diagnosis or surgical planning from various modalities typically involve the segmentation of anatomical structures as a preliminary step. Because of the huge amount of data and the complexity of these organs and structures, computer-based automatic segmentation methods are needed to fully exploit medical data.

Active contour model, since proposed in [1], has been extensively studied in this area. Level set methods, as an alternative of snake models, have been proposed in an effort to overcome some limitations of traditional parameterized active contour models. They can support complex topology naturally, extended to higher dimensions easily and are implicit, intrinsic and parameter free [2]. Among others, geodesic active contour[3], Chan-Vese model [4] and geodesic active region model [5] are three well-studied level set formulations for image segmentation which are based on gradients, region and the integration of boundary and region information, separately.

However, these common gradient or region based active contour models can not deal with occlusion problems or the presence of other missing information about the object which are common in many object extraction problems. Moreover, there are

Y. Liu, T. Jiang, and C. Zhang (Eds.): CVBIA 2005, LNCS 3765, pp. 61 – 71, 2005.
© Springer-Verlag Berlin Heidelberg 2005

many medical applications in which some prior knowledge about the object is available and useful. Therefore the incorporation of more specific prior information into to deformable models has received some attention. In [6], Leventon proposed an MAP formulation to incorporate shape prior using level set representation into segmentation process. Chen has employed an "average shape" to serve as the shape prior term in their energy functional [7]. However, neither the method of Leventon's nor the energy of Chen's can make use of region information of the image. On the other hand, Tsai[8] and Yang [9] have proposed their level set shape model ,separately, based on the integration of Leventon's level set shape representation idea and region based active contour models. However, both Tsai's and Yang's methods did not consider the boundary information. In [10], the authors have proposed a novel energetic form to introduce shape prior to level set representation and then applied to object extraction combined with geodesic active region model.

In this paper, we demonstrate a new theoretical interpretation of Mumford-Shah functional and arrive at a generalized level set formulation of the original Mumford-Shah functional based on a sound mathematical definition of line integral in [11]. After investigating the terms of level set method, we propose that by using a weighted length term, the new level set based variational formulation of the Mumford-Shah functional can provide a very general scheme where region homogeneity and boundary curve features (such as gradient or the shape of interested objects which are represented by evolving curves) can be incorporated into the segmentation process simultaneously. That is also the major novelty of the proposed method when compared with some related previous literatures, for example [12] and [13], where the variational formulation is just a heuristic combination of region, edge and shape terms. In our former paper [14], we have demonstrated that gradient information can be incorporated into this framework for brain MR image segmentation. In this paper, we show such a generalized formulation can also be effectively used to develop a level set shape model. Region-based forces make our method less sensitive to noise, gradient information allows for a better spatial localization, while the shape prior makes the model especially useful to recover objects of interest whose shape can be learned through statistical analysis. To be specific, our model not only exploits the region and gradient information of an image but also is a knowledge based method because it incorporates the shape of object for segmenting images.

The remainder of the paper is organized as follows. In section 2, we will briefly introduce the Mumford-Shah functional. The details of the new model and related numerical implementation will be discussed in section 3. Experimental results and conclusion will be given in section 4 and 5, separately.

2   Background

In the variational framework, an image I_0 is usually considered a real-valued bounded function defined on $\overline{\Omega}$, where Ω is a bounded and open subset of R^2 (in two dimension case) with $\partial\Omega$ its boundary. Let I be a differentiable function on Ω, Γ is a set of discontinuities (i.e. contours). In [15], Mumford and Shah proposed a functional to segment an image into homogeneous objects. A reduced form of this segmentation problem is simply the restriction of I to piecewise constant functions, i.e. I = constant c_i on each connected component Ω_i. Under this circumstance, the image segmentation problem, is solved through minimizing the following functional:

$$E_0^{MS}(I,\Gamma) = \sum_i \alpha_i \int_{\Omega_i} (I_0 - c_i)^2 d\vec{x} + v \bullet Length(\Gamma) \tag{1}$$

where α_i and v are scaling parameters, $|\Gamma|$ stands for the total length of the arcs making up Γ.

In [4], Chan and Vese formulated this functional in terms of the level set framework. Later, they generalized this method to treat multiple regions [16]. The similar work was also proposed by Tsai et al. [17]. However, both their methods did not consider the shape and gradient information of an image for segmentation problems.

3 Description of the Model

3.1 Shape Representation

The shape prior can be defined by many different methods in the literature, such as point distribution model [18], Fourier descriptor [19], and medial axis [20]. Following the lead of [6] and [7], in this paper, we adopt the implicit representation of the segmenting curve based on the level set method of Osher and Sethian [2] to build our statistical shape model. Specifically, the boundary curve of the object in a training set of n aligned images is embedded as the zero-level set of a higher dimensional function $\{\Phi_1, \Phi_2, ..., \Phi_n\}$ with negative distances assigned to the outside and positive distances inside the object. Then a distance map for each of the training image can be derived. As pointed out in [21], distance map is a dense descriptor capable of capturing an arbitrary shape whose bounded behavior in the presence of noise in the outline and in the object position makes it an attractive choice for image based statistical analysis. Furthermore, basic geometric properties such as curvature and the normal of evolving curves are easily derived. Finally, such a shape representation is also naturally consistent with level set based active contour models.

Using the technique developed in [6], we compute $\overline{\Phi}$, the mean level set function of the training shapes, as the average of these n signed distance functions $\overline{\Phi} = \frac{1}{n} \sum_{i=1}^{n} \Phi_i$. To extract the shape variabilities, Ψ_i is subtracted from each Φ_i to create the deviation form the mean. Each of the deviation Ψ_i is placed as a column vector to form a $N^d \times n$-dimensional shape-variability matrix S where d is the number of spatial dimensions and N^d is the number of samples of each level set function. Next using Singular Value Decomposition (SVD) to shape variance matrix:

$$\frac{1}{n}S \times S^T = V \sum V^T \tag{2}$$

where V is a matrix whose column vectors represent the orthogonal modes of variation in the shape and $\sum$ is an diagonal matrix whose diagonal elements are the corresponding eigenvalues. Now the most important modes of variations can be recovered
through Principle Component Analysis (PCA):

$$\phi(\lambda) = \overline{\Phi} + \sum_{j=1}^{k} \lambda_j \phi_j \tag{3}$$

where k is the number of selected principle modes of variation,
$\lambda = \{\lambda_1, \lambda_2, \ldots, \lambda_k\}$ are the linear weight factors for the k eigenshapes with the variances $\{\sigma_1^2, \sigma_2^2, \ldots, \sigma_k^2\}$ given by the eigenvalues calculated by the above SVD,
$\{\phi_1, \phi_2, \ldots, \phi_j\}$ are the corresponding principle modes(eigenvectors) and spatially
dependent. Note that a novel shape which is represented by the zero-level set of ϕ is
the function of vector λ. That's to say, by adjusting the values of vector λ, one varies ϕ which indirectly changes the shape.

In this paper, we used ellipse as our synthetic images. Specifically, we generated a
training set of 36 ellipses by changing the eccentricity with a Gaussian distribution
and applied PCA on the distance maps of training images. We thus select 1 principle
mode to fit 96% of the total variation (about the selection of k, please see 3.3). Fig.1
shows the shape of the mean and principle mode corresponding to the largest eigenvalue which is represented by the zero-level set.

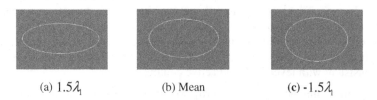

(a) $1.5\lambda_1$ (b) Mean   (c) $-1.5\lambda_1$

Fig. 1. Illustration of PCA : (b) is the mean shape,(a) and (c) demonstrate $\phi = \overline{\Phi} \pm 1.5\lambda_1\phi_1$
The shape is represented by the zero-level set of ϕ.

3.2 Generalization of the Mumford-Shah Functional

In this section, we present the generalized level set formulation of the Mumford-Shah
functional in bimodal case. According to level set theory originally proposed by
Osher and Sethian in [2], a geometric active contour can be represented by the zero-
level set of a real-valued Lipschitz function $\Psi : \Omega \subset R^2 \rightarrow R$ such that $\Psi > 0$ in-

side the evolving curve Γ and $\Psi < 0$ outside the curve. As in [4], the first term of Eq. (1) can be represented as follows (in bimodal case):

$$\alpha_1 \int_\Omega (I_0 - c_1)^2 H(\Psi) d\vec{x} + \alpha_2 \int_\Omega (I_0 - c_2)^2 (1 - H(\Psi)) d\vec{x} \qquad (4)$$

where c_1 and c_2 are the mean intensities inside and outside the active contour Γ, respectively, and $H(\Psi)$ is the Heaviside function defined as:

$$H(\Psi) = \begin{cases} 1, \Psi > 0 \\ 0, \ else \end{cases} \qquad (5)$$

Next let us consider the length term of the Mumford-Shah functional. In [11], the line integral of function $f(\vec{x})$ in R^2 is defined as the following formula:

$$\int_\Omega f(\vec{x}) \delta(\vec{x}) d\vec{x} \qquad (6)$$

where the region of integration is all of Ω, and $\delta(\vec{x})$ is the Delta function defined as follows:

$$\delta(\vec{x}) = \begin{cases} 1, \vec{x} = 0 \\ 0, \ else \end{cases} \qquad (7)$$

Because the Delta function prunes out everything except the boundary $\partial\Omega$ automatically, the one-dimensional Delta function can be used to rewrite the line integral in level set framework as (for more details, please see [11]):

$$\int_\Omega f(\vec{x}) \delta(\Psi) |\nabla\Psi| d\vec{x} \qquad (8)$$

Based on this definition of line integral, we propose to use the following weighted length to stand for the length term in Eq. (1) as:

$$\int_\Omega B(\vec{x}) \delta(\Psi) |\nabla\Psi| d\vec{x} \qquad (9)$$

where $B(\vec{x})$ is the weighted function which is used as boundary feature descriptor. In this paper, we exploit two kinds of function to drive the active contour towards the shape prior as well as high image gradients:

$$B(\vec{x}) = \beta_g g(\vec{x}) + \gamma_s d^2(s R \vec{x} + T, \phi(\lambda)) \qquad (10)$$

where β_g and γ_s are scaling parameters balancing the force of gradient and the shape prior. At the stationary point of the decent of Eq.(9), we expect the curve Γ to lie over points of high gradients and subject to shape prior driven by the boundary descriptor function.

Usually, $g(\vec{x})$ is defined as (in 2 dimension):

$$g(\vec{x}) = g(x,y) = \frac{1}{1 + |\nabla G_\sigma(x,y) * I_0(x,y)|^p}, p \geq 1 \tag{11}$$

where $G_\sigma * I_0$, a smoother version of I_0, is the convolution of the image I_0 with the Gaussian $G_\sigma(x,y) = \sigma^{-1/2} e^{-|x^2+y^2|/4\sigma}$. The function $g(\vec{x})$ is supposed to be positive in homogeneous regions and close to zero in high gradient of image.

$d^2(s\vec{R}x + T, \phi(\lambda))$ is used as a function to compute the distance between the evolving contour and the shape prior. In this paper, we only consider 2-D rigid transformation to capture pose variabilities (without the loss of generalization, affine transformation can also be considered in a similar way) where s is the scale factor, R is the rotation matrix in terms of the angle θ, and T is the translation factor. $\phi(\lambda)$ is the shape prior derived from PCA defined in Eq.(3) and d is the distance between a rigid transformed point of the evolving contour and its closest point on the zero-level set of $\phi(\lambda)$ which can be obtained by the fast marching method proposed in [22]. Such a distance function evaluates the shape differences between the evolving contour and the shape prior. Therefore the use of function d enables our implicit representation of shape to accommodate shape variabilities due to differences both in pose and in eigenshapes. Similar function d can also be found in [7] and [23]. However, both their methods can not make use of the region information of an image and are not derived from Mumford-Shah functional like here, either.

Taking into account of Eqs. (1), (9) and (4), the Mumford-Shah functional, using level set techniques, can be reformulated as follows:

$$E_{ms}^{new}(\Psi, s, R, T, \lambda) = \alpha_1 \int_\Omega (I_0 - c_1)^2 H(\Psi) d\vec{x}$$
$$+ \alpha_2 \int_\Omega (I_0 - c_2)^2 (1 - H(\Psi)) d\vec{x} + \int_\Omega B(\vec{x}) \delta(\Psi) |\nabla \Psi| d\vec{x} \tag{12}$$

where $B(\vec{x}) = \beta_g g(\vec{x}) + \gamma_s d^2(s\vec{R}x + T, \phi(\lambda))$ as in Eq.(10).The first two terms describe the attraction of region homogeneity forces ; the third term drives the contour according to the shape prior as well as the high gradient areas of the image. α_1, α_2, β_g and γ_s are four parameters used to adjust the weights of the region, gradient and shape forces in segmentation process. One can see that the new active contour model provides a general framework that unifies the region and boundary features (gradient and the shape prior) of an image for medical segmentation problems. Although the experiments part of this paper mainly demonstrate the influence of shape prior, we point out that the tradeoff between shape prior, gradient and region forces depends on how much faith one has in the prior shape model and the imagery for a specific application.

Using gradient decent method for the energy of Eq.(12), the evolution equations can be derived as follows (for the details, we refer to the Appendix of [14]):

$$
\frac{\partial \Psi}{\partial t} = \delta(\Psi)[\alpha_2(I_0 - c_2)^2 - \alpha_1(I_0 - c_1)^2 + \nabla \bullet (B\frac{\nabla \Psi}{|\nabla \Psi|})]
$$

$$
= \delta(\Psi)[\alpha_2(I_0 - c_2)^2 - \alpha_1(I_0 - c_1)^2 + \frac{\nabla B \bullet \nabla \Psi}{|\nabla \Psi|} + B\nabla \bullet \frac{\nabla \Psi}{|\nabla \Psi|}]
$$

(13)

$$
\frac{\partial s}{\partial t} = -2\gamma_s \int_\Omega \delta(\Psi)d\nabla d \bullet (R\vec{x})|\nabla \Psi|d\vec{x}
$$

(14)

$$
\frac{\partial \theta}{\partial t} = -2\gamma_s \int_\Omega \delta(\Psi)sd\nabla d \bullet (\frac{dR}{d\theta}\vec{x})|\nabla \Psi|d\vec{x}
$$

(15)

$$
\frac{\partial T}{\partial t} = -2\gamma_s \int_\Omega \delta(\Psi)d\nabla d |\nabla \Psi|d\vec{x}
$$

(16)

$$
\frac{\partial \lambda_i}{\partial t} = -2\gamma_s \int_\Omega \delta(\Psi)d\phi_i |\nabla \Psi|d\vec{x}
$$

$$
\lambda_i(0) = \lambda_{i_0}, \lambda_i \in [-3\sigma_i, 3\sigma_i], i = 1, 2, \dots, k \; [18]
$$

(17)

3.3 Implementation Techniques

The first issue is the choice of k, the number of modes of variation. In our experiments, we adopt the method described in [18] to compute the total variation in the image bases (for more details, please see [18]).

One important issue is the choice of the parameters of the region and boundary forces, In our experiments, we adopt an empirical way to choose parameters. When noise is high, we can choose a relatively higher value for the parameter of the length term, for example, β_g, γ_s in (10), in order to exert a strong regularization force. On the other hand, a high γ_s would indicate a more dependence on the statistical shape prior of the evolving contour.

About the possible regularization of the Heaviside function $H(\Psi)$ and $\delta(\Psi)$, we use in our experiments the same regularization form as in Chan-Vese model. c_1 and c_2 are computed with the method proposed in [4]. $\nabla B \bullet \nabla \Psi$ and $|\nabla \Psi|$ are discretized using up wind difference scheme [2] . The discretization of $\nabla \bullet \frac{\nabla \Psi}{|\nabla \Psi|}$ is with central difference scheme and the temporal derivative with a forward difference scheme. The Eqs. (14)-(17) are discretized using the methods introduced in [7]. When necessary, reinitializing the level set function at a few iterations using the fast marching method [22].

4 Experimental Results

In this section, we present the results obtained by our method when applied to synthetic, hand and medical images. The experimental results have achieved desirable performance and demonstrate the effectiveness of this new method.

4.1 Synthetic Images and Hand Images

In the first experiment, we used our segmentation method to recover an ellipse which is partially cut and placed with different pose (translation, rotation and scale) to the training images described in 3.1. In this experiment, we keep $\alpha_1 = \alpha_2 = 0.5$, $\beta_g = 0.25$ and $\gamma_s = 0.7$. The algorithm converged in a few seconds on a Pentium III PC. From Fig.2(c) and (d) one can see that compared to Chan-Vese model, our level set shape model successfully captured the missing part in noisy environment thanks to the prior shape information. Moreover, it can deal with shape variability due to pose.

The second experiment demonstrates that our model can recover the hand which is partially occluded by a vertical bar. The training set is composed by 35 human hand images and the number of principle mode is 5. In practice, we fixed $\alpha_1 = \alpha_2 = 0.5$, $\beta_g = 0.7$ and $\gamma_s = 0.8$. The algorithm converged in less than 1 minute . From Fig.3 (d) one can see that the new variational model can deal with occlusion problems.

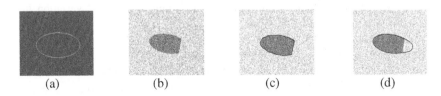

(a)   (b)   (c)   (d)

Fig. 2. Results for the synthetic ellipses: (a) the shape prior; (b) the object of interest; (c) results by Chan-Vese model ; (d) results obtained by our model

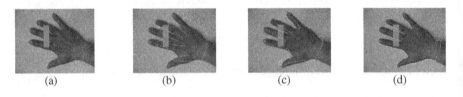

(a)   (b)   (c)   (d)

Fig. 3. Results for hand images: (a) original occluded hand; (b) the initial contour; (c) a middle step; (d) the final result, the occluded hand is recovered. The active contour is in white.

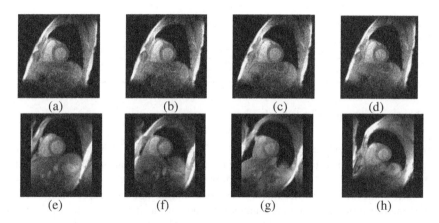

Fig. 4. Segmentation results for MR cardiac images: (a) is the original image for case 2, (b)~(d) are the three steps for the segmentation process; (e)~(h) are the final results for case 3,7,1 and 8, separately. The active contour is in red.

In sum, our variational level set shape model can extract objects with missing information, occlusion and local shape variability.

4.2 Medical Application

We have applied our algorithm to a lot of medical imagery problems. For simplicity, we only give the results for the extraction of left ventricles of 2-D cardiac MR images. The training base consists of 42 cardiac images whose outlines are traced by a doctor and the test sets are composed of 20 novel images. In implementation, we choose $\alpha_1 = \alpha_2 = 0.6$, $\beta_b = 0.8$ and $\gamma_s = 0.9$. In Fig.4 we show our results obtained by our model. One can see that the contours are able to converge on the desired boundaries even though some parts of the boundaries are too blurred to be detected only by gray level information. The algorithm usually converged in several minutes.

To validate the results, we computed the undirected Hausdorff distance [24] between the zero-level set A (N_A points) obtained by our algorithm and the manual segmentation results M (N_M points):

$$H(A,M) = \max(h(A,M), h(M,A)) \qquad (18)$$

where

$$h(A,M) = \frac{1}{N_A} \sum_{a \in A} \min_{m \in M} \|a - m\| \qquad (19)$$

The quantitative results for 14 cases are given in Table 1. One can see that virtually all the boundary points of the zero-level set lie in one ore two pixels of the manual segmentation.

Table 1. Distance between the results of our algorithm and manual segmentation (unit: pixel)

Case	1	2	3	4	5	6	7	8	9	10	11	12	13	14
Distance	1.9	0.9	0.8	1.2	0.7	1.3	0.8	1.1	1.0	1.5	0.9	1.3	1.2	1.0

5 Discussion and Conclusion

In this paper, we proposed a generalized level set formulation of Mumford-Shah functional for image segmentation with shape prior based on a sound mathematical definition of line integral in [11]. By embedding a weighted length term to the original Mumford-Shah functional, the novel variational model not only makes use of region homogeneities, but also provides a general framework to incorporate useful boundary features for image segmentation. In this paper, we have demonstrated that boundary information, such as shape prior as well as gradient information, can be efficiently incorporated into the segmentation process in this general framework.

The shape prior is represented by the zero-level set of signed distance maps in the attempt to avoid having to solve the point correspondence problem and is consistent with the curve evolution in a variational formulation well. The experiments indicate that our level set shape model can deal with missing information, occlusion problem and shape variation due to differences in pose and the eigenshapes. When applied to cardiac MR images, the variational contour model also achieved desirable performance. Although we did not give 3-D medical image illustration, the extension to 3-D medical image segmentation problems of the model is rather straightforward thanks to the level set representation of the evolving contour. Our method can also be extended to incorporate the prior image gray level information [25] or deal with multiple objects [16]. These will be the subjects of future research.

Acknowledgements. The authors Lishui Cheng and Xian Fan would like to particularly thank for the many helpful and stimulating discussions with Dr. Chenyang Xu and Dr. Yuanjie Zheng on medical image segmentation.

References

[1] M. Kass, A.Witkin, and D.Terzopoulos, "Snakes: Active Contour Models", *IJCV*, vol. 1, pp. 321-331, 1988.
[2] S. Osher, and J. A. Sethian, "Fronts propagating with curvature-dependent speed: algorithms based on Harmilton-Jacobi formulations", *J. Comp. Phys.*, vol. 79, pp. 12-49, 1988.
[3] V. Caselles, R. Kimmel, and G. Sapiro, "On geodesic active contours", *IJCV*, vol. 22(1), pp. 61-79,1997.
[4] T.F. Chan, and L.A. Vese, "Active contours without edges", *IEEE Trans. Image Processing*, vol. 10(2), pp. 266-277, 2001.
[5] N. Paragios, and R. Deriche, "Geodesic active regions: a new paradigm to deal with frame partition problems in computer vision", *J. Visual Communication and Image Representation*, vol. 13, pp. 249-268, 2002.

[6]   M. Leventon, W. Grimson and O. Faugeras, "Statistical shape influence in geodesic active contours", in *Proceeding of CVPR*, pp.316-323,2000.

[7]   Y. Chen, H.D. Tagare, S. Thiruvenkadam, et al., "Using prior shapes in geometric active contours in a variational framework", *IJCV*, vol.50(3), pp. 315-328, 2002.

[8]   A. Tsai, A. Yezzi, Jr., et al., "A Shape-Based Approach to the Segmentation of Medical Imagery Using Level Sets", *IEEE Trans. Medical Imaging*, vol. 22(2), pp. 137-153,2003.

[9]   J. Yang , L. H. Staib and J. S. Duncan, " Neighbor-Constrained Segmentation With Level Set Based 3-D Deformable Models", *IEEE Trans. Medical Imaging*, vol. 23(8), pp. 940-948,2004.

[10] M. Rousson , N. Paragios, "Shape priors for level set representation", in *Proceeding of ECCV*, pp. II: 78-93, 2002.

[11] S. Osher and R. Fedkiw, "Level Set Methods and Dynamic Implicit Surface", Springer-Verlag, pp. 13-15, ISBN: 0387954821, 2002.

[12] C.Pluempitiwiwiriyawei, et al., "STACS: New Active Contour Scheme for Cardiac MR I mage Segmentation", *IEEE Trans. Medical Imaging*, vol. 24(5), pp.593-603, 2005.

[13] M. Holtzman-Gazit, D. Goldsher, and R. Kimmel, "Hierarchial segmentation of thin structures in volumetric medical images", *MICCAI 2003, LNCS 2879*, pp.562-569, 2003.

[14] Lishui Cheng, Jie Yang, Xian Fan and Yuemin Zhu, "A Generalized Level Set Formulation of the Mumford-Shah Functional for Brain MR Image Segmentation", *IPMI 2005,LNCS 3565*,pp.418-430,2005.

[15] D. Mumford, and J. Shah, "Optimal approximations by piecewise smooth functions and associated variational problems", *Com. Pure and Applied Math.*, vol. 42, pp. 577-684, 1989.

[16] L. A. Vese and T. F. Chan, "A Multiphase Level Set Framework for Image Segmentation Using the Mumford and Shah Model", *IJCV*, vol.50 (3), pp. 271-293, 2002.

[17] A. Tsai, A. Yezzi, A. Willsky, "Curve evolution implementation of the Mumford-Shah functional for image segmentation, denoising, interpolation, and magnification," *IEEE Trans. Image Processing*, vol. 10(8), pp. 1169-1186, 2001.

[18] T. Cootes and C. Taylor, "Statistical Models of Appearance for Computer Vision", *Report*, Imaging Science and Biomedical Engineering, University of Manchester, 2004.

[19] L. H. Staib, J. S. Duncan, "Boundary finding with parametrically deformable models", *IEEE Trans. PAMI*, vol.14 (11), pp. 1061-1075, 1992.

[20] S. M. Pizer, P. T. Fletcher, S. Joshi, et al., "Deformable M-Reps for 3D Medical Image Segmentation", *IJCV*, vol. 55(2-3), pp. 85-106, 2003.

[21] P. Golland, "Statistical Shape Analysis of Anatomical Structures", PH.D. Dissertation, MIT, Department of Electrical Engineering and Computer Science, 2001.

[22] D. Adalsteinsson and J.Sethian, "A fast level set method for propagating interfaces", *J. Comp. Phys.*, vol. 118, pp. 269-277, 1995.

[23] X. Bresson, P. Vandergheynst and J.P.Thiran, "A prior information in image segmentation: energy functional based on shape statistical model and image information", in *Proceeding of ICIP*, pp. 425-428, 2003.

[24] D. Huttenlocher, G. Klanderman, W. Rucklidge, "Comparing images using the Hausdorff distance", *IEEE Trans. PAMI*, vol. 15(9), pp. 850-863, 1993

[25] J. Yang , J. S. Duncan, "3D image segmentation of deformable objects with joint shape-intensity prior models using level set", *Med. Image Analysis*, vol. 8(3), pp. 285-194,2004.

A Hybrid Eulerian-Lagrangian Approach for Thickness, Correspondence, and Gridding of Annular Tissues

Kelvin R. Rocha[1], Anthony J. Yezzi[1], and Jerry L. Prince[2]

[1] Georgia Institute of Technology, School of Electrical and Computer Engineering,
Atlanta, GA 30332-1100
{krocha, ayezzi}@ece.gatech.edu
[2] Johns Hopkins University, Department of Electrical and Computer Engineering,
Baltimore, MD 21218
prince@jhu.edu

Abstract. We present a novel approach to efficiently compute thickness, correspondence, and gridding of tissues between two simply connected boundaries. The solution of Laplace's equation within the tissue region provides a harmonic function whose gradient flow determines the correspondence trajectories going from one boundary to the other. The proposed method uses and expands upon two recently introduced techniques in order to compute thickness and correspondences based on these trajectories. Pairs of partial differential equations (PDEs) are efficiently computed within an Eulerian framework and combined with a Lagrangian approach so that correspondences trajectories are partially constructed when necessary. Results show that the proposed technique takes advantage of both the speed of the Eulerian PDE approach and the accuracy of the Lagrangian approach.

1 Introduction

Many parts of the human body have an annular tissue structure comprising two or more quasi-homogeneous tissues nested within one another. For example, the cerebral cortex is comprised of gray matter "sandwiched" between white matter on the inside and cerebrospinal fluid on the outside [1]. Another example is the left ventricular myocardium, which is intrinsically annular when viewed from cross-section images such as those obtained using magnetic resonance imaging (MRI) or computed tomography (CT) [2].

The thickness of such annular structures is often associated with functional performance or disease. For example, an increased thickness of the cerebral cortex may be associated with cortical dysplasias and lissencephaly [3], and decreased thickness may be related to Alzheimer's disease and anorexia nervosa [4]. In the heart, adequate thickening of the myocardium during systole is associated with a healthy heart, whereas overall thickening of the myocardium over time is associated with many cardiac diseases [5]. Sometimes it is also useful to subdivide (or grid) annular regions for regional characterization, labeling, or for finite element analysis [6].

A variety of methods have been described and used to measure thickness within annular regions. Most methods are ad hoc, often manually-assisted, and have accura-

Y. Liu, T. Jiang, and C. Zhang (Eds.): CVBIA 2005, LNCS 3765, pp. 72–81, 2005.
© Springer-Verlag Berlin Heidelberg 2005

cies that are highly dependent on the boundary shapes and on the person analyzing the images. Jones et al. [7] proposed an approach based on solving Laplace's equation that yields unique measures of thickness without paradoxes (see [8], [9]), and provides a strong initial basis for making thickness, correspondence, and gridding of annular regions unique, accurate, and repeatable. A faster, but less accurate, approach within an Eulerian framework was later presented in [8], [9]. In this newer approach partial differential equations (PDEs) are solved for the desired lengths thereby avoiding the explicit construction or tracing of any correspondence trajectory. In this paper we introduce a hybrid approach, in which the Eulerian approach is carefully modified so that it can use the Lagrangian approach where more precision is needed. The new method is significantly faster than the pure Lagrangian approach and more accurate than the Eulerian PDE approach.

In Section 2, we review how thickness and correspondence are defined and summarize both the Lagrangian and Eulerian PDE approaches. In Section 3, we describe in detail the proposed hybrid Eulerian-Lagrangian approach together with its numerical implementation. In Section 4, we compare the three approaches in terms of the precision of their results and their computational times using several images.

2 Thickness and Correspondences

Although there have been many attempts to properly define thickness within an annular region, most of them present certain problems [7]-[9]. For instance, the simple definition of thickness as the smallest Euclidean distance from a point in one surface to any point in the opposite surface has the problem that it lacks of reciprocity, that is, the thickness may be different in the case that the surfaces are interchanged. Jones *et al.* [7] defined thickness as the length of the flow lines of a harmonic function that is equal to 0 in one of the surfaces and equal to 1 in the other. The advantage of Jones' method is that these flow lines, which are called correspondence trajectories, have the highly desirable properties that they are orthogonal to each one of the surfaces, they do not intersect each other, and they are nominally parallel.

Let $R \subset \Re^n$ for $n = 2, 3$ be a spatial region with a simply connected inner boundary $\partial_0 R$ and outer boundary $\partial_1 R$ (see Fig. 1). These boundaries have a sub-voxel resolution and are usually given as level set representations of some given functions.

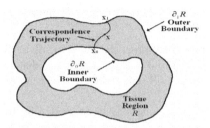

Fig. 1. Inner and outer boundaries of the tissue region R and a correspondence trajectory

Now let u be a harmonic function in R such that $u(\partial_0 R) = 0$ and $u(\partial_1 R) = 1$. The normalized gradient vector field of u coincides with the tangent vector field of the correspondence trajectories and is given by

$$\vec{T} = \nabla u/\|\nabla u\| . \tag{1}$$

For each point $\mathbf{x} \in R$ let the functions $L_0(\mathbf{x})$ and $L_1(\mathbf{x})$ be defined as the lengths of the correspondence trajectories that go from $\mathbf{x}$ to $\partial_0 R$ and from $\mathbf{x}$ to $\partial_1 R$, respectively. Accordingly, the thickness $W(\mathbf{x})$ of R at $\mathbf{x}$ is just

$$W(\mathbf{x}) = L_0(\mathbf{x}) + L_1(\mathbf{x}) . \tag{2}$$

In the Lagrangian approach proposed by Jones *et al.*, $L_1(\mathbf{x})$ is computed by integrating $\vec{T}$ from $\mathbf{x}$ to $\partial_1 R$, and $L_0(\mathbf{x})$ is computed by integrating $-\vec{T}$ from $\mathbf{x}$ to $\partial_0 R$. Then the thickness of R at $\mathbf{x}$ is obtained using (2). Integration can be carried out using a variety of methods such as Euler and Runge-Kutta integration.

Although very accurate and easy to implement, the Lagrangian approach is computationally intensive. This is the main reason why a faster method within and Eulerian framework was proposed in [8]. In the Eulerian PDE approach, thickness is computed by solving a pair of PDEs that are constructed from the geometry of the problem. From the differential structure of L_0 and L_1, the following set of PDEs must be satisfied for each point $\mathbf{x}$ in R

$$\nabla L_0 \cdot \vec{T} = 1, \text{ with } L_0(\partial_0 R) = 0 \ , \ -\nabla L_1 \cdot \vec{T} = 1, \text{ with } L_1(\partial_1 R) = 0 . \tag{3}$$

The characteristics of the first differential equation in (3) are (by design) equal to the correspondence trajectories; therefore the tangent field $\vec{T}$ determines the direction of its characteristic flow. Similarly, the negative of the tangent field, $-\vec{T}$, determines the direction of the characteristic flow of the second differential equation in (3). More specifically, if T_x, T_y, and T_z are the components of $\vec{T}$ at the grid point (i, j, k) in R, and if the grids are assumed to have spacing $\Delta x = \Delta y = \Delta z = 1$, it is shown in [8] that the numerical finite difference approximations for $L_0[i, j, k]$ and $L_1[i, j, k]$ using upwind schemes are

$$L_\alpha[i,j,k] = \frac{1 + |T_x| L_\alpha[i \oplus 1, j, k] + |T_y| L_\alpha[i, j \oplus 1, k] + |T_z| L_\alpha[i, j, k \oplus 1]}{|T_x| + |T_y| + |T_z|}, \text{ for } \alpha = 0, 1 , \tag{4}$$

where

$$\oplus = \begin{cases} \mp, & \alpha=0 \\ \pm, & \alpha=1 \end{cases}, \ i \pm 1 = \begin{cases} i+1, & T_x > 0 \\ i-1, & T_x < 0 \end{cases}, \ j \pm 1 = \begin{cases} j+1, & T_y > 0 \\ j-1, & T_y < 0 \end{cases}, \text{ and } k \pm 1 = \begin{cases} k+1, & T_z > 0 \\ k-1, & T_z < 0 \end{cases} . \tag{5}$$

Several iterative algorithms are proposed in [8] to solve (4). In all of them the initial values of L_0 and L_1 are set to 0 at all grid points so that values outside R serve as boundary conditions. Although all three methods yield the same solution, their convergence rates are different.

Besides computing thickness, one may be interested in finding the corresponding boundary points, that is, for any $\mathbf{x} \in R$ one wants to find the points $\mathbf{x}_0 \in \partial_0 R$ and $\mathbf{x}_1 \in \partial_1 R$ such that the correspondence trajectory going from $\mathbf{x}_0$ to $\mathbf{x}_1$ passes through $\mathbf{x}$ (see Fig. 1). Since the correspondence trajectories have the property that they do not intersect each other, there is only a pair of points, $\mathbf{x}_0$ and $\mathbf{x}_1$, satisfying this condition. Having unique corresponding boundary points in both $\partial_0 R$ and $\partial_1 R$ for every grid point in R allow us to generate anatomically shaped discrete grids within the tissue region. As described in [9], the Eulerian PDE approach can be also used to find correspondences. Let us define the correspondence functions $\phi_0 : \Re^n \rightarrow \Re^n$ and $\phi_1 : \Re^n \rightarrow \Re^n$, which map $\mathbf{x} \in R$ to the inner and outer boundaries of R, respectively. One of the two conditions that both ϕ_0 and ϕ_1 must satisfy is that they must remain constant along the correspondence trajectories, implying that their directional derivatives vanish along the direction given by $\vec{T}$. That is, we must have

$$(\nabla \phi_0)\vec{T} = (\nabla \phi_1)\vec{T} = \mathbf{0} , \tag{6}$$

where of $\nabla \phi_0$ and $\nabla \phi_1$ denote the Jacobian matrices of ϕ_0 and ϕ_1, respectively. In addition, each correspondence function must map a point on its own boundary to itself as well, which yields another set of conditions given by

$$\phi_0(\mathbf{x}) = \mathbf{x}, \forall \mathbf{x} \in \partial_0 R , \quad \phi_1(\mathbf{x}) = \mathbf{x}, \forall \mathbf{x} \in \partial_1 R . \tag{7}$$

Boundary correspondences can be computed by solving (6) subject to the boundary conditions in (7). In [9], the solution is found by using upwind schemes similar the ones used to solve (4) for computing the thickness of R. Specifically, for $\Delta x = \Delta y = \Delta z = 1$ the resulting finite difference equations are

$$\phi_\alpha[i,j,k] = \frac{|T_x| \phi_\alpha[i \oplus 1, j, k] + |T_y| \phi_\alpha[i, j \oplus 1, k] + |T_z| \phi_\alpha[i, j, k \oplus 1]}{|T_x| + |T_y| + |T_z|}, \text{ for } \alpha = 0,1 , \tag{8}$$

where the definitions in (5) hold. The same iterative procedures that can be used to solve L_0 and L_1 can also be used to solve for ϕ_0 and ϕ_1 above with the only difference being in the initialization procedure. In [9], the initialization is done by making $\phi_0[i, j, k]$ and $\phi_1[i, j, k]$ equal to (i, j, k) at grid points outside R that are next to the inner and outer boundaries, respectively.

Finally, as described in [9], pairs of PDEs similar to those in (8) can be used to find correspondences no just in the boundaries, but also in any level set of a function that is equal to 0 on $\partial_0 R$ and equal to 1 on $\partial_1 R$ such as the harmonic function u itself or the normalized length function $\overline{L}_0$ defined by $\overline{L}_0 = L_0 / (L_0 + L_1)$. These correspondences can then be used to generate shaped discrete grids within R.

3 A Hybrid Eulerian-Lagrangian Approach

The main advantage of the Eulerian PDE approach is its computational speed – several times faster than the Lagrangian approach, as shown in [8], [9]. On the other hand, as it is going to be shown in the next section, its main disadvantage is that it does not produce the highly accurate results that the Lagrangian approach yields. This is due to several factors. First, in the Eulerian PDE approach for thickness there is a lack of precision when setting up the boundary conditions as L_0 and L_1 are set to 0 at grid points in which they might have nonzero values. When doing this, the algorithm implicitly assumes an outer boundary that is shifted a little bit outward and an inner boundary that is shifted a little bit inward. As a result, the computed thickness tends to be larger than what it should be. This is especially problematic when there are just a few grid points between the inner and the outer boundary. Similarly, in the Eulerian PDE approach for correspondences, the boundary conditions for ϕ_0 and ϕ_1 at grid points are set up to be equal to their coordinate positions, creating a similar undesirable effect as above. We may encounter another problem when solving (8) as well. As illustrated in Fig. 2, it is possible to have the corresponding boundary points for grid point $\mathbf{x}$'s neighbors lying far apart on the boundary. Careful examination of (8) reveals that the computed values of ϕ_0 and ϕ_1 at $\mathbf{x}$ are convex combinations of ϕ_0 and ϕ_1 at grid points that are neighbors of $\mathbf{x}$. Therefore, it is possible for $\mathbf{x}$ to be mapped either far outside the boundary [Fig. 2(a)] or far inside the boundary [Fig. 2(b)], depending on the boundary's curvature.

It is logical to ask whether there is a way to naturally blend the Lagrangian and Eulerian PDE approaches so that the resulting method yields more accurate results than the Eulerian PDE approach, while requiring less computational time than the Lagrangian approach. Toward this end, we modify the previous Eulerian PDE approach to obtain a new hybrid algorithm with prescribable accuracy and the minimal possible sacrifice in speed. The first step to increase the accuracy of the Eulerian PDE approach is to improve the boundary conditions of the PDEs involved. We do this by using the Lagrangian approach to compute the values of L_0 and ϕ_0 at the grid points of R located immediately next to the inner boundary. Similarly, we use the Lagrangian approach to compute the values of L_1 and ϕ_1 at grid points immediately next to the outer boundary. Once we have computed these values, we use the Eulerian PDE approach to solve for L_0, L_1, ϕ_0, and ϕ_1 at the remaining grid points. In doing so, not only we obtain more accurate values near the boundaries, but also we avoid propagating larger computational errors throughout the whole region R. Since these grid points are at most one grid away from the boundary, the explicit computation of their correspondence trajectories does not require extensive computations.

Having improved the initial conditions for the Eulerian approach, the next step is to guarantee that points be mapped as closely as desired to the boundaries. This can be done by making some changes to the order transversal algorithm proposed in [8], which is very similar to the "fast marching method" used in solving the Eikonal equation [10]. In this algorithm points are visited in the order that they are reached by the correspondence trajectories as they flow away from the known boundary. As a result, only one full sweep through the grid points in R is required to solve for L_0 and ϕ_0 followed by one other sweep, but in a different direction, for L_1 and ϕ_1. Let λ be a chosen

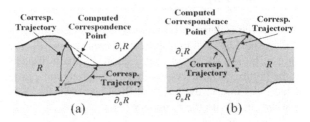

(a)   (b)

Fig. 2. Points mapped outside the annulus region due to a concavity (a) and to a convexity (b)

tolerance constant. As it will be explained shortly, λ will provide a mean to control the accuracy of the proposed hybrid approach. In the 2-D case, the idea consists in computing the value of the Euclidean distance between $\phi_\alpha[i\pm1, j]$ and $\phi_\alpha[i, j\pm1]$, where α could be either 0 or 1, before we consider $\phi_\alpha[i, j]$ to be solved. If this distance is less than λ, then we can assume that $\phi_\alpha[i, j]$ is very close to the boundary, otherwise we compute $\phi_\alpha[i, j]$ using another technique. One thing we can do is just to use the Lagrangian approach and follow the correspondence trajectory for this particular grid point until we reach the corresponding boundary. By doing so, we are taking full advantage of the Lagrangian approach and getting an accurate value. However, a faster way would be to follow the correspondence trajectory until it reaches a region between two grid points that have already been solved such that the distance between the two boundary maps is less than the tolerance λ. If they are close enough, we use the linear interpolation implicit in the discretized Eulerian PDE approach to estimate the value of $\phi_\alpha[i, j]$ at that point (since ϕ_α is constant along the correspondence trajectories, this is the value of ϕ_α at the original grid point), otherwise we continue following the trajectory and doing the same procedure until we find two correspondences that are close enough according to the desired tolerance.

We stress out that in the proposed hybrid approach we use the Lagrangian approach just when needed (e.g., whenever the Euclidean distance between $\phi_\alpha[i\pm1, j]$ and $\phi_\alpha[i, j\pm1]$ is greater than or equal to λ) otherwise we use the Eulerian PDE approach. Therefore, in general, we will not have to follow the whole correspondence trajectory. Consequently, depending on the value of λ, the proposed procedure can give us results as accurate as the Lagrangian approach or as fast as the Eulerian PDE approach. As it can be seen from (4), the values of L_0 and L_1 are computed in a similar way to those of ϕ_0 and ϕ_1. Consequently, it can be expected the computed values for L_0 and L_1 to be better approximations to the real values whenever the Euclidean distances between ϕ_0 and ϕ_1 at the grid points involved in the estimations are less than λ, than when they are greater than or equal to λ. Therefore, we can improve the precision of L_0 and L_1 if we compute them at the same time and in the same way as we compute ϕ_0 and ϕ_1 in the algorithm described above, taking into account that we have to add the arclength of the followed trajectory to the computed values. The hybrid Eulerian-Lagrangian approach to compute L_0 and ϕ_0 is summarized as follows:

Algorithm (Hybrid Eulerian-Lagrangian Approach):

{1} Initially tag all grid points in R as UNVISITED.

{2} Use the Lagrangian approach to compute the values of L_0 and ϕ_0 at grid points in R adjacent to the boundary $\partial_0 R$ and re-tag them as SOLVED.

{3} Use (4) and (8) to compute the values of L_0 and ϕ_0 at grid points in R next to the points already tagged as SOLVED, tag them as VISITED, and put them into a heap sorted by the values of u.

{4} Grab the grid point from the top of the current heap of VISITED points (i.e. the grid point with the smallest value of u). Remove this point from the heap and tag it as SOLVED.

{5} If the distance between the correspondence values of ϕ_0 at the neighboring grid points used in (8) is less than the desired tolerance λ, then compute ϕ_0 and L_0 using (4) and (8) and go to {7}, else set the arclength variable δ to 0.

{6} Follow the correspondence trajectory at the current grid point until it intersects the horizontal or vertical grid line between two grid points tagged as SOLVED and located one cell away from each other, record its arclength, and replace the value of δ with the sum of δ and the recorded arclength. If the distance between the values of ϕ_0 at these new grid points is greater than or equal to λ, then go to {6}, else compute ϕ_0 using linear interpolation and assign the resulting value to ϕ_0 of the original grid point of {5}. Compute L_0 using linear interpolation and add the value of δ to it. Assign this new computed value to L_0 of the original grid point of {5}.

{7} Update the values of L_0 and ϕ_0 using (4) and (8) for whichever neighbors of this grid point are not yet tagged as SOLVED. If any of these neighbors are currently tagged as UNVISITED, re-tag them as VISITED and add them to the current heap of VISITED grid points. Stop if all points in R have been tagged SOLVED, else go to {4}. ∎

The algorithm for computing L_1 and ϕ_1 is almost the same as above with minimal differences: in *{2}* we use the Lagrangian approach to compute the values of L_1 and ϕ_1 at points in R next to the boundary $\partial_1 R$ and in *{3}* the heap should be sorted by the values of $1 - u$ instead of u. For the 3-D implementation of the hybrid Eulerian-Lagrangian approach we note that there are three grid points involved in each one of (4) and (8), consequently we must compute the distances between the values of ϕ_0 (or ϕ_1) at each of these points and the others two (there are just three cases) and then compare the maximum of these distances with the desired tolerance λ. In addition, we must follow the trajectory until it intersects a square plane parallel to one of the three coordinate planes and formed by four neighbor grid points that are already solved. Besides computing thickness and correspondences at the same time and in a very fast way, the hybrid Eulerian-Lagrangian approach has two more important advantages. First, it terminates automatically so we do not have to keep testing for convergence. And second, the desired tolerance λ gives us a way to control the accuracy of the computed values. If λ is big enough, the hybrid Eulerian-Lagrangian approach will be nothing more than the Eulerian PDE approach with improved boundary conditions; whereas if λ is 0, the hybrid Eulerian-Lagrangian approach will yield the same results as the Lagrangian approach.

4 Results

In this section, we compare the performance of the hybrid Eulerian-Lagrangian approach with those of the Eulerian and the Lagrangian approaches in terms of accuracy and computational speed for three experimental regions. We used a novel numerical method that was presented in [11] to compute a very accurate estimation of the harmonic interpolant u within any annular region R. We then used this method, together with the Lagrangian approach with as much precision as possible, to compute highly accurate estimates of thickness and correspondences to serve as baseline for comparing the results of the three approaches on images for which the real values for thickness and correspondences are unknown in a simple closed form. To measure the accuracy of the computed correspondences in the experiments we define the correspondence distance error as the average over all grid points inside R of the Euclidean distances between ϕ_0 and the most accurately measured corresponding inner boundary point and between ϕ_1 and the most accurately measured corresponding outer boundary point. Unless otherwise stated, the tolerance value λ is set to 1 pixel for all experiments. We used the ordered traversal algorithm in our implementation of the Eulerian approach. All algorithms were implemented in C++ on a 2.52-GHz Pentium IV computer running Windows.

We tested the three different approaches on the annulus between two concentric circles of radii 40 and 80 (all units in pixels) shown in Fig. 3. Clearly, the thickness at any point in R is equal to 40 pixels. In addition, the corresponding boundary points for any $\mathbf{x}$ in R are just the intersections of the line passing through $\mathbf{x}$ and the center of the circles with the inner and outer circumferences. As a consequence, we can compare the computed thickness and correspondences with the exact values. The average computed thickness was equal to 40.01, 40.05, and 40.83 for the Lagrangian, hybrid Eulerian-Lagrangian, and Eulerian approach, respectively, whereas the correspondence distance error was 0.10, 0.12, 0.41 pixels, respectively. As expected, the accuracy of the hybrid Eulerian-Lagrangian approach was much better than that of the Eulerian approach, but not better than that of the Lagrangian approach. However, the computational times tell a different story, with the Eulerian approach being the fastest at 0.69 seconds and the Lagrangian approach being the slowest at 4.39 seconds. The Eulerian-Lagrangian approach took just 1.11 seconds. For this experiment, the proposed hybrid approach allowed us to get the best of both worlds: the precision of the Lagrangian approach with almost the same speed as the Eulerian approach. Fig. 3 shows the computed values of L_0 and L_1 using the hybrid Eulerian-Lagrangian approach. The computed thickness ranged from 39.98 to 40.15.

We again tested the three approaches with another synthetic region, shown in Fig. 4. This time, the region R was the annulus between a circle of radius 25 and an ellipse with minor and major radii of 50 and 90. Comparing to what we assumed to be the exact solution, we got an average relative thickness error, over the 12,148 pixels inside R, of 0.078%, 0.26%, and 2.24% for the Lagrangian, hybrid Eulerian-Lagrangian, and Eulerian approach. Additionally, the correspondence distance errors were 0.13, 0.14, and 0.52 pixels, respectively. The computational times were 3.97, 0.91, and 0.58 seconds, respectively. Again, the proposed approach required much less time than the Lagrangian approach, while the accuracy of the latter was better than that of the former.

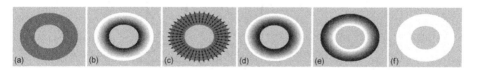

Fig. 3. Thickness computations for a synthetic annular region between two concentric circles. a) Circular annulus. (b) Harmonic interpolant. (c) Tangent field. (d) L_0. (e) L_1. (f) Thickness.

Finally, we applied all three methods to a 160 x 160 segmentation of the myocardium obtained from a short-axis MR image of the heart shown in Fig. 5, which also

depicts some correspondence trajectories, evidencing the need to form curved correspondence trajectories in some parts of the annular region R. The calculated thickness
using the proposed approach is shown in Fig. 5(e), in which brighter regions represent
thicker myocardium. Fig. 6 depicts the correspondence distance errors and the thickness relative errors for the three approaches, including the hybrid Eulerian-Lagrangian
approach with different values of tolerance λ. We note that for all cases the errors of
the Eulerian PDE approach are much greater than those of the other approaches. We
also observe that the performance of the proposed approach lies in-between those of
the Eulerian and the Lagrangian approaches. Particularly, when $\lambda = 0.5$ the errors of
the Lagrangian and hybrid Eulerian-Lagrangian approaches are very similar, despite
the fact that the hybrid approach required just about half the time required by the Lagrangian approach. Of course, this difference in computational time becomes much
more relevant when working with 3-D images.

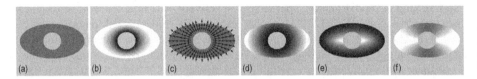

Fig. 4. Thickness computations for a synthetic annular region between a circle and an ellipse.
(a) Circular annulus. (b) Harmonic interpolant. (c) Tangent field. (d) L_0. (e) L_1. (f) Thickness.

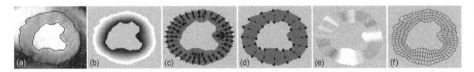

Fig. 5. Myocardial thickness from a short-axis MR image. (a) Endocardial and epicardial
boundaries. (b) Harmonic interpolant. (c) Tangent field. (d) Boundary correspondences for
some selected points. (e) Thickness. (f) Gridding of the region.

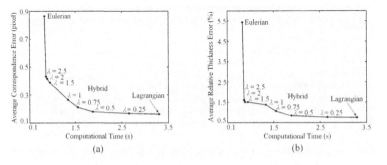

Fig. 6. Comparison of the different approaches in terms of the average correspondence distance
error, the average thickness relative error, and the computational time

5 Conclusions

We have presented a new hybrid Eulerian-Lagrangian algorithm for computing thickness, correspondences, and gridding in annular regions. These types of regions are of particular interest in medical imaging since their analysis can be used to early detect certain diseases or estimate functional performance of some parts of the human body. The innovation of the new method lies in the intricate way the Eulerian PDE approach and the Lagrangian approach are combined. These two earlier methods are completely different from each other and the way they can be efficiently and usefully blended is not straightforward at all as is evident from the description of the hybrid algorithm proposed. The whole purpose of this work was to create a practical approach that people would be more likely to use in contrast to the pure Lagrangian and pure Eulerian schemes previously published. The resulting technique possesses the best of both worlds, namely the speed of the Eulerian PDE approach and the accuracy of the Lagrangian approach, with the additional important (and practical) benefit of giving user precise control over the accuracy and maximum possible speed given that selected degree of accuracy. This makes the proposed method suitable for a much wider range of applications than either the Eulerian or Lagrangian approaches that are currently well known.

References

1. Henery, C., Mayhew, T.: The Cerebrum and Cerebellum of the Fixed Human Brain: Efficient and Unbiased Estimates of Volumes and Cortical Surface Areas. J. Anat., Vol. 167. (1989) 167-180
2. Park, J., Metaxas, D., Axel, L.: Analysis of Left Ventricular Wall Motion Based on Volumetric Deformable Models and MRI-SPAMM. Med. Imag. Analysis, Vol. 1. (1996) 53-71
3. Lef, J., et al.: Morphometric Analysis of Temporal Lobe in Temporal Lobe Epilepsy. Epilepsia, Vol. 7. (1998) 727-736
4. Fischl, B., Dale, A.M.: Measuring the Thickness of the Human Cerebral Cortex from Magnetic Resonance Images. Proc. Nat. Acad. Sci., Vol. 97. (2000) 1050–1055
5. DeBakey, M.E., Gotto, A.M., Jr.: The New Living Heart. Adams Media Corporation, Massachusetts (1997)
6. Pizer, S., Eberly, D., Fritsch, D., Morse, B.: Zoom-Invariant Vision of Figural Shape: The Mathematics of Cores. Comp. Vision Imag. Understanding, Vol. 69. (1998) 55–71
7. Jones, S.E., Buchbinder, B.R., Aharon, I.: Three-Dimensional Mapping of the Cortical Thickness Using Laplace's Equation. Hum. Brain Mapping, Vol. 11. (2000) 12–32
8. Yezzi, A.J., Prince, J.L.: An Eulerian PDE Approach for Computing Tissue Thickness. IEEE Trans. Med. Imag., Vol. 22. (2003) 1332-1339
9. Yezzi, A.J., Prince, J.L.: A PDE Approach for Thickness, Correspondence, and Gridding of Annular Tissues. Proc. Europ. Conf. Comp. Vision (ECCV), Copenhagen, 2002
10. Sethian, J.: Level Set Methods: Evolving Interfaces in Geometry, Fluid Mechanics, Computer Vision, and Material Science. Cambridge Univ. Press, U.K. (1996)
11. Duci, A., Yezzi, A.J., Mitter, S.K., Soatto, S.: Shape Representation via Harmonic Embedding. Proc. Intl. Conf. Comp. Vision, Vol. 1. (2003) 656-663

A Hybrid Framework for Image Segmentation Using Probabilistic Integration of Heterogeneous Constraints

Rui Huang, Vladimir Pavlovic, and Dimitris N. Metaxas

Deptartment of Computer Science, Rutgers University, Piscataway, NJ 08854
{ruihuang, vladimir, dnm}@cs.rutgers.edu

Abstract. In this paper we present a new framework for image segmentation using probabilistic multinets. We apply this framework to integration of region-based and contour-based segmentation constraints. A graphical model is constructed to represent the relationship of the observed image pixels, the region labels and the underlying object contour. We then formulate the problem of image segmentation as the one of joint region-contour inference and learning in the graphical model. The joint inference problem is solved approximately in a band area around the estimated contour. Parameters of the model are learned on-line. The fully probabilistic nature of the model allows us to study the utility of different inference methods and schedules. Experimental results show that our new hybrid method outperforms methods that use homogeneous constraints.

1 Introduction

Image segmentation is an example of a challenging clustering/classification problem where image pixels are grouped according to some notion of homogeneity such as intensity, texture, color, motion layers, etc. Unlike many traditional clustering/classification problems, where the class labels of different query points are inferred independently, image segmentation can be viewed as a *constrained* clustering/classification problem. It is reasonable to expect that class-labels of points that are in spatial proximity of each other will be similar. Moreover, the boundaries of segmented image regions are often smooth, imposing another constraint on the clustering/classification solution.

Markov Random Fields (MRFs) have long been used, with various inference techniques, in image analysis, because of their ability to impose the similarity constraints among neighboring image pixels and deal with the noise [1,2,3,4,5]. The MRF-based image segmentation method is an important representative of region-based segmentations, which assign image pixels to a region according to some image property (e.g., region homogeneity). The other major class of image segmentation methods are edge-based segmentations, which generate boundaries of the segmented objects. Among others, deformable models and their variants [6,7,8,9] are important representatives of this class.

Though one can label regions according to edges or detect edges from regions, the two kinds of methods are naturally different and have respective advantages and disadvantages. The MRF-based methods work well in noisy images, where edges are usually difficult to detect while the region homogeneity is preserved. The disadvantages of these

Y. Liu, T. Jiang, and C. Zhang (Eds.): CVBIA 2005, LNCS 3765, pp. 82–92, 2005.

methods are that they may generate rough edges and holes inside the objects, and they do not take account of the shape and topology of the segmented objects. On the other hand, in deformable model-based methods, a prior knowledge of object shape can be easily incorporated to constrain the segmentation result. While this often leads to sufficiently smooth boundaries, the oversmoothing may be excessive. And these methods rely on edge detecting operators, so they are sensitive to image noise and may need to be initialized close to the actual region boundaries. The real world images, especially medical images, usually have significant, often non-white noise and contain complex high-curvature objects with a strong shape prior, suggesting a hybrid method to take advantages of both MRFs and deformable models.

In this paper we propose a fully probabilistic graphical model-based framework to combine the heterogeneous constraints imposed by MRFs and deformable models, thus constraining the image segmentation problem. To tightly couple the two models, we construct a graphical model to represent the relationship of the observed image pixels, the true region labels and the underlying object contour. Unlike traditional graphical models, the links between contour and region nodes are not fixed; rather, they vary according to the state (position) of the contour nodes. This leads to a novel representation similar to Bayesian multinets [10]. We then formulate the problem of image segmentation under heterogeneous constraints as the one of joint region-contour inference and learning in the graphical model. Because the model is fully probabilistic, we are able to use the general tools of probabilistic inference to solve the segmentation problem. We solve this problem in a computationally efficient manner using approximate inference in a band area around the estimated contour.

The rest of this paper is organized as follows: section 2 reviews the previous work; section 3 introduces a new integrated model; detailed inference on the coupled model is described in section 4; section 5 shows the experimental results and comparison of alternative inference methods and schedules; and section 6 summarizes the paper and future work.

2 Previous Work

Because the exact MAP inference in MRF models is computationally infeasible, various techniques for approximating the MAP estimation have been proposed, such as MCMC [1], ICM [2], MPM [3], and two of the more recently developed fast algorithms: Belief Propagation (BP) [4] and Graph Cuts [5]. The estimation of the MRF parameters is often solved using the EM algorithm [11]. However, MRFs do not take account of object shape and may generate rough edges and even holes inside the objects. Since the introduction of Snakes [6], variants of deformable models have been proposed to address problems such as initialization (Balloons [7] and GVF Snakes [9]) and changes in model's topology [8]. One limitation of the deformable model-based method is its sensitivity to image noise, a common drawback of edge-based methods.

Methods for integration of region and contour models were studied in [12,13] using inside-outside and stochastic Gibbs models. The joint contour-region inference is accomplished using general energy minimization methods, without explicit model parameter learning. Chen et al. proposed a way of integrating MRFs and deformable mod-

The segmentation problem can now be viewed as a *joint* MAP estimation problem:

$$(\mathbf{c}, \mathbf{s}, \theta)_{MAP} = \arg\max_{\mathbf{c}, \mathbf{s}, \theta} P(\mathbf{c}, \mathbf{s}, \theta | \mathbf{y}) \tag{1}$$

where

$$P(\mathbf{c}, \mathbf{s}, \theta | \mathbf{y}) \propto P(\mathbf{y} | \mathbf{s}, \theta) P(\mathbf{s}, \mathbf{c}, \theta) P(\theta). \tag{2}$$

Note that we include the estimation of model parameters θ as a part of the segmentation process.

To define the joint distribution of the integrated model, we model the image likelihood term $P(\mathbf{y}|\mathbf{s})$ identical to the traditional MRF model (we drop the dependency on parameters θ when obvious):

$$P(\mathbf{y}|\mathbf{s}) = \prod_i P(y_i | s_i) = \prod_i p_i(s_i) = \prod_i \frac{1}{\sqrt{2\pi\sigma_{s_i}^2}} \exp\left(-\frac{(y_i - \mu_{s_i})^2}{2\sigma_{s_i}^2} \right) \tag{3}$$

where we assume the image pixels are corrupted by white Gaussian noise. The second term $P(\mathbf{s}, \mathbf{c})$ models a *joint* distribution of region labels and the contour. We represent this distribution in terms of two compatibility functions, rather than probabilities:

$$P(\mathbf{s}, \mathbf{c}) = \frac{1}{Z(\mathbf{s}, \mathbf{c})} \Psi_{sc}(\mathbf{s}, \mathbf{c}) \Psi_c(\mathbf{c}). \tag{4}$$

The first term models the compatibility of the region labels with the contour, defined as:

$$\begin{aligned}
\Psi_{sc}(\mathbf{s}, \mathbf{c}) &= \prod_{(i,j)} \Psi_{ss}(s_i, s_j) \prod_i \Psi_{sc}(s_i, c_{i'}) \\
&= \prod_{(i,j)} \psi_{ij}(s_i, s_j) \prod_i \psi_{ii'}(s_i, c_{i'}) \\
&= \prod_i \exp\left(\frac{\delta(s_i - s_j)}{\sigma^2} \right) \prod_i \psi_{ii'}(s_i, c_{i'})
\end{aligned} \tag{5}$$

where we incorporated a shape $\mathbf{c}$ to constrain the region labels $\mathbf{s}$, in addition to the original Gibbs distribution. Note that the dependency between the contour and the region labels is not deterministic. The uncertainty in region labels for a given contour can arise as an attempt to model, e.g., image aliasing and changes in region appearance at boundaries.

Since we only segment one specific region at a time, we need only consider the pixels near the contour, and label them either *inside* or *outside* the contour. We model the dependency between the contour $\mathbf{c}$ and the region labels $\mathbf{s}$ using the softmax function:

$$\psi_{ii'}(s_i = inside, c_{i'}) \sim 1 / \left(1 + \exp(-d^{(s)}(i, c_{i'})) \right) \tag{6}$$

induced by the signed distance of pixel i from the contour segment $c_{i'}$ (see Fig. 1(c)):

$$d^{(s)}(i, c_{i'}) = (d_{i'} - loc(i)) \times (d_{i'+1} - d_{i'}) / |d_{i'+1} - d_{i'}| \tag{7}$$

where $loc(i)$ denotes the spatial coordinates of pixel i. This equation only holds when the pixel is close to the contour, which accords with our assumption. When the contour nodes are ordered counter-clockwise, the sign is positive when pixel i is inside the contour and negative when it is outside.

The contour prior term $P(\mathbf{c})$ can be represented as:

$$\Psi_c(\mathbf{c}) = \prod_{i'} \Psi_{cc}(c_{i'-1}, c_{i'}) \prod_{i'} \Psi_b(c_{i'}) = \prod_{(i'-1,i')} \psi_{i'-1,i'}(c_{i'-1}, c_{i'}) \prod_{i'} \psi_{i'}(c_{i'}) \quad (8)$$

where $\psi_{i'-1,i'}(c_{i'-1}, c_{i'})$ is the contour smoothness term and $\psi_{i'}(c_{i'})$ is used to simulate the balloon force.

Despite the compact graphical representation of the integrated model, the exact inference in the model is computationally intractable. One reason for this is the large state space size of the contour nodes (the 2D image plane). To deal with this problem we restrict the contour searching to a set of normal lines along the current contour, as proposed in [16] (see Fig. 1(b)). That is, the state space of each contour node d_i is restricted to a small number, e.g., k, distinct values. In turn, the state space of each contour segment c_i is of size k^2. Now we can easily calculate the discretized contour smoothness term:

$$\psi_{i'-1,i'}(c_{i'-1}, c_{i'}) = e^{\left(-\omega_1 \frac{|d_{i'-1}-d_{i'+1}|^2}{4h^2} - \omega_2 \frac{|d_{i'-1}+d_{i'+1}-2d_{i'}|^2}{h^4}\right)} \quad (9)$$

and simulate the balloon force by defining $\psi_{i'}(c_{i'}) = [\psi_{i',1}, ..., \psi_{i',k}]$, where $\psi_{i',j}$ is the prior of each state j at the contour node $d_{i'}$.

Lastly, the parameter priors $P(\theta)$ are chosen from the appropriate conjugate prior families and are assumed to be uninformative. In this paper we primarily focus on the MRF parameters.

4   Model Inference Using Bp

The whole inference/learning algorithm for the hybrid model can now be summarized as below. The goal of our segmentation method is to find one specific region with a smooth and closed boundary. A seed point is arbitrarily specified and the region containing it is then segmented automatically. Thus, without significant loss of modeling generality, we simplify the MRF model and avoid possible problems caused by segmenting multiple regions simultaneously.

Initialize contour $\mathbf{c}$;
while (error > maxError) {
    1. Calculate a band area B around $\mathbf{c}$. Perform remaining steps inside B;
    2. Build links between the $\mathbf{s}$ and $\mathbf{c}$ layers according to the signed distances;
    3. Calculate the discretized states at each contour node along its normal;
    4. Estimate the MAP solution $(\mathbf{c}, \mathbf{s})_{MAP}$ using BP with schedule $\mathcal{S}$;
    5. Update model parameters θ_{MAP} and contour position $\mathbf{d}_{MAP}$;
}

As mentioned previously, the exact MAP inference even in the MRF model alone is often computationally infeasible. In our significantly more complex but probabilistic model, we resort to using the BP algorithm. BP is an inference method proposed by Pearl [17] to efficiently estimate Bayesian beliefs in the network by the way of iteratively passing messages between neighbors. It is an exact inference method in the network without loops. Even in the network with loops, the method often leads to good approximate and tractable solutions [18]. The implementation of BP in our model is slightly more difficult than the BP algorithm in a traditional pairwise MRF, since the model structure is more complicated. One can solve this by converting the model into an equivalent factor graph, and use the BP algorithm for factor graphs [19,20]. Here we give the straightforward algorithm for our specific model. Examples of the message passing rules are

$$
m_{ij}(s_j) = \max_{s_i} \left[\psi_i(s_i) \prod_{k \in \aleph(i) \backslash j} m_{ki}(s_i) m_{i'i}(s_i) \psi_{ij}(s_i, s_j) \right] \tag{10}
$$

$$
m_{i'i}(s_i) = \max_{c_{i'}} \left[\psi_{i'}(c_{i'}) \prod_{k' \in \aleph(i')} m_{k'i'}(c_{i'}) \prod_{k \in \aleph'(i') \backslash i} m_{ki'}(c_{i'}) \psi_{ii'}(s_i, c_{i'}) \right] \tag{11}
$$

with message definition given in Fig. 1(d). $\aleph$ denotes the set of neighbors from the same layer, and $\aleph'$ denotes the set of neighbors from a different layer. The rules are based on the max-product scheme. At convergence, the beliefs, e.g., of the pixel labels are

$$
b_i(s_i) \sim \psi_i(s_i) \prod_{k \in \aleph(i)} m_{ki}(s_i) m_{i'i}(s_i). \tag{12}
$$

A crucial question in this BP process is that of the "right" message passing schedule [19,20]. Different schedules may result in different stable/unstable configurations. For instance, it is widely accepted that short graph cycles deteriorate the performance of the BP algorithm. We empirically study this question in Section 5.3 and show that good schedules arise from understanding of the physical processes involved.

The BP is evoked only in a *band area* around current contour. A primary reason for the band-limited BP update is the computational complexity of inference. Moreover, the band-limited update can also be justified by the fact that the region labels of pixels far from the current contour have little influence on the contour estimates. When the BP algorithm converges, the model parameters (i.e., μ_{s_i} and σ_{s_i}) can be updated using following equations:

$$
\mu_l = \sum_i b(s_i = l) y_i / \sum_i b(s_i = l), \quad \sigma_l^2 = \sum_i b(s_i = l)(y_i - \mu_l)^2 / \sum_i b(s_i = l) \tag{13}
$$

where $l \in \{inside, outside\}$ and $b(\cdot)$ denotes the current belief.

Because the edges between the **s** layer and the **c** layer are determined by the distance between pixels and contour nodes, they also need to be updated in the inference process. This step follows directly after the MAP estimation.

5   Experiments

Our algorithm was implemented in MATLAB/C, and all the experiments were tested on a 1.5GHz P4 Computer. Most of the experiments took several minutes on the images of size 128×128.

5.1 Comparison with Other Methods

The initial study of properties and utility of our method was conducted on a set of synthetic images. The 64×64 perfect images contain only 2 gray levels representing the "object" (gray level is 160) and the "background" (gray level is 100) respectively. We then made the background more complicated by introducing a gray level gradient from 100 to 160, along the normal direction of the object contour to the image boundary (Fig. 2(a)). Fig. 2(b) shows the result of a traditional MRF-based method. The object is segmented correctly, however some regions in the background are misclassified. On the other hand, the deformable model slightly leaked from the high-curvature part of the object contour, where the gradient in the normal direction is too weak (Fig. 2(c)). Our hybrid method, shown in Fig. 2(d), results in a significantly improved segmentation.

We next generated a test image (Fig. 2(e)) by adding zero-mean Gaussian noise with σ 60 to Fig. 2(a). The result of the MRF-based method on the noisy image (Fig. 2(f)) is somewhat similar to that in Fig. 2(b), which shows the MRF can deal with image noise to some extent. But significant misclassification occurred because of the complicated background and noise levels. The deformable model either sticks to spurious edges caused by image noise or leaks (Fig. 2(g)) because of the weakness of the true edges. Unlike the two independent methods, our hybrid algorithm, depicted in Fig. 2(h), correctly identifies the object boundaries despite the excessive image noise. For visualization purposes we superimpose the contour on the original image (Fig. 2(a)) to show the quality of the result in Fig. 2(g) and Fig. 2(h).

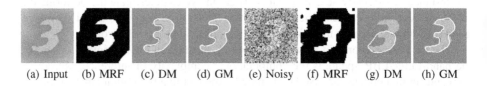

(a) Input   (b) MRF   (c) DM   (d) GM   (e) Noisy   (f) MRF   (g) DM   (h) GM

Fig. 2. Experiments on synthetic images

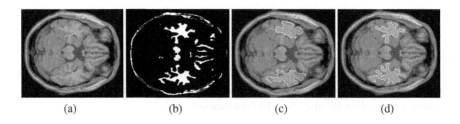

(a)   (b)   (c)   (d)

Fig. 3. Experiments on medical images

Experiments with synthetic images outlined some of the benefits of our hybrid method. The real world images (e.g., medical images) usually have significant, often non-white noise and contain multiple regions and objects, rendering the segmentation task a great deal more difficult. Fig. 3(a) is a good example of difficult images with complicated global properties, requiring the MRF-based method to automatically determine the number of regions and the initial values of the parameters. Fig. 3(b) is obtained by manually specifying the inside/outside regions to get an initial guess of the parameters for the MRF model. Our method avoids this problem by creating and updating an MRF model locally and incrementally. Another problem with MRF-based method is that we can not get a good representation of the segmented object directly from the model. The image is also difficult for deformable models because the boundaries of the objects to be segmented have many high-curvature parts. Fig. 3(c) exemplifies the over-smoothed deformable models. Our method's results, shown in Fig. 3(d) does not suffer from the problems. For the deformable model method, we started the balloon model at several different initial positions and use the best results for the comparison. On the other hand, our hybrid method is significantly less sensitive to the initialization of the parameters and the initial seed position.

5.2   Comparison of Different Inference Methods

We compared our proposed inference method (MAP by BP) with three other similar methods: maximum marginal posterior (MM), iterative conditional modes (ICM), and Gibbs sampling. In the MM method the inference process is accomplished using the sum-product belief propagation algorithm [20]. The algorithm yields approximate marginal posteriors, e.g., $P(s_i|\mathbf{y})$ that are then maximized on individual basis, e.g., $s_i* = \arg\max_{s_i} P(s_i|\mathbf{y})$. The ICM and Gibbs inference methods, respectively, maximize and sample from the local conditional models, e.g.,
$s_i* = \arg\max_{s_i} P(s_i|\text{Markov Blanket}(s_i))$, one variable at a time.

In all our experiments there was no substantial visible difference between the segmentation results of MAP and MM estimates, as exemplified by Fig. 4. Comparison of log likelihood profiles during inference revealed small differences—as expected, the sum-product inference outperforms the max-product in noisy situations. On the other hand, the use of ICM and Gibbs inference resulted in significantly worse final segmentation. For instance, when used only in the MRF layer, ICM and Gibbs-driven segmentation lead to final estimates shown in Fig. 4c and Fig.4d. Surprisingly, the differences in the log likelihood estimates appear to be less indicative of this final performance. The use of the two approximate inference methods, not shown here, in the DM layer resulted in very poor segmentation.

5.3   Comparison of Different Message Passing Schedules

The choice of the message passing schedule in the BP algorithm is an interesting and still open problem. We experimented with two different schedules. In the first schedule S_1 we first update messages $m_{ij}(s_j)$ in s-layer until convergence (this usually takes two or three iterations in our experiments), and then send messages $m_{ii'}(c_{i'})$ once (which is essentially passing messages from s-layer to c-layer). Next, we update messages $m_{i'j'}(c_{j'})$ in c-layer until convergence (usually in one or two iterations), and finally update messages $m_{i'i}(x_i)$, i.e., send messages back from c-layer to s-layer. In the other schedule S_2 we started from the top of the model, update all the messages $m_{ij}(s_j)$,

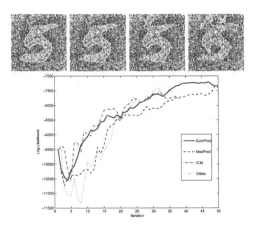

Fig. 4. Top: Final segmentation results of different inference schemes: (a) sum-product, (b) max-product, (c) ICM in MRF, sum-product in DM, and (d) Gibbs in MRF, sum-product in DM. Bottom: Changes in log likelihood during iterations of different inference schemes

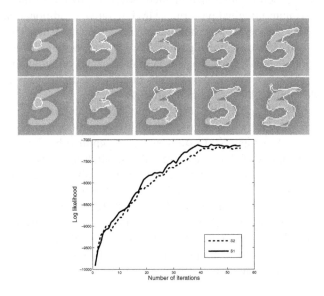

Fig. 5. Experiments with different message passing schedule. Top: $\mathcal{S}_1$, Center: $\mathcal{S}_2$, Bottom: Log likelihoods (computed at MAP estimates) using the two different schedules.

$m_{ii'}(c_{i'})$, $m_{i'j'}(c_{j'})$, and $m_{i'i}(s_i)$ in this sequence exactly once and repeat, until convergence.

The two message passing schedules were chosen to study the importance of within-model (e.g., inside MRF) local consistency (schedule $\mathcal{S}_1$) and between-models local consistency ($\mathcal{S}_2$). The former message passing schedule may be intuitively more appealing considering the physical difference of the two models (MRFs and deformable models) we are coupling. Traditional energy-based methods also point in the direction of this schedule; integration of forces is usually first computed in the individual horizontal layers. Moreover, S_1 leads to better experimental results. The upper two rows of Fig. 5 show, visually, the segmentation performance of the two schedules. The estimates of the likelihood resulting from the two schedule, displayed in the bottom row of Fig. 5, also indicate that S_1 is preferred to S_2. Again, the contour is superimpose on the perfect image for visualization purposes.

6 Conclusions

We proposed a new, fully probabilistic framework to combine two heterogeneous constraints, MRFs and deformable models, for the clustering/classification task of image segmentation. The framework was developed under the auspices of the probabilistic multinet model theory allowing us to employ a well-founded set of statistical estimation and learning techniques. In particular, we employed an approximate, computationally efficient solution to the otherwise intractable constrained inference of image regions. We showed the utility of our hybrid method and different inference schemes. We also presented two different message passing schedules. Finally, we point to the central role of inference schemes and message passing schedules in the segmentation process.

We are now working on including a stronger shape prior to the model, in additional to current smoothness term and balloon forces. In our future work we will consider similarity as well as dissimilarity constraints, specified by users or learned from data, to further reduce the feasible solution spaces in the context of image segmentation.

References

1. S. Geman and D. Geman. Stochastic Relaxation, Gibbs Distributions and the Bayesian Restoration of Images. *IEEE Transaction on Pattern Analysis and Machine Intelligence*, 6(6), 1984.
2. J. E. Besag. On the Statistical Analysis of Dirty Pictures. *Journal of the Royal Statistical Society B*, 48(3), 1986.
3. J. Marroquin, S. Mitter, and T. Poggio. Probabilistic Solution of Ill-posed Problems in Computational Vision. *Journal of American Statistical Association*, 82(397), 1987.
4. W.T. Freeman, E.C. Pasztor, and O.T. Carmichael. Learning Low-Level Vision. *International Journal of Computer Vision*, 40(1), 2000.
5. Y.Y. Boykov and M.P. Jolly. Interactive Graph Cuts for Optimal Boundary & Region Segmentation of Objects in N-D Images. *Proceedings of ICCV*, 2001.
6. M. Kass, A. Witkin, and D. Terzopoulos. Snakes: Active contour models. *International Journal of Computer Vision*, 1(4), 1987.
7. L.D. Cohen. On Active Contour Models and Balloons. *Computer Vision, Graphics, and Image Processing: Image Understanding*, 53(2), 1991.
8. T. McInerney and D. Terzopoulos. Topologically Adaptable Snakes. *Proceedings of ICCV*, 1995.
9. C. Xu and J.L. Prince. Gradient Vector Flow: A New External Force for Snakes. *Proceedings of CVPR*, 1997.
10. D. Geiger and D. Heckerman, Knowledge representation and inference in similarity networks and Bayesian multinets, *Artificial Intelligence*, 82:45-74, 1996.

11. Y. Zhang, M. Brady, and S. Smith. Segmentation of Brain MR Images Through a Hidden Markov Random Field Model and the Expectation-Maximization Algorithm. *IEEE Transaction on Medical Imaging*, 20(1), 2001.
12. U. Grenander and M. Miller. Representations of Knowledge in Complex Systems. *Journal of the Royal Statistical Society B*, 56(4), 1994.
13. S.C. Zhu and A.L. Yuille. Region Competition: Unifying Snakes, Region Growing, and Bayes/MDL for Multiband Image Segmentation. *IEEE Transaction on Pattern Analysis and Machine Intelligence*, 18(9), 1996.
14. T. Chen, D.N. Metaxas. Image Segmentation Based on the Integration of Markov Random Fields and Deformable Models. *Proceedings of MICCAI*, 2000.
15. R. Huang, V. Pavlovic, and D.N. Metaxas. A Graphical Model Framework for Coupling MRFs and Deformable Models. *Proceedings of CVPR*, 2004.
16. Y. Chen, Y. Rui, and T.S. Huang. JPDAF Based HMM for Real-Time Contour Tracking. *Proceedings of CVPR*, 2001.
17. J. Pearl, *Probabilistic Reasoning in Intelligent Systems: Networks of Plausible Inference*, Morgan Kaufmann Publishers, 1988.
18. Y. Weiss. Belief Propagation and Revision in Networks with Loops. *Technical Report MIT A.I. Memo 1616*, 1998.
19. F.R. Kschischang, B.J. Frey, and Hans-Andrea Loeliger. Factor Graphs and the Sum-Product Algorithm. *IEEE Transactions on Information Theory*, 47(2), 2001.
20. J.S. Yedidia, W.T. Freeman, and Y. Weiss. Understanding Belief Propagation and Its Generalizations. *IJCAI 2001 Distinguished Lecture track*, 2001

A Learning Framework for the Automatic and Accurate Segmentation of Cardiac Tagged MRI Images

Zhen Qian[1], Dimitris N. Metaxas[1], and Leon Axel[2]

[1] Center for Computational Biomedicine Imaging and Modeling (CBIM),
Rutgers University, New Brunswick, New Jersey, USA
[2] Department of Radiology, New York University, New York, USA

Abstract. In this paper we present a fully automatic and accurate segmentation framework for 2D tagged cardiac MR images. This scheme consists of three learning methods: a) an active shape model is implemented to model the heart shape variations, b) an Adaboost learning method is applied to learn confidence-rated boundary criterions from the local appearance features at each landmark point on the shape model, and c) an Adaboost detection technique is used to initialize the segmentation. The set of boundary statistics learned by Adaboost is the weighted combination of all the useful appearance features, and results in more reliable and accurate image forces compared to using only edge or region information. Our experimental results show that given similar imaging techniques, our method can achieve a highly accurate performance without any human interaction.

1 Introduction

Tagged cardiac magnetic resonance imaging(MRI) is a well known technique for non-invasively visualizing the detailed motion of myocardium throughout the heart cycle. This technique has the potential of early diagnosis and quantitative analysis of various kinds of heart diseases and malfunction. However, before it can be used in routine clinical evaluations, an imperative but challenging task is to automatically find the boundaries of the epicardium and the endocardium. (See Figure 1(a-c) for some examples.)

Segmentation in tagged MRI is difficult for several reasons. First, the boundaries are often obscured or corrupted by the nearby tagging lines, which makes the conventional edge-based segmentation method infeasible. Second, tagged MRI tends to increase the intensity contrast between the tagged and un-tagged tissues at the price of lowering the contrast between the myocardium and the blood. At the same time, the intensity of the myocardium and blood vary during the cardiac cycle due to the tagging lines fading in the myocardium and being flushed away in the blood. Third, due to the short acquisition time, the tagged MR images have a relatively high level of noise. These factors make conventional region-based segmentation techniques impractical. The last and the most

Y. Liu, T. Jiang, and C. Zhang (Eds.): CVBIA 2005, LNCS 3765, pp. 93–102, 2005.
© Springer-Verlag Berlin Heidelberg 2005

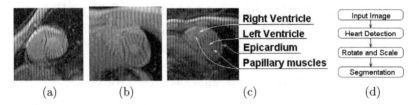

Fig. 1. (a-c) Some examples of tagged cardiac MRI images. The task of segmentation is to find the boundaries of the epicardium and endocardium (including the LV and RV and excluding the papillary muscles.) (d) The framework of our segmentation method.

important reason is that, from the clinicians' point of view, or for the purpose of 3D modeling, *accurate* segmentation based solely on the MR image is usually not possible. For instance, for conventional clinical practice, the endocardial boundary should exclude the papillary muscles for the purpose of easier analysis. However, in the MR images, the papillary muscles are often apparently connected with the endocardium and cannot be separated if only the image information is used. Thus prior shape knowledge is needed to improve the results of automated segmentation.

There have been some efforts to achieve tagged MRI segmentation. In [1], grayscale morphological operations were used to find non-tagged blood-filled regions. Then they used thresholding and active contour methods to find the boundaries. In [2], a learning method with a coupled shape and intensity statistical model was proposed. In [3,4], Gabor filtering was used to remove the tagging lines before the segmentation. These methods work in some cases. However they are still imperfect. In [1], morphological operations are sensitive to image noise, and the active contour method tends to get irregular shapes without a prior shape model. In [2], their intensity statistical model cannot capture the complex local texture features, which leads to inaccurate image forces. And in [3,4], the filtering methods blur the boundaries and decrease the segmentation accuracy.

In this paper, in order to address the difficulties stated above, we propose a novel and fully automatic segmentation method based on three learning frameworks: 1. An active shape model(ASM) is used as the prior heart shape model. 2. A set of confidence-rated local boundary criteria are learned by Adaboost, a popular learning scheme (see Section 2.2), at landmark points of the shape model, using the appearance features in the nearby local regions. These criteria give the probability of the local region's center point being on the boundary, and force their corresponding landmark points to move toward the direction of the highest probability regions. 3. An Adaboost detection method is used to initialize the segmentation's location, orientation and scale. The second component is the most essential contribution of our method. We abandon the usual edge or region-based methods because of the complicated boundary and region appearance in the tagged MRI. It is not feasible to designate one or a few edge or region rules to solve the complicated segmentation task. Instead, we try to use all possible information, such as the edges, the ridges, and the breaking points of tagging lines, to form a *complex rule*. It is apparent that at different locations on the heart boundary, this *complex rule* must be different, and our confidence in the *complex rule* varies too. It is impractical to manually set up each of these *complex rules* and weight their confidence ratings. Therefore, we implement Adaboost to learn a set of rules and confidence ratings at each landmark point on the shape model. The first and the second frameworks are tightly coupled. The shape model deforms under the forces from Framework 2 while controlled and smoothed by Framework 1. To achieve fully automatic segmentation, in Framework 3 the detection method automatically provides an approximate position and size of the heart to initialize the segmentation step. See Figure 1(d) for a complete illustration of the frameworks.

The remainder of this paper is organized as follows: in Section 2, we present the segmentation methodology, including Frameworks 1 and 2. In Section 3, we briefly introduce the heart detection technique of Framework 3. In Section 4 we give some details of our experiments and show some encouraging initial experimental results.

2   Segmentation Based on ASM and Local Appearance Features Learning Using Adaboost

There has been some previous research on ASM segmentation methods based on local features modeling. In [5], a statistical analysis was performed, which used sequential feature forward and backward selection to find the set of optimal local features. In [6], an EM algorithm was used to select Gabor wavelet-based local features. These two methods tried to select a small number of features, which is impractical to represent complicated local textures such as in tagged MRI. In [7], a simple Adaboost learning method was proposed to find the optimal edge features. This method didn't make full use of the local textures, and didn't differentiate each landmark point's confidence level. In our method, similarly using Adaboost, our main contributions are: the ASM deforms based on a more *complex* and robust rule, which is learned from the local appearance, not only of the edges, but also ridges and tagging line breakpoints. In this way we get a better representation of the local appearance of the tagged MRI. At the same time, we derive the confidence rating of each landmark point from their Adaboost testing error rates, and use these confidence ratings to weight the image forces on each landmark point. In this way the global shape is affected more by the *more confident* points and we eliminate the possible error forces generated from the *less confident* points.

2.1   ASM Shape Model

Since the shape of the mid portion of the heart in short axis (SA) images is consistent and topologically fixed (one left ventricle (LV) and one right ventricle (RV)), it is reasonable to implement an active shape model [8] to represent the desired boundary contours.

We acquired two image datasets each, from two normal subjects, using two slightly different imaging techniques. The datasets were acquired in the short axis plane. There are two sets of tagging line orientations ($0°$ and $90°$, or $-45°$ and $45°$) and slightly different tag spacings. Each dataset included images acquired at phases through systole into early diastole, and at positions along the axis of the LV, from near the apex to near the base, but without topological changes. An expert was asked to segment the epicardium (Epi), the left ventricle (LV) endocardium and the right ventricle (RV) endocardium from the datasets. In total, we obtained 220 sets (each set includes one LV, one RV, and one Epi) of segmented contours to use as the training data.

Segmented contours were centered and scaled to a uniform size. Landmark points were placed automatically by finding key points with specific geometric characteristics. As shown in Figure 2(a), the black points are the key points, which were determined by the curvatures and positions along the contours. For instance, $P1$ and $P2$ are the highest curvature points of the RV; $P7$ and $P8$ are on opposite sides of the center axis of the LV. Then, fixed numbers of other points are equally placed in between. In this way, the landmark points were registered to the corresponding locations on the contours. Here, we used 50 points to represent the shape.

For each set of contours, the 50 landmark points (x_i, y_i) were reshaped to form a shape vector $X = (x_1, x_2, ..., x_{50}, y_1, y_2, ..., y_{50})^T$. Then Principal Component Analysis was applied and the modes of shape variation were found. Any heart shape can be approximately modeled by $X = \bar{X} + Pb$, where $\bar{X}$ is the mean shape vector, P is the matrix of shape variations, and b is the vector of shape parameters weighting the shape variations.

After we find the image forces at each landmark point, as in Section 2.2, the active shape model evolves iteratively. In each iteration, the model deforms under the influence of the image forces to a new location; the image forces are then calculated at the new locations before the next iteration.

2.2 Segmentation Via Learning Boundary Criteria Using Adaboost

Feature Design. To capture the local appearance characteristics, we designed three different kinds of steerable filters. We use the derivatives of a 2D Gaussian to capture the edges, we use the second order derivatives of a 2D Gaussian to capture the ridges, and we use half-reversed 2D Gabor filters [9] to capture the tagging line breakpoints.

Assume $G = G((x - x_0)\cos(\theta), (y - y_0)\sin(\theta), \sigma_x, \sigma_y)$ is an asymmetric 2D Gaussian, with effective widths σ_x and σ_y, a translation of (x_0, y_0) and a rotation of θ. We set the derivative of G to have the same orientation as G:

$$G' = G_x \cos(\theta) + G_y \sin(\theta) \tag{1}$$

The second derivative of a Gaussian can be approximated as the difference of two Gaussians with different σ. We fix σ_x as the long axis of the 2D Gaussians, and set $\sigma_{y2} > \sigma_{y1}$. Thus:

$$G'' = G(\sigma_{y1}) - G(\sigma_{y2}) \tag{2}$$

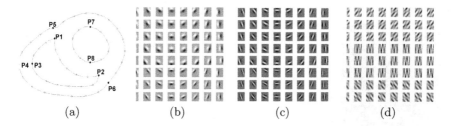

Fig. 2. (a) shows the automatic method used to place the landmark points. (b-d) are the sample sets of feature filters: (b) are the derivatives of Gaussian used for edge detection, (c) are the second derivatives of Gaussian used for ridge detection, and (d) are the half-reversed Gabor filters used for tag line breakpoint detection.

In the previous two equations, we set $x_0 = 0$, and tune y_0, θ, σ_x, σ_y, σ_{y1} and σ_{y2} to generate the desired filters.

The half-reversed 2D Gabor filters are defined as a 2D sine wave multiplied with the 2D derivative of a Gaussian:

$$F = G'(x,y) \cdot \mathbb{R}\{e^{-j[\phi+2\pi(Ux+Vy)]}\} \tag{3}$$

where G' is the derivative of a 2D Gaussian. U and V are the frequencies of the 2D sine wave, $\psi = arctan(V/U)$ is the orientation angle of the sine wave, and ϕ is the phase shift. We set $x_0 = 0$, $\sigma_x = \sigma_y = \sigma$, $-45° \leq \psi - \theta \leq 45°$, and tune y_0, θ, σ, ϕ, U and V to generate the desired filters.

For a 15x15 sized window, we designed 1840 filters in total. See Figure 2(b-d) for some sample filters.

Adaboost Learning. In the learning section, each training image is scaled proportionally to the scaling of its contours. At each landmark point of the contours, a small window (15x15) around it was cut out as a positive appearance training sample for this particular landmark point. Then along the normal of the contour, on each side of the point, we cut out two 15x15-sized windows as negative appearance training samples for this particular landmark point. Thus for each training image, at a particular landmark point, we got one positive sample and four negative samples (shown in Figure 3(a).) We also randomly selected a few common negative samples outside the heart or inside the blood area, which are suitable for every landmark point. For image contrast consistency, every sample was histogram equalized.

The function of the Adaboost algorithm [10,11] is to classify the positive training samples from the negative ones by selecting a small number of important features from a huge potential feature set and creating a weighted combination of them to use as an accurate strong classifier. During the boosting process, each iteration selects one feature from the total potential features pool, and combines it (with an appropriate weight) with the existing classifier that was obtained in the previous iterations. After many iterations, the weighted combination of the selected important features can become a strong classifier with high accuracy.

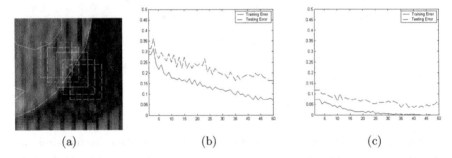

(a)   (b)   (c)

Fig. 3. (a) shows the method of setting the training data. The solid box is the positive sample around the landmark points. The four dashed line boxes along the normal are the negative samples. This way of setting the negative samples is chosen to make the classifier more adaptive to the particular landmark position. (b) and (c) show the training error (solid lines) and testing error (dash lines) of two landmark points versus Adaboost iteration times. (b) is a point on the LV, (c) is a point on the Epi. Note how the training and testing error decrease as Adaboost iterates. Also note the testing error of (b) is higher than (c): we are more confident of landmark point (c)'s classification result.

The output of the strong classifier is the weighted summation of the outputs of each of its each selected features, or, the weak classifiers: $F = \Sigma_t \alpha_t h_t(x)$, where α are the weights of weak classifiers, and h are the outputs of the weak classifiers.

We call F the boundary criterion. When $F > 0$, Adaboost classifies the point as being on the boundary. When $F < 0$, the point is classified as off the boundary. Even when the strong classifier consists of a large number of individual features, Adaboost encounters relatively few overfitting problems [12]. We divided the whole sample set into one training set and one testing set. The function of the testing set is critical. It gives a performance measure and a confidence level that tells us how much we should trust its classification result. Figure 3(b, c) shows the learning error curve versus the boosting iteration numbers at two selected landmark points. Note that every landmark point i has its own α, h and F_i.

Segmentation Based on Confidence Ratings. In the segmentation stage, we first select an initial location and scale, and then overlay the mean shape $\bar{X}$, which is obtained from ASM, onto the task image. In section 3 we describe an automatic initialization method.

At a selected landmark point i on the shape model, we select several equally spaced points along the normal of the contour on both sides of i, and use their F values to examine the corresponding windows centered on these points. In [12], a logistic function was suggested to estimate the relative boundary probabilities:

$$Pr(y = +1|x) = \frac{e^{F(x)}}{e^{F(x)} + e^{-F(x)}} \qquad (4)$$

We find a point j whose test window has the highest probability of being on the heart boundary. Thus an image force f should push the current landmark point

i toward j. Recall that, as discussed in the previous subsection, Adaboost gives the errors of the testing data e_i. We define the confidence rating as:

$$c_i = \ln \frac{1}{e_i};$$ (5)

Intuitively, when c_i is big, we trust its classification and increase the image force f, and conversely. Thus, we define the image force at landmark point i as:

$$f = \mu \cdot \frac{[\boldsymbol{x}(j) - \boldsymbol{x}(i)] \cdot c(i)}{||\boldsymbol{x}(j) - \boldsymbol{x}(i)||_2}$$ (6)

where μ is a scale as a small step size.

The detailed algorithm to update the parameters of the ASM model with the image force f can be found in [8].

3   Heart Detection Based on Adaboost Learning

The heart detection algorithm used is influenced by the Adaboost face detection algorithm developed by Paul Viola and Michael Jones [13]. The reason we adapt a face detection method is that these two problems are closely related. Often, there are marked variations between different face images, which come from different facial appearance, lighting, expression, etc. In heart detection, we have the similar challenges: the heart images have different tag patterns, shape, position, phase, etc.

We use the same Haar wavelet features as in [13]. The training data contained 297 manually cropped heart images and 459 randomly selected non-heart images. The testing data consisted of 41 heart images and 321 non-heart images. These data were resized to 24x24 pixels and contrast equalized. Adaboost training gave a strong classifier by combining 50 weak features. For an input task image, the detection method searched every square window over the image, and found a window with the highest probability as the final detection. If we rotate the task

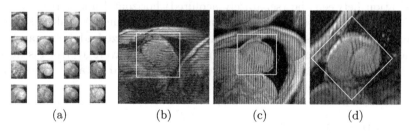

| (a) | (b) | (c) | (d) |

Fig. 4. (a) shows a few samples of the training data. (b), (c) and (d) are three detection results. For image (d), the image was rotated by a set of discrete angles before the detection, and the final detection is of the highest probability among all the discrete angles tested.

image by a set of discrete angles before the detection procedure, and compare the probabilities across the discrete angles, we are also able to detect hearts in rotated images (see Figure 4).

4   Representative Experimental Results and Validation

We applied our segmentation method to three data sets, one from the same subject and with the same imaging settings as the training data (but excluding the training data), and the other two novel data sets from two different subjects and with slightly different imaging settings. Respectively, the three data sets each contained 32, 48 and 96 tagged MRI images, with different phases, positions and tagging orientations. Each task image was rotated and scaled to contain a 80x80-pixel-sized chest-on-top heart, using the detection method before the segmentation. Each segmentation took 30 iterations to converge. Our experiment was coded in Matlab 6.5 and run on a PC with dual Xeon 3.0G CPUs and 2G memory. The whole learning process took about 20 hours. The segmentation process of one heart took 120 seconds on average. See Figure 5 for representative results.

For validation, we used the manual segmentation contours as the ground truth for the first and second data sets. For the third data set, because we don't have independent manual contours, we used cross validation, since we know that at the same position and phase, the heart shapes in the vertical-tagged and horizontal-tagged images should be similar. We denote the ground truth contours as T and our segmentation contours as S. We defined the average error distance as $\bar{D}_{error} = mean_{s_i \in S}(min||T - s_i||_2)$. Similarly the cross distance is defined as $\bar{D}_{cross} = mean_{s_i^{vertical} \in S^{vertical}}(min||S^{horizontal} - s_i^{vertical}||_2)$. In a 80x80 pixel-sized heart, the average error distances between the automatically segmented contours and the contours manually segmented by the expert for the first data set were: $\bar{D}_{error}(LV) = 1.12$ pixels, $\bar{D}_{error}(RV) = 1.11$ pixels, $\bar{D}_{error}(Epi) = 0.98$ pixels. For the second data set, $\bar{D}_{error}(LV) = 1.74$ pixels, $\bar{D}_{error}(RV) = 2.05$ pixels, $\bar{D}_{error}(Epi) = 1.33$ pixels. In the third dataset, the cross distances are: $\bar{D}_{cross}(LV) = 2.39$ pixels, $\bar{D}_{cross}(RV) = 1.40$ pixels, $\bar{D}_{cross}(Epi) = 1.94$ pixels. The larger distance in the cross validation arises in part from underlying mis-registration between the (separately acquired) horizontal and vertical images. Thus, the true discrepancy due to the segmentation should be smaller. From the above quantitative results, we find that for a normal-sized adult human heart, the accuracy of our segmentation method achieves an average error distance of less than 2mm. The cross validation results of the third data set suggest that our method is very robust as well.

5   Discussion

In this paper, we have proposed a learning scheme for fully automatic and accurate segmentation of cardiac tagged MRI data. The framework has three steps. In the first step we learn an ASM shape model as the prior shape constraint. Second, we learn a confidence-rated complex boundary criterion from the local

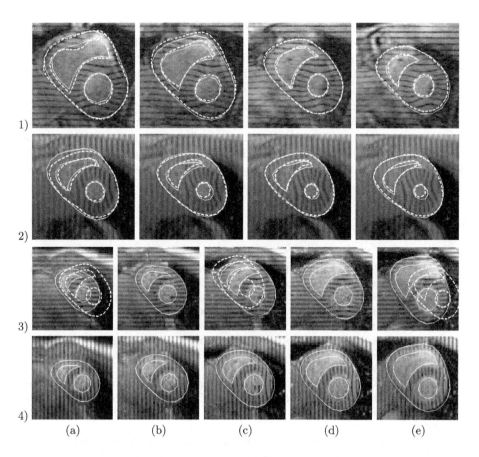

Fig. 5. The first and second rows of images come from the the first and second dataset, respectively. For better representation, the images in the first row vary in position and remain at the same phase, while the images in the second row vary in phase but remain at the same position. The solid contours are from our automatic segmentation method; the dashed contours are manual. Notice that the papillary muscles in LV are excluded from the endocardium. The third and fourth rows are from the third dataset. Manual contours are not available for this dataset, so we compare our segmentation results between the the horizontal and vertical tagged images that are at same position and phase. Qualitatively, the contours are quite consistent, allowing for possible misregistration between the nominally corresponding image sets. In (3a), (3c) and (3e) the dashed contours are testing examples of poor initializations, while the final contours are solid. Although the initialization is fay away from the target, the shape model moves and converges well to the target.

appearance features to use to direct the detected contour to move under the influence of image forces. Third, we also learn a classifier to detect the heart. This learning approach achieves higher accuracy and robustness than other previously available methods. Since our method is entirely based on learning, the way of choosing the training data is critical. We find that if the segmentation method is applied to images at phases or positions that are not represented in the training data, the segmentation process tends to get stuck in local minima. Thus the training data need to be of sufficient size and range to cover all possible variations that may be encountered in practice.

An interesting property of our method is that it is not very sensitive to the initialization conditions. As shown in Figure 5, even if the initial contours are far away from the target position, it can still eventually converge to the right position after a few iterations. This property makes automatic initialization feasible. The detection method gives only a rough approximation of the heart's location and size, but it is good enough for our segmentation purposes.

References

1. Montillo, A., Metaxas, D., Axel, L.: Automated segmentation of the left and right ventricles in 4d cardiac spamm images. In: Medical Imaging Computing and Computer-Assisted Intervention. (2002) 620–633
2. Huang, X., Li, Z., Metaxas, D.N.: Learning coupled prior shape and appearance models for segmentation. In: MICCAI (1). (2004) 60–69
3. Qian, Z., Huang, X., Metaxas, D., Axel, L.: Robust segmentation of 4d cardiac mri-tagged images via spatio-temporal propagation. In: Proceedings of SPIE Medical Imaging: Physiology, Function, and Structure from Medical Images. Volume 5746. (2005) 580–591
4. Metaxas, D., Chen, T., Huang, X., Axel, L.: Cardiac segmentation from mri-tagged and ct images. In: 8th WSEAS International Conf. on Computers, special session on Imaging and Image Processing of Dynamic Processes in biology and medicine. (2004)
5. Ginneken, B.V., Frangi, A.F., Staal, J.J., et al: Active shape model segmentation with optimal features. IEEE Trans. on Medical Imaging **21** (2002)
6. Jiao, F., Li, S., Shum, H., Schuurmans, D.: Face alignment using statistical models and wavelet features. In: IEEE Conf. on CVPR. Volume 1. (2003) 321–327
7. Li, S., Zhu, L., Jiang, T.: Active shape model segmentation using local edge structures and adaboost. In: Medical Imaging Augmented Reality. (2004)
8. Cootes, T., Taylor, C., Cooper, D., Graham, J.: Active shape models - their training and application. Computer Vision and Image Understanding **61** (1995) 38–59
9. Daugman, J.: Uncertainty relation for resolution in space, spatial frequency, and orientation optimized by two-dimensional visual cortical filters. Journal of the Optical Society of America A **2** (1985) 1160–1169
10. Freund, Y., Schapire, R.E.: A decision-theoretic generalization of on-line learning and an application to boosting. In: EuroCOLT '95: Proceedings of the Second European Conference on Computational Learning Theory. (1995) 23–37
11. Schapire, R.E.: The boosting approach to machine learning: An overview. In: In MSRI Workshop on Nonlinear Estimation and Classification. (2002)
12. R. E. Schapire, Y. Freund, P.B., Lee, W.S.: Boosting the margin: a new explanation for the effectiveness of voting methods. Annals of Statistics **26** (1998) 1651–1686
13. Viola, P., Jones, M.: Robust real-time object detection. Second International Workshop on Statistical and Computational Theories of Vision - Modeling, Learning, And Sampling. Vancouer, Canada, July 13 (2001)

A Local Adaptive Algorithm
for Microaneurysms Detection in Digital Fundus
Images

Ke Huang[1,*] and Michelle Yan[2]

[1] Department of Electrical and Computer Engineering,
Michigan State University East Lansing, MI48824, USA
`kehuang@egr.msu.edu`
[2] Siemens Corporate Research, 755 College Road East, Princeton, NJ08540, USA
`michelle.yan@siemens.com`

Abstract. Microaneurysms (MAs) detection is a critical step in diabetic
retinopathy screening, since MAs are the earliest visible warning of potential future problems. A variety of thresholding based algorithms have
been proposed for MAs detection in mass screening. Most of them process fundus images globally without a mechanism to take into account the
local properties and changes. Their performance is often susceptible to
nonuniform illumination and locations of MAs in different retinal regions.
To keep sensitivity at a relatively high level, a low grey value threshold
must be applied to the entire image globally, resulting in a much lower
specificity in MAs detection. Therefore, post-processing steps, such as,
feature extraction and classification, must be followed to improve the
specificity at the cost of sensitivity. In order to address this problem,
a local adaptive algorithm is proposed for automatic detection of MAs,
where multiple subregions of each image are automatically analyzed to
adapt to local intensity variation and properties, and furthermore prior
structural features and pathology, such as, region and location information of vessel, optic disk and hard exudate are incorporated to further
improve the detection accuracy. This algorithm effectively improves the
specificity of MAs detection, without sacrificing the achieved sensitivity.
It has potential to be used for automatic level-one grading of diabetic
retinopathy screening.

1 Introduction

Diabetic retinopathy is a widely spread eye disease that may cause blindness
in diabetic patients. Often patients may not be aware of being affected by the
disease until its late stage, thus annual screening of patients for possible diabetic
retinopathy is recommended. In the screening, microaneurysms (MAs), one of
the lesions that is the earliest visible in diabetic retinopathy, is an important

---

* This work was completed when K. Huang was an intern at Siemens Corporate Research.

Y. Liu, T. Jiang, and C. Zhang (Eds.): CVBIA 2005, LNCS 3765, pp. 103–113, 2005.

pathology to be detected and be followed-up closely. The number, density and location of MAs are important factors to quantify the progression of diabetic retinopathy. MAs are saccular outpouchings of the retinal capillaries, and their sizes range from 10 μm to 100 μm, but should always be less than 125 μm. As capillaries are too thin to be visible in digital fundus image, MAs appear to be isolated patterns that are disconnected from vessel structures. Hemorrhages are blood leaking from MAs and deposit in the retina. Small dotted hemorrhages are often hard to be visually differentiated from MAs. So like most of other publications, we make no distinction between small dotted hemorrhages and MAs. A digital fundus image with MAs is illustrated in the top figure of Fig. 5.

Manual identification of MAs is time consuming and subjected to inter- and intra-operator variability. Screening a large amount of diabetic patients annually poses a huge workload for ophthalmologists. Therefore, automatic detection of MAs and other lesions, and then referring only suspicious cases to ophthalmologists for further treatment attract much attentions from researchers. Most existing MAs detection techniques were developed with fluorescein angiogram, which is an image of the eye fundus obtained after a fluorescent dye was injected into the patient's body and passed through the blood vessels of the retina. MAs are then highlighted in fluorescein angiograms, which makes MAs detection easier. In recent years, the digital fundus image, which does not require dye injection, is getting more used for screenings. MAs are dark reddish small dots with a size of several pixels in digital fundus images, depending on image resolution. Although most techniques developed for angiogram can be directly applied to digital fundus images, care must be taken for the weaker contrast of MAs to surrounding pixels. In this paper, MAs detection in digital fundus images is addressed.

1.1 Related Work

The most widely used scheme for MAs detection contains a sequence of operations: image preprocessing, global thresholding, region grow and feature extraction, and then classification to discriminate true MAs from false detections [1,2,3,4,5,6]. An illustration of the procedure is shown in Fig.1. It has achieved success in MAs detection to some degree, however, several factors constrain further improvement of the detection accuracy.

First of all, local properties of retina and inhomogeneous illumination of different regions are not considered in this framework. Thus, a global processing method often generates considerable amount of false detections. Some preprocessing techniques, such as shade correction, can ease the severity of inhomogeneous imaging conditions, the problem associated with global thresholding still exists. Region grow, feature extraction and classification can remove some false detections, but these steps may also introduce extra errors. For example, as pointed out in [3,5], region growing of small objects such as MAs is not very reliable. The shape features in MAs detection are essential to classification [1,4,6]. However, due to the irregular shape of MAs [4], a classifier is usually trained to accept shapes varying in a large range, which leads to misclassification. These issues exist for MAs detection in fluorescein angiograms, and are likely to be

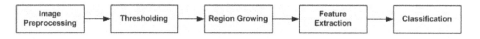

Fig. 1. Widely used scheme for MA detection

more severe in digital fundus images, where MAs appear to have much weaker contrast to their neighboring pixels. In addition, all parameters in this sequential procedure are coupled and affect each other - the parameters in a later processing step need to be adjusted according to the output of the previous one. As a result, the performance is more sensitive to parameter adjustment and less robust.

Another method based on normalized cuts [7] was proposed for MAs detection in [8], where two factors may hinder its success in real applications. Its performance is sensitive to the number of segments selected; and the computational complexity can be as high as $O(n^3)$, where n is the total number of pixels. It becomes impractical with a normal size of 1024×1280 digital fundus images.

1.2   Structure of the Paper

The rest of the paper is organized as follows. Section 2 proposes a new scheme for MAs detection that combines local adaptive detection with prior structural and lesion knowledge. It is then followed by a detailed description of the implementation. Section 2.1 describes the image division and enhancement techniques. Section 2.2 describes a local adaptive algorithm for MAs detection. Incorporation of prior knowledge, including detecting optic disk, vessel and hard exudate, is discussed in Section 2.3. Section 3 shows the results and comparison with the existing methods. Finally, Section 4 concludes the paper with possible future work.

2   New Scheme for MAs Detection

A new scheme is proposed for MAs detection based on analyzing the existing algorithms. The main goal is to (1) take into account the local properties and variations to improve the sensitivity of detection; (2) incorporate prior knowledge during detection, such as, no MAs would appear on vessels, to further reduce false detections; (3) be more robust to parameter selections, therefore to different imaging conditions. Fig. 2 illustrates the flowchart of our proposed scheme, where a fundus image is first automatically subdivided, and each subregion is then analyzed adaptively. Detections of optical disk, vessel and hard exudate are introduced in parallel to incorporate prior knowledge about locations where MAs would not appear.

In comparison with the scheme in Fig. 1, we believe that the new scheme contributes in the following aspects. A mechanism is introduced for including and analyzing the local properties of images in the detection. Instead of using

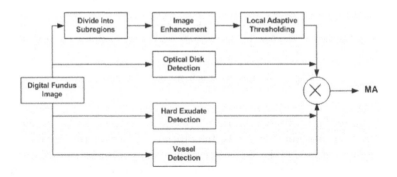

Fig. 2. Our proposed scheme for MAs detection

one global threshold, multiple automatically selected thresholds are used in MAs detection that is adapted to local variations, thus less false detections are generated. Reliable prior knowledge, such as locations of optic disk and vessel, is incorporated to improve the accuracy of detection, rather than employing region grow, feature extraction and classification that are often the sources of extra errors. Since most processing procedures in Fig. 2 are in parallel, the parameters in the scheme are less coupled, therefore less sensitive to the outputs of other procedures than the ones in Fig. 1.

2.1 Image Division and Enhancement

The first step in MAs detection is to divide an entire fundus image into multiple subregions such that in each subregion potential candidates of MAs can be robustly identified. Two options are available for image division: overlapping and non-overlapping. Neighboring subregions share common regions or pixels in an overlapping scheme, while as for a non-overlapping one, no regions or pixels are shared by two different subregions. In this paper, an overlapping division is used to avoid generating false candidates for MAs. An example of such a false candidate that could be generated by a non-overlapping division is given in Fig. 3, where part of another anatomical structure is cropped into a subregion and may be mistakenly identified as a MA candidate. In this implementation, the original fundus image is divided into subregions with a size $M_1 \times M_2$, where only the central $m_1 \times m_2 (m_1 < M_1, m_2 < M_2)$ region is of our interest. Given an image I with a size $N_1 \times N_2$, $\frac{N_1}{m_1} \times \frac{N_2}{m_2}$ subregions are obtained, and each subregion I_{n_1,n_2} is cropped from I as:

$$I_{n_1,n_2}(i,j) = I[m_1 n_1 - 0.5(M_1 - m_1) + i, m_2 n_2 - 0.5(M_2 - m_2) + j] \qquad (1)$$

where $0 \leq i \leq M_1 - 1$, $0 \leq j \leq M_2 - 1$, $0 \leq n_1 \leq \frac{N_1}{m_1} - 1$, $0 \leq n_2 \leq \frac{N_2}{m_2} - 1$. When $m_1 = N_1$ and $m_2 = N_2$, the local adaptive method becomes a global processing method. Large amounts of artifact may be generated when subregions are too

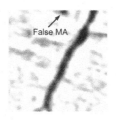

Fig. 3. False MA candidate caused by non-overlapping image division

small. For the size of 1024×1280, we found $M_1 = M_2 = 120$ and $m_1 = m_2 = 100$ is a good compromise.

Shading effect in digital fundus images presents slowly varying image intensity in background, which may be due to the different physiological properties in retina and the nonuniform illumination across the field of view. Usually an optic disk region is the brightest in a retinal image, and a macular region appears to be the darkest. The shading effect in MA detection is very undesirable, and needs to be compensated before detection. The correction is normally done by first estimating a background image and then subtracting the estimated background image from the original one to correct for background variations [9]. In this paper, the shade correction is applied to each subregion and a low-pass 2-dimensional (2D) Gaussian filter with 25×25 is used to estimate a background image. To enhance the visibility of small structures like MAs, contrast enhancement is applied to the difference image [10], where the following mapping function is used

$$u = \begin{cases} a_1 t^r + b_1, & if \ t \le \mu \\ a_2 t^r + b_2, & if \ t > \mu \end{cases} \tag{2}$$

where $a_1 = \frac{1}{2} \frac{u_{max} - u_{min}}{\mu^r - t_{min}^r}$, $b_1 = u_{min} - a_1 t_{min}^r$, $a_2 = \frac{1}{2} \frac{u_{max} - u_{min}}{t_{max}^r - \mu^r}$, $b_2 = u_{max} - a_2 t_{max}^r$ and μ is the mean gray value of all pixels to be enhanced. A low-pass 2D Gaussian filter is then applied to reduce the step effect in the image after shade correction and contrast enhancement. A sample of the contrast enhancement function, *i.e.*, equation (2), and the result from each processing step of shade correction are shown in Fig.4.

2.2 Local Adaptive MAs Detection

MAs appear to be small dark disks in the image after shade correction and contrast enhancement, while vessels and hard exudates also appear to be dark in the same image. Using the size information that any valid MA should not have more than 10 pixels in diameter with a resolution of 1024×1280, a filter called "Top-Hat" is used for identifying potential MAs from the shade corrected and enhanced image [1,3,4,5,6]. In the paper, a flat linear structure element with a length of 15 is chosen to perform morphological dilations on a subregion at each orientation, ranging from 0 to 170 degree with an interval of 10 degree.

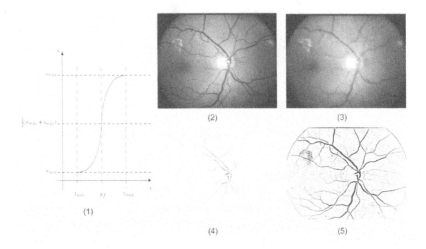

Fig. 4. Contrast enhancement function and shade correction. (1) mapping function for contrast enhancement; (2) green channel image; (3) estimated background; (4) difference image between green channel image and background; (5) difference image after contrast enhancement and smoothing.

Its output is defined as the minimum value of all orientations. So an image ΔI, defined as the difference between an output of the filter and its corresponding original image, responds much stronger at the areas where potential MAs are located. Pixel values are set to 0 where the differences are negative, thus, any disconnected bright disk like shapes will not produce strong responses to the filter.

To accurately identify MAs in a ΔI image, two factors should be taken into account: the area or size of a candidate covers and gray values in the area. Denote the area of a typical MA as ω pixels and the ω-th largest gray value in ΔI as $\Delta I(\omega)$, the threshold value T is set as:

$$T = \min\{\Delta I(\omega), T_{low}\} \qquad (3)$$

Note that a fast algorithm to extract the ω-th largest value from an unsorted array can be found in [11]. T_{low} is introduced here to avoid the threshold T is set too high, which may cause to miss potential candidates in the region. The situation could happen when there are multiple MAs in a subregion. T_{low} is a relatively high value, predefined to be the same for all subregions and $T_{low} > \Delta I(\omega)$ for most cases. A value of ω is set to be 25 in the paper. Thus each subregion associates with one threshold T that represents local characteristics of the subregion, and is adaptively analyzed for potential MA candidates. Each connected region in the thresholded image is then identified as a MA candidate region, denoted as mA_n. The mean of gray values in mA_n is computed to reflect the confidence how likely it corresponds to a true MA:

$$C(mA_n) = mean(\Delta I(i,j)), \ (i,j) \in mA_n \qquad (4)$$

The higher the value $C(mA_n)$, the more likely it is a true MA. So using the method, each candidate associates with a confidence value. The contrast enhancement in the previous stage sometime over-enhances some gray dotted areas, which may lead to high confidence values associated with them. To address this problem, the candidate generation procedure mentioned above is repeated on the corresponding original green channel subregion. The resulting confidence value is the product of the two confidence values. T_{low} is empirically set to 12 for each original green channel subregion. T_{low} for the corresponding enhanced subregion is set to 100, which reflects a much better contrast after enhancement.

2.3   Incorporation of Prior Knowledge for MAs Detection

It is known physiologically that MAs do not appear on the optical disk (OD), vessel (VS) and hard exudate (HE). Therefore, incorporating this important prior knowledge will help significantly reduce the number of false detections. An optic disk is the brightest part from which vessels are originated in a fundus image. Vessels appear to be a connected tree structure distributed over an entire fundus image. Hard exudate appears to be yellow waxy non-uniform regions with various sizes and shapes. These properties can be exploited further for detection, and some algorithms are given in literature, e.g., [12,13,14,15,16]. Once they are correctly identified and detected, the location information can be used to remove the MA candidates that are in those regions.

The algorithm described in [12] has been simplified and employed in the paper for OD detection. The shapes of detected ODs in the simplified way are not as accurate, but serve adequately the purpose of removing false MA detections that may appear on the central OD regions in our local adaptive candidate generation. We have developed a computationally efficient algorithm for vessel detection based on an adaptive multilevel image enhancement method [17]. It is applied to reduce false MAs on the vessels, and has produced very promising results. HE can be effectively separated using features in a color space [12,14]. However, large variations in a color space poses challenges. We combine both the color and texture features in this paper to detect HE . The waxy structure of HE produces a strong response to the "Top-Hat" filter, while other smooth yellow regions would not. This property is utilized in the HE detection for more robust performance.

3   Experiments

Experimental test is performed on 6 subjects, *i.e.* 12 digital fundus images with a size of 1024×1280. The first four images are taken from healthy eyes and should not have any MAs; the rest eight images are taken from patients who need medical attention.

Sensitivity and specificity are normally used to evaluate the performance of a MA detection system. Given an algorithm, changes in sensitivity are inversely

Table 1. Experiment results on MA detection: Global detection

Patient	1		2		3		4		5		6	
Without OD/VS/HE	25	23	10	16	68	56	60	43	20	15	62	72
With OD/VS/HE	14	12	4	9	45	42	41	32	13	8	27	23
True MA	0	0	0	0	26	28	28	22	8	4	20	16
False Detection	14	12	4	9	19	14	13	10	5	4	7	7

proportional to changes in specificity. In order to make meaningful and fair comparisons with global detection methods in general, the experiment is designed as follows. By making each subregion be equal to the size of an original image in the local adaptive algorithm, we obtain a global thresholding algorithm without the steps of region grow, feature extraction and classification, since this comparison is to demonstrate a local adaptive thresholding method produces less false detections than a global thresholding approach. To demonstrate the benefits of incorporating prior knowledge, such as locations of an optic disk, vessel and hard exudate, the results are compared with and without such *a priori* knowledge in the local and global algorithm.

All ground-truth are identified and labelled manually, and each of the local and global algorithm is asked to achieve 100% sensitivity, *i.e.*, detect all ground-truth labelled manually. Under this requirement, the total number of false MA detections is then compared for each algorithm with and without the detected OD/VS/HE regions. Results from the two methods are reported in Table 1 and Table 2, separately. The two tables have the same structure. The first row is the index of subjects and the following four rows are: (1) the total number of detected MAs without OD/VS/HE detection; (2) the total number of detected MAs with OD/VS/HE detection; (3) the total number of identified ground-truth; (4) the total number of false detections with OD/VS/HE detection.

Table 2. Experiment results on MA detection: Local Adaptive detection

Patient	1		2		3		4		5		6	
Without OD/VS/HE	5	6	2	3	39	38	40	30	10	7	48	49
With OD/VS/HE	0	1	0	0	29	30	31	25	8	4	21	18
True MA	0	0	0	0	26	28	28	22	8	4	20	16
False Detection	0	1	0	0	3	2	3	3	0	0	1	2

By comparing Table 1 and Table 2, the local adaptive method clearly generates much less false MA detections than the global method, ranging from 8 to 29 by looking at the numbers in the second rows from the two tables. The advantage

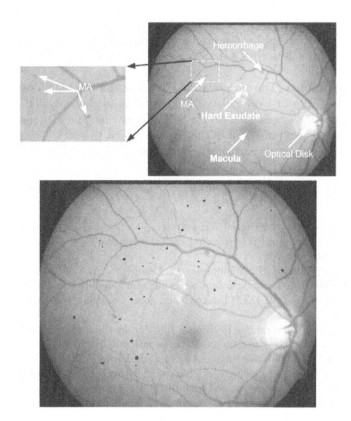

Fig. 5. Original digital fundus image with illustration of different structures (top) and the corresponding result from the local adaptive method (bottom). The detected MAs are labeled black in the bottom image.

of using prior information, *i.e.* locations from OD/VS/HE detection, is also obvious for the reduction of false detections, when comparing the second and third row of each table. We have observed some MA candidates generated on some OD and VS areas with nonuniform illumination and on the waxy textures of HE, using the prior information is able to remove them. The overall results clearly demonstrate that in combination with local adaptive detection, incorporating prior knowledge has significantly improved false detections without scarifying the sensitivity. A sample of the resulting detection with our proposed method is demonstrated in Fig. 5.

4   Conclusion and Future Work

A new local adaptive algorithm is proposed for improving overall performance of automatic MAs detection. It is achieved through the combination of local adaptivity and incorporating prior knowledge. The results clearly demonstrate that the new method effectively reduces the number of false detections, while keeping the detection sensitivity at a comparable level. Further clinical assessment is on going with ophthalmologists on much larger samples to study the sensitivity and specificity, and to validate its practical uses.

Acknowledgements. The authors would like to thank Dr. Juan Grunwald from Scheie Eye Institute of University of Pennsylvania for his valuable discussions and THS group of Siemens Medical HS SHC for providing us with digital fundus images evaluated and presented in the paper. Special thanks to the anonymous reviewers for their very constructive comments.

References

1. Cree, M., Olson, J., McHardy, K., Forrester, J., Sharp, P.: Automated microaneurysm detection. In: Proceedings of the International Conference on Image Processing. (1996) 699–702
2. Kamel, M., Belkasim, S., Mendonca, A., Campelho, A.: A neural network approach for the automatic detection of microaneurysms in retinal angiograms. In: Proceedings of the 2001 IEEE International Joint Conference on Neural Networks. (2001)
3. Mendonca, A., Campilho, A., Nunes, J.: Automatic segmentation of microaneurysms in retinal angiograms of diabetic patients. In: Proceedings of the 10th International Conference on Image Analysis and Processing. (2001) 728–733
4. Spencer, T., Olson, J., Mchardy, K., Sharp, P., Forrester, J.: An image-processing strategy for the segmentation and quantification of microaneurysms in fluorescein angiograms of the ocular fundus. Computers and Biomedical Reseearch **29** (1996) 284–302
5. Ege, B., Hejlesen, O., Larsen, O., Moller, K., Jennings, B., Kerr, D., Cavan, D.: Screening for diabetic retinopathy using computer based image analysis and statistical classification. Computer Methods and Programs in Biomedicine **62** (2000) 165–175
6. Goatman, K.: Automated detection of microaneurysms. (Online Document, http://www.biomed.abdn.ac.uk/Abstracts/A07890/)
7. Shi, J., Malik, J.: Normalized cuts and image segmentation. IEEE Transactions on Pattern Analysis and Machine Intelligence **22** (2000) 888–905
8. Pallawala, P., Hsu, W., Lee, M., Goh, S.: Automated microaneurysm segmentation and detection using generalized eigenvectors. In: Proceedings of IEEE Workshop on Application of Computer Vision (WACV). (2005)
9. Young, I., ed.: Shading Correction: Compensation for Illumination and Sensor Inhomogeneities. Current Protocols in Cytometry. Springer-Verlag, John Wiley and Sons, Inc., New York (2000)
10. Walter, T., Klein, J.: Automatic detection of microaneurysms in color fundus images of the human retina by means of the bounding box closing. In: Proceedings of the Third International Symposium on Medical Data Analysis. (2002) 210 – 220
11. Cormen, T., Leiserson, C., Rivest, R., Stein, C., eds.: Introduction to Algorithms (Second Edition). MIT Press (2001)
12. Li, H., Chutatape, O.: A model-based approach for automated feature extraction in fundus images. In: Proceedings of the International Conference on Computer Vision. (2003)

13. Hsu, W., Pallawala, P., Lee, M., Eong, K.: The role of domain knowledge in the detection of retinal hard exudates. In: Proceedings of the IEEE Conference on Computer Vision and Pattern Recognition. (2001)
14. Wang, H., Hsu, W., Goh, K., Lee, M.: An effective approach to detect lesions in color retinal images. In: Proceedings of the IEEE Conference on Computer Vision and Pattern Recognition. (2000)
15. Pinz, A., Bernogger, S., Datlinger, P., Kruger, A.: Mapping the human retina. IEEE Transactions on Medical Imaging **17** (1998) 606–619
16. Kirbas, C., Quek, F.: A review of vessel extraction techniques and algorithms. ACM Computing Surveys **36** (2004) 81–121
17. Huang, K., Yan, M.: A multi-level vessel detection algorithm. In: In Preparation. (2005)

A New Coarse-to-Fine Framework for 3D Brain MR Image Registration

Terrence Chen[1], Thomas S. Huang[1], Wotao Yin[2], and Xiang Sean Zhou[3]

[1] University of Illinois at Urbana Champaign,
Urbana, IL 61801, USA
{tchen5, huang}@ifp.uiuc.edu
[2] Columbia University,
New York, NY, USA
wy2002@columbia.edu
[3] Siemens Corporate Research,
Princeton, NJ 08540, USA
xzhou@scr.siemens.com

Abstract. Registration, that is, the alignment of multiple images, has been one of the most challenging problems in the field of computer vision. It also serves as an important role in biomedical image analysis and its applications. Although various methods have been proposed for solving different kinds of registration problems in computer vision, the results are still far from ideal when it comes to real world biomedical image applications. For instance, in order to register 3D brain MR images, current state of the art registration methods use a multi-resolution coarse-to-fine algorithm, which typically involves starting with low resolution images and working progressively through to higher resolutions, with the aim to avoid the local maximum "traps". However, these methods do not always successfully avoid the local maximum. Consequently, various rather sophisticated optimization methods are developed to attack this problem. In this paper, we propose a novel viewpoint on the coarse-to-fine registration, in which coarse and fine images are distinguished by different scales of the objects instead of different resolutions of the images. Based on this new perspective, we develop a new image registration framework by combining the multi-resolution method with novel multi-scale algorithm, which could achieve higher accuracy and robustness on 3D brain MR images. We believe this work has great contribution to biomedical image analysis and related applications.

1 Introduction

In medical image analysis, what is most often desired is a proper integration of the information provided by different images. Image registration, serving as the first step of the information integration process, is to bring various images into spatial alignment. In other words, it is a process of overlaying multiple images of the same type of objects taken at different times, by different modalities, and from different subjects. Image registration serves various functions in medical image applications: it can be used to obtain ampler information about the patient by registration images acquired from different modalities, to monitor and investigate tumor growth by images taken at

Y. Liu, T. Jiang, and C. Zhang (Eds.) CVBIA 2005, LNCS 3765, pp. 114–124, 2005.
© Springer-Verlag Berlin Heidelberg 2005

different times, to compare patients' data with anatomical atlases, to correct the motion of a series of data acquired continuously, etc. Despite the fact that registration is of great significance, fully automatic registration with high accuracy and robustness on 3D data is hardly achieved due to the difficulties of finding the most proper settings of the following factors: transformation, interpolation, similarity metric, and optimization. In this paper, we propose a multi-scale and multi-resolution coarse-to-fine (MMCTF) optimization method for 3D brain MR image registration, which can be used in conjunction with any transformation, interpolation method, and similarity metric to obtain consistent and accurate registration results.

1.1 Issues in Brain MRI Registration

In this section, we briefly introduce existing methods for medical image registration. A survey of more medical image registration methods, including semi-automatic registration methods using landmarks and interactive registration, can be found in [9]. Registration is the process to seek a transformation $T(\cdot)$ that registers the floating image F and the reference image R by maximizing their similarity:

$$T = \arg \max_T S(T(F(x)), R(x)),$$ (1)

where x are the coordinates of the voxel, and S is the similarity metric which measures the closeness of the two images. Determining the type of transformation is the first task of registration. It can be divided into linear transformation and nonlinear warping. Considering 3D linear transformation, it can be from 6 DOF (a rigid body transformation including 3 translations and 3 rotations) up to 12 DOF (an affine transformation including 3 translations, 3 rotations, 3 scales, and 3 skew parameters). Nonlinear warping encompasses a wide range of transformations, which can be up to millions of DOF and allow any geometric change between images. The most suitable type of transformation is determined based on factors such as the characteristics of the data, the need of a specific experiment or application, the dimensionality and the size of the data, and the tradeoff between speed and accuracy.

Interpolation methods are used to calculate the intensity of location between discrete points during transformation. There are several widely-practiced interpolation methods. Nearest neighbor decides the intensity of a location by taking the value from its nearest neighbor. Trilinear interpolation calculates the intensity from the 8 corner points of the 3D cube encompassing the specific location. Sinc interpolation calculates local intensity from much more than 8 neighbors. Although it is generally more accurate for registration between images with large transformations, Sinc interpolation requires much more computational time and is not widely used in 3D data.

Selecting the similarity metric is one of the most challenging problems in medical image analysis. Its purpose is to measure the closeness of different images. Similarity measurements of intra-modal and inter-modal registration of two images may be very different. In practice, mean absolute difference, least square difference, and normalized correlation are often used for intra-modal registration whereas mutual information [19], woods [20], and correlation ratio [16] are suitable for inter-modal cases.

Optimization method is used to search for the transformation that maximizes the similarity value given the cost function and the type of transformation. Although global maximum is always desired, it is not always worth doing exhaustive search due to unacceptable computational overhead, especially when the search is performed in high dimensional space. Powell's method [15] and gradient descent are two of the most well-known and widely-used local optimization methods. Multi-resolution methods, on the other hand, are often used to improve the robustness and speed up the registration process. A multi-resolution method is a coarse-to-fine method where images are registered progressively through lower resolutions to higher resolutions. Different resolutions of the image are obtained by different sub-samplings (fig. 2 (I)). Other optimization methods include apodization of the cost function [6], multi-start, etc. Apodization of the cost function gives greater weighting to the object region inside the FOV (Filed of View). Multi-start obtains several local maximums during the lowest resolution match and then passes these candidates to the next level to reduce the chance of missing the global maximum.

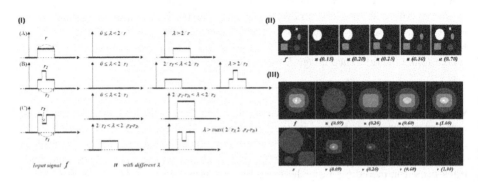

Fig. 1. (I) The TV-L-model on 1-d signal. Note that small scale signal can be separated from large scale signal using different λ according to their scale r ▷ —II— Original image f and different level of u when applying different (λ). (III) Additive signals with one included in the other can be extracted one by one using increasing values of (λ). s shows the original intensities of the four shapes before addition.

2 Methodology

In this section, we introduce the MMCTF framework and illustrate how it works for image registration. Before that, we first introduce the TV-L^1 model and extend it to 3D, which serves as the basis of the proposed framework. In the TV-based framework, an image f is modeled as the sum of image cartoon u and texture v, where f, u and v are defined as functions (or flow fields) in appropriate spaces. Cartoon contains background hues and important boundaries as sharp edges. The rest of the image, which is texture, is characterized by small-scale patterns. Since cartoon u is more regular than texture v, we can obtain u from image f by solving:

$$\min_{\Omega} \int |\nabla u| + \lambda \, \| t(u, f) \|_B, \tag{2}$$

where $\int_{\Omega}|\nabla u|$ is the total variation of u over its domain Ω, $\|t(u, f)\|_B$ can be any measure of the closeness between u and f, and λ is a scalar weight parameter. The choice of the measure $\|\cdot\|_B$ depends on applications. The first use of this model was the ROF model for image denoising [17], where $\|t(u, f)\|_B = \|f - u\|_{L^2}$. The essential merit of total variation based image model is the edge-preserving property [18]. First, minimizing the regularization measure $\int_\Omega |\nabla u(x)| dx$ only reduces the total variation of u over its support, a value that is independent of edge smoothness. Second, unless $\|t(u, f)\|_B$ specifically penalizes sharp edges, minimizing a fidelity term $\|t(u, f)\|_B$ (e.g., L^1 or L^2-norm of $f - u$) generally tends to keep u close to f, and thus, also keeps edges of f in u. Finally, minimizing $\int_\Omega |\nabla u| + \lambda \|t(u, f)\|_B$, with λ sufficiently big will keep sharp edges. ROF uses the L^2-norm, which penalizes big point-wise differences between f and u, so it removes small point-wise differences (noise) from f. Mainly due to this good edge-keeping property, this model has been adopted, generalized and extended in many way. One of them uses the L^1-norm as the fidelity term [2, 3, 11].

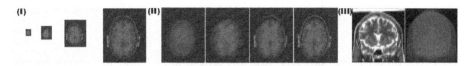

Fig. 2. (I) Traditional coarse-to-fine method uses different sub-samplings of the images. (II) Multi scales of the brain image obtained by the TV- L^1 model. (III) The contour image obtained by 3D TV-L^1 model (right) does not contain artifacts or noise in the original image (left).

2.1 The TV-L^1 Model for Scale-Driven Image Extraction

Formally, this TV-L^1 model is formulated as:

$$\min \int_\Omega |\nabla u(x)| dx \qquad s.t. \|f(x) - u(x)\|_{L^1} \leq \sigma, \tag{3}$$

where Ω is the image domain where functions f and u are defined on. Since (3) is a convex optimization problem, it can be reformulated as

$$\min_u \int_\Omega |\nabla u(x)| dx + \lambda |f(x) - u(x)| dx, \tag{4}$$

Just like the L^2-norm, the L^1-norm keeps u close to f (but under a different measure), so the edge-preserving property can be easily seen by following the similar argument of the ROF model. To concrete our claims, we give the TV-L^1 analytical results of some easy problems from $\Re$ to $\Re^3$. Fig.1 (I) illustrates the TV-L^1 method applied to 1-d signal. According to fig. 1 (I), with different values of λ, u keeps different signals according to their scales but not intensities. Now, we extend this to 2-d signal (i.e. an image). Chan and Esedoglu [3] have proved that solving equation (4) is equivalent to solving the following level-set-based geometrical problem:

$$\min_u \int_{-\infty}^{+\infty} Per(\{x : u(x) > u\}) + \lambda Vol(\{x : u(x) > u\} \oplus \{x : f(x) > u\}) du, \tag{5}$$

where $Per(\cdot)$ is the perimeter function, $Vol(\cdot)$ is the volume function, and $S1 \oplus S2 := (S1\backslash S2) \cup (S2\backslash S1)$, for any set $S1$ and $S2$. Using equation (5), Chan and Esedoglu [3] proved the following geometric properties of the solution $v(\lambda) = f - u(\lambda)$ in (4):

• Suppose $f = c_1 1Br(y)(x)$, a function with the intensity c_1 in the disk centered at y and with radius r, and the intensity 0 anywhere else. Then

$$u(\lambda) = \begin{cases} 0 \quad , & 0 \le \lambda \le 2/r \\ \{s1_{B_r(y)}(x) : 0 \le s \le c_1\} \quad , & \lambda = 2/r \\ c_1 1_{B_r(y)}(x) \quad , & \lambda > 2/r \end{cases} \tag{6}$$

By this property, when applying different values of λ, objects of different scales can be kept in either u or v. Fig. 1 (II) illustrates this property. Furthermore, we can extend this property to the following:

• Suppose $f = c_1 1Br_1(y)(x) + c_2 1Br_2(y)(x)$, where $0 < r_2 < r_1$ and $c_1, c_2 > 0$.

$$u(\lambda) = \begin{cases} 0 \quad , & \lambda < 2/r_1 \\ c_1 1_{B_{r_1}(y)}(x) \quad , & 2/r_1 < \lambda < 2/r_2 \\ (c_1 1_{B_{r_1}(y)} + c_2 1_{B_{r_2}(y)})(x) \quad , & \lambda > 2/r_2 \end{cases} \tag{7}$$

Fig. 1 (III) illustrates this property, which is proved in [4]. More discussions on 2D properties of the TV-L^1 model can be found in [21].

2.2 3D TV-ψ Model

The properties discussed in the previous section which has been developed and used for 2D image can be simply extended to 3D. First, we extend property (5) and claim that solving (2) in 3D is equal to solve the following equation:

$$\min_u \int_{-\infty}^{+\infty} Sur(\{x : u(x) > u\}) + \lambda Vol(\{x : u(x) > u\} \oplus \{x : f(x) > u\}) du, \tag{8}$$

where $Sur(\cdot)$ is the surface area function, and $Vol(\cdot)$ is the volume function. Using equation (8), we can extend previous geometric properties (6) and (7) to:

• Suppose $f = c_1 1B_r(y)(x)$, a function with the intensity c_1 in the ball centered at y and with radius r, and the intensity 0 anywhere else. Then

$$u(\lambda) = \begin{cases} 0 \quad , & 0 \le \lambda \le 3/r \\ \{s1_{B_r(y)}(x) : 0 \le s \le c_1\} \quad , & \lambda = 3/r \\ c_1 1_{B_r(y)}(x) \quad , & \lambda > 3/r \end{cases} \tag{9}$$

• Suppose $f = c_1 1B_{r1}(y)(x) + c_2 1B_{r2}(y)(x)$, where $0 < r_2 < r_1$ and $c_1, c_2 > 0$. Then

$$u(\lambda) = \begin{cases} 0 \quad , & \lambda < 3/r_1 \\ c_1 1_{B_{r_1}(y)}(x) \quad , & 3/r_1 < \lambda < 3/r_2 \\ (c_1 1_{B_{r_1}(y)} + c_1 1_{B_{r_2}(y)})(x) \quad , & \lambda > 3/r_2 \end{cases} \tag{10}$$

(9) is proved as follows and (10) can be easily proved by following the proof of (7).

Proof of property (9):
Proof. By assumption, $f = c11Br(y)(x)$. Without loss of generality, we assume $c_1 > 0$. Clearly, solution $u(x)$ of (4) is bounded between 0 and c_1, for all $x \in \Omega$. It follows that (8) is simplified to:

$$\min_u \int_0^{c_1} Sur(\{x : u(x) > u\}) + \lambda Vol(\{x : u(x) > u\} \oplus \{x : f(x) > u\})du, \quad (11)$$

Since $\{x : f(x) > u\} \equiv Br(y)$ for $u \in (0; c_1)$, $S(u) := \{x : u(x) > u\}$ must solve the following geometry problem:

$$\min_S Sur(S(u)) + \lambda Vol(S(u) \oplus B_r(y)), \quad (12)$$

for almost all $u \in (0; c_1)$. First, $S(u) \subseteq Br(y)$ holds because, otherwise, $S(u) := S(u) \cap Br(y)$ achieves lower objective value than $S(u)$. Then, it follows that

$$Vol(S(u) \oplus B_r(y)) = Vol(B_r(y) \setminus S(u)) \quad (13)$$

Therefore, to minimize (12) is to minimize the surface area of S while maximizing its volume. By extending the Isoperimetric Theorem into 3D, $S(u)$ must be either empty or a ball. Let r_S denote the radius of S, it follows that $r_S = r$ if $\lambda > 3/r$, $r_S = 0$ if

$$0 \leq \lambda < 3/r, \text{ and } r_S \ (\{0, r\} \text{ if } = 3/r. \quad \blacksquare$$

Based on the above properties, we can extract different scales of a brain by different λs, which is illustrated in fig. 2 (II). More precisely, if we select $\lambda \approx 3/r$, where r is close to the radius of the brain region, u will be close to the 3D contour of the brain.

2.3 The MMCTF Registration Algorithm

Traditional 3D brain MRI registration methods avoid local minimum and improve the efficiency of the registration process by a multi-resolution coarse-to-fine algorithm. This approach is not always sufficient for avoiding local minimum traps. To overcome this limitation, we propose a new viewpoint on coarse-to-fine registration – coarse and fine images can be distinguished by different scales of the objects (fig. 2 (II)). However, if we do a pure multi-scale coarse-to-fine registration, it may lose the efficiency of the traditional multi-resolution method. Hence, instead of using multi-scale method only, we develop a novel framework combining the two methods together to avoid the limitation of each other. Fig. 3 illustrates our final algorithm, a Multi-scale and Multi-resolution Coarse-To-Fine (MMCTF) framework. In order to simplify following discussions, we call the u obtained using $\lambda \approx 3/r$, which is the largest scale we used in the MMCTF framework, the *contour image* in this paper. In the MMCTF algorithm, the first step is to obtain the *contour images* of both the floating image and the reference image using 3D TV-L^1 model with λ ($3/r$, where r is the radius specifying the volume of interest. Second, we use a traditional coarse-to-fine (multi-resolution) method to register the two contour images. An initial search for translation, rotation, and global scaling parameters is applied at the beginning of the lowest resolution registration to speed up the search. The initial search includes matching the COM (center of mass) of the two images and finding the best initial rotation by searching every 30 degree in all directions. Since it is in the lowest resolution, this initial search can be done efficiently. After the initial search, the Powell's local optimization method [15] is used to search for the maximum of the similarity measurement in each level. Followed by the registration of the contour images, the final parameters can be used to register the floating and reference images. We would like to point out that although we can do more scales in between the contour image and the original image by increasing the value of ((fig. 2 (II)), empirically only two scale levels are enough for robust and accurate registration. Besides, it is much more efficient to perform the registration with only two scale levels. There are several advantages of this combination framework: 1.) The multi-resolution method is used for initial registration, which finds a good registration efficiently at the beginning. 2.) Since the multi-resolution is performed on the contour images, which consist of only the contours without detailed features, the chance that the gross features in the low resolution images mislead further registration is much smaller. 3.) By a multi-scale registration, a good registration can be easily found based on the contour images. 4.) Noise or other artifacts, which may degrade the registration performance and cause local maximum/minimum, barely exist in the contour images. (fig. 2 (III)) 5.) Empirically, only two scale levels are enough to obtain satisfying results. Besides, since the registration of the contour images is mostly very close to the final registration, step 10 in fig. 3 normally costs only a little more computational time than pure multi-resolution method.

1. $F^1 \leftarrow$ Normalize(input floating image)
2. $R^1 \leftarrow$ Normalize(reference image)
3. $F_c^1 \leftarrow \arg\min_u \int_\Omega \|\nabla u(x)\| + \frac{3}{r_F}\|F(x) - u(x)\| \, dx$
4. $R_c^1 \leftarrow \arg\min_u \int_\Omega \|\nabla u(x)\| + \frac{3}{r_R}\|R(x) - u(x)\| \, dx$
5. $\Theta \leftarrow$ calculate initial parameters based on F_1^8 and R_1^8
6. $\Theta \leftarrow \arg\max_\Theta$ Registration(F_c^8, R_c^8, Θ)
7. $\Theta \leftarrow \arg\max_\Theta$ Registration(F_c^4, R_c^4, Θ)
8. $\Theta \leftarrow \arg\max_\Theta$ Registration(F_c^2, R_c^2, Θ)
9. $\Theta \leftarrow \arg\max_\Theta$ Registration(F_c^1, R_c^1, Θ)
10. $\Theta \leftarrow \arg\max_\Theta$ Registration(F^1, R^1, Θ)
11. Output $\leftarrow$ Transformation(F^1, Θ)

F^i: sub-sampling of F to i mm in thickness.
r_F: radius of the brain in image F.
r_R: radius of the brain in image R.
I_c: the *contour image* of image I.
Normalize($\cdot$): normalize image to 1mm in thickness.
Registration(A, B, Θ): Register A to B by parameter set Θ.
Transformation(A, Θ): Transform A by parameter set Θ.

Fig. 3. The MMCTF algorithm

3 Experimental Results

In this section, we compare the proposed MMCTF algorithm with one of the famous brain MR image registration methods, FLIRT [6], and with the traditional pure multi-resolution (PMR) coarse-to-fine method. For fair comparison, the following settings are used in all methods throughout the experiments. Transformation: 3D affine transformation with 12 DOF (3 translations, 3 rotations, 3 scales, and 3 skews). Cost function: although any similarity metric can be used in our framework, correlation ratio is adopted for inter-modal registration since it is suggested in [6], which we aim to compare to. In addition, normalized correlation is used for intra-modal registration. Interpolation: Trilinear interpolation. The step sizes used to search for each parameters are: translation: $\Delta t = 0.5$, rotation: $\Delta\theta = 0.3°$, scale: $\Delta s = 0.005$, and skew: $\Delta k = 0.005$. The number of intensity bins used per image for correlation ratio is $256/n$, where n is the resolution in *mm*. Some other optimization settings used by FLIRT (i.e. apodization of the cost function, multi-start, etc.) to improve robustness and efficiency are not implemented in PMR and MMCTF. The T_1 weighted images we use are real 3D brain MR images. The T_2 weighted image is obtained from brainweb [8].

3.1 Accuracy Evaluation

Although the quantitative assessment of registration methods is quite difficult, a method can be affirmed as relatively more accurate than others if it consistently obtains higher similarity values, under the circumstances that all other settings are the same. In the first experiment, we evaluate the registration accuracy between 6 high resolution T_1 weighted MR images with size 207×255×207. 15 total registrations between each pair of the six images are evaluated. Normalized correlation is chosen as the similarity measurement. Fig. 4 shows the results. In fig. 4, the three methods achieve similar and consistent results, which means that the traditional multi-resolution method is good enough for high resolution intra-modal registration. Next, we evaluate the inter-modal registration accuracy between images with different resolution. In this experiment, we register one low resolution 181×217×30, T_2 weighted MR image with voxel dimension 1×1×5 mm^3 to six different high resolution 207×255×207, T_1 weighted MR images with voxel dimension 1×1×1 mm^3. Correlation ratio is used to measure the similarity. Fig. 5 illustrates the results. In this more complicated and difficult case, although all methods register the images well, the strength of MMCTF is demonstrated by the higher similarity of images. Fig. 5 shows that the MMCTF algorithm reaches higher maximum value of the correlation ratio, which proves that the proposed algorithm has a much higher chance to reach global

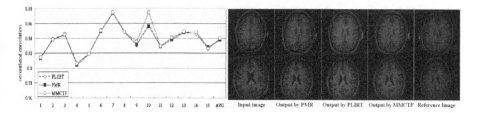

Fig. 4. Left: Normalized correlation between registered and reference images (intra-modal registration). Right: An example (2D slice from 3D data).

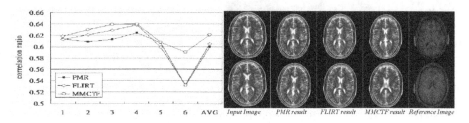

Fig. 5. Left: Correlation ratio between registered and reference images (inter-modal registration). Right: An example (2D slice from 3D data).

maximum. It can also be observed by human eyes that the registration results of the MMCTF are closer to the reference images (fig. 5 (right)).

3.2 Robustness Evaluation

The robustness evaluation of the registration method is originally purposed by Jenkinson and Smith [7]. In this paper, we use a similar way to evaluate the robustness of the registration algorithm. Similar to the inter-modal experiment in the accuracy evaluation, we register the same low resolution T_2 weighted MR image with voxel dimension $1\times1\times5$ mm^3 to six different high resolution T_1 weighted MR images with voxel dimension $1\times1\times1$ mm^3. However, for each registration, we operate ten different initial transformations on the T_2 weighted low resolution image before the registration process, including four global scalings of 0.7, 0.8, 0.9, and 1.1, four different rotations of -10, -2, 2, and 10 degrees about the anterior-posterior (y) axis, and two extreme cases with rotations of -10 and 10 degrees about y axis plus the second skew factor = 0.4. The ten transformed images are then registered to the reference image. To evaluate the robustness, we compare the ten registration results to the registered image which obtained directly from the original floating image to the reference image. If the registration algorithm is robust, these 10 values should show little difference. Fig. 6 shows the results. In fig. 6 (I), the variance between the results obtained by the MMCTF model is much smaller than the variances of FLIRT and PMR. In fact,

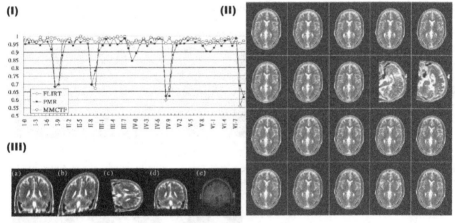

Fig. 6. (I) Normalized correlation between registered images with different initial transformations and the registered image without initial transformation. 6 cases (I~VI) in total and each with 10 different initial transformations (0~9). (II) The first two rows: Registration results of the same image with different initial transformations by FLIRT. The last two rows: Same results by MMCTF. 10 initial parameters from left to right, top to down are global scalings: 0.7, 0.8, 0.9, and 1.1, rotation about y-axis, 2, -2, 10, and -10 degrees, and rotation of -10 and 10 degrees plus 2nd skew factor = 0.4. (III) (a): Floating image; (b): (a) after initial transformation, rotation = -10 and 2nd skew factor = 0.4. (e): Reference image; (c): Result of registering (b) to (e) by FLIRT; (d): Result of registering (b) to (e) by MMCTF.

FLIRT and PMR fail to register some images correctly after large initial transformations. On the contrary, the MMCTF algorithm always gets consistent and good registration results throughout the experiments. Fig. 6 (II) shows one sample of the registration results obtained by FLIRT and MMCTF. While FLIRT fails to register the images in the last two cases, all results registered by the proposed MMCTF algorithm are very consistent. Fig. 6 (III) illustrates the coronal view. The floating image is first transformed by -10 degrees about the y axis and 0.4 of the second skew parameter.

4 Summary and Conclusion

In this paper, we try to improve the accuracy and robustness of biomedical image registration using a novel coarse-to-fine image registration framework. The results show that by integrating the novel multi-scale idea into original multi-resolution registration framework, we can improve both consistency and accuracy of both intermodal and intra-modal registrations on 3D brain MR images. The proposed framework is also expected to be useful for registration of other types of biomedical images and may also contribute to high dimensional non-linear warping, which normally requires much more computation. Although the computation overhead of the TV-L^1 model on 3D data is high, it is fully parallel computable, which greatly alleviates this problem. Our future work includes comparing our method with other famous works such as mutual information based methods [14, 19] and extending the capability of our model to handle local affine transformation.

References

1. F. Alizadeh, and D. Goldfarb. "Second-order cone programming" Mathematical Programming 95(1), pp. 3-51, 2003.
2. S. Alliney "Digital filters as absolute norm regularizers" IEEE Trans. on Signal Processing, vol. 40, pp. 1548-1562, 1992.
3. T. F. Chan, and S. Esedoglu, "Aspects of Total Variation Regularized L1 Function Approximation" UCLA CAM Report 04-07, Feb, 2004.
4. T. Chen, W. Yin, X. S. Zhou, D. Comaniciu, T. S. Huang, "Illumination Normalization for Face Recognition and Uneven Background Correction Using Total Variation Based Image Models" CVPR, 2005.
5. D. Goldfarb, and W. Yin, "Second-order cone programming methods for total variation-based image restoration" Columbia CORC TR-2004-05, May, 2004.
6. M. Jenkinson, P. Bannister, J. M. Brady, and S. M. Smith, "Improved Optimisation for the Robust and Accurate Linear Registration and Motion Correction of Brain Images," NeuroImage, 17(2), 825-841, 2002.
7. M. Jenkinson, P. Bannister, J. M. Brady, and S. M. Smith, "Improved Optimisation for the Robust and Accurate Linear Registration and Motion Correction of Brain Images," NeuroImage, 17(2), 825-841, 2002.
8. R. K. -S. Kwan, A. C. Evans, and G. B. Pike, "MRI simulationbased evaluation of image-processing and classification methods",IEEE Trans. Med. Img, 18(11):1085-1097, 1999.
9. J. B. A. Maintz and M. A. Viergever, "A survey of Medical Image Registration," Medical Image Analysis, 2(1), 1-36, 1998.

10. Y. Meyer, "Oscillating patterns in image processing" Univ. Lecture Series 22, AMS, 2000.
11. M. Nikolova, "Minimizers of cost-functions involving nonsmooth data-fidelity terms" SIAM Journal on Numerical Analysis, vol. 40:3, pp. 965-994, 2002.
12. P. Oenev, and J. Atick, "Local feature analysis: A general statistical theory for object reperesentation" Network: Computation in Neural System, Vol. 7, pp. 477-500, 1996.
13. S. Osher, and O. Scherzer, "G-norm properties of bounded variation regularization" UCLA CAM Report 04-35, 2004. 13. W. Press, S. Teukolsky, W. Vetterling, and B. Flannery, "Numerical Recipies in C," Cambridge University Press, 2nd Edition, 1995.
14. J.P.W. Pluim, J. B. A. Maintz, and M. A. Viergever, "Mutual information based registration of medical images: a survey", IEEE Med. Img. 22:986-1004, 2003.
15. W. Press, S. Teukolsky, W. Vetterling, and B. Flannery, "Numerical Recipies in C," Cambridge University Press, 2nd Edition, 1995.
16. A. Roche, G. Malandain, X. Pennec, and N. Ayache, "The corrlation ratio as a new similarity measure for multi-modal image registration," MICCAI, 1998.
17. L. Rudin, S. Osher, and E. Fatemi, "Nonlinear total variation based noise removal algorithms" Physica D, vol. 60, pp. 259- 268, 1992.
18. D. Strong, and T. Chan, "Edge-preserving and scaledependent properties of total variation regularization" Inverse problems 19, pp.S165-S187, 2003.
19. P. Viola, and W. Wells, " Alignment by maximization of mutual information" ICCV, 1995.
20. R. Woods, J. Mazziotta, and S. Cherry, "MRI-PET registration with automated algorithm," Journal of Computer Assisted Tomography, 17(4), pp. 536-546, 1993.
21. W. Yin, T. Chen, X.-S. Zhou, and A. Chakraborty, "Background correction for cDNA microarray images using the TV+L1 model", Bioinformatics, 21(10), pp 2410-2416, 2005.

A New Vision Approach for Local Spectrum Features in Cervical Images Via 2D Method of Geometric Restriction in Frequency Domain

Viara Van Raad

STI Medical Systems, Honolulu, HI 96813, USA
viarav@ieee.org

Abstract. Digital colposcopy is an emerging new technology, which can be used as adjunct to the conventional Pap test for staging of cervical cancer and it can improve the diagnostic accuracy of the test. Computer aided diagnosis (CAD) in digital colposcopy has as a goal to segment and outline abnormal areas on the cervix, one of which is an important anatomical landmark on the ectocervix - the transformation zone (TZ). In this paper we proposed a new method for estimation of the local spectrum features of cervical cancer in vivo. We used a 2D method to estimate the energy of the local frequency bands, using a geometric restriction (GR). In the current work we reported up to 12 dB difference between the local power spectral density content of the region of interest (ROI) and (ROI)complimentary for the mid-frequency band. We devised a method to present pseudo-color visual maps of the cervical images, useful for CAD and successful ROI segmentation.

1 Introduction to Cervical Image Features

Cervical cancer is the most frequent cancer in women under 35 years of age [1]. It is a preventable disease, one in which the neoplastic changes grow slowly and they can often be treated effectively in the early stages of neoplasia. Visual impression of the cervix are highly correlated with the accuracy of staging and diagnosis of cancer [2], hence a computer-aided diagnosis (CAD) is a promising tool for prevention of cervical cancer [3]. In medical practice it is essential to diagnose the abnormal cervical tissue and this often is performed by medical experts. Simulating the "trained expert approach," our method aims to evaluate automatically the transformation zone (TZ), where 90% of the cancers occur. Punctuation, mosaicism and abnormal vessels are diagnostic features of precancer. These can be evaluated and assessed quantitatively using signal processing methods [3]. The cervical cancer precursors are located within the TZ. Here, we propose to evaluate the vascularity within the TZ in terms of texture. The vascularity and cervical texture is a clinical phenomena, expressed as vascular punctuation, vascular mosaics, columnar epithelium (CE) and CE's metaplasia - all rich in texture. There is no previous attempt to use joint-time-frequency analysis (JTFA) for textural features on the cervix. The advantage of JTFA

Y. Liu, T. Jiang, and C. Zhang (Eds.): CVBIA 2005, LNCS 3765, pp. 125–134, 2005.
© Springer-Verlag Berlin Heidelberg 2005

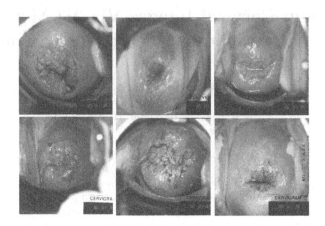

Fig. 1. Illustration of various types of maturing TZ with a different textural content. The degree of metaplasia (transformation from a columnar epithelium (CE)) to squamous epithelium (SE) is different amongst normal cervices.

is its independency from color perception and variations in illumination. JTFA does not need color calibration. To demonstrate the texture in TZ, a variety of colposcopic images are depicted in Figure 1 with the centrally located TZ surrounding the dark cervical canal. Computerized detection of diagnostic features for CAD in cervical imagery (using both reflectance and hyperspectral imaging) started in early 90'es. B. Pogue et al. [4] studied color as a diagnostic feature to differentiate high grade (HG) squamous intraepithelial lesions (SIL) form normal squamous metaplasia (SM), using pixelwise measurements of chromaticity and found that *the color has no statistical significance* to discriminate the HG SIL from the SM. B. Pogue et al. used also the Euler number to study cervical textures as diagnostic feature. They found that the Euler number is statistically significant to discriminate the HG SIL from the SM. Ji et al. explored further texture, studying six diagnostic textural patterns of the HG SIL, accumulating 24-dimensional feature vectors. These vectors were used to measure objectively two different grades of cancer. Each texture pattern represented a specific characteristic of the particular neoplasia. Ji et al. reported that the densities of the line intersections in thresholded images, the entropies and the local statistical moments (the zeroth to the third moment) are the most significant discriminant features. Using the 24 dimensional vectors, a classifier was built, classifying the HG SIL with 95% accuracy [5]. Although Ji et al. algorithm was successful for the task, the described texture classification scheme has not been assessed in terms of scale-space. The classification was performed only at a single scale which is useful under constrained conditions. In real, the texture parameters are dependent on the focal distance, that varies during patient examination. In case of a change in these conditions, the scale of the texture and the texture metrics will vary accordingly for each patient and the scheme described in [5] could be obso-

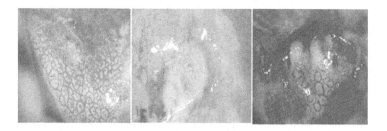

Fig. 2. Three images that depict magnified coarse mosaic formation from blood vessels within the TZ. The coarse mosaics is related to HG SIL.

lete. Scale independent TZ texture features were studied in [6] and [7] these were assessed independently from the grain of the texton [6] using various scales [7] via Gabor decomposition. These schemes are valuable for analyzing the various textures depicted in Figure 1. For example - a mosaics is a important sign of HG SIL, it has degrees of coarseness as it is depicted in Figure 2. Currently, in this paper we are proposing a 2D local power spectrum estimation method via Geometric Restriction (GR) in the 2D frequency domain for texture's quantitative measurement.

The paper is organized as follows: Section 1 introduces us to the core of the problem in cervical cancer feature detection *in vivo*. Section 2 contains the background theory of PSD and windowing, including the Welch algorithm in 1D. Section 3 shows our 2D method of PSD with GR. In Section 4 we briefly discuss the achieved visual discrimination as gray scale images; the evaluations of the band separation in the gray scale images in measures; the pseudo-color map for gray scale images and the segmentation of ROI by automatic thresholding. In Section 5 we discuss the introduced methods and suggest further work.

2 Previous Methods for Local Power Spectral Density Estimation

There are several methods for power spectral density (PSD) estimation. The most prevalent non-parametric methods are the Bartlett, the Welch and the Blackman-Tukey methods. A powerful parametric methods is the autocorrelation method (eq. 1 aka Burg's algorithm).These and many other valuable methods in 1D were described in [11] and elsewhere. These are the Maximum Entropy estimations, Prony's method, Pisarenko harmonic decomposition and the minimum-variance spectral estimation. It is important to underline that not all of the 1D methods can be used in image analysis (2D) due to restrictions such as shift and phase invariance and Nyqust's limits. One of the prominent methods that can be transferred from 1D to 2D is the Welch algorithm for PSD [13] which is relatively simple frequency-based algorithm. The Wiener-Khinchin theorem [9] states that the inverse Fourier Transform or the absolute square of $F(\omega)$ as the power spectrum of a signal $f(t)$ yields the same as the autocorrelation function $R_{XX}(t)$ of $f(t)$ and it represents the "full (theoretical) power" of $f(t)$:

$$R_{XX}(t) = \int\limits_{-\infty}^{+\infty} \overline{f}(\tau)f(t+\tau)d\tau = \mathcal{F}_\omega^{-1}[|F(\omega)|^2](t) \tag{1}$$

The autocorrelation of $f(t)$ is maximum at the origin, hence, the $R_{XX}(t)$ in (1) is always limited by the energy of the signal, as the signal $f(t)$ must have a finite energy. The $S_{XX}(\omega) = |F(\omega)|^2$ is called the *power spectrum* of the signal and it is always real.

The simplest and the one with no phase distortion JTFA method for local frequency features estimation on images is the STFT. This method is using a Gaussian window in time and frequency domains (GW) (eq. 2), optimal in both time and frequency domains.

$$g(t) = \exp(-\frac{1}{2}\frac{t^2}{\sigma_t^2}); \ G(\omega) = \sqrt{\frac{2\pi}{\sigma_u^2}} \exp(-\frac{1}{2}\frac{\omega^2}{\sigma_u^2}) \tag{2}$$

Therefore, using GW for windowing, the proposed 2D method is similar to the Welch method for local power spectral estimation in 1D [13].

2.1   The Welch Algorithm for PSD Estimation

During the last 30 years, devoted in spectral estimation, the Welch algorithm in 1D [13] is the most used method for practical applications. The algorithm is based on the modified periodogram averages ([10] and [14]). The essence of the Welch algorithm is that for a data stream $f[n]$ (a discrete signal) a sliding windowed portion of the signal $f[n]$ is used as series of steps, segmenting the signal into K overlapping sequences, each one of length L. The ith sequence of the signal is defined by the relation:

$$f[i,m] = f[m + i(1-r)L], \tag{3}$$

where the indices are $i = 0, 1, ...K - 1$, and $m = 0, 1, 2...L - 1$ (L even) and r represents the percentage of overlap. The most often use percentage of overlap is $r = 1$ for 100% overlap and $r = 0.5$ for 50% overlap. The data can be windowed using various windows and the effects of the application of these windows are discussed in specialized parts of many signal processing books and articles: [15] and elsewhere. Windowing is applied to prevent a spectral leakage or distortions (aliasing) from the highest frequencies of the "all-or-nothing" window.

3   Proposed PSD Estimation Via Geometric Restriction

We propose to manipulate the separation of the bands in 2D without filtering. This is performed using a Euclidean distance restriction in frequency, ensuring

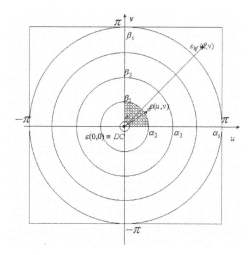

Fig. 3. The density estimation for $s-$band partition of the local frequency domain in a bandlimited windowed portion of the signal $[-\pi, \pi]$, adjacent to image point. In the center is the zero frequency DC. The most distant point (α_s, β_s) is the highest frequency $[-\tau, \tau]$.

highest accuracy of the calculated PSD. The number of boundaries in the frequency domain is s (Figure 3). In this way we avoid the drawbacks of creating very narrowband 2D filters, eliminating distortions in their frequency response.

We directly manipulated the frequency transformed window in 2D. The bandlimited signal (with boundaries $[-\pi, \pi]$) have spectral signatures in each of the 2D 'stripes' for each window at all image points. We defined the bounds of each frequency band as a stripe, using 2D Euclidian distance criteria, limiting them with $s + 1$ circular bounds, forming s-bands. Thus, the PSD of each image point (windowed with GW) has a representative window in the frequency domain. PSD is an average of the band's energy, normalized by the stripe's area. The scheme is illustrated in Figure 3). We predefined the boundaries of each band using an Euclidian distance from each point of the 2D "window" with central point the DC (Figure 3). The PSD within k^{th} band $(B_k \subset B = [B_1, B_2, ... B_s])$, is expressed in equation (4), thus representing the PSD or the energy distribution for band B_k with area A_k. The PSD of kth stripe is:

$$PSD_k = \frac{1}{A_k} \int\limits_{\alpha_{k-1}}^{\alpha_k} \int\limits_{\beta_{k-1}}^{\beta_k} \varepsilon(u, v) du dv \qquad (4)$$

By calculating each PSD for all bands we can form a PSD-based image similar to RGB image - each channel will contain the "energy" in one of the s bands - $I_{PSD}^{(s)}$. This feature image reflects the local frequency content at each point at a [Y,I,Q]–color transformed gray scale image I_{colp}. By this means we can have separate bandpassed feature images $I_{PSD}^{(1)}$, $I_{PSD}^{(2)}$....$I_{PSD}^{(s)}$, representing a subset for the energy content that belong to the original image I_{colp}. We can analyze this using one gray scale image at a time, for example - the luminance Y.

4   Results

We demonstrate the effectiveness of the current method for visual discrimination based on the tristimulus theories of the Human Visual System (HVS) [17] decomposing the gray scale image in three frequency bands, in a similar fashion as the ear perceives pitch. We also evaluate the differences of ROI discrimination to underline the differences in signal power for both regions (ROI's PSD power versus ROI^C), mimicking HVS discrimination in the "simple cells" of the cortex.

We processed 70 color images (512 x 512) by the proposed method using gray scale images only [Y] [17]. We varied the GW using different cutoff frequencies. Here we present only the results form GW with three cutoff frequencies (Figure 4). Each image depicted there is one of the three band-passed images (column-wise) and cutoff frequencies (row-wise). Whilst the first band has high values for centrally located ROI, ROI^C has also strong content low frequencies. The second band shows a clear outline of the TZ (ROI) and large attenuation of the area of ROI^C. Figure 4 demonstrated a well-defined TZ using GW with $\sigma_k \geq 0.45\pi$ and $\sigma_k \leq 0.65\pi$. The gray scale images in the second band shows the best feature separation. Hence, band 2 is the best candidate for texture feature detection.

4.1   Visual Discrimination of ROI in Gray Scale Images

Figure 4 reinforced that band 2 is the most suitable for textural feature detection. Features in band 3 exhibit strong presence of specular reflection (SR) - an artifact in endoscopy and colposcopy images. Band 3 contains mostly the outline of SR.

4.2   Evaluation of Band Separation in ROI

The pooled average values of ROIs and its complement - the ROI^C was estimated as well, studying the impact of the scale-space parameters of the GW (σ_{u_1,u_2}) for ROI vs. ROI^C discrimination, changing σ_{u_1,u_2} from 0.15π. to 0.5π. The differences in pooled average values for Band 1 to Band 3 reached the maximum of 20dB in Band 2. The absolute differences for the pixel set of ROI was compared to the adjacent set of pixels of ROI^C for each σ_k depicted by the graphs in 4. The results were evaluated automatically using Matlab. The evaluation was performed using "ground truth" binary masks for ROI and ROI^C (read for more details in [8]). Binary mask of the "ground truth" was applied automatically for experiments with different σ_k.Analysis of these values shows that the values for ROI in band 2 are *all positive*, while the values of ROI^C for the band 3 *are all negative*, resulting in twofold difference (shown on the Figure 5) for the location-wise PSD difference estimates differentiating between the ROI and ROI^C (see

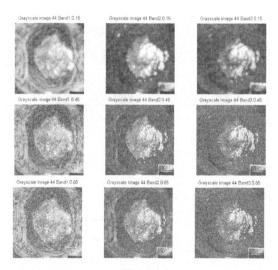

Fig. 4. Gray scale images that illustrate the formation of separate PSD-based images into three bands using a geometric restriction. The upper row troika are calculated with $\sigma_k = 0.15\pi$ for band$_1$, band$_2$ and band$_3$. The second row is a set of three band specific images when $\sigma_{k=0.25}$ is used. The images on the lowest row are calculated for $\sigma_k = 0.45\pi$.

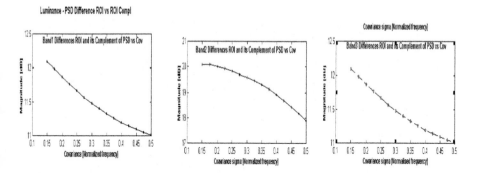

Fig. 5. Luminance(Y)-based differences of PSD values $[dB]$ of ROI and ROI^C for three bands with varying covariance of the applied Gaussian filter

Figure 5). Luminance only results are displayed of Figure 5), but the data from the both chrominance channels [I, Q] yielded lower difference values, evaluated against the "ground truth" $(\mathcal{A}\{|ROI - ROI^C|\})$, taken set-wize for band separation. The results for the chrominances reached 5-6 dB difference for Band 2 for either chromaticity, while the Y -based results reached 20dB difference for Band 2.The differences within the ROI and ROI^C yields a further possibility to find the ideal threshold for bimodal segmentation of these images, which we demonstrate this further in Figure 6.

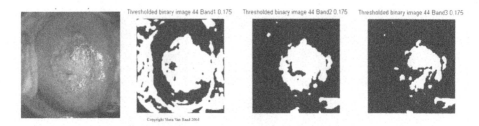

Fig. 6. Depicts the original RGB image and the binary image at three bands

4.3   Pseudo-Color Maps Based on HVS

Representing each of the three bands as tri-stimuli of the HVS we will mimic the frequency band separation from the proposed method. Thus, we show that texture can be perceived in a similar as the pitch of the sound by the ear. This enhances also the Human-Computer Interaction concept of diagnosis. Assigning color to a particular combination of frequency values to a location from image can reveal important frequency structure. This concept is presented on Figure 7. The green color is associated with the small grain texture, whilst the red color shows relative constancy (low frequency) for that particular location. This color is assigned automatically.

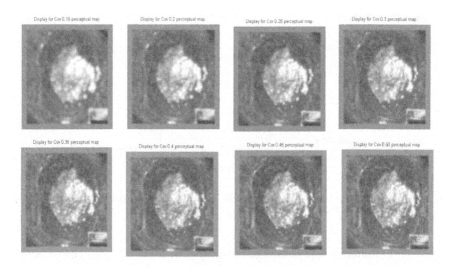

Fig. 7. Illustrates a pseudo-color map in scale-space-frequency via sliding Gaussian window. The window σ_k varies form 0.15π to 0.5π in normalized frequency.

We created the pseudo color map as we "combined" the quantitative information using one type of source image: e.g. using only Y, or only I or only Q components. In a case where we will be looking for multidimensional feature, each of the (Y,I,Q) 3-band separation will lead to 9-dimensional feature. In the current case, we are presenting the pseudo-color images from 3-band separation based on the luminance (Y) information only. The pseudo-color map, illustrated on Figure 7 represents a 3-tuple image formed by $band_1$, $band_2$ and $band_3$, whilst we varied the variance of the Gaussian window σ_k starting from 0.15π to 0.65π (step of 0.05π) with $\sigma_k = 0.15\pi$ shown to be the upper left image. The idea of the pseudo-color map is to collate an unique combination of values in 3D color space, that be created from the three bands ($Band_1$, $Band_2$, $Band_3$), presented as multi-dimensional data, using the perceptual ability of the Human Visual System (HVS) that view the surrounding world hypothesized by the tri-stimuli theory [17]. The unique combination of the response in the three band at each point can be associated with a specific color, that could point to "normality" or "disease."

5   Concluding Remarks

We devised a new method that analyzes textural features in joint-time frequency space. We showed that the method can be developed further and it can be used for an accurate estimation of ROI. We proposed this method offering an increased accuracy of the band-wise estimates for ROIs in gray scale cervical images. An advantage of this method is that the averaged energy per band is useful for non-oriented texture evaluation, combined with flexible and specific 2D frequency-based boundary placement. The method can be very precise in estimation of parameters, although the Matlab implementation carries a heavy computational load.

In addition, a HVS concept using a tristimulus vision and perception can be applied to distinguish textures with different diagnostic content. The reported experimental results demonstrated the merits of the method as an effective way to discriminate features either visually and by using metrics. The so proposed visual discrimination methods for pseudo-color image feature matching can be applied either for CAD in colposcopy or in other image modalities.

In our future work we will emphasize on developing a training unsupervised algorithm for automatic vascular texture detection or detection of lesions and areas such as TZ, ectropion and abnormal vessels networks. We will continue work on implementing an algorithm useful for real-time applications with an increased computational speed.

Acknowledgements. The author would like to thank the administrative and research staff at STI-Medical Systems, Honolulu, HI, USA for the financial and the research support given. My gratitude is extended to G. Bignami (Science and Technology International) for his suggestions and comments.

References

1. V. Beral and M. Booth, "Precision of cervical cancer incidence and mortality in England and Wales," Lancet, Vol. 1, pp. 495, 1986.
2. M. L. Steward and Y. C. Collins, "Strength of Correlations Between Colposcopic Impressions and Biopsy Histology," Gynecol. Oncol.,Vol. 89, pp.424-428, 2003.
3. V. Van Raad and A. Bradley, "Emerging Technologies, Signal Processing and Statistical Methods for Screening of Cervical Cancer *in vivo* - Are they good candidates for Cervical Screening?," IEEE - IEE Proceedings of Advances in Biomed. Signal and Information Processing, Vol. 2, pp.210-217, 2004.
4. B. W. Pogue, Marry-Ann Mycek, D. Harper, "Image Analysis for Discrimination of Cervical Neoplasia," J. BioMed. Optics, Vol. 5(1), pp. 72-82, 2000.
5. Q. Ji, J. Engel and E. R. Craine, "Texture Analysis for Classifications of Cervix Lesions," IEEE Trans. Medical Imaging, Vol. 19 (11), pp. 1144 - 1149, 2000.
6. V. Van Raad, "Gabor Wavelet Design for Analysis of Cervical Images". Proc. of the World Congress of BioMed Eng., Vol (4), pp. 16-20, 2003.
7. V. Van Raad, "Frequency Space Analysis of Cervical Images Using Short Time Fourer Transform". Proc. of the IASTED In. Conf. of BioMed Eng., Vol (1), pp. 77-81, 2003.
8. V. Van Raad, "Design of Gabor Wavelets for Analysis of Texture Features in Cervical Images," IEEE Silver Anniversary Conference of BioMed. Eng., Cancun, Mexico, 17-21 Sept. 2003.
9. A. I. Khinchin, "Mathematical Foundations of Information Theory," Dover Publications, 1957.
10. T. S. Durani and J. M. Nightingale, "Probability Distributions fo Discrete Fourier Spectra," Proc. Inst. Elect. Eng., Vol.120(2), pp. 299-311, 1973.
11. J. G. Proakis and D. G. Manolakis, "Digital signal Processing: Principles, Algorithms and Applications," Prentice Hall 1996.
12. D. Gabor, "Theory of Communications," Journal of IEE, Vol. 93, pp. 429-457, 1946.
13. P.D. Welch, "The Use of the Fast Fourier Transfrom for the Estimation of Power Spectra," IEEE Trans. Audio Elctroacoust., Vol.(AU-15), pp.70-73, 1967.
14. P. E. Johnson and D. G. Long, " The Probability Density of Spectral Estimates Based on Modified Periodogram Averages," IEEE TRanscations on Signal processing, Vol.47(5), pp. 1255-1261, 1999.
15. A. V. Oppenheim and R. W. Schafer, "Discrete Time Signal Processing," Chapter 11,Prentice Hall Signal Processing Series, 1989.
16. N. Otsu, "A Threshold Selection Method from Gray-Level Histogram," IEEE Trans. Systems, Man, and Cybernetics, Vol. 8, pp. 62-66, 1978.
17. G. Wyszecki and W. S. Stiles, "Color Science," John Wiley, New York, 1967.

Active Contours Under Topology Control
Genus Preserving Level Sets

Florent Ségonne[1,2], Jean-Philippe Pons[3], Eric Grimson[1], and Bruce Fischl[1,2]

[1] M.I.T. Computer Science and Artificial Intelligence Laboratory
[2] Athinoula A. Martinos Center - MGH/NMR Center
[3] I.N.R.I.A - Projet Odyssée

Abstract. We present a novel framework to exert topology control over a level set evolution. Level set methods offer several advantages over parametric active contours, in particular automated topological changes. In some applications, where some *a priori* knowledge of the target topology is available, topological changes may not be desirable. This is typically the case in biomedical image segmentation, where the topology of the target shape is prescribed by anatomical knowledge. However, topologically constrained evolutions often generate topological barriers that lead to large geometric inconsistencies. We introduce a topologically controlled level set framework that greatly alleviates this problem. Unlike existing work, our method allows connected components to merge, split or vanish under some specific conditions that ensure that no topological defects are generated. We demonstrate the strength of our method on a wide range of numerical experiments and illustrate its performance on the segmentation of cortical surfaces and blood vessels.

1 Introduction

Active contours constitute a general technique of matching a deformable model onto an image by means of energy minimization. Curves or surfaces deform within a 2-dimensional or 3-dimensional image subject to both internal and external forces and external constraints. Since their introduction by Kass et al. in [9], active contours have benefited many computer vision research areas.

Geometric active contours, which represents the manifold of interest as level sets of functions defined on higher-dimensional manifolds [13,3], offer many advantages over parametric approaches. In addition to their ease of implementation, level sets do not require any parameterization of the evolving contour. Self-intersections, which are costly to prevent in parametric deformable models, are naturally avoided and topological changes are automated. Also, the geometric properties of the contour, such as the normal or the curvature, are easily computed from the level set function.

The ability to automatically change topology is often presented as an advantage of the level set method over explicit deformable models. However, this behavior is not desirable in some applications. This is typically the case in biomedical image segmentation, where the topology of the target shape is prescribed by anatomical knowledge. In order to overcome this problem, a topology-preserving variant of the level set method has been proposed [7]. The level set function is iteratively updated with a modified

Y. Liu, T. Jiang, and C. Zhang (Eds.): CVBIA 2005, LNCS 3765, pp. 135–145, 2005.

procedure based on the concept of *simple point* from digital topology [1]; the final mesh is obtained with a modified topology-consistent marching cubes algorithm. This method ensures that the resulting mesh has the same topology as the user-defined initial level set.

While such topological preservation is desired in some applications, it is often too restrictive. Because the different components of the contour are not allowed to merge or to split up, the number of connected components will remain constant throughout the evolution. This number must be known by the user *a priori* and the initial contour must be designed accordingly. Also, the sensitivity to initial conditions, which already limits the applicability and efficiency of active contour methods, is considerably increased. The initial contour must both have the same topology as the target shape and be close enough to the final configuration, otherwise the evolution is likely to be trapped in topological dead-ends including large geometric inconsistencies (*cf* Fig.1 b&e).

In this paper, we propose a method to exert a more subtle topological control on a level set evolution. Some *a priori* knowledge of the target topology can be integrated without requiring that the topology be known exactly. Our method greatly alleviates the sensitivity to initial conditions by allowing connected components to merge, split or vanish without introducing any topological defects (such as handles). For example, an initial contour with a spherical topology may split into several pieces, go through one or several mergings, and finally produce a certain number of contours, all of which will be topologically equivalent to a sphere. A subset of these components may then be selected by the user as the desired output (typically the largest component if one spherical contour is needed, the others being caused by noise).

Our approach is based on an extension of the concept of *simple point* to "multi-label" images, that we have called *multisimple point*. This criterion ensures that no topological defects are generated while splitting or merging the components of the object. This algorithm fills the gap between the original level set framework and topology-preserving level set methods. We apply our method to the segmentation of cortical surfaces in Magnetic Resonance Imaging (MRI) and of blood vessels in Magnetic Resonance Angiography (MRA).

2   Background

2.1   Topology

Topology is a branch of mathematics that studies the properties of geometric figures that are preserved through deformations, twistings and stretchings, hence without regard to size, absolute position.

Here, we focus on closed contours (i.e. compact surfaces) in three dimensions. Any compact connected orientable surface is homeomorphic to a sphere with some number of handles. This number of handles is a topological invariant called the *genus*. For example, a sphere is of genus 0 and a torus is of genus 1. The genus g is directly related to another topological invariant called the *Euler characteristic* χ by the formula $\chi = 2 - 2g$. The Euler characteristic is of great practical interest because it can be calculated from any polyhedral decomposition of the surface by $\chi = V - E + F$, where V, E and F denote respectively the number of vertices, edges and faces of the polyhedron.

Homeomorphisms are used to define the *intrinsic* topology of an object, independently of the embedding space. For example, a knotted solid torus has the same genus as a simple torus, or a hollow sphere as two spheres. In order to topologically differentiate these surfaces, one needs a theory that considers the embedding space. Homotopy, which defines two surfaces to be homotopic if one can be continuously transformed into the other, is such a theory that provides a measure of an object's topology (see [8] for an excellent course in algebraic topology).

2.2 Digital Topology

Digital topology provides an elegant framework, which transposes the continuous concepts of topology to discrete images. In this theory, binary images inherit a precise topological meaning. In particular, the concept of homotopic deformation, necessary to assign a topological type to a digital object, is clearly defined through the notion of *simple point*. An extensive discussion of these concepts can be found in the work of Mangin et al [12]. In this section, some basic notions of digital topology are presented. All definitions are from the work of G. Bertrand, which we refer to for more details [1].

A 3D binary digital image I is composed of a foreground object X and its inverse, the complement $\overline{X}$. We first need the concept of *connectivity*, which specifies the condition of adjacency that two points must fulfill to be regarded as connected. Three types of connectivity are commonly used in 3D: 6-, 18- and 26-connectivity. Two voxels are 6-adjacent if they share a face, 18-adjacent if they share at least an edge and 26-adjacent if they share at least a corner. In order to avoid topological paradoxes, different connectivities, n and $\overline{n}$, must be used for X and $\overline{X}$. This leaves us with four pairs of compatible connectivities, (6,26), (6,18), (18,6) and (26,6). We note that digital topology does not provide a consistent framework for multi-label images, since no compatible connectivities could be chosen for neighboring components of the same object. Digital topology is strictly limited to binary images.

We then go to the definition of a *simple point*. This concept is central to the method of [7] and to our method. A point of a binary object is *simple* if it can be added or removed without changing the topology of both the object and its background, i.e. without changing the number of connected components, cavities and handles of both X and $\overline{X}$. A simple point is easily characterized by two *topological* numbers with respect to the digital object X and a consistent connectivity pair $(n, \overline{n})$. These numbers, denoted $T_n(x, X)$ and $T_{\overline{n}}(x, \overline{X})$, have been introduced by G. Bertrand in [1] as an elegant way to classify the topology type of a given voxel. The values of $T_n(x, X)$ and $T_{\overline{n}}(x, \overline{X})$ characterize isolated, interior and border points as well as different kinds of junctions. In particular, a point is simple if and only if $T_n(x, X) = T_{\overline{n}}(x, \overline{X}) = 1$. Their efficient computation, which only involves the 26-neighborhood, is described in [2].

2.3 Topology-Preserving Level Sets

Han et al. [7] have used the concept of simple point to design a topology-preserving variant of the level set framework. The binary object of interest is the interior of the contour, i.e. the domain where the level set function is strictly negative: $X=\{x|\Phi(x) < 0\}$.

The digital topology of X is preserved during the evolution by the means of a modified update procedure detailed in Algorithm 1, below. This approach prevents digital non-simple grid points from changing sign, therefore retaining the initial digital topology throughout the level set evolution.

Algorithm 1 Topology-preserving level sets. Han et al. [7]

---

for all iterations **do**
  for all grid points **do**
    Compute the new value of the level set function
    if the sign does not change **then**
      Accept the new value
    else {sign change}
      Compute the topological numbers
      if the point is simple **then**
        Accept the new value
      else
        Discard the new value
        Set instead a small value of the adequate sign

For this method to be useful, it must be complemented with a topology-consistent isocontour extraction algorithm. Standard marching squares or marching cubes algorithm [11] do not generate topologically consistent tessellations. In order to alleviate this problem, Han et al. have designed a modified connectivity-consistent marching contour algorithm, by building a specialized case table for each type of digital topology. Using the topology-preserving level set algorithm and the topology-consistent marching contour algorithm in conjunction, with the same digital topology $(n, \overline{n})$ throughout the process, guarantees that the output mesh is topologically equivalent to the user-defined initial level set.

3 Methods

The simple point condition is a very efficient way to detect topological changes during a level set evolution. However, in many applications, the topology-preserving level set method of Han et al. is too restrictive.

The primary concern is topological defects such as handles, which are difficult to retrospectively correct [6,4,5,10]. On the other hand, changes in the number of connected components during the evolution are less problematic. Different connected components are easily identified using standard region growing algorithms. A subset of them may be selected by the user as the final output, typically the largest one if a single component is needed, the others being imputable to noise in the input data. Unexpected cavities, which can be interpreted as background $\overline{n}$-connected components, might generate large geometrical inaccuracies in level set evolutions that prevent their formation. This might be of particular importance when dealing with noisy data or in medical imaging, when unexpected medical structures, such as tumors, might exist in the volume to be segmented.

We extend the concept of simple point to allow distinct connected components to merge and split while ensuring that no additional handle is generated in the object. For example, an initial contour with spherical topology may split into several pieces, generate cavities, go through one or several mergings, and finally produce a specific number of surfaces, all of which are topologically equivalent to a sphere.

3.1   From Simple Points to Multisimple Points

The different values of T_n and $T_{\overline{n}}$ characterize the topology type of a given point x, providing important information with regards to its connectivity to the object X. In particular, isolated points are characterized by $T_n = 0$ and $T_{\overline{n}} = 1$, while different junctions by $T_n > 1$ and $T_{\overline{n}} = 1$. This additional information can be used to carefully design a multi-label digital framework, which allows different connected components to split, merge or vanish under topology control.

We say that a point is *multisimple* if it can be added or removed without changing the number of handles of the object X. Contrary to the case of simple points, the addition of a multisimple point may merge several connected components, and its removal may split a component into several parts. We note $C_n(x, X)$ the set of n-connected components of $X \setminus \{x\}$ that are n-adjacent to x. If the cardinality of this set is strictly greater than one, the addition or removal of x involves a merge or a split respectively. By duality, the generation of one or several cavities in X can be interpreted as a split of connected components of $\overline{X}$.

Formally, a point is said to be multisimple if and only if:

$$T_{\overline{n}}(x, \overline{X}) = 1$$
$$\forall\, C \in C_n(x, X),\ T_n(x, C) = T_{\overline{n}}(x, \overline{C}) = 1$$

or

$$T_n(x, X) = 1$$
$$\forall\, C \in C_{\overline{n}}(x, \overline{X}),\ T_n(x, \overline{C}) = T_{\overline{n}}(x, C) = 1$$

When merging or splitting connected components by adding or removing a multisimple point, the total genus (i.e. the total number of handles) of the different components is preserved. We note that, under this condition, an isolated point is a multisimple point, which allows components to be created or to disappear.

3.2   Level Set Evolution Under Topology Control

With the concept of multisimple point in hand, we are now ready to describe our new level set framework. Similarly to the approach of Han et al. [7], we exploit the binary nature of the level set function that partitions the underlying digital image into strictly negative inside points and positive outside points. During the evolution, we maintain a map L of labels coding for the different connected components of X and $\overline{X}$.

The update procedure for each grid point at each iteration is concisely described in Algorithm 2. The simple point condition, more restrictive, is checked first, because it is computationally cheaper. If the point is non-simple, then $C_n(x, X)$ and $C_{\overline{n}}(x, \overline{X})$ are computed in order to check the multisimple criterion. We refer to the technical report [14] for more details.

Interestingly, if x is part of the background (resp. foreground) object and is a candidate for addition, $C_n(x, X)$ (resp. $C_{\overline{n}}(x, \overline{X})$) can be deduced directly from the map L. If x is a candidate for removal in X (resp. in $\overline{X}$), the complete set $C_n(x, X)$ (resp. $C_{\overline{n}}(x, \overline{X})$) must be computed. However, when dealing with components that do not possess any handles, the most common situation in practice, the computation of $C_n(x, X)$ and $C_{\overline{n}}(x, \overline{X})$ only involves local computations.

Some care must be taken in order to ensure that the map of labels L is correctly updated. The more complex case is the removal of a multisimple point involving a split: in this case, some unused labels must be assigned to the new connected components. The first equation of each condition guarantees that sign changes do not generate ambiguous label changes. For each point $x \in X$ changing sign, only one single connected component C of the inverse object $\overline{X}$ is adjacent to the point x; unambiguously, the newly assigned label of x is the one of the component C.

Algorithm 2 Genus Preserving Level Sets

Compute the new value of the level set function
if the sign does not change **then**
    Accept the new value
else {sign change}
    Compute the topological numbers
    if the point is simple **then**
        Accept the new value
    else {non-simple point}
        if the point is multisimple **then**
            Accept the new value
            Update $L(x)$
        else
        Discard the new value
        Set instead a small value of the adequate sign

The resulting procedure is an efficient level set model that prevents handles from being created during the evolution, allowing the number of connected components (including cavities) to vary. We insist on the fact that digital topology does not provide a consistent framework for multi-label images. However, by ensuring that no components of the same object X or $\overline{X}$ are adjacent, topological inconsistencies can be eliminated.

4   Experiments and Applications

In this section, we present some experiments illustrating the performance of our approach and introduce some potential applications. We first apply our level set framework to two synthetic examples to demonstrate its ability to handle disconnected components and cavities. Next, two segmentation tasks are presented: the generation of cortical surfaces from MRI images and the extraction of blood vessels from MRA images.

4.1   Experiments

'C' shape: First, we consider the segmentation of a simple 'C' shape under two different initializations (*cf* Fig.1 *a-c* & *d-f*). Our method, columns *c,f*, is compared to the

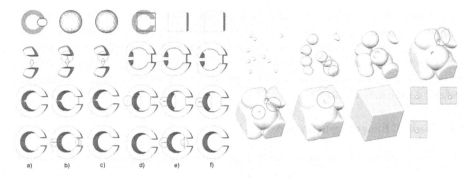

Fig. 1. Left: Segmentation of a 'C' shape using a spherical initialization a-c and a rectangular initialization d-f. The top row shows cuts of the 3D shape locating the initial component. a,d: Traditional level set evolution. b,e: Topology-preserving level set evolution. c,f: level set evolution under topology control. Differences of behavior are circled in the images. Note that in both cases, our level set framework is able to correctly segment the shape of interest, without generating invalid topology during the evolution. Right: Segmentation of a cubic shape containing 3 cavities. 10 initial seed points were randomly selected. Note how components split, merge and disappear during the evolution, and how the active contour encloses cavities.

original level set formulation, columns *a,d*, and the topology-preserving model introduced by Han et al. [7], columns *b,e*. In the case of this simple example, standard level sets produce accurate segmentations. However, they do not provide control over the final topology, as illustrated by the second initialization, column *d*. During the evolution, the level set automatically changes topology, temporarily generating a toroïdal shape.

On the other hand, topology-preserving level sets, while guaranteeing the correct topology, might easily be geometrically inaccurate (see Fig.1 *b,e*). Topological barriers, generated during the evolution to prevent topological changes, generate incorrect contour configurations which are difficult to retrospectively correct. We note that even close initializations (*cf* column *e*) can lead to inaccurate segmentations.

The behavior of our approach corresponds to a trade-off in between the previous two methods. Our level set framework, which offers more flexibility during the evolution, greatly alleviates the sensitivity to initialization. It provides a control over the topology of all connected components, without enforcing strong topological constraints. The first initialization (*cf* column *c*) produces a level set evolution, which splits the active contour into three distinct components with a spherical topology. While one of these components vanishes, the two other components merge, closing the 'C' shape. In this case, topologically controlled level sets behaved in exactly the same way traditional level sets do. Our method is still sensitive to topological barriers, in the sense that it will not allow component to generate handles. However, it is less likely to be trapped into topological dead-ends than a strict topology-preserving model. This is illustrated in Fig.1 *f*, where the spherical component is prevented from generating a handle until it gets separated into two distinct components.

Formation of cavities: The second experiment illustrates the ability of our approach to generate cavities during the evolution. The object to be segmented is a synthetic cube, containing 3 large cavities. 10 seed points, randomly selected inside and outside the volume, were used to initialize the level set evolution reported in Fig.1-right. During the evolution, components merge, vanish and produce cavities, generating a final accurate representation constituted of 3 spherical cavities and the main object. We note that all the components are easily extracted, since they carry distinct labels that are iteratively updated during the evolution.

4.2   Medical Image Segmentation

Two segmentation tasks are presented that illustrate the potential benefits of our novel level set framework : the segmentation of cortical surfaces from MRI and the extraction of blood vessels from MRA data sets. The level set evolution is naively guided by a simple intensity-based velocity term and a curvature term:

$$\partial_t\phi(x,t) = [\alpha(I(x) - T(x)) - \kappa]|\nabla\phi|,$$

where $I(x)$ and κ represents the image intensity and mean curvature respectively at location x, T is a threshold computed locally from image intensities, α a weighting coefficient equal to $\alpha = 0.1$.

Cortical segmentation: Excluding pathological cases, the cortex, which corresponds to a highly-folded thin sheet of gray matter, has the topology of a sphere. The extraction of accurate and topologically correct cortical representations is still an active research area [4,6]. In this example, the cortical surface is initialized with 55 spherical components, automatically selected in a greedy manner, such that every selected point is located at a minimal distance of $10mm$ from the previous ones (see Fig.2). During the evolution, the components progressively merge together and enclose cavities, resulting in a final surface composed of one single spherical component with 5 cavities. The same evolution without topology constraint produces a final cortical surface with 18 topological defects (i.e. handles).

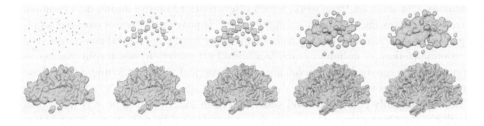

Fig. 2. Segmentation of the cortex from an anatomical MRI. The initial level set was constituted of 55 connected components. The final surface has a spherical topology, corresponding to an Euler number of 2. The same level set evolution without topological control results in a final surface with 18 topological defects (Euler number of $\chi = -34$).

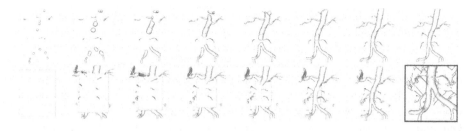

Fig. 3. Segmentations of blood vessels in a 3D angiography under two different initializations. Top row: 20 seed points were selected to initialize the active contour, which generates 3 components. Bottom row: An enclosing contour is used to initialize the level set. After 9 mergings and 99 splittings, the final segmentation is constituted of 91 components, 53 of which were due to random noise. The last image in the black frame shows the final segmentation produced by a topologically constrained evolution under the same initialization.

Segmentation of blood vessels: Finally, we show how our method could be applied to the segmentation of blood vessels from Magnetic Resonance Angiography. Because these vessels do not split and merge, their topology is the one of several distinct components with no handles (i.e. each component has the topology of a sphere). While traditional level sets produce segmentations that could include topological defects, topologically constrained level sets would result in a slow and laborious segmentation. Since the simultaneous evolution of several components, which cannot be merged together, can easily be trapped in topological dead-ends, each component would need to be iteratively initialized, when the evolution of the previous one has terminated.

On the other hand, our method offers the possibility to concurrently evolve multiple components that can merge, split and . The initial contour can be initialized by a set of seed points, manually or automatically selected, or by a single enclosing component, without affecting much the final representation.

Figure 3 shows the segmentation of an angiography under two different initializations. In a first experiment (*cf* top row), 20 seed points were automatically selected at the brightest locations in the MRA. The level set evolution iteratively merged most of the components, generating a final segmentation with 3 spherical components. In the second experiment (*cf* bottom row), one single global component, enclosing most of the object of interest, was used to initialize the active contour. During the evolution, 9 components merged and 99 split producing a final segmentation composed of 91 components, 53 of which were single voxel components due to random noise in the imaging process.

5   Discussion and Conclusion

We introduce a new level set framework that offers control over the topology of the level set components during the evolution. Previous approaches either do not constrain the topology or enforce a hard topological constraint. Our method exerts a subtle control over the topology of each component to prevent the formation of topological defects. Distinct components can merge, split or disappear during the evolution, but no handles will be generated. In particular, a contour solely composed of spherical components will only produce spherical components throughout the evolution. In this case, which is the most common situation in practice, all computations are local and the multisimple point checking can be done efficiently. The only computational complexity comes from the generation of new components, as new labels need to be assigned to each of them.

While the original level set model does not provide any topological control, topology-preserving level sets enforce a strong constraint that is often too restrictive. Our framework establishes a trade-off in between the two models. It offers a subtle topological control that alleviates most problems of methods that enforce a strong topological constraint (i.e. sensitivity to initialization and noise, simultaneous evolution of multiple components and speed of convergence). The experiments presented in this paper illustrate some potential applications that could greatly benefit from our approach.

References

1. G. Bertrand. Simple points, topological numbers and geodesic neighborhoods in cubic grids. *Pattern Recognition Letters*, 15(10):1003–1011, 1994.
2. G. Bertrand. A boolean characterization of three-dimensional simple points," pattern recognition letters. *Pattern recognition letters*, 17:115–124, 1996.
3. V. Caselles, R. Kimmel, and G. Sapiro. Geodesic active contours. *The International Journal of Computer Vision*, 22(1):61–79, 1997.
4. B. Fischl, A. Liu, and A.M. Dale. Automated manifold surgery: Constructing geometrically accurate and topologically correct models of the human cerebral cortex. *IEEE Transaction on Medical Imaging*, 20:70–80, 2001.
5. I. Guskov and Z. Wood. Topological noise removal. *Graphics Interface Proceedings*, pages 19–26, 2001.
6. X. Han, C. Xu, U. Braga-Neto, and J.L. Prince. Topology correction in brain cortex segmentation using a multiscale, graph-based approach. *IEEE Transaction on Medical Imaging*, 21(2):109–121, 2002.
7. X. Han, C. Xu, and J.L. Prince. A topology preserving level set method for geometric deformable models. *IEEE Transactions on Pattern Analysis and Machine Intelligence*, 25(6):755–768, 2003.
8. Allen Hatcher. *Algebraic Topology*. Cambridge University Press, 2002.
9. M. Kass, A. Witkin, and D. Terzopoulos. Snakes: Active contour models. In *First International Conference on Computer Vision*, pages 259–268, London, June 1987.
10. N. Kriegeskorte and R. Goeble. An efficient algorithm for topologically segmentation of the cortical sheet in anatomical mr volumes. *NeuroImage*, 14:329–346, 2001.
11. William E. Lorensen and Harvey E. Cline. Marching cubes: A high resolution 3d surface construction algorithm. In M.C. Stone, editor, *Proceedings of the SIGGRAPH*, pages 163–169, Anaheim, CA, July 1987. in Computer Graphics, Volume 21, Number 4.
12. J.-F. Mangin, V. Frouin, I. Bloch, J. Regis, and J. Lopez-Krahe. From 3d magnetic resonance images to structural representations of the cortex topography using topology preserving deformations. *Journal of Mathematical Imaging and Vision*, 5:297–318, 1995.

13. S. Osher and J.A. Sethian. Fronts propagating with curvature-dependent speed: Algorithms based on Hamilton–Jacobi formulations. *Journal of Computational Physics*, 79(1):12–49, 1988.
14. F. Ségonne, J.-P. Pons, F. Fischl, and E. Grimson. A novel active contour framework. multi-component level set evolution under topology control. *CSAIL Publications - AI memos*, AIM-2005-020, 2005.

A Novel Multifaceted Virtual Craniofacial Surgery Scheme Using Computer Vision

A.S. Chowdhury[1,*], S.M. Bhandarkar[1], E.W. Tollner[2], G. Zhang[2],
J.C. Yu[3], and E. Ritter[3]

[1] Department of Computer Science,
The University of Georgia, Athens GA 30602 -7404, USA
{ananda, suchi}@cs.uga.edu
[2] Dept. of Biological & Agricultural Engg,
The University of Georgia, Athens, GA 30602 – 4435, USA
{btollner, gzhang}@engr.uga.edu
[3] Dept. of Plastic Surgery,The Medical College of Georgia,
Augusta, GA 30912, USA
{jyu, eritter}@mcg.edu

Abstract. The paper addresses the problem of virtual craniofacial reconstruction from a set of Computer Tomography (CT) images, with the multiple objectives of achieving accurate local matching of the opposable fracture surfaces and preservation of the global shape symmetry and the biomechanical stability of the reconstructed mandible. The first phase of the reconstruction, with the mean squared error as the performance metric, achieves the best possible local surface matching using the Iterative Closest Point (ICP) algorithm and the Data Aligned Rigidity Constrained Exhaustive Search (DARCES) algorithm each used individually and then in a synergistic combination. The second phase, which consists of an angular perturbation scheme, optimizes a composite reconstruction metric. The composite reconstruction metric is a linear combination of the mean squared error, a global shape symmetry term and the surface area which is shown to be a measure of biomechanical stability. Experimental results, including a thorough validation scheme on simulated fractures in phantoms of the craniofacial skeleton, are presented.

1 Motivation

In modern society, craniofacial fractures are encountered very frequently with the two most prominent causes being gunshot wounds and motor vehicle accidents [1]. These frequently encountered fractures possess some distinct patterns. Sometimes, the patterns imply a single fracture, and, in some other cases, there can be a combination of single fractures [2]. From the surgical standpoint, fractures are fixated one at a time in the operating room and thus can and must be so decomposed in the pre-surgical planning as well. Thus, practically speaking, in almost all the cases, reconstruction

---

* Corresponding author's e-mail: ananda@cs.uga.edu

Y. Liu, T. Jiang, and C. Zhang (Eds.): CVBIA 2005, LNCS 3765, pp. 146 – 159, 2005.

from a single mandibular fracture assumes paramount importance. The plastic surgeon in the operating room restores the form and function of the fractured bone elements in the craniofacial skeleton typically by first exposing all the fragments, then returning them to their normal configuration, and finally maintaining these reduced bone pieces with rigid screws and plates. However, there are several critical and inherent limitations to this current, standard approach. To visualize the fragments in order to reduce them necessitates their exposure which consequently reduces the attached blood supply. To improve the blood supply, one can decrease the extent of dissection. However this means not being able to visualize the entire fracture, which could lead to potential misalignments of the bone fragments. Additionally, the cost of surgery becomes prohibitive with the increased operating time necessary to ensure an accurate reconstruction, especially in complex cases [3]. An elaborate virtual reconstruction scheme involving a single mandibular fracture is proposed in this work which can potentially reduce the operating time and consequently, the cost of surgery without sacrificing surgical precision, thus drastically reducing the operative and post-operative patient trauma.

2   Literature Review and Our Contribution

A lot of interesting research has been performed over the past decade in various aspects of craniofacial/maxillofacial surgery. Because of space limitations, only a few representative works are mentioned here. The mass tensor model is used for fast soft tissue prediction in [4] whereas the mass-spring model is used for fast surgical simulation from CT data in [5]. The problem of building a virtual craniofacial patient from CT data has been addressed in [6] whereas a reconstruction approach involving complete 3D modeling of the solid high-detailed structure of the craniofacial skeleton, starting from the information present in the 3D diagnostic CT images can be found in [7]. The *Iterative Closest Point (ICP)* [8] algorithm is seen to be a popular computer vision algorithm for surface registration in the field of medical imaging. Some variants of the ICP algorithm that incorporate certain statistical concepts such as Expectation Maximization (EM) in the context of medical imaging can be found in [9]. The basic benefit of the ICP algorithm is that it gives an accurate result given a good initial starting point. Another surface registration algorithm called the *Data Aligned Rigidity Constrained Exhaustive Search (DARCES)* which incorporates a *Random Sample Consensus (RANSAC)* model fitting approach [10], is popular because of its robustness to outliers and has also been used in medical imaging [11].

In this paper, we address the problem of single fracture craniofacial reconstruction from broken solid fragments. Our principal contribution is the formulation of a novel two-phase virtual reconstruction scheme. The first phase of our proposed reconstruction scheme employs the *ICP* and *DARCES* algorithms first individually and then in a novel synergistic combination. The ICP algorithm in our implementation solves the 3D correspondence problem using Bipartite Graph Matching. The synergetic combination of the two algorithms, where the output of the DARCES algorithm is fed as an input to the ICP algorithm, is observed to result in an improved surface matching algorithm with a considerable reduction in both, the mean squared error (MSE) and the execution time. We briefly describe the first phase of reconstruction in this paper and refer the interested reader to our previous work in [12]. The anatomy of the human mandible clearly exhibits bilateral symmetry. Furthermore, basic biophysical principles indicate that the most stable state for a solid body is the state with minimum energy [13] and this fact should be applicable to the human mandible as well. Since both the ICP and DARCES algorithms are essentially data driven and are purely local in nature, the first phase cannot explicitly guarantee the preservation of either the global shape symmetry or the biomechanical stability of the reconstructed human mandible. The incorporation of anatomical shape knowledge in medical image registration has been discussed in [14, 15]. However, we go one step further in the second phase of our reconstruction paradigm. In the second phase, a composite reconstruction metric is introduced and expressed as a linear combination of three different terms, namely (a) the MSE, (b) a global shape symmetry term and (c) a surface area term (which is shown to be a measure of biomechanical stability). An angular perturbation scheme is used to optimize the composite reconstruction metric. Thus the second reconstruction phase enables us to explore and address, in an innovative manner, the anatomical shape preservation as well as biophysical stability issues in the reconstruction paradigm (which may not be always possible in the operating room). As shown in this paper, the second phase of reconstruction integrates computer vision algorithms with ideas from biophysics and mathematics to generate a more accurate reconstruction.

3   Image Preprocessing

The input to the system (Fig.1) is a sequence of 2D grayscale images of a fractured human mandible, generated via Computer Tomography (CT). Each image slice is 150 mm x 150 mm with an 8-bit color depth. A simple thresholding scheme is used to binarize each CT image slice (Fig. 2b). A 2D Connected Component Labeling (CCL) algorithm in conjunction with an area filter is used to remove some unwanted artifacts (Fig. 2c). The results of the 2D CCL algorithm are propagated across the CT image slices, resulting in a 3D CCL algorithm. Interactive contour detection is then performed on all the 2D CT slices. The contour points from the CT image stack are assembled to form a 3D surface point data set. The data sets resulting from two opposable fracture surfaces are denoted as the sample dataset and the model dataset.

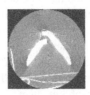

Fig. 1. A sequence of CT images (where higher intensity values represent mandible fragments and artifacts and lower intensity values represent soft tissue)

Fig. 2. (a) A typical 2D CT slice. (b) The CT slice after thresholding. (c) The CT slice after Connected Component Labeling and Size Filtering. In (b) and (c), the lower intensity values represent mandible fragments and artifacts.

4 Reconstruction Phase I - Surface Matching Algorithms

The first phase of the virtual reconstruction consists of applications of the ICP, DARCES and hybrid DARCES-ICP algorithms. For the ICP algorithm [8], the matching point pairs (forming the *closest set*) are determined in a novel fashion using the Maximum Cardinality Minimum Weight (MCMW) Bipartite Graph Matching algorithm [16] based on the Hungarian Marriage method proposed by Kuhn [17]. The 3D sample and model data sets correspond to the two disjoint vertex sets (V_1, V_2) in a bipartite graph $G(V, E)$. The edge-weight $(W_{ij} \in E)$ between any two nodes i and j (such that $i \in V_1$ and $j \in V_2$) is deemed to be the Euclidean distance between them. Note that the Euclidean distance is invariant to a 3D rigid body transformation. The bipartite graph matching implicitly preserves the local shape of the two surfaces (to be registered) with arbitrary orientation, without necessitating their pre-alignment. The edge weights are given by:

$$W_{ij} = ((x_i - x_j)^2 + (y_i - y_j)^2 + (z_i - z_j)^2)^{1/2} \tag{1}$$

The MSE (ξ^2) is given by:

$$\xi^2 = (1/N) \sum_{i=1}^{N} \|c_i - (Rs_i + T)\|^2 \tag{2}$$

where R denotes the rotation matrix, T, the translation vector, s_i, a point in the sample data set and c_i, the corresponding point in the closest set. A pre-specified error convergence criterion of 0.001 was used. A RANSAC-based approach for the DARCES algorithm was adopted [10]. All the 3D rigid body transformation parameters were computed using the Singular Value Decomposition (SVD) algorithm [18]. A novel synergistic combination of the DARCES and ICP algorithms, where the inputs to the ICP algorithm are the original model set and, the sample set transformed by the DARCES algorithm, was employed [12]. The ICP algorithm yields an accurate 3D rigid body transformation but is sensitive to outliers in the input data. The DARCES algorithm, on the other hand, enables outlier rejection but the computed transformation is only approximate. In the DARCES-ICP hybrid algorithm, the pairs of matched points generated by the DARCES algorithm serve to reduce the cardinalities of the two data sets to be matched (using bipartite graph matching) in the ICP algorithm. Consequently, the dense bipartite graph used to determine the *closest set* in the ICP algorithm is reduced to a sparse bipartite graph with fewer nodes and edges. Thus, the subsequent MCMW bipartite graph matching procedure in the ICP algorithm has a lower execution time since it is run on a more meaningful (in terms of the number of pairs of matching points in the two vertex sets V_1 and V_2) sparse bipartite graph. Also, a much lower MSE is achieved by the ICP algorithm for the matching of the two fracture surfaces, since the DARCES algorithm provides a better starting point to the ICP algorithm by virtue of outlier removal. We have also achieved further improvement in local surface matching with suitable modeling of surface irregularities and their incorporation in the reconstruction scheme [19].

5 Identification of the Plane of Bilateral Symmetry

In order to ensure preservation of the global shape of the reconstructed human mandible, the plane of bilateral symmetry [20] – [24] is determined for the reconstructed human mandible. We assume the general equation of a three-dimensional plane to be:

$$F(x, y, z) = Ax + By + Cz - D = 0 \qquad (3)$$

It is well known that the planes of reflection symmetry for any rigid body pass through its centre of mass and that their coefficients are the components of the eigenvectors of the real symmetric moment of inertia matrix/tensor [13]. This fact allows us to determine the possible candidates for the planes of reflection symmetry without recourse to exhaustive search [23]. The elements of the 3x3 moment of inertia matrix/tensor are the second order centralized moments for the rigid body under consideration. Once the coefficients of the three symmetry planes are determined, the entire mandible is reflected about each of these planes. For each point *f(x, y, z)* in the reconstructed mandible, there exists a corresponding point $f_R(x, y, z)$ in the reflected mandible, given by the following equation [21]:

$$f_R(x, y, z) = \begin{cases} f(x, y, z) - 2 \dfrac{F(f)}{\|\nabla F\|} \dfrac{\nabla F}{\|\nabla F\|} \ if \ F(f) > 0 \\ f(x, y, z) + 2 \dfrac{F(f)}{\|\nabla F\|} \dfrac{\nabla F}{\|\nabla F\|} \ otherwise \end{cases} \qquad (4)$$

where the F is computed using equation (3). There are various measures of symmetry to be found in the literature such as the sum of absolute distance and the normalized cross- correlation [20 - 23]. The proposed metric is a linear combination of the normalized cross-correlation and a novel set-theoretic measure. If one treats the reconstructed mandible *g* and the reflected mandible *h* as two N-dimensional vectors, the normalized cross-correlation γ between *g* and *h* is given by [20, 21, 24]:

$$\gamma(g, h) = \frac{(g - \overline{g}u).(h - \overline{h}u)}{\|g - \overline{g}u\| \ \|h - \overline{h}u\|} \qquad (5)$$

where $\bar{g}$ and $\bar{h}$ are the means of the elements of g and h respectively and u is an N-dimensional unit vector. Alternatively, g and h can be considered as two 3D data sets of cardinality n. A novel set theoretic term β is introduced as a measure of overlap between the sets g and h:

$$\beta = 1 - \frac{|g \; \Delta \; h|}{|g \; \cup \; h|} \qquad (6)$$

where Δ denotes the symmetric difference between and $\cup$ represents the union of the reconstructed mandible set g and the reflected mandible set h. Interestingly, β lies between 0 (when there is no overlap between g and h) and 1 (when there is perfect overlap between g and h). The proposed metric for global shape symmetry, denoted by GM, is given by:

$$GM = \lambda_1 * \gamma + \lambda_2 * \beta \qquad (7)$$

$$\text{where } \sum_{i=1}^{2} \lambda_i = 1 \qquad (8)$$

Depending on the problem structure and image representation, different values of λ_1 and λ_2 can be chosen. We assume $\lambda_1 = \lambda_2 = 0.5$ for our present problem. The plane with the largest value of GM is deemed to be the plane of bilateral symmetry.

6 Estimation of Biomechanical Stability

Surface energy minimization is modeled along the well accepted principle of strain potential minimization, which, in turn, is based on minimization of the strain energy of an isotropic solid. The strain potential (U) can be defined as follows:

$$U = \iiint_V f \text{(normal and shear strains, Young's and shear moduli, Poisson ratio)} \, dv \qquad (9)$$

Details of the functional form of f for an isotropic solid may be found in [25]. The normal and shear strains occurring in response to a force field are represented by a displacement field u and resisted by forces arising from the Young's and shear moduli. A body force B (operating on a volume V with surface area S) and surface shear forces T will result in a deformation pattern that minimizes U. Further, it can be shown that the following criterion must be satisfied under equilibrium conditions [25]:

$$\iint_S T.\delta u \, \delta a + \iiint_V B.\delta u \, \delta v - \delta U = 0 \qquad (10)$$

The integral on the left in equation (10) is a surface energy term. For the purpose of this discussion, we may assume near zero resistance to movement resulting from a force of unity, thus the energy related to volumetric response is near zero. Hence it can be concluded that a minimum potential energy state results in minimum surface energy. Further, minimum surface energy in the context of moving fragments with constant surface force is consistent with minimum surface area. So, a biomechanically stable state (i.e. a state with minimum potential energy) is guaranteed by a state with minimum surface area. Only the top and bottom curved surfaces (of the six possible surfaces) of the human mandible in the CT image stack, that account for the maximum contribution to the total surface area, are considered. Each surface (S) can be modeled of as an aggregation of disjoint surface patches (SP) [26]:

$$S = \bigcup_{i=1}^{n} SP_i \tag{11}$$

$$SP_i \cap SP_j = \phi \quad \text{if} \quad i \neq j \tag{12}$$

The determinant (gm) of the first fundamental form matrix $\mathbf{G}$ [26, 27] for each surface patch is computed using techniques of differential geometry. The area of each surface (SA), in terms of its constituent surface patch areas (SPA) and metric determinants (gm), is given by the following equation:

$$SA = \sum_{i=1}^{n} gm_i^{1/2} * SPA_i \tag{13}$$

where n is the number of surface patches comprising a given surface. Each digital surface (patch) is approximated by an analytic surface (patch) using a least-squares surface fitting technique [26, 27]. Discrete bi-orthogonal Chebyshev polynomials are used as the basis functions for each such surface patch within an N x N window (where $N = 5$ in our case). The surface function estimate that minimizes the sum of squared surface fitting error within the window is given by:

$$\hat{f}(u,v) = \sum_{i,j=0}^{3} a_{i,j} \varphi_i(u) \varphi_j(v) \tag{14}$$

where the φ_i's are the basis functions for the Chebyshev polynomials. Coefficients of the functional approximation are given by:

$$a_{i,j} = \sum_{(u,v)=(-M,-M)}^{(u,v)=(M,M)} f(u,v) b_i(u) b_j(v) \tag{15}$$

where $M = (N-1)/2$ and the b_i's are the normalized versions of the above polynomials. From the estimated coefficients, the first and second order partial derivatives of the fitted surface patch are computed. These partial derivatives are used to compute the elements of the first fundamental form matrix $\mathbf{G}$ of the fitted surface patch. Finally, the determinant gm of the matrix $\mathbf{G}$ for that surface patch is computed [26, 27].

7   Reconstruction Phase II - Angular Perturbation Scheme

The rationale behind the second phase of the reconstruction scheme, which consists of an angular perturbation scheme, is to arrive at a reconstruction that minimizes the

MSE between the matched fracture surfaces and also yields the best possible shape symmetry and biomechanically, the most stable configuration. A normalized composite reconstruction metric (*CRM*), which is a linear combination of the MSE, the inverse of the global shape symmetry (since the optimization problem is formulated as one of minimization) and the surface area (as a measure of surface energy, which, in turn, determines biomechanical stability) is proposed as a performance measure for the perturbation scheme and is given by:

$$CRM = \alpha_1 * \xi^2 + \alpha_2 * GM^{-1} + \alpha_3 * ((TSA + BSA)/2) \tag{16}$$

where ξ^2 is the MSE, *GM* is given by equation (7), and *TSA* and *BSA* denote the top and bottom surface areas respectively and are estimated using equation (13). The α_i 's are determined using the following equation:

$$\frac{\alpha_1}{|\partial(\xi^2)|} = \frac{\alpha_2}{|\partial(GM^{-1})|} = \frac{\alpha_3}{|\partial((TSA + BSA)/2)|} ; \sum_{i=1}^{3} \alpha_i = 1 \tag{17}$$

where $|\partial(t)|$ denotes the normalized absolute difference (i.e. difference of the maximum and minimum values, divided by the maximum value) of the term t over the range of perturbation. One of the rationales behind model generation is to exploit certain key anatomical measurements to fine tune the coefficients in the equation (16). However, presently, these coefficients are computed based on the normalized absolute differences of the associated factors over the range of angular perturbations (see Fig. 5). The perturbations are applied to the fracture site in steps of 0.2^0 from -1^0 to $+1^0$ about each of the x, y and z axes. In each perturbed state, a new *CRM* is estimated after re-computing all the three components in equation (16). The small range of angular perturbations is justified based on a reasonable expectation that the locally best (minimum MSE yielding) solution generated by the DARCES-ICP hybrid algorithm is not very far off from the best overall solution (resulting the minimum *CRM* value). The choice of angular quantization (0.2^0) is a judicious compromise between execution time and accuracy. The smaller the angular quantization, higher the execution time of the algorithm. On the contrary, making the angular quantization too large may prevent the algorithm from arriving at the best possible solution. The state generating the minimum *CRM* value is deemed to be the desired reconstruction.

8   Experimental Results and Analysis

The reconstructed images for the DARCES, ICP and hybrid DARCES-ICP algorithms are presented in Fig. 3. In Fig. 4, the projections, along each of the coordinate axes, of the 3D reconstruction obtained using the hybrid DARCES-ICP algorithm are visually compared with the projections of the original mandible.

The quantitative reconstruction results (i.e., the MSE), obtained by using the various surface matching algorithms (described in Section 4) are shown in Table 1. Table 2 shows typical values for the parameters γ, β and *GM* (in the equations (5), (6)

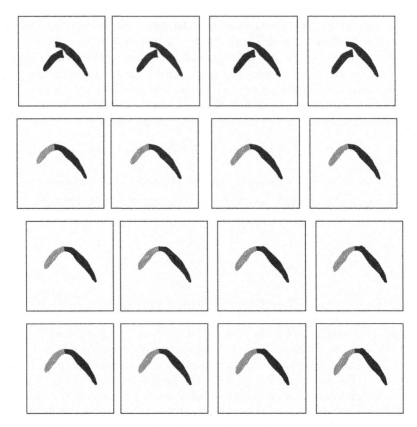

Fig. 3. The first row represents broken mandible fragments in typical CT slices. The second, third and fourth rows respectively represent reconstruction resulting from ICP, DARCES and hybrid DARCES-ICP algorithms.

and (7) respectively) for the three different candidate symmetry planes in the unperturbed state. The variations of the mean squared error, the inverse global metric for the plane of the bilateral symmetry, the average surface area and the normalized composite reconstruction metric as a function of angular perturbations along all the three major axes are graphically portrayed in Figs. 5(a)-5(d) respectively. The ranges of variations for these parameters along with their coefficients in equation (17) are shown in Table 3. Interestingly, with the incorporation of very small angular perturbations, it is possible to attain a reconstruction state, which not only yields better results in terms of the average surface area and shape symmetry, but also significantly reduces the local MSE. This is clearly revealed in Table 4, where the first and the second row respectively show the values of different terms of equation (16) for the unperturbed configuration (i.e. the reconstruction generated by the hybrid DARCES-ICP algorithm) and the optimal configuration (for a perturbation of -0.4^0 about the x-axis, yielding the minimum normalized *CRM* value). These results show the effectiveness of the novel second phase of the proposed virtual reconstruction.

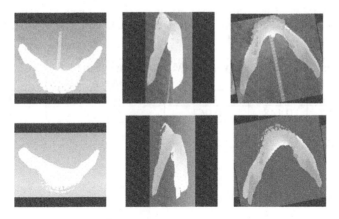

Fig. 4. Comparison of the original and reconstructed mandibles. The top row is the original mandible and the bottom row is the reconstructed mandible obtained using DARCES-ICP hybrid algorithm. The first, second and the third columns represent the 3D projections along the x, y and z axes respectively.

Table 1. A comparison of MSE values obtained by applying various surface matching algorithms [12, 19]

Surface Matching Scheme	MSE (mm^2)
ICP	0.91
DARCES	0.33
Hybrid DARCES-ICP	0.25

Table 2. Symmetry plane determination for a typical unperturbed state resulting from phase-I of the reconstruction

γ	β	GM	Equation of the Plane	Comment
0.79	0.88	0.83	0.98x – 0.16y + 0.12z = 65.42	Plane of Bilateral Symmetry
0.27	0.72	0.50	-0.20x + 0.87y – 0.45 z = 58.78	-
0.35	0.82	0.59	-0.03x + 0.47y + 0.88z = 50.95	-

Table 3. Comparison of the normalized variations of the different terms in eqn. (16) and their coefficients in eqn. (17)

	MSE	Inverse Global Symmetry	Average Surface Area
Variations	0.86	0.07	0.12
Coefficients	0.82	0.06	0.11

The experimental results and subsequent analysis presented in this section are for a typical single fracture reconstruction which is carried out using our developed software *InSilicoSurgeon* [12], which is built on top of *ImageJ*, the imaging software from *NIH* [28]. Our software contains a simple but elegant Graphical User Interface

Table 4. Comparison of the performance measures associated with the optimal state (-0.4^0 rotation about x-axis) and the unperturbed state (the MSE, Inverse_GM, Average Surface Area and CRM values are all normalized).

Axis	Angle	MSE	Inverse_GM	Average Surface Area	CRM
x	-0.4^0	0.138	0.952	0.892	0.275
-	-	0.148	0.964	0.982	0.293

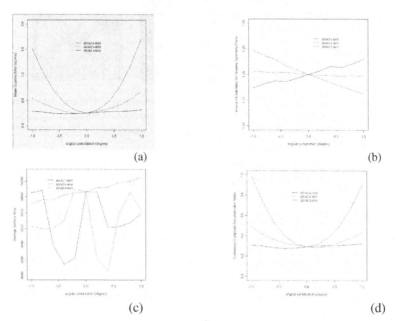

(a)　　　　　　　　　　(b)

(c)　　　　　　　　　　(d)

Fig. 5. Variations in the (a) mean squared error (ξ^2) (b) Inverse Global Metric for the Plane of Bilateral Symmetry (GM^{-1}) (c) Average Surface Area ((TSA + BSA/2)) (d) Normalized *CRM*, with angular perturbation along all the three major axes

InSilicoSurgeon 1.0			
Image PreProcessing	Thresholding	CCL	Boundary Extraction
Reconstruction Phase-I	DARCES	ICP	Hybrid DARCES-ICP
Reconstruction Phase-II	Shape Symmetry	Biomechanical Stability	Angular Perturbation
Geometric Transformation and Help	Rotation	Translation	Help

Fig. 6. A snapshot of the developed GUI where the extreme left column describes various stages of the reconstruction and each button performs a dedicated task (is evident from the name of the button)

(GUI) which can be of substantial help for virtual surgery as well as surgical training purposes. A *Help* button is provided for general guidance. The *Geometric Transformation* button (see Fig. 6) is used to finally bring the various bone fragments into registration.

9   Model Generation and Validation of the Virtual Reconstruction

In addition to the visual comparison and qualitative estimation of the accuracy of the virtual craniofacial reconstruction, we used solid modeling for further validation. The serial images of the reconstructed human mandible were loaded into the 3D Doctor software [29] which builds the virtual solid model from the serial CT scans and facilitates initial processing and 3-D viewing. Solid models were saved in the STL file format for prototype development and further analyses. The solid models were printed on a StratoSys rapid prototype printer (model: Dimension, software: Catalyst 3.4)[1], which reproduces a solid model by layering high density polyethylene plastic in 4 nm layers with repeated passes. A comparison of key anatomical measurements between the reference and reconstructed mandible were made. The STL files were transformed via AutoCAD into a Pro/E compatible file format for Finite Element (FE) analyses. Research is also currently underway for assigning appropriate material properties and for identifying a suitable constitutive model for the mandible material.

10   Conclusions and Future Work

The paper addressed the important problem of virtual craniofacial reconstruction with multiple objectives of obtaining accurate local surface matching as well as ensuring global shape preservation and biomechanical stability of the reconstructed human mandible. The present application can be used as a pre-surgical planning tool and as a training tool for surgical residents. In phase-I of the reconstruction, two different classes of algorithms namely the ICP and the DARCES were first applied individually and then in a cascaded manner for accurate surface matching. The combination of the two algorithms resulted in an improved MSE, and a considerable reduction in the execution time compared to the ICP algorithm used in isolation. The plane of bilateral symmetry was computed for the best possible reconstruction resulting from the first phase, using a novel combination of the normalized cross-correlation and a set theoretic measure. Minimization of surface area was shown to be mathematically equivalent to minimization of surface energy and used as a measure of biomechanical stability. The average surface area was estimated for the best reconstructed mandible resulting from the first phase. A composite reconstruction metric, expressed as a linear combination of the mean squared error, global shape symmetry and surface area, was introduced as a performance measure in the second phase of the reconstruction. A local search in this phase, based on an angular perturbation scheme, was shown to result in a solution that minimizes the composite reconstruction metric instead of just the MSE alone. A validation scheme was proposed to measure the effectiveness of the entire reconstruction by generation of a solid model of the reconstructed mandible. It is important to note that although the experiments thus far have been performed on phantom data sets (experiments on real data sets are ongoing), our reconstruction paradigm, with the statistically robust RANSAC-based DARCES algorithm, as an integral component, is adequate to handle the issue of outliers and missing data in case of real data sets. The hybrid DARCES-ICP algorithm could be expected to provide an accurate reconstruction (with lower MSE) followed by the

---

[1] 14950, Martin Dr. Eden Prairie, MN 55344, USA.

second reconstruction phase to guarantee a minimum *CRM* value on real data sets. Future research will involve (i) model guided feedback to fine tune the coefficients of the different terms in the composite metric in equations (16) and (17) to result in an even better reconstruction, and (ii) extending the present single fracture reconstruction framework to multiple fractures using a combinatorial optimization approach.

References

1. R. E. King, J.M. Scianna and G.J. Petruzzelli, Mandible fracture patterns: a suburban trauma center experience: *American Journal of Otolaryngology.* 25(5), pp. 301-307, 2004.
2. B.O. Ogundare, A. Bonnick and N. Bayley, Pattern of mandibular fractures in an urban major trauma center: *Journal of Oral & Maxillofacial Surgery.* 61(6), pp. 713-718, 2003.
3. C. Zahl, D. Muller, S. Felder and K.L. Gerlach, Cost of miniplate osteosynthesis for treatment of mandibular fractures: a prospective evaluation. *Gesundheitswesen,* 65(10): pp. 561-565, 2003.
4. W. Mollemans, F. Schutyser, N. Nadjmi and P. Suetens, Very fast soft tissue predictions with mass tensor model for maxillofacial surgery planning systems: *Proc. of 9th Annual Conference of the International Society for Computer Aided Surgery*, pp. 491 – 496, 2005.
5. E. Keeve, S. Girod and B. Girod, Craniofacial Surgery Simulation: *Proc. of Visualization in Biomedical Computing,* pp. 541 – 546, Springer 1996.
6. R. Enciso, A. Memon, U. Neumann, and J. Mah, The Virtual Cranio-Facial Patient Project: *Proc. of 3D Imaging*, (Medical Imaging Session) 2003.
7. A. Sarti, R. Gori, C. Marchetti, A. Bianchi and C. Lamberti, Maxillofacial Virtual Surgery from 3D CT Images: *VR in medicine*, Ed. by M. Akay and A. Marsh, IEEE EMBS Series, IEEE Press. 1999.
8. P.J. Besl and N.D. McKay, A Method for Registration of 3-D Shapes, *IEEE Trans. PAMI,* Vol. 14(2), pp. 239 – 256, 1992.
9. S. Granger, X. Pennec, and A. Roche, Rigid Point-Surface Registration Using an EM variant of ICP for Computer Guided Oral Implantology: *Proc. of the Int. Conf. on Medical Image Computing and Computer Assisted Intervention (MICCAI),* LNCS Vol. 2208, pp. 752-761, Utrecht, The Netherlands, 2001.
10. C.S. Chen, RANSAC-Based DARCES: A New Approach to Fast Automatic Registration of Partially Overlapping Range Images, *IEEE Trans. PAMI,* 21(11), pp. 1229 – 1234, 1999.
11. M. Rogers and J. Graham, Robust Active Shape Model Search for Medical Image Analysis, *Proc. of Int. Conf. on Medical Image Understanding and Analysis (MIUA),* Portsmouth, UK, 2002.
12. S.M. Bhandarkar, A.S. Chowdhury, Y. Tang, J. Yu and E.W. Tollner: Surface Matching Algorithms for Computer Aided Reconstructive Plastic Surgery: *Proc. of IEEE Int. Symposium on Biomedical Imaging (ISBI)*, pp. 740 - 743; Arlington, USA. 2004.
13. H. Goldstein, *Classical Mechanics,* Chapter 5, Addison-Wesley, 1982.
14. Y. Wang, B. Peterson and L. Staib, Shape-based 3D Surface Correspondence Using Geodesics and Local Geometry. *IEEE Conf. on Computer Vision and Pattern Recognition (CVPR),* Vol. II, pp. 644- 651, 2000.
15. K.M. Pohl, S.K. Warfield, R. Kikinis, W.E.L. Grimson and W.M. Wells, Coupling Statistical Segmentation and PCA Shape Modeling: *Proc. of the Int. Conf. on Medical Image Computing and Computer Assisted Intervention MICCAI,* Vol. I, pp. 151- 159, Saint-Marlo, France, 2004.

16. W.Y. Kim and A.C. Kak, 3-D Object Recognition Using Bipartite Matching Embedded in Discrete Relaxation, *IEEE Trans. PAMI,* 13(3), pp. 224 – 251, 1991.
17. H.W. Kuhn, The Hungarian method for the assignment problem, *Nav. Res. Log.* Quart. 2, 1955.
18. K.S. Arun, T.S. Huang and S.D. Blostein, Least-Squares Fitting of Two 3-D Point Sets, *IEEE Trans. PAMI,* Vol. 9(5), pp. 698 – 700, 1987.
19. S.M. Bhandarkar, A.S. Chowdhury, E.W. Tollner, J.C. Yu, E.W. Ritter and A. Konar: Surface Reconstruction for Computer Vision-based Craniofacial Surgery. *Proc. of IEEE Int. Workshop on Applications of Computer Vision (WACV),* pp. 257 – 262, Breckenridge, USA. 2005.
20. S. Prima, S. Ourselin, and N. Ayache. Computation of the Mid-Sagittal Plane in 3D Brain Images. *IEEE Trans. on Medical Imaging,* 21(2), pp. 122-138, 2002.
21. B. Ardekani, J. Kershaw, M. Braun and I. Kanno, Automatic Detection of the Mid-Sagittal Plane in 3-D Brain Images, *IEEE Trans. Medical Imaging,* Vol. 16(6), 1997, 947- 952.
22. A. Tuzikov, O. Colliot and I. Bloch, Brain Symmetry plane computation in MR images using inertia axes and optimization, *Intl. Conf. on Pattern Recognition,* Vol. 1, pp. 10516-10519, 2002.
23. S. Gefan, Y. Fan, L. Bertrand and J. Nissanov, Symmetry-based 3D Brain Reconstruction, *IEEE Symp. Biomedical Imaging,* pp. 744 – 747, 2004.
24. L. Junck, J.G. Moen, G.D. Hutchins, M.B. Brown, and D.E. Kuhl, Correlation methods for the centering, rotation and alignment of functional brain images, *Journal of Nuclear Medicine.,* Vol. 31(7), pp. 1220- 1226, 1990.
25. I.H. Shames, *Mechanics of deformable solids.* Prentice-Hall Inc., Englewood Cliffs, NJ, 1964.
26. P.J. Besl, Surfaces in Early Range Image Understanding. *PhD Thesis,* Chapter 3, Univ. of Michigan. 1986.
27. M. Suk and S.M. Bhandarkar, *Three-dimensional Object Recognition from Range Images,* Chapter 7, Springer-Verlag, Tokyo. 1992.
28. *ImageJ* Website: http://rsb.info.nih.gov.
29. *3D Doctor* Website: http://www.ablesw.com/3d-doctor/3ddoctor.html.

A Novel Unsupervised Segmentation Method for MR Brain Images Based on Fuzzy Methods

Xian Fan[1], Jie Yang[1], Yuanjie Zheng[1], Lishui Cheng[1], and Yun Zhu[2]

[1] Institute of Image Processing and Pattern Recognition,
Shanghai Jiao Tong University (SJTU), Shanghai, 200030, P.R.China
[2] Department of Biomedical Engineering, Yale University, New Haven, CT, USA

Abstract. Image segmentation is an important research topic in image processing and computer vision community. In this paper, we present a novel segmentation method based on the combination of fuzzy connectedness and adaptive fuzzy C means (AFCM). AFCM handles intensity inhomogeneities problem in magnetic resonance images (MRI) and provides effective seeds for fuzzy connectedness simultaneously. With the seeds selected, fuzzy connectedness method is applied. As fuzzy connectedness method makes full use of the inaccuracy and 'hanging togetherness' property of MRI, our new method behaves well in both simulated and real images.

1 Introduction

Image segmentation is one of the most important step or research topics of computer vision. It is also the foundation of medical image analysis and clinical planning. Due to the great amount of data and the high requirement of segmentation result, automatic segmentation has aroused increasing interest.

Images are by nature fuzzy [1]. This is especially true to the biomedical images. The fuzzy property of images is usually made by the limitation of scanners in the ways of spatial, parametric, and temporal resolutions. The heterogeneous material composition of human organs also adds to the fuzzy property in magnetic resonance images (MRI). As the objective of image segmentation is to extract the object from the other parts, segmentation by hard means may despoil the fuzziness of images, and lead to bad results. By contrast, using fuzzy methods to segment biomedical images would respect the inherent property fully, and could retain inaccuracies and uncertainties as realistically as possible [2].

Although the object regions of biomedical images manifest themselves with heterogeneity of intensity values due to their fuzzy property, knowledgeable human observers could recognize the objects easily from background. That is, the elements in these regions seem to "hang together" to form the object regions in spite of their heterogeneity of intensity.

In 1973, Dunn[3] firstly developed "fuzzy c-means" (FCM) which is a fuzzy clustering method to allow one piece of data to belong to two or more clusters. In [4], Bezdek improved the algorithm so that the objective function minimizes in an iterative procedure. The method is nearly unsupervised, and is computationally fast.

Y. Liu, T. Jiang, and C. Zhang (Eds.): CVBIA 2005, LNCS 3765, pp. 160–169, 2005.

However, FCM does not address the problem of intensity inhomogeneities. Therefore, it does not work well in the presence of great noise. As intensity inhomogeneities are caused by non-uniformities in the RF field during acquisition, they often happen to MRI. In 1999, Pham and Prince [5] improved FCM and proposed a new method AFCM, which behaves well to overcome the problem of intensity inhomogeneities. But AFCM may perform poorly in the presence of extreme noise [5].

In [6], Rosenfeld developed fuzzy digital topological and geometric concepts. He defined fuzzy connectedness by using a min-max construct on fuzzy subsets of 2-D picture domains. Based on these, Udupa [7] introduces a fundamental concept called affinity, which combined fuzzy connectedness directly with images and utilized it for image segmentation. Thus the properties of inaccuracy and hanging togetherness are made full use of. However, the step of manual selection of seeds, although onerous and time-consuming, is unavoidable in the initialization of fuzzy connectedness. Moreover, it is hard to select effective seeds in the presence of extreme noise, especially when the object is not connected.

This paper proposes a novel segmentation method based on the combination of fuzzy connectedness and AFCM, and applies it to segment MR brain images. The proposed algorithm first simultaneously achieves inhomogeneity compensation and automatic seed selection through AFCM, then fuzzy connectedness method is applied using the selected seeds. The contribution of this paper is as follows. 1). The proposed segmentation method is robust to intensity inhomogeneities. 2). The procedure is unsupervised since the seeds for fuzzy connectedness are automatically selected. 3). Accuracy of result is further enhanced due to the good behavior of fuzzy connectedness. Experiments on simulated and real MR brain images prove that this new method behaves well.

The remainder of this paper is organized as follows. Section 2 briefly introduces the fuzzy connectedness method and AFCM. Section 3 describes our fuzzy connectedness and AFCM based method in detail. Section 4 presents the experimental results. Conclusions are given in Section 5.

2   Background

This section briefly describes the two fuzzy methods, fuzzy connectedness method and AFCM.

2.1   Fuzzy Connectedness

First, we summarize the fuzzy connectedness method for segmentation proposed by Udupa[7].

Let X be any reference set. A *fuzzy subset* of $\mathcal{A}$ is a set of ordered pairs where $\mu_{\mathcal{A}} : X \rightarrow [0,1]$. $\mu_{\mathcal{A}}$ is called the *membership function* of $\mathcal{A}$ in X.

Let Z^n be the set of all spels (space elements) in n-dimensional Euclidean space R^n. A fuzzy relation α in Z^n is said to be a *fuzzy adjacency* if it is both reflexive and symmetric. It is desirable that α be such that is a non increasing function of the distance $\| c - d \|$ between c and d .We call the pair (Z^n, α), where α is a fuzzy adjacency, a *fuzzy digital space*.

A *scene over* a fuzzy digital space (Z^n, α) is a pair $\mathcal{C} = (C, f)$ where $C = \{c \mid -b_j \leq c_j \leq b_j$ for some $b \in Z_+^n\}$; Z_+^n is the set of n -tuples of positive integers; f , called *scene intensity*, is a function whose domain is C . C is called the *scene domain*, whose range $[L, H]$ is a set of numbers (usually integers).

Let $\mathcal{C} = (C, f)$ be any scene over (Z^n, α) . Any fuzzy relation κ in C is said to be a *fuzzy spel affinity* (or, *affinity* for short) *in* $\mathcal{C}$ if it is reflexive and symmetric. In practice, for κ to lead to meaningful segmentation, it should be such that, for any $c, d \in C$, $\mu_\kappa(c, d)$ is a function of 1) the fuzzy adjacency between c and d ; 2) the homogeneity of the spel intensities at c and d ; 3) the closeness of the spel intensities and of the intensity-based features of c and d to some expected intensity and feature values for the object. Further, $\mu_\kappa(c, d)$ may depend on the actual location of $\mu_\kappa(c, d)$ (i.e., μ_κ is shift variant).

Path strength is denoted as the strength of a certain path connecting two spels. Saha and Udupa[7] have shown that under a set of reasonable assumptions the minimum of affinities is the only valid choice for path strength. So the path strength is

$$\mu_{\mathcal{N}}(p) = \min_{1 < i \leq l_p} \left[\mu_\kappa(c_{i-1}, c_i) \right], \tag{1}$$

where p is the path $< c_1, c_2, ..., c_{l_p} >$ and $\mathcal{N}$ is denoted as the fuzzy κ -net in C . Every pair of (c_{i-1}, c_i) is a link in the path while c_{i-1} and c_i may not always be adjacent.

For any scene $\mathcal{C}$ over (Z^n, α) , for any affinity κ and κ –net $\mathcal{N}$ in $\mathcal{C}$, fuzzy κ -connectedness K in $\mathcal{C}$ is a fuzzy relation in C defined by the following membership function. For any $c, d \in C$

$$\mu_K(c, d) = \max_{p \in P_{cd}} \left[\mu_{\mathcal{N}}(p) \right]. \tag{2}$$

Combined with eq.(1), eq.(2) shows the min-max property of the fuzzy connectedness between each two spels, as is illustrated in Fig.1.

As in Fig.1., a physical analogy one may consider is to think that there are a lot of strings connecting spels A and B , each with its own strength (called path strength as to a certain path). Imagine A and B are pulled apart. Under the force the strings will break one by one. As to a certain string, the link where the string breaks is denoted as the path strength of this string (the path strength is defined as the minimum affinity of

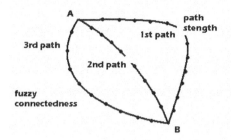

Fig. 1. Illustration of the path strength and fuzzy connectedness described in fuzzy connectedness method

all the links in the path). When all but one string are broken, the last string behave as the strongest one and it's path strength is denoted as the fuzzy connectedness between spels A and B.

Let S be any subset of C. We refer to S as the set of seed spels and assume throughout that $S \neq \varnothing$. The fuzzy $k\theta$ -object of $\mathcal{C}$ containing S equals

$$O_{K\theta}(S) = \left\{ c \mid c \in C \text{ and } \max_{s \in S}[\mu_K(s,c)] \geq \theta \right\}. \tag{3}$$

With eq.(3), we could extract the object we want given θ and S. This could be computed via dynamic programming [7].

2.2 AFCM

We now briefly describe the objective function for AFCM. Detailed and complete descriptions of steps are provided in [5]. The objective function for AFCM is as follows.

$$
\begin{aligned}
J_{AFCM} &= \sum_{i,j} \sum_{k=1}^{C} u_k(i,j)^2 \left\| y(i,j) - m(i,j)v_k \right\|^2 \\
&+ \lambda_1 \sum_{i,j} \left(\left(D_i * m(i,j) \right)^2 + \left(D_j * m(i,j) \right)^2 \right) \\
&+ \lambda_2 \sum_{i,j} \left(\left(D_{ii} * m(i,j) \right)^2 + 2 \left(D_{ij} * m(i,j) \right)^2 + \left(D_{jj} * m(i,j) \right)^2 \right)
\end{aligned}
\tag{4}
$$

In which $u_k(i,j)$ is the membership value at pixel location (i,j) for class k. $y(i,j)$ is the observed image intensity at location (i,j), and v_k is the centroid of class k. The total number of classes C is assumed to be known. D_i and D_j are the standard forward finite difference operators along the rows and columns, and $D_{ii} = D_i * D_i$, $D_{jj} = D_j * D_j$, and $D_{ij} = D_i * *D_j$ are second-order finite differences. The symbols '$*$' and '$**$' denote the one and two-dimensional discrete convolution operators, respectively. The last two terms is the first-order and second-order regularization, respectively and λ_1, λ_2 is the parameters. The major difference between FCM and AFCM is $m(i, j)$, which is assumed to be smooth and slowly varying. It is by multiplying the centroids by $m(i, j)$ that AFCM could compensate intensity inhomogeneities.

3 Proposed Method

In this section, we propose a new segmentation method which is unsupervised and robust, based on the combination of fuzzy connectedness and AFCM.

Intensity inhomogeneities are the common problem to most of real MRI. There are two ways to compensate them. The first is to preprocess the images with the correction algorithm followed by the segmentation one. The second is to correct and segment the image simultaneously. In the proposed method, AFCM is applied to the images first so that not only the intensity inhomogeneities are compensated, but also the images are segmented. Since AFCM may perform poorly in the presence of extreme noise [5], this segmentation result is only used as the pre-segmentation one.

On the other hand, as Udupa has been trying to utilize the fuzzy nature of the biomedical images in both aspects of inaccuracy and hanging togetherness, users' identifying seed spels belonging to the various objects is always left to be an onerous task. Therefore, automatic selection of seeds becomes important in our research work.

Our new method combines the two fuzzy methods organically. In the proposed method, while seed selection is made automatic, the intensity inhomogeneities could be overcome, and the accuracies of the result are guaranteed. Our goal is to both implement automatic seed selection and guarantee the segmentation quality.

The outline of the new method is as follows. First, AFCM is used to pre-segment the MR brain image, through which the scope of the seeds is obtained. Since the number of seeds within the scope is much more than that we need, the seeds within the scope are automatically eliminated according to their spatial information. With the left seeds as an initialization, the MR brain image is segmented by fuzzy connectedness. Here are the detailed steps of our proposed algorithm applied to MR brain images.

Step 1. Preprocess the MR brain images, including denoising, intensity correction. In intensity correction, a standardized histogram of MR brain image is acquired, and all the other images' is corrected so that their histogram would match the standardized one as best as possible [8].

Step 2. Set the cluster number C to 4, and pre-segment the image by AFCM, so that the expected segmented objects will be white matter, grey matter, CSF and background.

Step 3. After the convergence of AFCM, compute each cluster's centroid v_k, $k = 1, 2, 3, 4$.

Step 4. Compute the variance δ_k of the k th cluster. The scope of the seeds is defined by the equation

$$v_k \pm 0.3\,\delta_k . \tag{5}$$

in which 0.3 is the heuristic parameter.

Step 5. Define N as the number of seeds in fuzzy connectedness.

Step 6. Take the spatial information of the spels within the scope into account, and class them into N clusters. Make the center spels of each cluster the seeds as initialization.

Step 7. Segment the image precisely with selected seeds by fuzzy connectedness method.

With step 1, we get the standardized histogram of each MR brain image, which guarantees that the parameter 0.3 in eq.(5) will work. Then according to the average and variance intensity of the object of interest, the scope of the seeds could be gotten with the eq.(5). Although this is a heuristic algorithm, it could be noticed in section 4 that it does work in different situations. What's more, since the spatial information of these spels is taken into account, the automatically selected seeds are effective.

4 Experimental Results

In this section, we give the experimental results with both simulated and real MR brain images.

To simulated images, as the reference result is the "ground truth", accuracy is described with three parameters: true positive volume fraction (TPVF), false positive volume fraction (FPVF), and false negative volume fraction (FNVF). These parameters are defined as follows:

$$FPVF(V,V_t) = \frac{|V - V_t|}{|V_t|}, FNVF(V,V_t) = \frac{|V_t - V|}{|V_t|} . \tag{6}$$

Where V_t denotes the set of spels in the reference result, V denotes the set of spels resulting from the users' algorithms. $FPVF(V,V_t)$ denotes the cardinality of the set of spels expressed as a fraction of the cardinality of V_t that are in the segmentation result of the method but not in V_t. Analogously, $FNVF(V,V_t)$ denotes a fraction of V_t that is missing in V. We use probability of error (PE) to evaluate the overall accuracy of the simulated image segmentation. PE [9] could be described as

$$PE = FPVF(V,V_t) + FNVF(V,V_t) . \tag{7}$$

The larger PE is, the poorer the accuracy of the segmentation method is.

To the real images, as the reference result is made manually, the inaccuracy of the reference segmentation result should be taken into account. Zijdenbos's[10] Dice Similarity Coefficient (DSC), which has been adopted for voxel-by-voxel classification agreement, is proper to evaluate the segmentation result of real images. We now describe it as follows. For any type T, assuming that V_m denotes the set of pixels assigned for it by manual segmentation and V_α denotes the set of pixels assigned for it by the algorithm, DSC is defined as follows:

$$DSC = 2 \; \frac{|V_m \cap V_\alpha|}{|V_m| + |V_\alpha|} . \tag{8}$$

Since manual segmentations are not "ground truth", DSC provides a reasonable way to evaluate automated segmentation methods.

4.1 Simulated Images

We applied our method on simulated MR brain images provided by McConnell Brain Image Center [11]. As the brain database has provided the gold standard, validation of the segmentation methods could be carried out. The experimental images in this paper were imaged with T1 modality, 217 * 181 (spels) resolution and 1mm slice thickness. 5% noise has been put up and the intensity-nonuniformity is 40%.

We take the 81th to 100th slices of the whole brain MRI in the database, and segment them with fuzzy connectedness (FC), AFCM and the proposed method respectively. The evaluation values are listed in table 1 according to the gold standard.

It could be noticed in table 1 that our method behaves best, and the second is AFCM, the last fuzzy connectedness. That is because when faced with relatively high noise, it is hard to select fine seeds manually for fuzzy connectedness, especially to grey matter and CSF. However, when the intensity inhomogeneities are compensated by AFCM, fuzzy connectedness works well, showing that the automatically selected

Table 1. Average value of 20 simulated images using three segmentation methods (%)

Study	TPVF	FPVF	FNVF	PE
AFCM	97.31	2.30	2.69	4.99
FC	96.23	2.02	3.77	5.79
Proposed Method	98.68	1.23	1.32	2.55

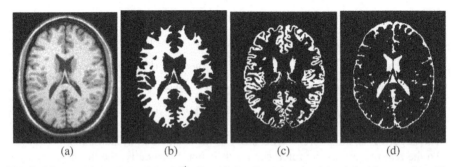

(a)   (b)   (c)   (d)

Fig. 2. Segmentation result of the 90th slice of simulated images (a) original image; (b) white matter; (c) grey matter; (d) CSF

seeds are effective. Thus, the proposed method behaves best, with the high accuracy obtained by fuzzy connectedness and compensated intensity inhomogeneities by AFCM. Fig.2 shows the 90th slice of the simulated database. Fig.2 (b), (c) and (d) are white matter, grey matter and CSF, respectively.

4.2 Real Images

We applied our method to twelve real MRI brain data sets. They were imaged with a 1.5 T MRI system (GE, Signa) with the resolution 0:94 *1.25*1.5 mm (256* 192* 124 voxels). These data sets have been previously labeled through a labor-intensive (usually 50 hours per brain) manual method by an expert. We first applied our method on these data sets and then compared with expert results. We give the results from the 5th to the 12th of them gained by our method in Table 2 and Fig. 3.

Table 2. Average DSC of the 5th to 12th real cases using three segmentation methods (%)

	1	2	3	4	5	6	7	8
FC	74	75	78	76	75	78	76	78
AFCM	77	78	80	81	82	83	82	81
Proposed Method	83	84	85	83	84	86	83	82

According to table 2, the rank of DSC of three methods is the same as that in simulated image experiments. There are several data sets corrupted badly by noise, and the intensity inhomogeneities are rather common in these real images. As AFCM has the function of compensate intensity inhomogeneities, it behaves better than fuzzy connectedness. However, fuzzy connectedness shows high accuracy when the selected seeds are effective. Thus, through the compensation of intensity inhomogeneities and automatic selection of seeds by AFCM, the proposed method segments the images with the highest accuracy of the three.

We segment the white matter, grey matter and CSF, respectively, using proposed method, fuzzy connectedness and AFCM. Take the 8th case as an illustration. Fig.3 is the segmentation result of the 70th slice of the whole brain. As the automatically

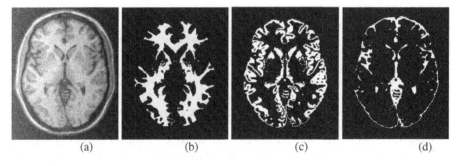

(a)   (b)   (c)   (d)

Fig. 3. Segmentation result of real images (a) original image; (b) white matter; (c) grey matter; (d) CSF

selected seed number is defined beforehand, we choose 10 for white matter, 25 fore grey matter and 30 for CSF. That's because in grey matter and CSF, the objects are not connected due to noise and heterogeneous composition of human organs. And because fuzzy connectedness segments one object of one seed in it, the last step of the proposed method need more seeds for grey matter and CSF.

5 Conclusion

Accuracy and automation are the two main goals in image segmentation. The proposed method is designed especially to aim at these two goals. The experiments illustrate that the proposed method is unsupervised, and more accurate than both AFCM and fuzzy connectedness method.

Fuzziness is the nature of images. When images are segmented by fuzzy means, the inaccuracy property of the elements is adopted. AFCM makes use of fuzzy clustering techniques, and compensates the intensity inhomogeneities of the images. On the other hand, fuzzy connectedness is a method which takes both the inaccuracies and hanging-togetherness of the elements into consideration. That is, it takes into account not only the intensity information, but the location of spels and their mutual relationship as well. Although fuzzy connectedness method behaves well, the selection of seeds takes operators time and energy. And in the case of great noise, it is so hard to select enough effective seeds for an ordinary operator. In our fuzzy connectedness and AFCM based method, the intensity inhomogeneities problem is solved by AFCM, and at the same time automatic seed selection is implemented. Our method is robust due to the high accuracy of fuzzy connectedness. Moreover, as the number of automatically selected seeds could be controlled, automatic seed selection is as manageable as manual one. Through simulated and real image experiments, we could see that the proposed method could not only automatically select seeds, but has a relatively high accuracy.

References

1. Udupa, J.K., Saha, P.K.: Fuzzy Connectedness and Imaging Segmentation. Proceedings of The IEEE. Vol.91, No.10, pp: 1649-1669, 2003
2. Saha, P.K., Udupa, J.K. and Odhner, D.: Scale-based fuzzy connected image segmentation: Theory, algorithms, and validation. Computer Vision and Image Understanding. Vol.77, pp: 145-174, 2000
3. Dunn, J.C. A Fuzzy Relative of the ISODATA Process and Its Use in Detecting Compact Well-Separated Clusters. Journal of Cybernetics. Vol.3, pp: 32, 1973
4. Bezdek, J.C.: Pattern Recognition with Fuzzy Objective Function Algorithms. Plenum Press. 1981
5. Pham, D.L., Prince, J.L.: An Adaptive Fuzzy C-Means Algorithm for Image Segmentation in the Presence of Intensity Inhomogeneities. Pattern Recognition Letters. Vol.20, No.1, pp: 57-68, 1999.
6. Rosenfeld, A. Fuzzy digital topology. Information and Control. Vol.40, No.1, pp: 76, 1979

7. Udupa, J.K. Samarasekera, S. Fuzzy Connectedness and Object Definition: Theory, Algorithms, and Applications in Image Segmentation. Graphical Model and Image Processing. Vol.58, No.3, pp: 246, 1995
8. Nyul, L.G., Udupa, J.K.: On standardizing the MR image intensity scale. Magn Reson Med. Vol.42, pp: 1072-1081, 1999
9. Dam, E.B.: Evaluation of diffusion schemes for multiscale watershed segmentation. MSC. Dissertation, University of Copenhagen, 2000
10. Zijdenbos, A.P., Dawant, B.M., Margolin, R.A., Palmer, A.C. : Morphometric analysis of white matter lesions in MR images: Method and validation. IEEE Transactions on Medical Imaging. Vol.13, No.4, pp: 716, 1994
11. Cocosco, C.A., Kollokian, V., Kwan, R.K.-S., Evans, A.C.: BrainWeb: Online Interface to a 3D MRI Simulated Brain Database. NeuroImage. Vol.5, No.4, pp: part 2/4, S425, 1994

A Pattern Classification Approach to Aorta Calcium Scoring in Radiographs

Marleen de Bruijne

IT University of Copenhagen, Denmark
marleen@itu.dk

Abstract. A method for automated detection of calcifications in the abdominal aorta from standard X-ray images is presented. Pixel classification based on local image structure is combined with a spatially varying prior that is derived from a statistical model of the combined shape variation in aorta and spine.

Leave-one-out experiments were performed on 87 standard lateral lumbar spine X-rays, resulting in on average 93.7% of the pixels within the aorta being correctly classified.

1 Introduction

Calcifications in the abdominal aorta were shown to correlate with the presence — or future development — of calcifications at other sites such as the coronary arteries, and are an important predictor for future cardiovascular morbidity and mortality [7,12,13]. Accurate and reproducible measurement of the amount of calcified deposit in the aorta is therefore of great value in diagnosis, treatment planning, and the study of drug effects. Several automatic and semi-automatic calcium scoring methods have been proposed for CT [2,9].

This paper aims at automatically detecting calcified plaques in the lumbar aorta from standard radiographs. Although CT is better suited for identifying and quantifying atherosclerosis, standard X-rays have the advantage that they are cheap and fast. Several approaches to manually quantifying the severity of aortic calcification in radiographs have been proposed, of which the antero-posterior severity score by Kauppila et al. [10] is the most popular. For this score, the lumbar part of the aorta is divided in four segments adjacent to the four vertebra L1-L4, and the severity of the anterior and posterior aortic calcification are graded individually for each segment on a 0-3 scale. The results are summed in a composite severity score ranging from 0 to 24. Such manual scoring systems have been successfully applied in epidemiological studies, but can not describe subtle changes in disease progression and are labor-intensive and prone to inter- and intra-observer variations.

An automated calcification detection scheme would allow for automatic scoring according to the current semi-quantitative standards as well as for continuous and likely more precise quantification by for instance counting the number of calcified pixels or assessing the density of separate calcifications [3]. To our knowledge, no method currently exists for automatic detection of calcified plaques from standard radiographs.

Calcifications show up in X-ray images as small and usually elongated bright structures. One of the main problems in automatic detection of calcification is that many

Y. Liu, T. Jiang, and C. Zhang (Eds.): CVBIA 2005, LNCS 3765, pp. 170–177, 2005.

other structures in the image, e.g. bone and image artifacts, have a similar appearance. If the location of the aorta is known in the image the detection becomes easier, but aorta segmentation is a difficult problem as well since the non-calcified parts of the aorta are not visible in X-ray. However, the shape and position of the aorta are strongly correlated to the shape and position of the spine, which is much easier detected in the image. In this work we use knowledge of the shape of the spine to aid appearance-based calcification detection.

We combine pixel classification on the basis of local intensity features with a spatially varying calcium prior that is dependent on the position of a pixel with respect to the spine. The spatially varying prior is derived from a statistical model of combined spine and aorta shape variation, together with a model of how the calcium is distributed within the aorta. The method requires the localization of the corner and midpoints of the first four lumbar vertebra. Currently manual input is used here — obtained from a vertebral morphometry study on the same dataset — but these point positions could also be derived from an automatic spine segmentation, see e.g. [6,11].

Section 2 of this paper deals with modelling the distribution of calcium inside the aorta as well as modelling the distribution of calcium in relation to the vertebrae. Our approach to calcium detection, combining appearance-based pixel classification and the models of calcium distribution, is described in Section 3. Section 4 presents experiments on 87 digitized X-ray images, and a discussion and conclusion are given in Section 5.

2   Estimating Calcium Prior Probability

It is well known that the distribution of calcification in the aorta is not uniform. The number of plaques increases towards the aortic bifurcation, and due to the projection imaging the majority of the plaques is visible along the anterior and posterior aortic walls and not in between.

If a large training set of example images with annotated aorta and calcifications was available, the probability of presence of calcium in each pixel could be estimated by labelling calcified pixels as 1 and non-calcified as 0, warping all aortas on top of each other, and computing the average labelled aorta image.

If the training set is limited the above procedure will lead to incorrect results; pixels inside the aorta may coincidentally have a very high or low probability of being calcified. As a trade-off between generalizability and specificity, in this work we model the cross-sectional and longitudinal presence of calcium separately.

In a set of labelled training images, the part of the aorta adjacent to the first four lumbar vertebrae is selected and intensity profiles are sampled perpendicular to the vessel axis, reaching from the anterior to the posterior wall. All profiles are normalized to equal length and averaged to form a cross-sectional calcium prior distribution. For each image, one longitudinal profile is formed by summing the values in the individual profiles. An average longitudinal profile is computed by length normalizing and averaging the longitudinal profiles of all images.

For a given aorta shape, a calcium prior probability map can then be constructed by sweeping the cross-sectional prior profile along the axis, modulated with the longitudi-

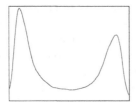 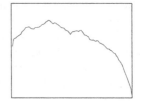

Fig. 1. Cross-sectional profile (left) and longitudinal profile (right) of calcium distribution inside the aorta. Prevalence of calcium is higher at the aortic walls and near the aortic bifurcation.

nal profile. The two profiles and an example of a calcium probability map are given in Figures 1 and 2.

2.1   Estimating the Location of Aortic Walls

In general, the shape and location of the aorta will not be known a priori, and since the aortic walls are only visible if calcium is present, automatic aorta segmentation can not be used as a first step to guide calcium detection. However, the shape and location of the aorta are strongly correlated with the shape and location of the spine [4]. In the following we will use a set of training images in which the aorta and the vertebrae have been annotated to model the probability density function of aorta shape and location conditional on the spine shape.

To constrain the shapes of possible aortas, any kind of shape model from which samples can be drawn can be inserted here. We will use the popular linear point distribution models (PDM) as proposed by Cootes and Taylor [5] to model the object shape variations observed in the training set.

In PDMs, shapes are defined by the coordinates of a set of landmark points which correspond between different shape instances. A collection of training shapes are aligned using for instance Procrustes analysis [8] and a principal component analysis (PCA) of the aligned shapes yields the so-called *modes of shape variation* which describe a joint displacement of all landmarks. Each shape can then be approximated by a linear combination of the mean shape and these modes of variation. Usually only a small number of modes is needed to capture most of the variation in the training set.

To construct a conditional shape model of the aorta given the spine, the spine and aorta landmarks are combined into one shape vector. The Procrustes alignment must be done only on the spine part of the combined shapes. The distribution $P(S_1|S_2)$, the probability distribution of the expected aorta shape and pose S_1 for a given spine S_2, can be then modelled as the Gaussian conditional density

$$P(S_1|S_2) = \mathcal{N}(\mu, K)$$

with

$$\mu = \Sigma_{12}\Sigma_{22}^{-1}S_2$$
$$K = \Sigma_{11} - \Sigma_{12}\Sigma_{22}^{-1}\Sigma_{21}$$

and Σ_{ij} are obtained from the covariance matrix of the combined model

$$\Sigma = \begin{bmatrix} \Sigma_{11} & \Sigma_{12} \\ \Sigma_{21} & \Sigma_{22} \end{bmatrix}$$

as

$$\Sigma_{ij} = \frac{1}{n-1} \sum_n (S_{in} - \bar{S}_i)(S_{jn} - \bar{S}_j)^T.$$

An example of the modes of variation of such a conditional model is given in Figure 3.

2.2 Spatially Varying Prior

To derive a spatial calcium prior, the aorta shape distribution is represented by a random sample of N shapes drawn from the Gaussian conditional shape model. The final calcium probability map is then constructed by averaging the N individual prior maps. Note, that to get a true probability the 'prior' would need to be normalized so that the probabilities of the two classes sum to 1. We here omit this normalization.

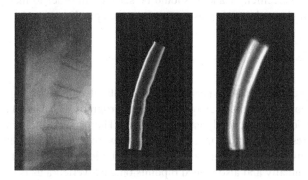

Fig. 2. From left to right: Original image, inverted for better visibility of calcium (left); annotated aorta with constructed calcium probability map; calcium probability map from 50 random samples of the aorta conditional shape model

3 Calcification Detection

A pixel classifier is trained to distinguish between calcium and background pixels on the basis of local image descriptors. We have chosen a general scheme in which pixels are described by the outputs of a set of Gaussian derivative filters at multiple scales, and a k-NN classifier is used for probability estimation. The probability that a pixel with feature vector $\mathbf{x}$ belongs to class ω is thus given by

$$P(\omega|\mathbf{x}) = \frac{k_\omega}{k}, \tag{1}$$

where k_ω among the k nearest neighbors belong to class ω.

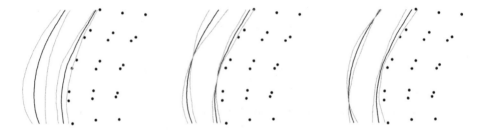

Fig. 3. Modes of variation of the aorta (gray and black lines) given the known positions of vertebrae corner- and mid-points (black points). The mean aorta shape is given in black, the mean shape ± 3 standard deviations in gray. From left to right the first three modes of variation are shown.

The spatial prior can be applied simply as a multiplication of the soft classification from Equation 1 with the calcium prior map as computed in Section 2.

For classification with as well as without spatial prior, a threshold defining the desired sensitivity/specificity tradeoff should be selected in order to make a final binary decision of whether calcium is present or not in each pixel.

4 Experiments

Leave-one-out experiments are performed on 87 lateral spine radiographs taken from a combined osteoporosis-atherosclerosis screening program. The dataset is diverse, ranging from uncalcified to severely calcified aortas. The original radiographs have been scanned at a resolution of 0.1 mm per pixel and were inverted for better visibility of calcific deposits. A medical expert outlined all calcifications adjacent to vertebrae L1 through L4 manually and also placed 6 points on each vertebra as is routinely done in vertebral morphology studies.

4.1 Parameter Settings

Before further analysis the images were normalized to zero mean and unit variance. The appearance features used include the original image and the derivatives up to and including the third order computed at three different scales. Training pixels were selected randomly from a region of interest including the aorta and its surroundings. The set of samples is normalized to unit variance for each feature, and k-NN classification is performed with an approximate k-NN classifier [1] with k=25. In all cases, results reported are accuracies of hard classification with the overall optimal threshold that is kept constant for all 87 images.

In the conditional shape model, 6 manually placed landmarks on each of the vertebrae are used and 50 aorta landmarks are selected on each aortic wall by equidistant sampling along the manual outlines. The first 5 modes of shape variation are selected for the conditional shape model, and $N = 100$ aorta shapes are sampled randomly from the model to form the calcium prior probability map.

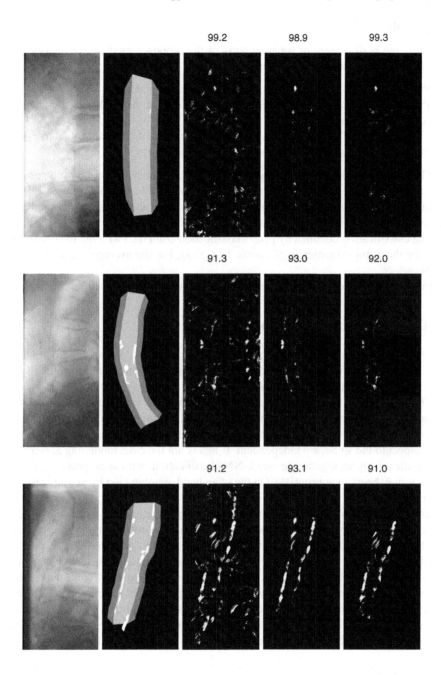

Fig. 4. Examples of classifications obtained for images of varying degree of calcification. Each row gives the different results for one image, from left to right: Original image (inverted for improved visibility of calcium); Manual segmentation; Pixel classification alone; Pixel classification combined with calcium prior for manually segmented aorta; Pixel classification and calcium prior from conditional shape model. The numbers above each image denote the classification accuracy.

4.2   Results

To assess the performance of separate parts of the proposed method, we measure the accuracy in three different experiments:

1. Pixel classification on the basis of appearance features alone
2. Pixel classification on the basis of appearance features combined with calcium prior for a known aorta
3. The complete scheme; pixel classification on the basis of appearance features combined with calcium prior from the conditional model

The pixel classification alone yields an average accuracy, defined as the percentage of correctly classified pixels *inside the aorta*, of 93.8%. Combining this with the spatially varying prior based on the manually drawn aorta shape results in a small, but significant ($p = 0.0004$ in a paired t-test) improvement to 94%.

The classification obtained by pixel classification combined with the fuzzy calcium prior for the aorta estimates is of course less good, but the average accuracy is still 93.7%.

Figure 4 shows examples of the classification results by the three different schemes.

5   Discussion and Conclusion

We propose an automated method for detection of calcified deposits in radiographs of the lumbar aorta, which may be used as an inexpensive screening tool for quantifying atherosclerosis and cardiovascular risk.

The results of a standard pixel classification were improved by combination with a spatially varying prior. The assumption underlying the proposed combination by multiplication is that the two individual probabilities, based on appearance and on position with respect to the spine, are independent. If this is not the case, modelling appearance and position features together in one k-NN classification, with appropriate scaling of features, may be more appropriate. On the other hand, combination by multiplication is much faster.

The current approach, in which the calcification detection task is guided by samples of an aorta shape model, can be extended to a joint optimization of aorta shape distribution and calcification detection. A likelihood weight for each of the aorta shape samples can be defined on basis of how well the expected calcium distribution coincides with the measured calcifications, and subsequently a new shape set — with smaller variance — can be constructed through weighted resampling from the current set. In such an iterative optimization in which the spatial prior is updated in each iteration, the advantage of combination by multiplication instead of using one large k-NN classifier becomes obvious. We are currently investigating the feasibility of such methods.

Acknowledgements

We would like to thank L.B. Tánko and C. Christiansen of the Center for Clinical and Basic Research (CCBR A/S), Denmark, for providing the data sets and manual segmentations used in this study, L.A. Conrad-Hansen and M.T. Lund of the IT University of Copenhagen, Denmark, for providing the software to perform the manual segmentations, and CCBR A/S, Denmark, for funding.

References

1. S. Arya, D.M. Mount, N.S. Netanyahu, R. Silverman, and A.Y. Wu. An optimal algorithm for approximate nearest neighbor searching. *Journal of the ACM*, (45):891–923, 1998.
2. C. Hong C, K.T. Bae, and T.K. Pilgram. Coronary artery calcium: Accuracy and reproducibility of measurements with multi-detector row CT — assessment of effects of different thresholds and quantification methods. *Radiology*, 227:795–801, 2003.
3. L.A. Conrad-Hansen, M. de Bruijne, F.B. Lauze, L.B. Tánko, and M. Nielsen. Quantizing calcification in the lumbar aorta on 2-D lateral X-ray images. In *Proceedings of the ICCV workshop Computer Vision for Biomedical Image Applications: Current Techniques and Future Trends*, Lecture Notes in Computer Science, 2005.
4. L.A. Conrad-Hansen, J. Raundahl, L.B. Tánko, and M. Nielsen. Prediction of the location of the posterior aortic wall using the first four lumbar vertebrae as a predictor. In *Medical Imaging: Image Processing*, volume 5370 of *Proceedings of SPIE*. SPIE Press, 2004.
5. T.F. Cootes, C.J. Taylor, D.H. Cooper, and J. Graham. Active shape models – their training and application. *Computer Vision and Image Understanding*, 61(1):38–59, 1995.
6. M. de Bruijne and M. Nielsen. Shape particle filtering for image segmentation. In *Medical Imaging Computing & Computer-Assisted Intervention*, volume 3216 of *Lecture Notes in Computer Science*, pages I:186–175. Springer, 2004.
7. D.A. Eggen, J.P. Strong, and H.C.J. McGill. Calcification in the abdominal aorta: relationship to race, sex, and coronary atherosclerosis. *Archives of pathology*, 1964.
8. C. Goodall. Procrustes methods in the statistical analysis of shape. *Journal of the Royal Statistical Society B*, 53(2):285–339, 1991.
9. I. Isgum, B. van Ginneken, and M. Olree. Automatic detection of calcifications in the aorta from CT scans of the abdomen. *Academic Radiology*, 11(3):247–257, March 2004.
10. L.I. Kauppila, J.F. Polak, L.A. Cupples, M.T. Hannan, D.P. Kiel, and P.W. Wilson. New indices to classify location, severity and progression of calcific lesions in the abdominal aorta: a 25-year follow-up study. *Atherosclerosis*, 25(132(2)):245–250, 1997.
11. P.P. Smyth, C.J. Taylor, and J.E. Adams. Vertebral shape: Automatic measurement with active shape models. *Radiology*, 211(2):571–578, 1999.
12. P.W.F. Wilson, L.I. Kauppila, C.J. ODonnell, D.P. Kiel, M. Hannan, J.M. Polak, and L.A. Cupples. Abdominal aortic calcific deposits are an important predictor of vascular morbidity and mortality. *Circulation*, 103:1529 – 1534, 2001.
13. J.C.M. Witteman, J.L.C. Van Saase, and H.A. Valkenburg. Aortic calcification as a predictor of cardiovascular mortality. *Lancet*, 2:11201122, 1986.

A Topologically Faithful, Tissue-Guided, Spatially Varying Meshing Strategy for Computing Patient-Specific Head Models for Endoscopic Pituitary Surgery Simulation

M.A. Audette, H. Delingette, A. Fuchs, O. Astley, and K. Chinzei

AIST, Surgical Assist Group, Namiki 1-2, Tsukuba, 305-8564, Japan
m.audette@aist.go.jp

Abstract. This paper presents a method for tessellating tissue boundaries and their interiors, given as input a tissue map consisting of relevant classes of the head, in order to produce anatomical models for finite element-based simulation of endoscopic pituitary surgery. Our surface meshing method is based on the simplex model, which is initialized by duality from the topologically accurate results of the Marching Cubes algorithm, and which features explicit control over mesh scale, while using tissue information to adhere to relevant boundaries. Our mesh scale strategy is spatially varying, based on the distance to a central point or linearized surgical path. The tetrahedralization stage also features a spatially varying mesh scale, consistent with that of the surface mesh.

1 Introduction

Virtual reality (VR) based surgical simulation involves the interaction of a user with an anatomical model representative of clinically relevant tissues and endowed with realistic constitutive properties, through virtual surgical tools. This model must be sufficiently descriptive for the interaction to be clinically meaningful: it must afford advantages over traditional surgical training in terms of improving surgical skill and patient outcome. Our simulation application, *endoscopic transnasal pituitary surgery*, is a procedure that typically involves removing mocusa, enlarging an opening in the sphenoid sinus bone with a rongeur, making an incision in the dura mater, and scooping out the pathology with a curette, while avoiding surrounding critical tissues [4]. This entails anatomical meshing capable of an accurate depiction of the pituitary gland and of the arteries and cranial nerves surrounding it, as well as the brain, relevant sinus bones, dura mater, and any imbedded pathology, as shown in figure 1. This paper presents a method for tessellating tissue boundaries and their interiors, featuring surface and volume meshing stages, as part of a *minimally supervised* procedure for computing patient-specific models for neurosurgery simulation.

Our clinical application, in light of the presence of surrounding critical tissues and the correlation between lack of experience and surgical complications [5], is a good candidate for simulation. Furthermore, this application requires dense

Y. Liu, T. Jiang, and C. Zhang (Eds.): CVBIA 2005, LNCS 3765, pp. 178–188, 2005.

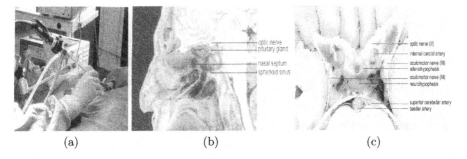

Fig. 1. Illustration of endoscopic trans-nasal pituitary surgery: (a) OR setup; (b) sagittal image of the head featuring the pituitary gland, parasellar bones, brain and cranium; (c) oblique image featuring pituitary gland and surrounding critical tissues (reproduced with permission [4])

shapes in the field of view of the endoscope, while limiting the number of elements overall and still maintaining the conformality of the mesh. This argument justifies the application of a spatially varying mesh strategy. Furthermore, an important objective of ours is the recruitment of finite element (FE) modeling in our simulation, because of the rigorous treatment and the material descriptiveness afforded by the method. Specifically, we want to apply a recent *hierarchical multirate* FE software architecture [1] designed for surgical simulation. As shown on figure 2, this architecture partitions the underlying volume into a sparse, linearly elastic parent mesh as well as one or more dense, possibly nonlinear child meshes. It then decouples the subregions in a manner analogous to the Norton equivalent in circuit analysis: for each subregion, parent or child, it expresses the other subregion(s) encountered at each node as *one* equivalent impedance and force. A FE system composed of a parent and n children, characterized by a relatively large stiffness matrix $\mathbf{K}$, is then reduced to decoupled systems with significantly smaller stiffness matrices $\hat{\mathbf{K}}_i$, $i = 1 \ldots n + 1$.

The implications of our objectives for anatomical meshing are as follows.

1. Assuming that we have a sufficiently descriptive patient-specific tissue map as input, such as illustrated in figure 3 [3], the *meshing must be rigourously tissue-guided*, with the proviso that for the sake of the simulation, it may be allowable, even preferable from a computational standpoint, to consider some tissue boundaries together. Also, it must specifically account for critical tissues in order to penalize gestures that cause damage to them. In constrast, existing meshing methods have been demonstrated typically on imaging data consisting of 2-class problems [14]: inner tissue and outer background, whereas our simulation requires a far more descriptive anatomical mesh.

2. The method must produce as *few elements as possible*, to limit the complexity of the real-time problem, while meeting our requirements for haptic, visual and constitutive realism. Therefore, *mesh scale must be spatially flexible*, to allow small elements near the surgical target, particularly if an

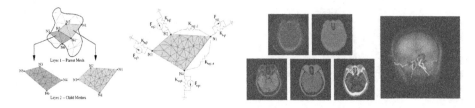

Fig. 2. Partition of FE domain into parent and child meshes; parent Norton equivalents, seen by child (reproduced with permission [1])

Fig. 3. Tissue map computation from CT and MR, exploiting tubular structure of critical tissues and embedded structure of other soft tissues (from [3])

endoscopic view is required, while producing significantly larger elements far away, thereby limiting the number of elements overall, and still maintaining the conformality of the mesh. The hierarchical multirate FE model of [1] suggests a way of treating this mesh that alleviates adverse effect on the condition number of the system, provided that parent and child systems are not themselves too ill-conditioned.

3. The *meshing must reflect the topology* of the underlying tissue: if a tissue features one or more inner boundaries, as well as an outer boundary, these boundaries must be accounted for, if the clinical and constitutive realism of the simulation requires it. Proceeding this way gives us the option of modeling the ventricles, filled with corticospinal fluid, as well as sinuses of arbitrarily complex topology, on a patient-specific basis.

4. Next, the method should *afford both 2D and 3D elements*, as some tissues are better modeled as collections of surface elements, such as the dura mater, thin cranial bones and vasculature [1], while others are inherently volumetric. Existing methods that are purely volumetric [14] suffer from their inability to model tissues that are inherently curviplanar: rather than use just a few shell elements that feature no short edges, they are condemned to using a needlessly large number of small tetrahedra or hexahedra to limit the proportion between the longest and shortest edge of each for numerical stability [11].

5. Last, the meshing method must *produce high-quality triangles and tetrahedra*: within each 2D or 3D element the edges should be of near-equal length, as opposed to 1 or 2 edges significantly shorter than the others, for the sake of rapid convergence of the FE method [11]. Also, wherever smooth anatomical boundaries are involved, the surface visible to the user should be continuous, except where surgical interaction invalidates this assumption. Existing methods can also achieve continuous surfaces as well as high-quality triangles [6], but have not yet demonstrated a mesh scale strategy sufficiently flexible to meet our endoscopic simulation requirements.

---

[1] The latter might be simplified as a curvilinear element, were it not for the requirement that cutting through it should appear realistic and be appropriately penalized in our simulation.

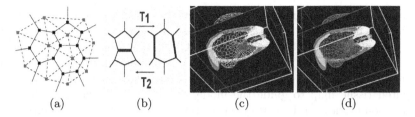

Fig. 4. Illustration of tissue-guided simplex models: (a) 2-simplex mesh and dual triangulation; (b) T_1 and T_2 Eulerian operators defined on 2-simplex mesh; prior results [2]: (c) radially varying simplex and (d) dual triangulated surface, topologically equivalent to a sphere. This topological limitation is addressed by this paper.

The goal of the surface meshing procedure is to establish the topologically faithful tissue surfaces bounding each class or contiguous subset of classes, where each surface mesh exhibits the required edge scale pattern. Given our objectives, we have opted for a surface model-based approach to tessellating anatomical boundaries, featuring the well-known *simplex* model [7], illustrated in figure 4 (a). Its topological operators, specifically the Eulerian T_1 and T_2, as illustrated figure 4 (b), as well as the edge swap T_7[7], provide explicit control over individual faces and edges. This surface meshing stage is followed by a tetrahedralization stage that also meets our mesh scale objectives and that *uses as input the triangular boundaries produced by the surface meshing stage*.

1.1 Topologically Accurate Tissue-Guided Simplex Meshing with Spatially Varying Edge Scale

As shown in figure 4 (a), the *m-simplex* mesh (black) is a discrete active surface model [7], characterized by each vertex being linked to each of $m+1$ neighbours by an edge. A surface model in 3D is realized as a 2-simplex, where each vertex has 3 neighbours, and this representation is the dual of a triangulated surface (blue), with each simplex vertex coinciding with a center, and each simplex edge being bisected by an edge, of a triangle. A balloon force can act on this mesh to cause it to expand until some image-based force halts this expansion. Furthermore, this surface model also features other *internal forces* [7] that nudge each simplex face, and consequently each dual triangle, towards having edges of equal or locally consistent length, and towards C_0, C_1 or C_2 continuity, for example. The edge scale can be constant, within some tolerance, as in figure 4 (c), or spatially varying as in figure 4 (d), consistent with a decomposition into parent (top, in white) and child (blue) subsystems, and leading to a triangulated surface of comparable scale.

This model has been limited by its topological equivalence with a sphere, in the absence of topological adaptivity. While topological adaptivity is achievable, based on operators published in [7], the convergence of the surface to the intended boundary, involving hundreds of iterations of a model integrating internal and image forces, is fraught with local extrema, a situation exacerbated by the capability of splitting or fusing. To alleviate this issue, we instead initialize the simplex model with a dense surface mesh of high accuracy and topological fidelity, resulting from Marching Cubes (MC) [9], based on the duality between a triangular surface and a 2-simplex mesh. We then decimate the simplex mesh in a highly controlled, spatially varying manner, while exploiting a previously computed tissue map to guide the model on a tissue-specific basis. The final simplex boundaries can be converted to triangulated surfaces by duality.

This way of proceding allows us more control over the decimation than existing algorithms not based on surface models, as our spatially varying control over mesh scale allows us to resolve the relevant anatomical surfaces densely enough for endoscopic simulation, while still limiting the number of triangles and tetrahedra enough to make real-time interaction feasible. Control over mesh size is typically implemented through the T_1 and T_2 operators, as triggered by geometric measurements of each simplex face or edge. For example, if the smallest edge of a face is smaller than the edge scale objective at that position, in order to produce a sparser mesh we delete that edge by a T_1 operation. Also, if a simplex face has more than k vertices ($k = 7$ usually), coinciding with a triangular mesh vertex with more than k incident, typically elongated, triangles, we also use T_1 and T_2 to reduce the number of simplex vertices and improve surface mesh quality.

It should also be emphasized that our procedure identifies anatomical surfaces prior to volumetric meshing, rather than proceed directly from the classification to tissue-guided volumetric meshing, because some tissues are inherently curviplanar rather than volumetric and are more efficiently modeled by shell elements than tetrahedra or hexahedra. Also, a purely volumetric approach will in general not produce a mesh that is as smooth and that closely agrees with the anatomical boundary: from a haptic and visual rendering standpoint, an anatomical model with jagged or badly localized boundaries would detract from the realism and clinical relevance of a surgical simulator as well as confuse the user.

We start from a densely triangulated surface produced by Marching Cubes, post-processed by an existing, topology-preserving, decimation method [10], which is somewhat more computationally efficient than ours and in order to reduce the number of triangles to a manageable number, as well as with identification and area-thresholding of contiguous structures, all VTK-based [13]. This stage produces a set of triangulated surfaces that we convert to simplex meshes by duality. From geometric tests to ascertain the shortest edge of each face, we iteratively perform T_1 operations on those faces whose shortest edge are furthest from their respective objective. We can use *heap-sorting* to fix the "worst" edge first. We note that when the curvature of the boundary may be sufficiently pronounced, with respect to the edge scale objective, T_1 operations lead to faces whose center lies too far from the boundary (only the vertices of each face are attracted to the boundary by image forces). At that point, the optimal representation may be a trade-off between the desired edge scale and the desired proximity of the face center to the boundary (a parameter). This trade-off entails the recruitment of T_2 operators to partition each ill-fitting face into two.

1.2 Spatially Varying Edge Scale Strategies: Radial and Surgical Path-Based Distance

As demonstrated in figure 4, control over simplex mesh edge scale can be exercised with a *Radially Varying Surface Mesh Scale* function $\mathcal{L}_{sm}\left(d_R(\mathbf{x}, \mathbf{p}_c)\right)$. This function is defined at any $\mathbf{x}$ in the volume spanned by the mesh, based on the Euclidian distance $d_R(\mathbf{x}, \mathbf{p}_c) = \|\mathbf{x} - \mathbf{p}_c\|$ from a *user-provided central point* $\mathbf{p}_c$ (e.g.: on the pituitary gland). For example, we may define

$$\mathcal{L}_{sm}(d_R(\mathbf{x})) = \begin{cases} \mathcal{L}_{sm,min} & \text{if } d_R(\mathbf{x}) <= d_{min} \\ \mathcal{L}_{sm,min} + (\mathcal{L}_{sm,max} - \mathcal{L}_{sm,min})\left\{1 - \exp\left[\frac{-(d_R(\mathbf{x}) - d_{min})}{d_{scale}}\right]\right\} & \text{otherwise,} \end{cases} \quad (1)$$

where $\mathcal{L}_{sm,min}$ and $\mathcal{L}_{sm,max}$ specify smallest and largest edge scales of the simplex mesh, and d_{min} and d_{scale} determine the behaviour of the function bridging the two values: an exponential function of the distance of the midpoint of the edge e_i to the central point. This scale function thereby produces consistently small edges near the pituitary gland and, beyond a transition whose abruptness is controlled by the parameter d_{scale}, longer edges away from it. We can also enforce a face area scale function, which can be derived from the edge scale.

Alternately, we can specify at any $\mathbf{x}$ a *Surgical Path Based Mesh Scale* function $\mathcal{L}(d_{SP}(\mathbf{x}, S))$, substituting d_{SP} for d_R in expression (1), where $S = \{E_i(\mathbf{p}_i, \mathbf{p}_{i+1})\}$ is a set of linear edges E_i. Each edge E_i connects 2 user-provided points $\mathbf{p}_i$ and $\mathbf{p}_{i+1}$, and together they approximate an intended surgical path:

$$d_{SP}(\mathbf{x}, S) \equiv \min_{E_i \in S} d_{edge}(\mathbf{x}, E_i)) \quad \text{where} \quad d_{edge}(\mathbf{x}, E_i)) \equiv \min_{u+v=1} \|u\mathbf{p}_i + v\mathbf{p}_{i+1} - \mathbf{x}\|, \quad (2)$$

where $u, v \in [0, 1]$. This expression defines the minimum distance from $\mathbf{x}$ to the set of edges S that is a linearized approximation of the intended surgical path.

This notion of using proximity to a point or to an intended surgical path to optimize mesh size can be extended to choices about constitutive and clinical realism. For example, within a distance threshold ε_d from a point or a path[2], we may elect to model soft tissues as *nonlinearly elastic*, beyond which we are content with *linearly elastic* behaviour. Or, for any $\mathbf{x}$ where $d_{SP}(\mathbf{x}, S) > \varepsilon_d$, we may model skin, muscle, fat and bone as having a *prescribed null displacement*, thereby effectively eliminating them from the real-time FE problem, whereas closer to the surgical path, we can account for the material properties of mucosa, muscle and even bones, as in the case of the sphenoidal sinus. Finally, far away from the path, it is expedient to *not account for critical tissues*, which can be obtained based on processing of MRI data with the method in [3] and of MRA data with a method such as [12], as this subset of critical tissues is less relevant to the simulation and otherwise would only add to computational overhead.

---

[2] This threshold need not be constant along a path: if for example we had to model a cranial procedure, as the inwards arclength s of the path increases, $\varepsilon_d(s)$ would tend to be larger at the surface (s=0) and become smaller along the path.

1.3 Almost-Regular Volumetric Meshing with Spatially Varying Resolution Control

The last stage in our procedure partitions each volume bounded by a triangulated mesh, coinciding with a tissue class or contiguous subset of tissue classes, into tetrahedral elements consistent with the FE method. The volumetric meshing stage is a published technique [8] that automatically produces an optimal tetrahedralization from a given polygonal boundary, such as a triangulated surface. In this case, optimality is defined as near-equal length of the tetrahedral edges, along with a sharing of each inner vertex by a nearly consistent number of edges and tetrahedra. This method features the optimal positioning of inner vertices, expressed as a minimization of a penalty functional, followed by a Delaunay tetrahedralization. The resulting near-regularity is important for FE stability and efficiency [11]. Moreover, based on the relationship between the number of simplex and triangle vertices $V_t \approx V_{sm}/2$ [7] and after some manipulation, a target simplex mesh size of $\mathcal{L}_{sm}(\mathbf{x})$ works out to a triangle or a tetrahedral mesh size of $\mathcal{L}_t(\mathbf{x}) \approx \sqrt{2}\mathcal{L}_{sm}(\mathbf{x})$. We modify this technique by integrating into the penalty functional the now-familiar spatially varying scale function, which is specified as a target edge length $\mathcal{L}_t(\mathbf{x})$ for each tetrahedron.

2 Results and Discussion

Figures 5 and 6 contrast an existing, curvature-sensitive (but otherwise spatially consistent), decimation algorithm [10] with our spatially varying, simplex-based surface mesh decimation. Figure 5 displays a synthetic cube with 4 tubular openings through it, along axes x and y, to which we've added a synthetic hemispherical "gland" in its inner ceiling: (a) surface as originally identified by MC, (b) as decimated by the existing method. Its dual, featuring 1224 faces, initializes our spatially varying method, whose results are shown in (c), featuring 585 faces and dense faces on the gland, where edge colour from white to fully saturated red indicates a tissue proximity varying between 0 and 3 mm, and

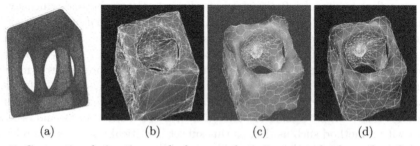

(a)   (b)   (c)   (d)

Fig. 5. Contrasting decimation methods on synthetic invaginated cube surface, featuring a hemispheric inner gland: (a) wireframe of MC results; (b): existing decimation method [10] displayed as a 3D wireframe overlaid on a surface rendering; (c) and (d): radially varying simplex mesh, featuring final simplex and dual triangular results

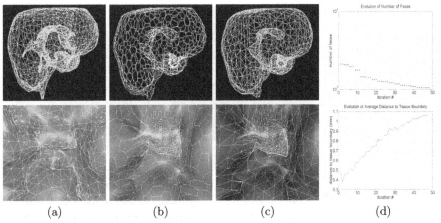

(a)   (b)   (c)   (d)

Fig. 6. Contrasting decimation methods on brain surface: (a) existing method, featuring wireframe of overall brain surface mesh and closeup of wireframe overlaid on rendering of brain surface, centered on pituitary gland; (b) radially varying simplex mesh, featuring wireframe and overlay closeup views as in (a); (c) radially varying triangular surface, dual to simplex mesh in (b). (d) Decimation statistics: top, number of faces, and bottom, average distance to boundary, versus simplex iteration respectively, in going from the dual of (a) to (b) (2618 to 1051 faces).

whose dual triangulated surface appears in (d). We choose a proximity threshold that is tight at the gland and looser far away. A halt is triggered here by a near-constant number of faces, where scale-based T_1 and proximity-based T_2 operations offset each other. Figure 6 shows results for a brain surface, going from the prior method in (a) to the results of our method in (b) and (c). The graphs (d) illustrate the evolution in terms of the number of simplex faces and average distance to the tissue boundary: the reduction of the number of faces is traded off against proximity to the boundary, especially far from the area of surgical interaction. Here, T_1 and T_2 operations are applied every 3 iterations.

Next, figure 7 illustrates the flexibility and clinical applicability of the surface meshing method, in its ability to characterize relevant critical tissues, which are currently modeled as hollow and meshed at constant density. Blood vessels irrelevant to the simulation are not considered.

Figure 8 depicts how a combination of path-based ($\varepsilon_{d,SP}$ =10mm) and radial ($\varepsilon_{d,R}$ =25mm) distance allows us to convert "distant" extra-cranial tissue to "null displacement" tissue to exclude it from the real-time biomechanical problem. These two distances are then used to determine the mesh scale.

Finally, figure 9 illustrates our topologically accurate, radially varying tetrahedralization results, on the cube and brain volumes. The former meshing is visualized as a wireframe composed of all tetrahedral edges. The brain tetrahedral meshing is shown a semi-transparent volume whose intersection with a clipping plane is shown as a set of triangles, as well as a wiremesh of all edges in a manner comparable to the cube.

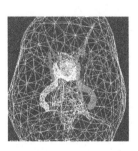

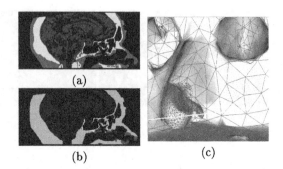

Fig. 7. Clinically useful meshing: superposition of relevant critical tissue meshes with brain surface: basilar arteries, optic and oculomotor nerves, shown as triangular mesh.

Fig. 8. Illustration of use of radial and path-based distance to convert "distant" extra-cranial soft tissue to tissue of null displacement and determine edge scale: (a) original tissue map [3]; (b) null-displacement tissue in orange; (c) final wireframe and rendering of triangulated surface, with dense results visible within 10mm of path.

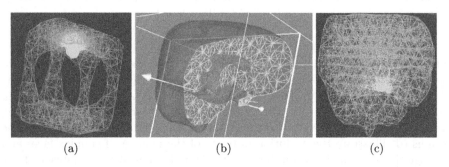

Fig. 9. Illustration of topologically accurate, radially varying brain volume tetrahedralization: (a) invaginated cube visualized as 3D wireframe of all tetrahedral edges, with child mesh in pink and parent mesh in turquoise; brain mesh visualized as: (b) semi-transparent boundary of clipped volume, where triangular intersections of tetrahedra with clipping plane shown as white wireframe, and (c) 3D wireframe rendering.

3   Conclusions

This paper presented a new meshing strategy for computing patient-specific anatomical models comprised of triangles and tetrahedra coinciding with, or for computational efficiency idealized as, homogeneous tissue, in a manner that addresses the requirements of endoscopic pituitary surgery simulation. Our surface mesh method combines the strengths of Marching Cubes and the simplex mesh model for computing triangulated boundaries, in terms of topological fidelity and control of mesh characteristics such as edge scale. While each method, on its own, is well researched, the combination of the two, and in particular the edge scale strategy, is novel. Our strategy offers promise for dealing with the conflicting requirements of narrowly focused, and especially endoscopic, visualization and haptic rendering as well as the computation of body forces and displacements over large volumes, particularly if combined with hierarchical multirate finite elements. Our notion of edge scale extends flexibly to decisions about constitutive and clinical realism, such as which subset of tissues to consider as having null displacement. This method is conceived to be extensible to surgery simulation in general, and it appears able to deal with any tissue shape as well as most practical requirements for tissue mesh size.

In the near future, the particular choice of parameters for our application will be settled in conjunction with improvements to the prior tissue classification and with the application of HMFEs to our models. We will also investigate a conformality-preserving simplex force, which would cause two contiguous boundaries to share vertices wherever desirable. A more thorough validation of these methods will follow, based on a refinement of the MNI digital head phantom to account for bone and critical tissues.

References

1. O. Astley & V. Hayward, Multirate Haptic Simulation Achieved by Coupling Finite Element Meshes Through Norton Equivalents, *IEEE Int. Conf. Rob. Auto.*, 1998.
2. M.A. Audette et al., Towards Patient-specific Anatomical Model Generation for Finite Element-based Surgical Simulation, *Int. Symp. Surg. Sim. & Soft Tis. Model. IS4TM*, LNCS 2673, pp. 356-361, 2003.
3. M.A. Audette and K. Chinzei, The Application of Embedded and Tubular Structure to Tissue Identification for the Computation of Patient-Specific Neurosurgical Simulation Models, *Int. Symp. Med. Sim*, LNCS 3078, PP. 203-210, 2004.
4. P. Cappabianca et al., *Atlas of Endoscopic Anatomy for Endonasal Intracranial Surgery*, Springer, 2001.
5. I. Ciric et al., Complications of Transsphenoidal Surgery: Results of a National Survey, Review of the Literature, and Personal Experience, *Neurosurg.*, Vol. 40, No. 2., pp. 225-236, Feb. 1997.
6. P.W. de Bruin et al., Improving Triangle Mesh Quality with Surface Nets, *Med. Image Comput. & Comput. Assist. Interv. MICCAI 2000*, pp 804-813, 2000.
7. H. Delingette, General Object Reconstruction Based on Simplex Meshes, *Int. J. Comp. Vis.*, Vol. 32, No. 2, pp. 111-146, 1999.
8. A. Fuchs, Almost Regular Triangulations of Trimmed NURBS-Solids, *Eng. w. Comput.*, Vol. 17, pp. 55-65, 2001.
9. W. Lorensen & H. Cline, Marching Cubes: a High Resolution 3D Surface Construction Algorithm, *Computer Graphics*, Vol. 21, No. 4, pp. 163-170, July 1987.
10. W. Schroeder et al., Decimation of Triangle Meshes, *Comput. Graph. SIGGRAPH '92*, 26(2):65-70, Oct. 1992.
11. J.R. Shewchuk, What is a Good Linear Element? Interpolation, Conditioning and Quality Measures, *11th Int. Meshing Roundtbl. Conf.*, pp. 115-126, 2002.

12. A. Vasilevskiy & K. Siddiqi, Flux Maximizing Geometric Flows, *IEEE Trans. Patt. Anal. & Mach. Intel.*, Vol. 24, No. 2, pp. 1565-1578, 2002.
13. VTK: Visualization Toolkit, *http://public.kitware.com/VTK*.
14. Y. Zhang, C. Bajaj & B.S. Sohn, 3D Finite Element Meshing from Imaging Data, *Computer Method in Applied Mechanics and Engineering*, to appear, 2005.

Applying Prior Knowledge in the Segmentation of 3D Complex Anatomic Structures

Hong Shen[1], Yonggang Shi[2], and Zhigang Peng[3]

[1] Siemens Corporate Research, Inc., 755 College Road East, Princeton, NJ,
shenh@scr.siemens.com
[2] Electrical and Computer Engineering Department, Boston University, MA
[3] Department of Electrical & Computer Engineering and Computer Science,
University of Cincinnati, OH

Abstract. We address the problem of precise segmentation of 3D complex structure from high-contrast images. Particularly, we focus on the representation and application of prior knowledge in the 3D level set framework. We discuss the limitations of the popular prior shape model in this type of situations, and conclude that shape model only is not complete and effective if not augmented by high-level boundary and context features. We present the principle that global priors should not compete with local image forces at the same level, but should instead guide the evolving surface to converge to the correct local primitives, thus avoiding the common problems of leakage and local minima. We propose several schemes to achieve this goal, including initial front design, speed design, and the introduction of high-level context blockers.

1 Introduction

The segmentation of objects such as anatomies and pathologies from 3D medical volume data poses a challenging problem. The challenges include inhomogeneous intensity and strong edges within the object, and weak or broken boundaries. To cope with these challenges, high-level prior knowledge or global priors needs to be incorporated.

A 3D complex structure has complex surface boundaries and strong high-level features. A good example is the human vertebra, as shown in Figure 1. We believe this is a type of segmentation problem that is not well addressed in the literature, especially when it is from a high-contrast data such as multi-slice CT images. First, such a structure is too complex to be segmented by 2D methods on a slice-by-slice basis. On the other hand, inter-slice resolution is high enough to provide the inter-slice correlation needed for 3D methods. Second, it differs from the objects shown in many literatures on medical image segmentation, such as organs in MR or Ultrasound data, in which the shape is often unclear. A 3D complex structure in high-contrast data has relatively well-defined shape, at least for a human, who can perform consistent delineation of the object boundaries on 2D slice images. On the other hand, the boundaries, when viewed locally, are not clear at all. There are gaps, weak or diffused boundaries everywhere. Further, such a structure is usually adjacent or even connected to a neighbor-

Y. Liu, T. Jiang, and C. Zhang (Eds.): CVBIA 2005, LNCS 3765, pp. 189–199, 2005.

ing structure with similar image properties. A special challenge is, since the shape looks clearly defined for a human, the segmentation result has to closely match the consistent human perception.

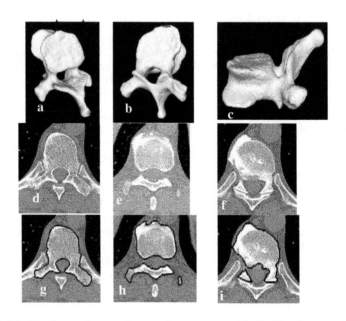

Fig. 1. (a)-(c): 3D views of a complex vertebra structure. (d)-(f): Vertebra on selected axial slices, with its neighboring vertebra and rib structures. While the shape looks well defined for a human, local boundaries are weak at many locations. Also notice the pathological abnormal shape on the top-left corner of the vertebra in (e)&(f). (g)-(i): 2D contours delineated by a human. Regions not enclosed by black contours belong to other vertebras and ribs.

In the past decades, the level set method [1,2] received much attention. However, level set only reacts to local properties. It truthfully conforms to whatever local information it encounters. Since a 3D complex structure usually also has very complex local image properties, level set is bound to fail when no prior knowledge is applied.

1.1 Prior Work: Surface Model

Recent works provide schemes for representing prior knowledge—particularly global shape priors. Leventon et al. [3] followed by others [4,5] proposed the PCA model that uses global shape priors to augment the level set framework. This approach uses signed distance functions to represent a shape, and applies PCA analysis on a set of registered training samples. A model is therefore allowed to vary within the linear space spanned by eigenvector shapes. To constrain the surface evolution process, the difference between the current surface and a matched shape in the model space is applied as a penalty force. This term is summed with the local image force term to com

pute the speed map. A multiplier is introduced between the two terms, the modifica
tion of which will adjust the strength of the model term. This type of scheme provides
a unified solution to the issue of incorporating prior shape knowledge, and has shown
to be successful in many applications, especially when the shape is not well defined in
image data and therefore requires a strong shape model.

The linear PCA model on signed distance function is only valid within the limited
space [3,4] centered at the mean shapes. Therefore usually only small coefficients are
allowed. Further, for practical purpose, the number of modes or dimensions is also
small; otherwise the search of model space for the most similar shape will be intractable. This issue becomes prominent in the segmentation of a 3D complex structure,
which usually has high variations in shape. A large number of modes are needed, resulting in a high-dimensional model space. At the same time, a shape can be far away
from the mean shape, leading to high values of the coefficients, which will drive the
algorithm out of the linear range. We cannot afford to have a full representation of
most structure variations, even at the theoretical level. Above all, there are high variations due to age, gender, race, and especially countless pathological abnormalities.
From the practical side, to obtain a large and representative set of training samples
poses a challenging problem. Aside from selecting samples, the manual segmentation
of a 3D complex structure is an arduous task. Even if we have all the offline time and
resource to set up such a model space, it would be too large for the system to search
under any reasonable online performance requirement.

The above problem combines with the inherent issue from the same-level competition between prior knowledge and local image properties in the PCA framework.
Since the surface model cannot even roughly cover the variations of 3D complex
structures, we need to rely on the surface evolution of level set to converge to local
boundaries. The problem is, at many locations the two pieces of information will not
agree. Obviously, this cannot be completely addressed by adjusting the multiplier.
The not-well-fit model shape will compete with local primitives to pull the evolving
surface away from these strong features and the abnormal boundaries. This can be
seen from the limited literatures covering vertebra segmentation [3]. Converged surface was quite far way from the object boundaries that would be easily delineated by a
human observer.

1.2 Our Approach

Merely the surface model is not a sufficient representation of prior knowledge. This is
not just because an affordable and practical shape model space will not even roughly
cover the spectrum of variations, but also because any surface model is extracted from
the training data by some kind of averaging operations, which leads to the loss of high
frequency information. High-level features such as abrupt edges, ridges, etc., can only
be explicitly represented rather than embedded in a shape model.

In the surface evolution process, global priors should not be simply added to local
image forces, creating competition at the same level. It should serve as a guidance to
help the surface selectively converge to the "correct" local properties, avoiding local

minima and preventing leak-out. Since the convergence of level set depends on the initial front as well as local speed, we will spend our effort mainly in the design of the initial front and the speed map. Beside this, high-level context features will be a major help in preventing leakage. A prior knowledge representation should include a small set of surface models, augmented by the explicit description of a set of known high-level features. For the sake of clarity, we exemplify the general principles for such a situation in the context of vertebra segmentation from chest CT volume data.

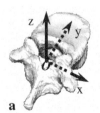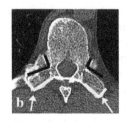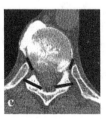

Fig. 2. Global prior representation. (a) The mean shape and the common coordinate system. (b)(c) Parametric planes representing high-level boundary features (4 in total) and context features (6 in total). Their cross-sections within the axial plane are marked white (also pointed by arrows) and black, respectively.

2 Prior Knowledge Representation

2.1 The Mean Shape Template

A small number of vertebras are selected and their surfaces are manually segmented by 2D contour delineation. At the same time, the spinal channel and the two roughly parallel inter-vertebra planes are also segmented. These features are used to register the samples with a common coordinate system such that the centroid of the spinal channel is at the origin, the normal of the two planes align with the z-axis, and the spinal channel is roughly symmetric with respect to the plane $x=0$. Following Leventon et al. [3], we then construct from the transformed surfaces a set of signed distance functions $S = \{\phi_1, \phi_2, ..., \phi_n\}$ such that the surface of the ith sample is represented as $\Gamma = \{\mathbf{x} \mid \mathbf{x} \in R^3, \phi(\mathbf{x}) = 0\}$. We define the mean shape as

$$\bar{\phi} = \frac{1}{n} \sum_{i=1}^{n} \phi_i,$$

(1)

an example of which is shown in Fig. 2(a). It has the essential shape and structure that characterize a vertebra. Certainly, we do not intend to cover large variations. The mean shape is used as a rough guide or template. This low requirement allows a small sample size, corresponding to a much smaller manual task. For a more general scheme, a small number of PCA shapes can be stored. In the case of vertebra, we only store the mean shape.

2.2 High-Level Features

Linear primitives include intensity edges, ridges, and valleys. If the locations of the strong and same-type primitives in a local neighborhood roughly form a flat surface, we can fit a simple parametric model and describe it as a high-level feature.

If a high-level feature is based on the *ridges* or *edges* from the object boundary, then it is a high-level *boundary* feature. A high-level *context* feature, on the other hand, comes from the intensity *valleys* located at the interface between the object and a neighboring structure. Both types of high-level features are recorded with reference to the common coordinate system. Without loss of generality, we use the plane models

$$\mathbf{B}_i^T \mathbf{x} = 0, \quad i = 1 \cdots m \tag{2}$$

$$\mathbf{C}_j^T \mathbf{x} = 0, \quad j = 1 \cdots n \tag{3}$$

to describe the high-level boundary and context features, respectively. Here $\mathbf{x}$ is the homogeneous coordinate vector, m and n are the number of high-level boundary and context features, respectively. As will be discussed later, high-level context features will be crucial in the prevention of leakages. We record in total 4 boundary planes and 6 context planes for each vertebra, as shown in Fig.2(b)&(c).

3 Speed Map Design for Level Set Evolution

The surface evolvement of level set depends on speed that is computed from local image properties [6], which can be region-based [7] or primitive-based. In many situations, neither of the methods is sufficient.

3.1 Speeds Based on Sub-region Division

The image properties of a 3D complex structure are usually non-uniform within the object. Therefore we can divide the object into sub-regions. For each sub-region, we choose the proper type of speed, either region-based or primitive-based. One piece of prior knowledge we did not present in Section 2 is the division of sub-regions within the object. We record a set of planes in the common coordinate system to describe sub-region boundaries, as illustrated in Fig. 3.

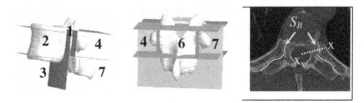

Fig. 3. (a)(b) Dividing the mean shape into sub-regions.(c) Definition of blocker region. All points that are on different sides of x_v with respect to surface S_B is in the blocker region.

Sub-regions 1, 2, 3, and 7 have blurred boundaries and high intensity variations. Noise is also strong and cannot be easily smoothed lest the boundary will be further blurred. The average intensities in these regions are higher than the background, which suggests the usage of region-based intensity speed. Following Chan-Vese [7],

$$F_{\text{Im} age}(\mathbf{x}) = \alpha \left[(I(\mathbf{x}) - c_{1i})^2 - (I(\mathbf{x}) - c_{2i})^2 \right], \mathbf{x} \in R_i, \ i = 1, 2, 3, 7 \tag{4}$$

is used to describe the speed, where c_{1i} and c_{2i} are the estimated average intensity inside and outside the vertebra, respectively.

Sub-regions 4 and 6 both have relatively strong edges, despite the blurred and broken boundaries. We compute $g(\mathbf{x})$ as the combined response term of edges and ridges. Its gradient is projected on the normal of the level set function ϕ.

$$F_{\text{Im} age}(\mathbf{x}) = \beta \nabla g(\mathbf{x}) \cdot \nabla \phi(\mathbf{x}, t), \quad \mathbf{x} \in R_i, i = 4, 6, \tag{5}$$

For sub-region 5 there are both the high intensity variation and strong edges, and we design the speed to be based on both edge and region:

$$F_{\text{Image}}(\mathbf{x}) = \gamma \left[(I(\mathbf{x}) - c_{1i})^2 - (I(\mathbf{x}) - c_{2i})^2 \right] + (1 - \gamma) \nabla g(\mathbf{x}) \cdot \nabla \phi(\mathbf{x}, t), \quad \mathbf{x} \in R_5 \tag{6}$$

The speed map is unified, although the types of speeds vary with respect to locations. The speed of all types are normalized to be at the same range and made continuous at boundaries of sub-regions.

3.2 Blocker Speed Based on Context Features

Suppose the similarity transformation from model to data is described as $\mathbf{x}_{image} = \mathbf{T} \mathbf{x}_{model}$, where $\mathbf{T}$ is the transformation matrix, the high-level contexts features in Eq.3 and are mapped as

$$\mathbf{C}_j^T \mathbf{T}^{-1} \mathbf{x}_{image} = 0, \quad j = 1 \cdots n \tag{7}$$

which remain as planes.

The detection of high-level feature in the image is obviously different from that of low-level features. We search the correspondent plane in the small parametric space:

$$\mathbf{P} \in (\mathbf{C}_j^T \mathbf{T}^{-1} - \Delta \mathbf{P}, \mathbf{C}_j^T \mathbf{T}^{-1} + \Delta \mathbf{P}) \tag{8}$$

in which the plane is only allowed limited variation $|\Delta \mathbf{P}|$. The search is via model-fitting techniques such as the Hough transform. After primitive detection in the local neighborhood, each primitive votes with its strength $e(\mathbf{x})$. The vote for a candidate plane $\mathbf{P}$ is therefore

$$U(\mathbf{P}) = \sum_{|\mathbf{P}\mathbf{x}| < \varepsilon} e(\mathbf{x}) \tag{9}$$

where ε is a minor distance value. The winner is then

$$\mathbf{P}_{final} = \underset{\mathbf{P}\in(\mathbf{C}_j^T\mathbf{T}^{-1}-\Delta\mathbf{P},\ \mathbf{C}_j^T\mathbf{T}^{-1}+\Delta\mathbf{P})}{\arg\max} U(\mathbf{P}) \tag{10}$$

Certainly the bin size for voting needs to be carefully chosen. This method is very robust as long as the local primitives are in majority over noises and outliers.

The detected parametric plane is an approximation of the actual surface S_B, as shown in Fig. 2(a)&(b). Therefore primitive detection is again applied on the close neighborhoods of $\mathbf{P}_{final}$, along its normal direction. The strongest and closest primitives are accepted as the points that form S_B.

A high-level context feature belongs to the background, and hence intensity valleys are detected as the primitive to vote in the Hough transform. These valleys also form the refined surface S_B. For high-level boundary features, intensity edges and ridges are detected instead.

We here introduce a blocker speed term that is built up from a high-level context feature to prevent leakage. Let S_B be an oriented surface, and hence it partitions the 3D space into two sides. We further assume that the line connecting any two points on the different sides of S_B, only makes one intersection with it. Using a fixed point $\bar{x}_v$ inside the transformed mean shape as an anchor, we define the blocker region including all points on the other side of S_B:

$$\Omega_B = \{\mathbf{x} \mid (\overline{\mathbf{xx}}_v \cap S_B) \in \overleftrightarrow{\mathbf{xx}}_v\} \tag{11}$$

If there are n blocker regions, we combined them:

$$\Omega_B = \Omega_{B1} \cup \Omega_{B2} \cup \cdots \cup \Omega_{Bn} \tag{12}$$

Specifically, we set $F_{Block}(\mathbf{x}) = -1$ for $\mathbf{x} \in \Omega_B$, which overrides $F_{Image}(\mathbf{x})$ defined in Section 3.1. The above definition of blocker region is illustrated in Fig. 3(c). Obviously, the blocker region prevents the surface from evolving into it. The surface is forced to converge to local properties outside the blocker region. By using a high-level context feature blocker we can prevent leakage but still allow the surface to converge freely to local boundaries that belong to the object.

3.3 Level Set Formulation

In addition to the image-dependent speed and blocker speed, we also use the smooth speed, κ, the mean curvature of the surface. Also, we define a field

$$v_B(\mathbf{x}) = \begin{cases} 1, & \mathbf{x} \in \Omega_B \\ 0, & else \end{cases} \tag{13}$$

to denote if a point is inside the blocker region. Thus the final speed is defined as

$$F_{Final}(\mathbf{x}) = (1 - v_B(\mathbf{x}))F_{Image} + v_B(\mathbf{x})F_{Blocker} + \varepsilon\kappa \tag{14}$$

According to [10], the evolution of the surface is embedded in the evolution of a level set function $\phi(t)$:

$$\frac{\partial \phi}{\partial t} = F_{Final}(\mathbf{x}) \left|\nabla \phi\right| = ((1 - V_B(\mathbf{x}))F_{Image} - V_B(\mathbf{x}) + \varepsilon \kappa) \left|\nabla \phi\right| \tag{15}$$

where $\kappa = \nabla \cdot \dfrac{\nabla \phi}{|\nabla \phi|}$ is the mean curvature of the level set.

4 Initial Front Design

The initial front of level set greatly affects the evolution and convergence of the surface. Works on level set segmentation often use such simple shape as a circle or a sphere as the initial front, and rely on level set to recover the object shape and topology. The results often prove the power and flexibility of level set. In the segmentation of 3D complex shapes, however, it is crucial to carefully design the initial front so as to avoid local minima. A well-designed initial front will have similar shape and topology as object surface, and be close to the desired boundaries.

With this in mind, we map the mean shape on to the image. To estimate a similarity transformation between the mean shape and the image, we detect the spinal channel and the two inter-vertebra planes, as shown in Fig. 4(a). The plane normal $\mathbf{n}$ of the mean shape is first rotated to align with that of the object. The mean shape is then rotated around $\mathbf{n}$ such that the long and short axes of the spinal channel in the axial plane are aligned with those of the object. The mean shape is then scaled so that the area of the spinal channel in the axial plane equals that of the object. Finally the mean shape is shifted so that the centroid of spinal channel coincides with that of the object. This mapping is application-specific. However, a transformation can be estimated with other more general methods to map the initial shape, and we have seen examples in the literature [8].

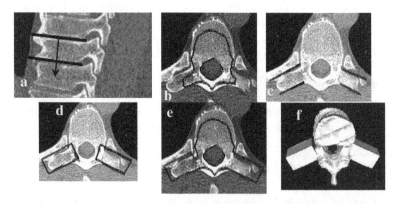

Fig. 4. Initial front design. (a) Inter-vertebra planes. (b) The mapped mean shape. (c) High level context and boundary features on the two sides of the transverse processes. (d) The rectangular parallelepipeds that contain the high-level features. (e) The initial front contour (f) 3D shape of initial front.

The cross-section of the surface of the mapped mean shape model is illustrated in Fig. 4(b). It possesses most of the desired properties of initial front. However, since it is only an average of shape of limited samples, it is not yet a good initial front. As shown in Fig. 4(b), the surface of the mean shape is quite far away from the actual image boundary at the two transverse processes. Such an initial front will be captured by local minima and not converge to the outside true boundaries.

A costly option is to search for a higher order PCA shape to use as the initial front. Instead, we adjust the mean shape with high-level features. We define Π as the set that contain all points inside the mean shape. As described in Section 3.3, we detect the planes that represent the high-level features on the two sides of the transverse processes, the cross-section of which is shown in Fig. 4(c). Having detected the two planes

$$P_i = \{\mathbf{x} \mid \mathbf{a}_i \cdot \mathbf{x} = 0\}, i = 1,2 \tag{16}$$

where $\mathbf{x}$ is the homogeneous coordinate vector. Take an arbitrary shape Σ such that

$$P_i \subset \Sigma, i = 1,2 \text{ and } \Sigma \cap \Pi \neq \phi \tag{17}$$

where ϕ is the empty set. We then merged the regions:

$$\Lambda = \Pi \cup \Sigma \tag{18}$$

from which we construct the signed distance function as the implicit representation of the new surface. As shown in Fig.4(c), the dark lines are the cross-sections of detected high-level features P_i with the axial plane, and we fit an arbitrary shape Σ that contains these features and at the same time connected to the mean shape Π. In this case we constructed two rectangular parallelepipeds as shown in Fig.4(d). The new front Λ is shown in Fig. 4(e) and Fig. 4(f).

5 Results

The cross-section contours of converged surfaces in axial, coronal and sagittal planes are shown in Fig. 5. We show in alterative rows the original image and segmentation results. The images in the result columns are dimmed in order to clearly show the contours. The cases include all types of complications, such as weak boundary, crowed and connected neighboring structures, partial volume effects, pathological abnormalities, and high intensity variations. On the other hand, a trained human observer would still be able to consistently delineate the boundaries. Although we did not show human-drawn contours here, it is clear that our segmentation result should closely match what a human would have drawn.

We tested on 5 chest CT data sets, each with 300-400 slices of 512×512 images, and with in-plane and inter-plane resolutions of (0.5~0.8) mm and 1mm, respectively. Each data set contains around 9 vertebras of different shapes covered in the chest portion. The results are generally satisfactory, as shown in Fig. 5. The algorithm heavily

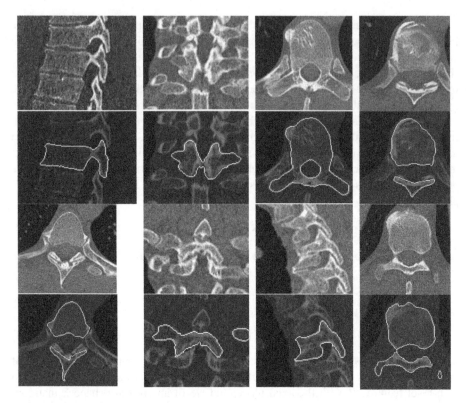

Fig. 5. Selected 3D segmentation results shown as the cross-section contours in axial, sagittal and coronal planes. The first and third rows show original image, and the other two rows show the contours. The result rows have the image dimmed to show the contours more clearly.

depends on the correct detection of high-level features. Although the detection scheme is robust by itself, we are still working on its improvement.

6 Conclusions

We have proposed a scheme for incorporating prior knowledge into the level set segmentation of 3D complex structure. The prior knowledge includes shape and high-level features. The design of speed and initial front comes from prior knowledge and guides the local surface to converge to the correct object boundaries. We introduced the concept of context blocker speed, which is crucial in the prevention of leakage. We also attempted to combine several types of speeds according to location.

We exemplify our scheme with the human vertebra segmentation because it is one of most complicated 3D structures. We also chose high-contrast CT as the data type. This is because a vertebra has well-defined shape only in CT data, from which precise segmentation is possible.

Acknowledgements

We would to thank our colleagues at Siemens Corporate Research-- Greg Slabaugh and Gozde Unal for their most valuable comments, discussions, and encouragements.

References

[1] R. Malladi, J. A. Sethian, and B. C. Vemuri. Shape modeling with front propagation: a level set approach, *IEEE Transactions on Pattern Analysis and Machine Intelligence*, 17(2), 158-75, 1995.

[2] D. Adalsteinsson, and J. Sethian, A fast level set method for propagating interfaces, *Journal of Computational Physics*, 118, 269-277, 1995.

[3] M. E. Leventon, W. E. Grimson, and O. Faugeras, Statistical shape influence in geodesic active contours, *Proceedings IEEE Conference on Computer Vision and Pattern Recognition*, 1(1), 316-323. 2000.

[4] A. Tsai, A. Yezzi, W. Wells, C. Tempany, D. Tucker, A. Fan, W. E. Grimson, and A. Willsky, A shape-based approach to the segmentation of medical imagery using level sets, *IEEE Transactions on Medical Imaging*, 22(2), 137-154, 2003.

[5] J. Yang, H., S. Staib, and J., S., Duncan, Neighbor-constrained segmentation with level set based 3-D deformable models, *IEEE Transactions on Medical Imaging*, 23(8), 940-948, 2004.

[6] J. S. Suri, K. Liu, S. Singh, S.N. Laxminarayan, X. Zeng, and L. Reden, Shape recovery algorithm using level sets in 2-D/3-D medical imagery, a state-of-the-art review, *IEEE Transactions on Information Technology in Biomedicine*, 6(1), 8-28, 2002.

[7] T. Chan, and L. Vese, An active contour model without edges, *IEEE Transactions on Image Processing*, 10(2), 266-277, 2001.

[8] C. Baillard, P. Hellier, and C. Barillot, Segmentation of brain images using level sets and dense registration, *Medical Image Analysis*, 5, 185-194, 2001.

Automatic Extraction of Femur Contours from Hip X-Ray Images*

Ying Chen[1], Xianhe Ee[1], Wee Kheng Leow[1], and Tet Sen Howe[2]

[1] Dept. of Computer Science, National University of Singapore,
3 Science Drive 2, Singapore 117543
{chenying, eexianhe, leowwk}@comp.nus.edu.sg
[2] Dept. of Orthopaedics, Singapore General Hospital,
Outram Road, Singapore 169608
tshowe@sgh.com.sg

Abstract. Extraction of bone contours from x-ray images is an important first step in computer analysis of medical images. It is more complex than the segmentation of CT and MR images because the regions delineated by bone contours are highly nonuniform in intensity and texture. Classical segmentation algorithms based on homogeneity criteria are not applicable. This paper presents a model-based approach for automatically extracting femur contours from hip x-ray images. The method works by first detecting prominent features, followed by registration of the model to the x-ray image according to these features. Then the model is refined using active contour algorithm to get the accurate result. Experiments show that this method can extract the contours of femurs with regular shapes, despite variations in size, shape and orientation.

1 Introduction

Extraction of bone contours from x-ray images is an important first step in computer analysis of medical images. For example, to detect fractures in femur bones from x-ray images [1,2,3], it is necessary to first determine the contours of the femurs within which features are to be extracted for fracture detection. In the work of [4], contours of carpal bones are determined followed by extracting features within the bone region for skeletal age assessment. Interestingly, most of the existing work on medical image segmentation has been focused on CT and MR images. Much less work has been done on the segmentation of x-ray images.

Classical image segmentation algorithms assume that the regions to be segmented contain homogeneous features. With this assumption, the segmentation algorithms attempt to segment the input image into regions based on feature homogeneity criteria. Unfortunately, such homogeneity criteria are not satisfied for large and complex bones in x-ray images. For instance, in a femur x-ray image (Fig. 1), the femoral head region contains nonuniform texture pattern due to the trabeculae (Fig. 1b), and the femoral shaft region has nonuniform intensity due

---

* This research is supported by NMRC/0482/2000.

Y. Liu, T. Jiang, and C. Zhang (Eds.): CVBIA 2005, LNCS 3765, pp. 200–209, 2005.

to the hollow interior within solid bony walls (Fig. 1a). Moreover, the femoral head overlaps with the pelvis bone. In this case, the extraction of bone contours becomes a more complex problem than classical image segmentation problem. This paper describes a model-based approach for automatically extracting femur contours from standard hip x-ray images used in clinical practice (Fig. 1a).

2 Related Work

As discussed in Section 1, classical image segmentation algorithms that rely on region homogeneity criteria are not applicable for the extraction of femur contours in x-ray images. These algorithms include thresholding, region growing, region splitting and merging, watershed, classifier, clustering, etc. [5,6].

Deformable models such as active contour [7], active shape [8], and level set method [9] have also been used for medical image segmentation [6]. These methods are contour-based instead of region-based. So, they have the potential of extracting contours of body parts that do not contain homogeneous features. An important weakness of these approaches is that they typically require good initialization of the model contour. If the model is poorly initialized, these approaches can be easily affected by noise and extraneous edges in the image, resulting in incorrect segmentation of the regions.

The atlas-based approach [6] can overcome the weakness of deformable models by roughly aligning a spatial map called atlas to the image before applying deformable model methods. That is, it attempts to solve the initialization problem of deformable models by using prior knowledge such as spatial relationships between the body parts in the images. This approach is very promising but it is typically application specific. That is, segmentation of different images of different body parts typically require different kinds of atlas that contain different prior knowledge. This approach has been applied to the segmentation of brain MR images [10,11] and abdominal CT images [12].

In our application, the atlas-based approach can still face difficulties because the femurs in different images can be oriented differently (Fig. 4) due to variations in the patients' standing postures resulting from femur fractures. Incorporating articulation of body parts in the atlas-based approach may help to solve the problem of model initialization but it makes the atlas very complex and difficult to use. Instead, we apply a simpler model-based approach specific to the femur bone that can handle variations in shape, size, as well as the orientation of the femur in different images.

3 Overview of Algorithm

Our algorithm takes a standard hip x-ray image (Fig. 1a) as the input and automatically extracts femur contours in the x-ray image. It is a model-based algorithm that consists of three main stages:

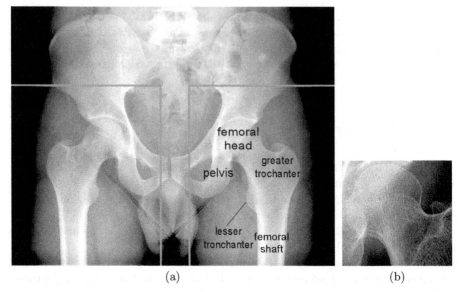

Fig. 1. (a) A standard hip x-ray image. The dark lines delineate the regions that contain the femurs. (b) Close-up view of femoral head.

1. Delineation of the regions that contain the left and the right femurs.
2. Registration of a 2D model femur contour to femur regions in the image.
3. Application of the active contour algorithm with shape constraints to refine the femur model to accurately identify the femur contour in the image.

The first stage is easy to automate because the pose of the patients are similar when the hip x-ray images are taken. The femurs always fall in the left and right bottom corners of the images. Based of 50 training samples, it is determined that the femur region falls within a bounding box of size 990 × 1160 pixels.

The second and third stages are described in the following sections.

3.1   Registration of Femur Model

This stage applies prior knowledge about the femur to register a model of the femur contour to the one in the image. It consists of four main steps:

1. Detection of candidate femoral shafts represented by pairs of parallel lines.
2. Detection of candidate femoral heads represented by circles.
3. Detection of candidate turning points near the base of the greater trochanter.
4. Piecewise registration of model femur contour.

1. Detection of Candidate Femoral Shafts

The outer contours of the femoral shaft consists of two approximately parallel straight lines. So, the natural way to detect femoral shaft is to find a pair of long parallel straight lines.

Femoral shaft detection is performed as follows. First, up to 8 points near the bottom of the image with the largest horizontal intensity gradient components are identified. These are good candidate feature points because the points of the shaft contours have very large intensity gradients. The directions of the intensity gradients at these points should not be larger than 30° (determined from training samples) because the shafts are roughly vertical in the images.

Next, contour following method is applied to identify approximately straight lines starting at the points detected above. The points along a line should have roughly the same intensity gradient direction, and fit well onto a straight line.

After identifying all candidate lines, they are paired up to form candidate femoral shaft contours. The lines are paired based on the following criteria:

- The width w_i between a pair i of lines should fall within an acceptable range. From training samples, it is found the width has a unimodal distribution which can be modeled by a Gaussian G_s with a mean μ_s of 44.64 pixels and a standard deviation σ_s of 4.67. So, given the width w_i, the probability that the pair of lines is the shaft contour is given by $G_s(w_i|\mu_s, \sigma_s)$.
- The lines in a pair i have the correct intensity gradient directions. Specifically, the intensity gradient of the line on the left of the femur should change from dark to bright along the positive x-axis, and that of the line of the right of the femur should change in the opposite direction. Moreover, they should also have large intensity gradient magnitudes M_i, which is computed as the mean of the intensity gradient magnitudes of the points along the lines.
- Thus, the probability P_i that a pair i of lines is indeed the shaft contour is proportional to the product $M_i G_s(w_i|\mu_s, \sigma_s)$, assuming the intensity gradient magnitude and the shaft width are independent factors. The intensity gradient magnitude is based on x-ray absorption, while the shaft width is based on the patient's body size. These two factors are thus independent.

So, each candidate femoral shaft i is associated with a probability measure P_i. The top candidates, at most three, with the largest probability measures are kept. Figure 2(a) illustrates an example with two candidate femoral shaft contours.

2. Detection of Candidate Femoral Heads

The femoral head is approximately circular. Usually, the contour of the femoral head is not very distinctive. On the other hand, the femur socket of the hip bone appears as strong edges in x-ray images, and the points on these strong edges have very large horizontal or vertical intensity gradient components. So, such points are detected at the top left corner of the femur region in the image. Next, circles are fitted over these points using circular Hough transform.

For a particular patient, the size of the femoral head is positively related to that of the femoral shaft. From training samples, it is found that the ratio of the radius of the femoral head to the width of the femoral shaft has a unimodal distribution which can be modeled by a Gaussian G_h with a mean μ_h of 0.91 and a standard deviation σ_h of 0.11. Given a fitted circle i with radius r_i and a

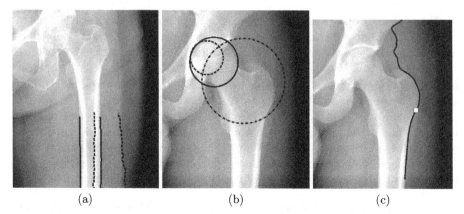

Fig. 2. (a) Candidate femoral shafts. (b) Candidate femoral heads. (c) Turning point (white dot) at greater trochanter.

candidate shaft with width w_i, the probability that circle i falls onto the femoral head is given by $G_h(r_i/w_i|\mu_h, \sigma_h)$. For each candidate shaft found in the previous step, the top femoral head candidates, at most three, with the largest probabilities are kept. This produces at most nine shaft-head combinations. Fig. 2(b) illustrates an example with 3 candidate femoral heads.

3. Detection of Candidate Turning Points

In addition to the candidate femoral shafts and heads, an important feature point which we call the "turning point" is also extracted (Fig. 2c). This feature point is required to correctly initialize the model feature contour for running the active contour algorithm. It is obtained as follows:

- For each candidate femoral shaft, the line on the right side of the parallel pair is extended upward using contour following method with the straight line condition relaxed. So, the line now traces a curve that goes along the boundary of the greater trochanter.
- Next the second derivatives of the points along the curve is computed. The locations of the zero crossings of the second derivatives are identified.
- For each shaft-head combination, the candidate turning points along the shaft and below the center of the head are identified.
- The lowest candidate turning points, at most three, are kept for each shaft-head combination. This produces at most 27 shaft-head-turning point combinations.

4. Piecewise Registration of Femur Model

The model femur contour is divided by five feature points into five segments (Fig. 3a). The corresponding features points in the image are obtained as follows.

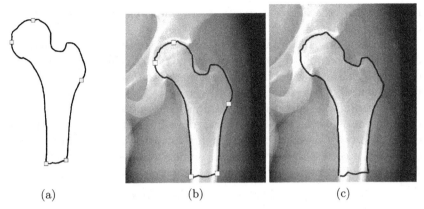

(a)   (b)   (c)

Fig. 3. (a) Model femur contour divided into 5 segments. (b) Piecewise registered femur model used as the initial configuration of the snake algorithm. (c) Extracted femur contour after running the snake algorithm.

The two feature points on the head contour are obtained from the top-most and left-most points of a candidate femoral head. The two feature points at the bottom of the shaft contour are obtained from a candidate femoral shaft. The last feature point is a candidate turning point.

The model femur contour is placed onto the image by piecewise registration of the segments based on each of the 27 possible shaft-head-turning point combinations. The registration of each segment is performed by computing the scaling factor s, rotation matrix $\mathbf{R}$ and translation vector $\mathbf{T}$ that maps a model feature point $\mathbf{p}$ to the corresponding image feature point $\mathbf{q}$:

$$\mathbf{q} = s\mathbf{R}\mathbf{p} + \mathbf{T}. \tag{1}$$

All other points along the model contour are mapped in the same way onto the image. Figure 3(a) illustrates a model femur contour that is registered onto the image and to be used as the initial configuration of the active contour algorithm.

3.2   Active Contour with Curvature Constraints

The original active contour [7], or snake, algorithm is too flexible for this application and has a high tendency of being attracted to noise and extraneous edges instead of the desired femur contour. To allow the snake to avoid noise and extraneous edges, shape constraints are added to the snake model.

The snake is represented by a parametric contour $\mathbf{v}(s) = (x(s), y(s))$, $0 \leq s \leq 1$. Its internal energy $E_i(\mathbf{v}(s))$ is defined as

$$E_i(\mathbf{v}(s)) = \frac{1}{2} \left(\alpha \|\mathbf{v}'(s)\|^2 + \beta \|\mathbf{v}''(s)\|^2 \right) \tag{2}$$

where α and β controls the stretching and bending of the snake contour. It is attracted to image features such as edges and lines. The image features are represented by the external energy E. In our application, the gradient vector flow field [13] is used for E.

The shape of a snake can be constrained by constraining its curvature. The curvature of a contour is proportional to the rate of change of the tangent of the contour, which is a second derivative of the contour point. So, the curvature can be represented by the second derivative vector $\mathbf{v}''(s) = (x''(s), y''(s))$.

To constrain the curvature, we introduce a spring force that is proportional to the difference between the actual curvature $\mathbf{v}''(s)$ of the snake and the reference curvature $\boldsymbol{\omega}(s)$ of the model. The reference curvature is obtained by averaging the curvature of corresponding points in training samples. Then, the spring energy $E_c(\mathbf{v}(s))$ is given by

$$E_c(\mathbf{v}(s)) = \frac{\xi}{2}\|\mathbf{v}''(s) - \boldsymbol{\omega}(s)\|^2 \tag{3}$$

where ξ is a constant parameter that controls the stiffness of the snake. The larger the ξ, the more stiff is the snake, and thus, the better is the snake in preserving its reference shape encoded by the reference curvature $\boldsymbol{\omega}(s)$.

The snake's total energy E_T is

$$E_T = \int \left[E_i(\mathbf{v}(s)) + E_c(\mathbf{v}(s)) + E(\mathbf{v}(s)) \right] ds. \tag{4}$$

When E_T is minimized, $\mathbf{v}(s)$ satisfies the following Euler-Lagrange equation, which can be obtained using variational calculus:

$$-(\alpha \mathbf{v}'(s))' + (\beta \mathbf{v}''(s))'' + (\xi \mathbf{v}''(s) - \xi \boldsymbol{\omega}(s))'' + \nabla E(\mathbf{v}(s)) = 0. \tag{5}$$

Denote the vectors $\nabla E = \mathbf{F} = (F_x, F_y)$ and $\boldsymbol{\omega} = (\omega_x, \omega_y)$. Discretizing Eq. 5 and rewriting in matrix form yields

$$\begin{aligned} \mathbf{A}_x\,\mathbf{x} + \mathbf{F}_x &= 0 \\ \mathbf{A}_y\,\mathbf{y} + \mathbf{F}_y &= 0. \end{aligned} \tag{6}$$

Let the snake be a closed contour with n points such that $\mathbf{v}(n+1) = \mathbf{v}(1)$. Then, the matrix $\mathbf{A}_x$ is given by

$$\mathbf{A}_x = \begin{bmatrix} c_1 & d_1 & e_1 & 0 & \cdots & 0 & a_1 & b_1 & f_1 \\ b_2 & c_2 & d_2 & e_2 & 0 & \cdots & 0 & a_2 & f_2 \\ \vdots & \vdots & \vdots & \vdots & \vdots & \vdots & \vdots & \vdots & \vdots \\ d_n & e_n & 0 & \cdots & 0 & a_n & b_n & c_n & f_n \\ 0 & 0 & 0 & 0 & \cdots & 0 & 0 & 0 & 1 \end{bmatrix} \tag{7}$$

where

$$\begin{aligned} a_i = e_i &= \beta + \xi \\ b_i = d_i &= -\alpha - 4\beta - 4\xi \\ c_i &= 2\alpha + 6\beta + 6\xi \\ f_i &= \xi(-\omega_{x,i-1} + 2\omega_{x,i} - \omega_{x,i+1}). \end{aligned} \tag{8}$$

Compared to the original snake, $\mathbf{A}_x$ has an additional column of constants f_i that capture the second derivatives of the reference curvature at points $\mathbf{v}(i)$.

Moreover, an extra row of n zeros followed by a 1 is added to make the matrix square and invertible. The matrix $\mathbf{A}_y$ is the same as $\mathbf{A}_x$ except ω_x in f_i is replaced by ω_y.

Equation 6 can be solved iteratively by regarding $\mathbf{x}$ and $\mathbf{y}$ as functions of time t, yielding the iterative update equations:

$$\begin{aligned}
\mathbf{x}(t) &= (\mathbf{A}_x + \gamma \mathbf{I})^{-1}(\gamma \mathbf{x}(t-1) - \mathbf{F}_x(t-1)) \\
\mathbf{y}(t) &= (\mathbf{A}_y + \gamma \mathbf{I})^{-1}(\gamma \mathbf{y}(t-1) - \mathbf{F}_y(t-1)).
\end{aligned} \tag{9}$$

The constrained snake algorithm is applied onto each of the candidate shaft-head-turning point combinations. After the snake algorithm has converged, the shape difference between the candidate resultant snake and the reference model is computed in terms of the mean squared error of rigid registration between them. The candidate result with the smallest shape difference is regarded as the extracted femur contour.

Existing methods that also incorporate geometric constraints in the snake include [11,14]. Shen et al. [11] embedded geometric information as attribute vector into a snake. The attribute vector contains the areas of triangles formed by each point on the snake and their two neighboring points. During the snake's evolution process, the areas of the triangles are constrained. However, triangles of different shapes can have the same area. So, this method may not reliably constrain the snake's shape.

Foulonneau et al. [14] includes Legendre moments in the snake. The shortcoming of this method is that moments provide global description of a reference shape. Large local deformations such as size variations of parts of the femur and orientation variations of femurs in different images (Fig. 4) would change the moments significantly even though the overall shape remains roughly the same. Moreover, this method will become very complex if rotation invariance, left out in [14], is to be considered as well.

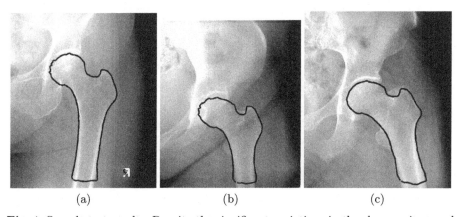

| (a) | (b) | (c) |

Fig. 4. Sample test results. Despite the significant variations in the shapes, sizes, and orientations of the femurs in the images, correct femur contours are extracted. The errors are: (a) 0.98 pixel (b) 3.27 pixels (c) 3.92 pixels.

In comparison, our method not only allows the snake to handle shape and size variations but also variations in the orientations of the femurs.

4   Tests and Discussion

A training set of 100 femur images with manually extracted contours were used to determine the shaft width model and the femoral head radius model. A different set of 172 femur images were used to test the contour extraction method. The size of all training and testing images was 297×348. A simple model femur is used by the algorithm to extract the femur contours in the test images. The error of an extracted contour is measured in terms of the mean error between the points on the extracted contour and their corresponding points on the manually marked contour. Success rate is the fraction of testing samples whose femur contours are extracted accurately. A femur contour is considered successfully extracted if the error is less than 8 pixels, which is only 2% of the image size.

Of the 172 testing samples, 81.4% of the femur contours were successfully extracted, despite the variations in shapes, sizes and orientations of the femurs in the images (Fig. 4). The mean and standard deviation of the errors of the successful samples are 3.88 pixels and 1.50 pixels.

Among the failed cases, 31.3% are such that at least one of the candidate solution is acceptable but not the top ranking solution (e.g., Figure 5a). If we consider these cases as successful cases, the success rate becomes 87.2%.

The other 68.7% of the failed cases do not have acceptable results among the candidate results. Failed samples are either fracture cases such as Figure 5(b) or healthy femurs with odd shapes such as Figure 5(c) or images that contain artifacts such as extraneous straight lines caused by the analogue imaging process. Odd shaped femurs have very short neck or shaft or both, due to the unusual standing postures of the patients with fractures on the other femurs.

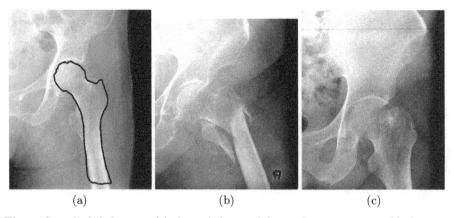

(a)	(b)	(c)

Fig. 5. Sample failed cases. (a) One of the candidate solution is acceptable but not ranked at the top. (b) Fractured femur with severe shape distortion. (c) Healthy femur with an odd shape. There is almost no neck or shaft.

5 Conclusion

This paper presented a method for automatically extracting femur contours from x-ray images. The method detects the positions of the femoral shaft, head and turning points. Then, a model femur contour is registered piecewise to the x-ray image according to these detected features. Finally, active contour with shape constraints is applied to accurately identify the femur contour. Experiments show that this method can successfully extract the contours of femurs with regular shapes, despite variations in size, shape, and orientation. Our continuing research is to extend the method to the extraction of the contours of femurs with severe shape distortions and of other body parts in x-ray images.

References

1. Chen, Y., Yap, W.H., Leow, W.K., Howe, T.S., Png, M.A.: Detecting femur fractures by texture analysis of trabeculae. In: Proc. ICPR. (2004)
2. Lim, S.E., Xing, Y., Chen, Y., Leow, W.K., Howe, T.S., Png, M.A.: Detection of femur and radius fractures in x-ray images. In: Proc. 2nd Int. Conf. on Advances in Medical Signal and Information Processing. (2004)
3. Lum, V.L.F., Leow, W.K., Chen, Y., Howe, T.S., Png, M.A.: Combining classifiers for bone fracture detection in x-ray images. In: Proc. ICIP. (2005)
4. Lin, P., Zhang, F., Yang, Y., Zheng, C.: Carpal-bone feature extraction analysis in skeletal age assessment based on deformable model. J. of Computer Science and Technology (2004)
5. Rogowska, J.: Overview and fundamentals of medical image segmentation. In Bankman, I.N., ed.: Handbook of Medical Imaging, Processing and Analysis. Academic Press (2000) 69–85
6. Pham, D.L., Xu, C., Prince, J.L.: Current methods in medical image segmentation. Annual Review of Biomedical Engineering 2 (2000) 315–337
7. Kass, M., Witkin, A., Terzopoulos, D.: Snakes: active contour models. Int. J. of Computer Vision 1 (1987) 321–331
8. Cootes, T.F., Hill, A., Taylor, C.J., Haslam, J.: The use of active shape models for locating structures in medical images. Image and Vision Computing 12 (1994) 355–366
9. Sethian, J.A.: Level Set Methods. Cambridge University Press (1996)
10. Aboutanos, G.B., Nikanne, J., Watkins, N., Dawant, B.M.: Model creation and deformation for the automatic segmentation of the brain in MR images. IEEE Trans. on Biomedical Engineering 46 (1999) 1346–1356
11. Shen, D., Herskovits, E.H., Davatzikos, C.: An adaptive-focus statistical shape model for segmentation and shape modeling of 3-D brain structures. IEEE Trans. on Medical Imaging 20 (2001)
12. Park, H., Bland, P.H., Meyer, C.R.: Construction of an abdominal probabilistic atlas and its application in segmentation. IEEE Trans. on Medical Imaging 22 (2003) 483–492
13. Xu, C., Prince, J.L.: Gradient vector flow: A new external force for snakes. In: Proc. IEEE Conf. on CVPR. (1997)
14. Foulonneau, A., Charbonnier, P., Heitz, F.: Geometric shape priors for region-based active contours. In: Proc. ICIP. (2003)

Automatic Landmarking of $2D$ Medical Shapes Using the Growing Neural Gas Network

Anastassia Angelopoulou[1], Alexandra Psarrou[1],
José García Rodríguez[2], and Kenneth Revett[1]

[1] Harrow School of Computer Science, University of Westminster,
Harrow HA1 3TP, United Kingdom
{agelopa, psarroa, revettk}@wmin.ac.uk
[2] Departamento de Tecnología Informática y Computación, Universidad de Alicante,
Apdo. 99. 03080 Alicante, Espana,
{jgarcia}@dtic.ua.es

Abstract. MR Imaging techniques provide a non-invasive and accurate method for determining the ultra-structural features of human anatomy. In this study, we utilise a novel approach to segment out the ventricular system in a series of high resolution T1-weighted MR images. Our approach is based on an automated landmark extraction algorithm which automatically selects points along the contour of the ventricles from a series of $2D$ MRI brain images. Automated landmark extraction is accomplished through the use of the self-organising network the growing neural gas (GNG) which is able to topographically map the low dimension of the network to the high dimension of the manifold of the contour without requiring *a priori* knowledge of the structure of the input space. The GNG method is compared to other self-organising networks such as Kohonen and Neural Gas (NG) maps and an error metric is applied to quantify the performance of our algorithm compared to the other two.

1 Introduction

The cerebral ventricles are buried within the centre of the brain parenchyma and are the source of cerebral spinal fluid, which provides nutritive and cushioning support to the brain and spinal cord. Neuropathologies involving the ventricles range from severe hypertrophy diagnostic for hydrocephalus, to mild and diffuse enlargements associated with AIDS, Alzheimer's Disease and Schizophrenia [4,7]. Currently, MRI techniques are employed routinely in the diagnosis of ventricular related diseases. In many cases, the extent of disease progression can be determined by quantifying the extent of the change in ventricular morphology and/or volume [4]. The usual practise in a clinical setting is to perform a high resolution T1-weighted MRI followed by laborious post-processing steps. The first stage in the post-processing step is to segment out the ventricles, which can be difficult in many cases if the patient is not properly aligned in the scanner. Next, the ventricles must be segmented followed by volumetric quantification. These post-processing steps are laborious and must be very accurate if the purpose of the

Y. Liu, T. Jiang, and C. Zhang (Eds.): CVBIA 2005, LNCS 3765, pp. 210–219, 2005.

scan is to help determine the extent of disease progression. In very overburdened medical facilities, performing this task manually may not be feasible. In addition, in a multi-centre study or when a patient visits multiple medical facilities, there is little assurance that the post-processing steps will be performed in an identical fashion. An automated procedure may provide the means of yielding objective and consistent results across various institutions. It is imperative therefore that an accurate, rapid and automated algorithm be developed and deployed. That is the subject of the rest of this paper.

There are several algorithms that have been employed to perform automatic segmentation. These algorithms can be broadly classified into landmark and non-landmark based approaches. Typical non-landmark based techniques have been published using region-growing algorithms [15], level set [1], and rough sets based [17] techniques have been applied in the medical imaging domain.

Landmark based techniques can be classified as manual, semi-automatic and automatic. Because the first two are laborious and subjective especially when applied to 3D images, various attempts have been made to automate the process of landmark based image registration and correct correspondences among a set of shapes. Sousa's *et al.* [16] method, which uses the landmarks of the mean shape of an MRI foot data set as a reference to automatically generate the landmarks to the training set by locally searching the distance between the given landmark point from the mean shape and the nearest strong edge in the image, is arbitrary since the mean shape can be defined only for closed boundaries and for set of images that are mainly aligned and have small variations.

Davies *et al.* [3] method of automatically building statistical shape models by re-paremeterising each shape from the training set and optimising an information theoretic function to assess the quality of the model has received a lot of attention recently. The quality of the model is assessed by adopting a minimum description length (MDL) criterion to the training set. This is a very promising method and the models that are produced are comparable to and often better than the manual built models. However, due to very large number of function evaluations and nonlinear optimisation the method is computationally expensive.

Recently, Fatemizadeh *et al.* [5] have used modified growing neural gas to automatically correspond important landmark points from two related shapes by adding a third dimension to the data points and by treating the problem of correspondence as a cluster-seeking method by adjusting the centers of points from the two corresponding shapes. This is a promising method and has been tested to both synthetic and real data, but the method has not been tested on a large scale for stability and accuracy of building statistical shape models.

In this work, we introduce a new and computationally inexpensive method for the automatic selection of landmarks along the contours of 2D MRI slices of human brain. The incremental neural network, the growing neural gas (GNG) is used to automatically annotate the training set without using *a priori* knowledge of the structure of the input patterns. Unlike other methods, the incremental character of the model avoids the necessity to previously specify a reference shape. The method is used for the representation of two-dimensional outline of the ventricles, which can be extended to three dimensions. As will be discussed in Section 3, GNG does not use any *a priori* knowledge, as its adaptation process is incremental based on competitive hebbian learning. To evaluate the accuracy of the method we have tested it with other self-organising models such as Kohonen maps and Neural Gas (NG) maps and global distance error have been applied to measure the quality of the adaptation of the network.

The remaining of the paper is organised as follows. Section 2 introduces the statistical shape models and its application to automated ventricular segmentation. Section 3 provides a detailed description of the topology learning algorithm GNG and the error measurement used for the adaptation process. A set of experimental results is presented in Section 4, followed by our major conclusions and future work.

2   Statistical Shape Models

When analysing biological shapes it is convenient and usually effective to describe them using statistical shape models. The most well known statistical shape models are Cootes *et al.* [2] 'Point Distribution Models' (PDMs) that models the shape of an object and its variation by using a set of n_p landmark points from a training set of S_i shapes. In this work, PDM represents the ventricles as a set of n_p automatically extracted landmarks (in our case 64, 100, 144 and 169 neurons) in a vector $\mathbf{x} = [x_{i0}, x_{i1}, ..., x_{in_{p-1}}, y_{i0}, y_{i1}, ..., y_{in_{p-1}}]^T$. In order to generate flexible shape models the S_i shapes are aligned (translated, rotated, scaled) and normalised (removing the centre-of-gravity and placing it at the origin) to a common set of axes. The modes of variations of the ventricles are captured by applying principal component analysis (PCA). The ith shape in the training set can be back-projected to the input space by a linear model of the form:

$$\mathbf{x} = \overline{\mathbf{x}} + \Phi\beta_i \tag{1}$$

where $\overline{\mathbf{x}}$ is the mean shape, Φ describes a set of orthogonal modes of shape variations, and β_i is a vector of weights for the ith shape. To ensure that the above weight changes describe reasonable variations we restrict the weight β_i to the range $-2\sqrt{\lambda} \leq \beta_i \leq 2\sqrt{\lambda}$ and the shape is back-projected to the input space using Equation (1). PCA works well as long as good correspondences exist. To obtain the correspondences and represent the contour of the ventricles a self-organising network GNG was used.

3   Topology Learning

One way of selecting points of interest along the contour of $2D$ shapes is to use a topographic mapping where a low dimensional map is fitted to the high dimensional manifold of the contour, whilst preserving the topographic structure of the data. A common way to achieve this is by using self-organising neural networks where input patterns are projected onto a network of neural units such that similar patterns are projected onto units adjacent in the network and vice versa. As a result of this mapping a representation of the input patterns is achieved that in postprocessing stages allows one to exploit the similarity relations of the input patterns. Such models have been successfully used in applications such as speech processing [9], robotics [14,11] and image processing [13]. However, most common approaches are not able to provide good neighborhood and topology preservation if the logical structure of the input patten is not known *a priori*. In fact, the most common approaches specify in advance the number of neurons in the network and a graph that represents topological relationships between them, for example, a two-dimensional grid, and seek the best match to the given input pattern manifold. When this is not the case the networks fail to provide good topology preserving as for example in the case of Kohonen's algorithm.

The approach presented in this paper is based on self-organising networks trained using the Growing Neural Gas learning method [6]. This is an incremental training algorithm where the number of units in the network are determined by the unifying measure for neighborhood preservation [8], the topographic product. The links between the units in the network are established through competitive hebbian learning [10]. As a result the algorithm can be used in cases where the topological structure of the input pattern is not known *a priori* and yields topology preserving maps of feature manifold [12].

3.1 Growing Neural Gas

With Growing Neural Gas (GNG) [6] a growth process takes place from minimal network size and new units are inserted successively using a particular type of vector quantisation [9]. To determine where to insert new units, local error measures are gathered during the adaptation process and each new unit is inserted near the unit which has the highest accumulated error. At each adaptation step a connection between the winner and the second-nearest unit is created as dictated by the competitive hebbian learning algorithm. This is continued until an ending condition is fulfilled, as for example evaluation of the optimal network topology based on the topographic product [8]. This measure is used to detect deviations between the dimensionalities of the network and that of the input space, detecting folds in the network and, indicating that is trying to approximate to an input manifold with different dimensions. In addition, in GNG networks learning parameters are constant in time, in contrast to other methods whose learning is based on decaying parameters.

In the remaining of this Section we describe the growing neural gas algorithm and ending condition as used in this work. The network is specified as:

- A set N of nodes (neurons). Each neuron $c \in N$ has its associated reference vector $w_c \in R^d$. The reference vectors can be regarded as positions in the input space of their corresponding neurons.
- A set of edges (connections) between pairs of neurons. These connections are not weighted and its purpose is to define the topological structure. An *edge aging scheme* is used to remove connections that are invalid due to the motion of the neuron during the adaptation process.

The GNG learning algorithm to map the network to the input manifold is as follows:

1. Start with two neurons a and b at random positions w_a and w_b in R^d.
2. Generate at random an input pattern ξ according to the data distribution $P(\xi)$ of each input pattern. In our case since the input space is $1D$, the input pattern is the (x, y) coordinate of the edges. Typically, for the training of the network we generated 1000 to 10000 input patterns depending on the complexity of the input space.
3. Find the nearest neuron (winner neuron) s_1 and the second nearest s_2.
4. Increase the age of all the edges emanating from s_1.
5. Add the squared distance between the input signal and the winner neuron to a counter error of s_1 such as:

$$\Delta error(s_1) = \|w_{s_1} - \xi\|^2 \qquad (2)$$

6. Move the winner neuron s_1 and its topological neighbours (neurons connected to s_1) towards ξ by a learning step ϵ_w and ϵ_n, respectively, of the total distance:

$$\Delta w_{s_1} = \epsilon_w(\xi - w_{s_1}) \qquad (3)$$

$$\Delta w_{s_n} = \epsilon_w(\xi - w_{s_n}) \qquad (4)$$

for all direct neighbours n of s_1.
7. If s_1 and s_2 are connected by an edge, set the age of this edge to 0. If it does not exist, create it.
8. Remove the edges larger than a_{max}. If this results in isolated neurons (without emanating edges), remove them as well.
9. Every certain number λ of input patterns generated, insert a new neuron as follows:
   - Determine the neuron q with the maximum accumulated error.
   - Insert a new neuron r between q and its further neighbour f:

$$w_r = 0.5(w_q + w_f) \qquad (5)$$

   - Insert new edges connecting the neuron r with neurons q and f, removing the old edge between q and f.
10. Decrease the error variables of neurons q and f multiplying them with a consistent α. Initialize the error variable of r with the new value of the error variable of q and f.
11. Decrease all error variables by multiplying them with a constant γ.
12. If the stopping criterion is not yet achieved (in our case the stopping criterion is the number of neurons), go to step 2.

The algorithm was tested with different number of neurons so that the best topological map can be achieved. The testing involved two cases were the number of neurons were too few or too excessive for the training set of the images. In the former the topological map is lost, not enough neurons to represent the contour of the ventricles and in the later an overfit is performed.

3.2   Error Minimisation

The goal of training a network is to minimise the expected *quantisation or distortion error*. In our case is to find the values of the reference vectors $w_c, c \in R^d$ of the input pattern distribution $P(\xi)$ such that the error:

$$E = \sum_{\forall \xi \in R^d} \| w_{s\xi} - \xi \|^2 \, P(\xi) \qquad (6)$$

is minimised, where s_ξ is the nearest neuron to the input pattern ξ.

Figure 1 shows the quantisation error for the three self-organising maps (SOMs) for different number of neurons. From Figure 1 one can see that the distortion error for Kohonen is very big compared to NG and GNG but for NG the results are slightly better to GNG, since it has less distortion error thus better topology preservation, but the learning time is 20 times higher compared to GNG (Figure 6). However, as the number of neurons increases the distortion error decreases and stabilises for both networks. For both Kohonen and NG in the adaptation rule it is assumed that the numbers of weights are known and are not allowed to change. GNG overcomes this as it is a growth mechanism and new neurons are inserted based on local error measurements. Thus GNG can give better preservation compared to the other two and when tested to a larger scale of data set (the above algorithms have been tested to hand shapes).

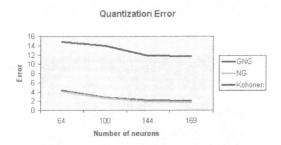

Fig. 1. Quadratic error for different SOMs and neurons

4   Experiments

The data that we used in this study was obtained from the MNI BIC Centre for Imaging at McGill University, Canada. These images are 1 mm thick, 181x217 pixels per slice ($1.0mm^2$ in-plane resolution), 3% noise and 20% INU. These images are used as our gold standard for segmentation, as every voxel in the entire volume has been correctly labelled to a tissue class by the McGill Institute. The entire brain volume consisted of 181 slices, from which we extracted those that contained ventricles (slices 49-91). The images are 16 bit grey scale, which were thresholded out manually to remove all but the outline of the ventricles. Since most typical clinical MRI volumes are on average 5 mm thick, we selected 4

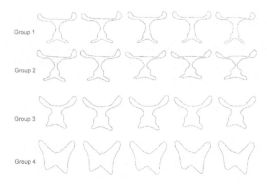

Fig. 2. The first mode ($m = 1$) of variation for the four groups of 5 contiguous slices taken from MR brain data. Range of variation $-2\sqrt{\lambda} \leq \beta_i \leq 2\sqrt{\lambda}$.

groups of 5 contiguous slices to produce our point distribution model. In Figure 2 the modes of variation for all four groups are displayed by varying the first shape parameter $\beta_i\{\pm 2\sigma\}$ over the training set. The qualitatively results show that GNG leads to correct extraction of corners of anatomical shapes and are compact when the topology preservation of the network is achieved (Figure 4).

In Figure 3 two shape variations from the automatically generated landmarks were superimposed to groups 4 and 3 from the training set. These modes effectively capture the variability of the training set and present only valid shape instances.

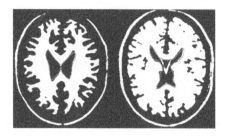

Fig. 3. Superimposed shape instances to groups 4 and 3 from the training set

Table 1 shows the total variance achieved by maps containing varying number of neurons (64, 100, 144, 169) used for the automatic annotation (Figure 4). The map of 100 neurons is the most compact since it achieves the least variance compared to 64, 144 and 169 neurons among the four groups. It is interesting to note that whilst there is significant difference between 64, and 169 neurons -not enough neurons to represent the object (Image A) and too many neurons (Image D)- the mapping with 100 is good and has no significant difference with the mapping of 144 neurons. The reason is that for the current size of the images the distance between the neurons is short enough so adding extra neurons does not

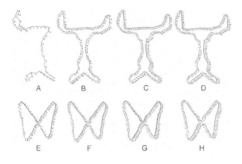

Fig. 4. Automatic annotation with network size of 64 (Image A, E), 100 (Image B, F), 144 (Image C, G) and 164 (Image D, H) neurons for two groups of the MRI volumes of the ventricles

Table 1. A quantitative comparison of various neurons adapted to the ventricle model with total variance per group

Groups	64 (neurons)	100 (neurons)	144 (neurons)	169 (neurons)
V_{T_1}	9.8340	1.9385	3.9668	3.9235
V_{T_2}	13.1873	1.7284	4.3672	3.1617
V_{T_3}	6.7822	2.0109	3.2260	4.0057
V_{T_4}	2.2567	1.6198	2.8398	3.5861

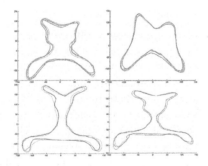

Fig. 5. The means of the four groups and for different neurons. The blue outlines represent the means of the 64, 144 and 169 neurons. The red outline represents the most compact mean achieved with the mapping of 100 neurons.

give more accuracy in placement. Figure 5 shows superimposed the mean shapes of each group and for all neurons. The red shape referring to the 100 neurons is the most compact mean shape. We have tested and compared our method with two other SOMs, the Kohonen map and the NG map. The quantitative results show that GNG is significantly faster compared to Kohonen and NG, and the learning time is not so significant in GNG with the insertion of neurons

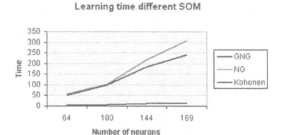

Fig. 6. Learning time for various SOMs and at various neurons

compared to the other two where the adaptation process slows dramatically as
the number of neurons increases.

Figure 6 shows a comparative diagram of the learning time of various SOMs
and at different number of neurons. The adaptation with 64 neurons is only 3 sec
with GNG compared to the 57 sec and 52 sec with Kohonen and NG, but with
64 neurons the topology preservation in most of the shapes is lost independent
of the selection of the SOM. A good adaptation with 100 and 144 neurons takes
6 and 11 seconds respectively at 1000 patterns to adapt to the contour of the
ventricles.

5   Conclusions

In this paper, we have used an incremental self-organising neural network (GNG)
to automatically annotate landmark points on a training set of ventricle outlines. We have shown that the low dimensional incremental neural model (GNG)
adapts successfully to the high dimensional manifold of the contour of the ventricles, allowing good eigenshape models to be generated completely automatically
from the training set. With the current formulation of our algorithm, we can
calculate the volume of the ventricles by integrating the area of the ventricles
across each slice. The accuracy of our automated segmentation algorithm is better compared to the self-organising networks NG and Kohonen both in quality
(Figure 1) and in execution time (Figure 6). In addition, we have shown that the
optimum number of neurons required to represent the contour depends mainly
on the resolution of the input space and if it is not sufficient then the topology
preservation is lost or overfit.

In future work, we could extend this technology so that it will generate
3D models directly. In addition, the generalisability of this model needs to be
determined by applying it to various phantoms and other MRI standards. In
addition, we will investigate what is the most suitable number of neurons for
classifying ventricles. Lastly, we will investigate applying this technology to other
brain tissue components in an effort to generate a complete MRI segmentation
utility.

References

1. C. Baillard, P. Hellier, and P. Barillot. Segmentation of 3D brain structures using level sets and dense registration. *IEEE Workshop on mathematical Methods on Biomedical Image Analysis*, pages 94–101, 2000.
2. T. F. Cootes, C. J. Taylor, D. H. Cooper, and Graham J. Training models of shape from sets of examples. *3rd British Machine Vision Conference*, pages 9–18, 1992.
3. H. Rhodies Davies, J. Carole Twining, F. Tim Cootes, C. John Waterton, and J. Chris Taylor. A minimum description length approach to statistical shape modeling. *IEEE Transaction on Medical Imaging*, 21(5):525–537, 2002.
4. Y. Ding, J.P. McAllister II, B. Yao, N. Yan, and A.I. Canady. Axonal damage associated with enlargement of ventricles during hydrocepahlus: A silver impregnation study. *Neurological Research*, 23(6):581–587, 2001.
5. E. Fatemizadeh, C. Lucas, and H. Soltania-Zadeh. Automatic landmark extraction from image data using modified growing neural gas network. *IEEE Transactions on Information Technology in Biomedicine*, 7(2):77–85, 2003.
6. B. Fritzke. A growing neural gas network learns topologies. *In Advances in Neural Information Processing Systems 7*, pages 625–632, 1995.
7. B. Gelman, S. Dholakia, S. Casper, T.A. Kent, MW. Cloyd, and D. Freeman. Expansion of the cerebral ventricles and correlation with acquired immunodeficiency syndrome neuropathology in 232 patients. *Arch Pathol Lab Med*, 120(9):866–871, 1996.
8. J. Geoffrey, F. Goodhill, and J. Terrence. A unifying measure for neighbourhood preservation in topographic mappings. *Proceedings of the 2nd Joint Symposium on Neural Computation*, 5:191–202, 1997.
9. T. Kohonen. *Self-organising maps*. Springer Verlag, 2001.
10. T. Martinez. Competitive hebbian learning rule forms perfectly topology preserving maps. In *ICANN.*, 1993.
11. T. Martinez, H. Ritter, and K. Schulten. Three dimensional neural net for learning visuomotor-condination of a robot arm. *IEEE Transactions on Neural Networks*, 1:131–136, 1990.
12. T. Martinez and K. Schulten. Topology representing networks. *The Journal of Neural Networks*, 7(3):507–522, 1994.
13. M. Nasrabati and Y. Feng. Vector quantisation of images based upon kohonen self-organizing feature maps. In *Proc. IEEE Int. Conf. Neural Networks.*, pages 1101–1108, 1988.
14. H. Ritter and K. Schulten. Topology conserving mappings for learning motor tasks. In *Neural Networks for Computing, AIP Conf. Proc.*, 1986.
15. HG. Schnack, PHE. Hulshoff, WFC. Baare, MA. Viergever, and RS. Kahn. Automatic segmentation of the ventricular system from mr images of the human brain. *NeuroImage*, 14:95–104, 2001.
16. A. Souza and J.K. Udupa. Automatic landmark selection for active shape models. *Proccedings of SPIE*, 2005.
17. S. Widz, K. Revett, and D. Slezak. An automated multi-spectral MRI segmentation algorithm using approximate reducts. *Rough Sets and Current Trends in Computing*, pages 815–824, 2004.

Biomedical Image Classification with Random Subwindows and Decision Trees

Raphaël Marée, Pierre Geurts, Justus Piater,
and Louis Wehenkel

GIGA Bioinformatics Platform / CBIG, Department of EE & CS,
Institut Montefiore, University of Liège, B-4000 Liège, Belgium

Abstract. In this paper, we address a problem of biomedical image classification that involves the automatic classification of x-ray images in 57 predefined classes with large intra-class variability. To achieve that goal, we apply and slightly adapt a recent generic method for image classification based on ensemble of decision trees and random subwindows. We obtain classification results close to the state of the art on a publicly available database of 10000 x-ray images. We also provide some clues to interpret the classification of each image in terms of subwindow relevance.

1 Introduction

Image classification is an important problem which appears in many application domains. Manual classification of images is time-consuming, repetitive, and could not always be considered reliable. Therefore, there is an important need for automatic image classification tools. Given a set of training images labelled into a finite number of classes, the goal of an automatic image classification method is to build a model that will be able to predict accurately the class of new, unseen images.

In biomedical applications, such automatic techniques could help to organize large-scale image databases into image categories before further retrieval or diagnostic [LGD+05]. A class could for example denote a code [LSK+03] corresponding to an imaging modality and direction, a body part, and a biological system examined, in order to organize images in a general way without limitation to a specific diagnostic study. The annotation of such images is usually done automatically by medical equipments and/or manually adapted by physicians or radiologists. However, [GKK+02] has examined reliability of the encoded information from past clinical routines and the authors observed that some entries are missing, or are false, or do not describe the anatomic region precisely. Automatic image classification systems are thus an important, complementary, first step in medical imaging.

Image classification methods have also been proposed to setup clinical diagnosis tools based on functional magnetic resonance [ZST+05, LTC+04] or optical tomography [BH05] images. Another interesting application is the study of the

Y. Liu, T. Jiang, and C. Zhang (Eds.): CVBIA 2005, LNCS 3765, pp. 220–229, 2005.

phenotypic effects of drugs in human cells [KDN01] where a class could for example denote stomatocytes, discocytes, or echinocytes. It is also desirable to setup high-throughput cell phenotype screening [CEW+04] where the goal of an automatic image classification method could be to identify classes of subcellular phenotypes, for example cytoplasm, mitochondria, nucleoli, ... In histological image classification [ZCC05], a class could represent a tissue from an organ and part of the body: pancreas, lung, thyroid, ...

1.1 Related Work

Till recently, image classification systems usually relied on a pre-processing step, specific to the particular problem and application domain, which aims at extracting a reduced set of "interesting" features from the initially huge number of pixels. This reduced set is then used as new input variables (or "signatures") for traditional learning algorithms (for example a nearest neighbor or neural network classifiers), possibly tuned for the specific application ([GMT+96], [AZC01], [ALTS03]).

The limitation of this approach is clear: When considering a new application or when new image classes appear, it is often necessary to manually adapt the pre-processing step by taking into account the specific characteristics of the new task. However, a more recent trend is to consider combining several different types of features that describe different aspects of an image. For example, in [LGD+05], image recognition rates are improved by combining global texture measures and local pixel neighborhood information. In [CEW+04], 448 different image features are extracted corresponding to textures descriptions, intensity distributions, edges, ... Other recent computer vision studies [MTS+05] suggest that current feature detectors are complementary (some being more adapted to structured scenes while others to textures) and that all of them should ideally be used in parallel, what would likely increase robustness to different types of image transformations.

In [MGPW05b], we have proposed a generic approach to image classification. Indeed, as we generally don't know in advance what is useful in images to classify them, we proposed to describe images by the combination of a large number of square patches randomly extracted from images ("Random Subwindows"). This process has the advantage to provide a rich representation of images corresponding to various overlapping regions both local and global, whatever the task and content of images. Moreover, to avoid discarding useful information and to be able to classify a large number of classes, we proposed to use a highly informative representation that is basically the pixel values of these subwindows. This representation is also normalized to improve robustness to scale changes. To handle this high-dimensional data and to extract useful information, we rely on recent tree-based machine learning ensemble methods [MGPW05a]. These methods are indeed able to handle more and more complex problems (high-dimensional data) without requiring any a priori information about the application. This approach has been evaluated on various image classification datasets involving the classification of digits, faces, objects, buildings, photographs, ...

1.2   This Work

In this paper, we propose to apply and slightly adapt our general approach [MGPW05b] to a specific biomedical application: the classification of a database of 10000 grey-level x-ray images into 57 categories.[1] For image classification methods, this is a very challenging task because of the intra-class variability of such images. But thanks to the generality of the approach, only some minor adaptations have been required to tackle specific issues of this dataset and to obtain results comparable to the state of the art. In this paper, we also propose an interpretation of the classification results by focusing on the test subwindows that contribute to the classification of one image.

The biomedical dataset we used is described in Section 2. The main steps of the approach and its adaptation are described in Section 3. Our empirical results, and the interpretation of the results are given in Section 4.

2   IRMA X-Ray Dataset

The IRMA dataset contains 10000 anonymous x-ray images, which have been arbitrarly selected from clinical routine at Aachen University of Technology Hospital (RWTH), Germany. These images were acquired using different imaging techniques and modalities (plain radiography, fluoroscopy, angiography) with different relative directions of the device and the patient (coronal, sagittal, axial, other). They represent different anatomic body parts (cranium, spine, arm, chest, abdomen, leg, pelvis, breast, hand, ...) and biological systems (muscu-loscetal, uropoietic, gastrointestinal, reproductive, cardiovascular) of patients of various ages, genders, and pathologies. All images are in grey levels and were downscaled to fit into a 512×512 bounding box maintaining the original aspect ratio. All images were classified according to the IRMA code [LSK+03]. Based on this code, 57 classes were defined. As mentionned by [PG04], in addition to natural variations between different patients, the intra-class variability is high for that kind of task, caused in particular by varying orientation and alignment, and/or by the presence of cloths, jewels, artificial-implants and medical instruments, and/or because images are characterized with contrast variation, non-uniform intensity background and various sources of noise. The task is thus non-trivial for image classification methods. Figure 2 exhibits some images of the dataset with intra-class variability, but also images from different classes that may look similar for non-experts.

3   Method

In this section, we briefly describe the framework that we proposed in [MGPW05b] with an emphasis on minor changes for the purpose of the task considered in this paper.

---

[1] IRMA database courtesy of TM Lehmann, Dept. of Medical Informatics, RWTH Aachen, Germany, http://www.irma-project.org.

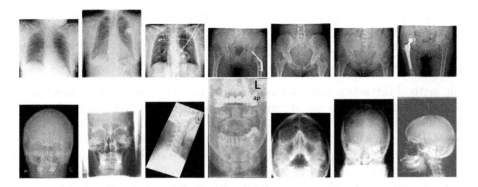

Fig. 1. Some plain radiographies. On the first line, the three first images are from the same class (chest), the four following ones are from another class (pelvis). On the second line, all images are from 7 different classes related to cranium or cervical spine. Note that all these images are correclty classified by our method.

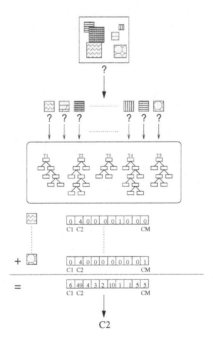

Fig. 2. Recognition: randomly-extracted subwindows are propagated through the trees (here $T = 5$). Votes are aggregated and the majority class is assigned to the image.

During the training phase, subwindows are randomly extracted from training images (3.1), and a model is constructed by machine learning (3.2). Classification of a new test image (3.3) similarly entails extraction and description of subwindows, and the application of the learned model to these subwindows. Aggregation of subwindow predictions is then performed to classify the test image, as illustrated in Figure 2.

3.1 Subwindows

The method extracts a large number (N_w) of possibly overlapping, square subwindows of random sizes and at random positions from training images. Subwindows are resized to a fixed scale (16×16 pixels) and encoded by their grey-value pixels. Each subwindow is thus described by a feature vector of 256 integer values. The same random process and descriptors are used for test images.

For the specific x-ray task, the method has to cope with a learning dataset with very unbalanced class distributions. For example, a "chest" class is represented by more than 2500 images while several other classes have less than 20 images. For example, an "abdomen" class has only 9 training images. In order to have an equal number of subwindows in each class, we extract from each training image a number of subwindows inversely proportional to the number of images in its class. More precisely, from each training image of class c, we extract $N_w/(m * nb_c)$ subwindows where m is the number of classes and nb_c the number of training images of class c. For testing, we extract a fixed number of subwindows in each image, $N_{w,test}$, as in the original method.

3.2 Learning

At the learning phase, a model is automatically built using subwindows extracted from training images. First, each subwindow is labelled with the class of its parent image. Then, any supervised machine learning algorithm can be applied to build a subwindow classification model. Here, the input of a machine learning algorithm is thus a training sample of N_w subwindows, each of which is described by 256 integer input variables and a discrete output class. The learning algorithm should consequently be able to deal efficiently with a large amount of data, first in terms of the number of subwindows and classes of images in the training set, but more importantly in terms of the number of values describing these subwindows. In this context, and following our previous comparative study [MGPW05a], we use the Tree Boosting [FRS96] and Extra-Trees [GEW05] algorithms. Their advantages are the computational efficiency (especially Extra-Trees) and their good accuracy.

3.3 Recognition

In this approach, the learned model is used to classify subwindows of a test image. To make a prediction for a test image with an ensemble of trees grown from subwindows, each subwindow is simply propagated into each tree of the ensemble. Each tree outputs conditional class probability estimates for each subwindow. Each subwindow thus receives T class probability estimate vectors where T denotes the number of trees in the ensemble. All the predictions are then averaged and the class corresponding to the largest aggregated probability estimate is assigned to the image.

4   Experiments

4.1   Protocol and Method Parameters

To be able to directly compare our results with other methods, we used the standard protocol defined in the context of the ImageCLEF 2005 Automatic Annotation Task [iCS05]. The learning set is composed of 9000 images and the remaining 1000 images are used for testing.

The parameters of our method were fixed to $N_w = 800000$ learning subwindows (which corresponds approximately to 14000 subwindows per class), $T = 25$ trees, and $N_{w,test} = 500$ subwindows are randomly extracted from each test image. To minimize contrast variations between images, we have applied the contrast enhancement technique of ImageMagick[2] (-normalize option) to each image which transforms it to span the full range of grey values.

For each machine learning method within the framework, the values of several parameters need to be fixed.

Extra-Trees. With Extra-Trees, the only parameter is the number K of attributes randomly selected at each test node. To fix its value, we used an internal cross validation in the learning sample to determine the best of $K \in \{1, 16, 128, 256\}$. The best result was obtained with $K = 256$ and then we used this value to build a model on the whole learning set.

Tree Boosting. Boosting requires that the learning algorithm does not give perfect models on the learning sample (so as to provide some misclassified instances). Hence, with this method, we used with decision trees the stop-splitting criterion described by [Weh97]. It uses a hypothesis test based on the G^2 statistic to determine the significance of a test. In our experiments, we fixed the nondetection risk α to 0.005, as in our previous study for object recognition [MGPW05a].

4.2   Accuracy Results

Our results using the standard protocol are reported in Table 1 in terms of misclassification error rates on the independent test set, as well as several results obtained by 11 other research units. [3] Among the 46 methods evaluated on this dataset, a majority of them yield more than 20% error rate where each 0.1% corresponds to 1 misclassification. The Random Subwindows combined with Tree Boosting method yields 140 errors among 1000 test images (14%) and compares very well with the best result on this dataset (12.6%). Combining Random Subwindows with Extra-Trees also yields good results with 14.7% error rate. Table 2 also gives results when the correct class occurs among the first r classes, and we observe that the error rate could be reduced downto 6.6% with Tree Boosting if the correct class is only required to be within the top three classes.

---

[2] http://www.imagemagick.org/

[3] All results are available on http://www-i6.informatik.rwth-aachen.de/~deselaers/imageclef05_aat_results.html.

Table 1. Error rates on IRMA dataset (our results *italic*) [iCS05]

Method	error rate
1-NN + IDM [KGN04]	12.6%
1-NN + CCF + IDM + Tamura	13.3%
Discriminative patches [DKN05]	13.9%
Random Subwindows + Tree Boosting	14.0 %
MI1 Confidence	14.6%
Random Subwindows + Extra-Trees	14.7%
Gift 5NN8g	20.6%
...	...
Nearest Neighbor, 32 × 32, Euclidian	36.8%
...	...
Texture directionality	73.3%

Table 2. Error rates for rank $r = 1, ..., 5$

Method	$r = 1$	$r = 2$	$r = 3$	$r = 4$	$r = 5$
RSw + Tree Boosting	14.0 %	9.0%	6.6%	6.5%	6.5%
RSw + Extra-Trees	14.7%	9.4%	7.0%	7.0%	7.0%

4.3   Computational Efficiency

Even though our current implementation has not been fully optimized, some indications can be given about computational requirements. For example, on a standard 2.4Ghz computer it took us about 75 hours to build a tree ensemble by boosting, and 18 hours to build an ensemble of 25 Extra-Trees (without counting the pre-processing tasks[4] such as subwindow sampling, extraction and normalization). With these models, the CPU time needed to classify a single new image was of about 1.125s (without taking into account the time needed to extract the 500 subwindows).

Notice that the computational complexity of the training algorithm is on the order of $TN_w \log N_w$, and that of the testing stage is essentially proportional to $TN_{w,test} \log N_w$. These numbers could thus be adjusted in order to comply with the desired requirements. For example, with Tree Boosting, using $N_{w,test} = 100$ instead of 500 reduced classification time to 0.225s, at the price of a negligible increase in error rate (which increased from 14% to 14.1%).

4.4   Relevant Subwindows

Beyond misclassification error rates, it could be interesting to observe how the proposed method classifies images, or in other words which subwindows contribute to the correct classification of one image. As mentionned before and illustrated by Figure 2, for one test image, each subwindow is propagated into

---

[4] For the pre-processing tasks, we used ImageMagick.

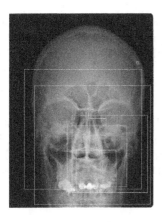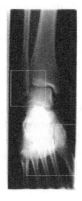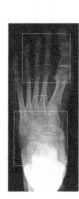

Fig. 3. Subwindows with the highest number of correct votes for three test images (from classes cranium, ankle joint, and foot).

the T trees of the ensemble and thus receives T votes. Consequently, we have for each subwindow the distribution of votes for all classes. The subwindows that receive the highest number of votes for a given class can then be considered as the most specific ones for that class and their visualization on the top of the image can bring potentially useful information about that class.

This functionality could be very helpful if the goal of the biomedical image classication task is for example to detect and classify diseased regions. The most relevant regions for a given class could then be shown to experts for further analysis.

In Figure 3, we simply provide some examples of subwindows receiving a high number of correct votes when using Random Subwindows combined with Tree Boosting. We observe that both small and large regions are among the best classified subwindows of many test images. It seems to confirm that it is not straigthforward to determine in advance what is useful in images to classify them and thus both local and global regions should be used by image classification methods.

5   Conclusions

In this paper we evaluated the applicability of our image classification method based on ensemble of decision trees and random subwindows [MGPW05b], for a specific biomedical task: x-ray image classification. We obtained results comparable to the state of the art with around 14% error rate on a 57 class dataset involving large intra-class variability and very unbalanced class distributions. For the task of retrieving the correct class within the third best classes, our method yields 6.6% error rate. We also provide a novel simple way to understand how the method classifies images which may be of high interest for biomedical applications.

Our results confirm the potential of the approach for a wide range of applications. Many biomedical applications could benefit from this approach especially since it is directly applicable without tedious adaptation. We plan to apply the method to other biomedical applications as soon as such image datasets will be publicly available. Possible applications are for example the classification of pharmaceutical powders, human cells, histological tissues, . . .

Acknowledgments

Raphaël Marée is supported by the GIGA-Interdisciplinary Cluster for Applied Genoproteomics, hosted by the University of Liège. Pierre Geurts is a Postdoctoral Researcher at the National Fund for Scientific Research (FNRS, Belgium). IRMA database courtesy of TM Lehmann, Dept. of Medical Informatics, RWTH Aachen, Germany.

References

[ALTS03]   S. Antani, LR. Long, G. Thoma, and RJ. Stanley. Vertebra shape classification using mlp for content-based image retrieval. In *Proc. International Joint Conference on Neural Networks (IJCNN)*, pages 160–165, July 2003.

[AZC01]   M.-L. Antonie, O. R. Zaïane, and A. Coman. Application of data mining techniques for medical image classification. In *Proc. of Second Intl. Workshop on Multimedia Data Mining (MDM/KDD'2001) in conjunction with Seventh ACM SIGKDD*, pages 94–101, August 2001.

[BH05]   V. Balasubramanyam and A. H. Hielscher. Classification of optical tomographic images of rheumatoid finger joints with support vector machines. In *Proc. SPIE Advanced Biomedical and Clinical Diagnostic Systems III*, volume 5692, pages 37–43, April 2005.

[CEW+04]   C. Conrad, H. Erfle, P. Warnat, N. Daigle, T. Lörch, J. Ellenberg, R. Pepperkok, and R. Eils. Automatic identification of subcellular phenotypes on human cell arrays. *Genome Research*, 14:1130–1136, 2004.

[DKN05]   T. Deselaers, D. Keysers, and H. Ney. Discriminative training for object recognition using image patches. In *Proc. International Conference on Computer Vision and Pattern Recognition (CVPR)*, volume 2, pages 157–162, June 2005.

[FRS96]   Y. Freund and E. Robert Schapire. Experiments with a new boosting algorithm. In *Proc. Thirteenth International Conference on Machine Learning*, pages 148–156, 1996.

[GEW05]   P. Geurts, D. Ernst, and L. Wehenkel. Extremely randomized trees. *Submitted*, 2005.

[GKK+02]   MO. Güld, M. Kohnen, D. Keysers, H. Schubert, BB. Wein, J. Bredno, and TM. Lehmann. Quality of dicom header information for image categorization. In *Proceedings SPIE*, pages 280–287, 2002.

[GMT+96]   M. Goldbaum, S. Moezzi, A. Taylor, S. Chatterjee, J. Boyd, E. Hunter, and R. Jain. Automated diagnosis and image understanding with object extraction, object classification, and inferencing in retinal images. In *Proc. IEEE International Conference on Image Processing (ICIP)*, volume 3, pages 695–698, 1996.

[iCS05]   Springer Lecture Notes in Computer Science, editor. *Proc. of Cross Language Evaluation Forum (CLEF), to appear*, 2005.

[KDN01]   D. Keysers, J. Dahmen, and H. Ney. Invariant classification of red blood
            cells. In *Proc. Bildverarbeitung für die Medezin (BVM)*, pages 367–371,
            March 2001.

[KGN04]   D. Keysers, C. Gollan, and H. Ney. Classification of medical images
            using non-linear distortion models. In *Bildverarbeitung für die Medizin
            (BVM)*, pages 366–370, March 2004.

[LGD⁺05]   TM. Lehmann, MO. Güld, T. Deselaers, D. Keysers, H. Schubert,
            K. Spitzer, H. Ney, and BB Wein. Automatic categorization of medi-
            cal images for content-based retrieval and data mining. *Computerized
            Medical Imaging and Graphics*, 29(2):143–155, 2005.

[LSK⁺03]   TM. Lehmann, H. Schubert, D. Keysers, M. Kohnen, and BB. Wein.
            The irma code for unique classification of medical images. In *SPIE*,
            volume 5033, pages 109–117, 2003.

[LTC⁺04]   Y. Liu, L. Teverovskiy, O. Carmichael, R. Kikinis, M. Shenton, C.S.
            Carter, V.A. Stenger, S. Davis, H. Aizenstein, J. Becker, O. Lopez, ,
            and C. Meltzer. Discriminative MR image feature analysis for automatic
            schizophrenia and alzheimer's disease classification. In *Proc. of the 7th
            International Conference on Medical Image Computing and Computer
            Aided Intervention (MICCAI '04)*, pages 393–401, October 2004.

[MGPW05a]   R. Marée, P. Geurts, J. Piater, and L. Wehenkel. Decision trees and ran-
            dom subwindows for object recognition. In *ICML workshop on Machine
            Learning Techniques for Processing Multimedia Content (MLMM2005)*,
            2005.

[MGPW05b]   R. Marée, P. Geurts, J. Piater, and L. Wehenkel. Random subwindows
            for robust image classification. In Cordelia Schmid, Stefano Soatto,
            and Carlo Tomasi, editors, *Proceedings of the IEEE International Con-
            ference on Computer Vision and Pattern Recognition (CVPR 2005)*,
            volume 1, pages 34–40. IEEE, June 2005.

[MTS⁺05]   K. Mikolajczyk, T. Tuytelaars, C. Schmid, A. Zisserman, J. Matas,
            F. Schaffalitzky, T. Kadir, and L. Van Gool. A comparison of affine
            region detectors. *International Journal of Computer Vision, to appear*,
            2005.

[PG04]   A. Pinhas and H. Greenspan. A continuous and probabilistic framework
            for medical image representation and categorization. In *Proc. of SPIE
            Medical Imaging*, volume 5371, 2004.

[Weh97]   L. Wehenkel. *Automatic Learning Techniques in Power Systems*. Kluwer
            Academic Publishers, Boston, November 1997.

[ZCC05]   D. Zhao, Y. Chen, and H. Correa. Statistical categorization of human
            histological images. In *Proc. of Internation Conference on Image Pro-
            cessing (ICIP)*, 2005.

[ZST⁺05]   L. Zhang, D. Samaras, D. Tomasi, N. Volkow, , and R. Goldstein.
            Machine learning for clinical diagnosis from functional magnetic reso-
            nance imaging. In *Proc. International Conference on Computer Vision
            (CVPR)*, volume 2, pages 1211–1217, 2005.

Combining Binary Classifiers for Automatic Cartilage Segmentation in Knee MRI

Jenny Folkesson[1], Ole Fogh Olsen[1], Paola Pettersen[2], Erik Dam[1,2], and Claus Christiansen[2]

[1] Image Analysis Group, IT University of Copenhagen, Denmark
jenny@itu.dk
[2] Center for Clinical and Basic Research, Ballerup, Denmark

Abstract. We have developed a method for segmenting tibial and femoral medial cartilage in MR knee scans by combining two k Nearest Neighbors (kNN) classifiers for the cartilage classes with a rejection threshold for the background class. We show that with this threshold, two binary classifiers are sufficient compared to three binary classifiers in the traditional one-versus-all approach. We also show that the combination of binary classifiers produces better results than a kNN classifier that is trained to partition the voxels directly into three classes. The resulting sensitivity, specificity and Dice volume overlap of our method are 84.2%, 99.9% and 0.81 respectively. Compared to state-of-the-art segmentation methods, our method outperforms a fully automatic method and is comparable to a semi-automatic method.

1 Introduction

One of the most common health defects among elderly today is osteoarthritis (OA), a disease which most often affect weight bearing joints such as knees and hips and is characterized by the degeneration of the articular cartilage. As of today, the treatment is restricted to symptom control because there are no disease-modifying drugs [1]. Therefore, much effort is put into OA drug development and consequently for finding quantitative measures of disease progression.

Magnetic resonance imaging (MRI) allows for quantitative evaluation of the articular cartilage [2], and cartilage deterioration can be detected using this technique [3]. Recently it has been shown that low-field dedicated extremity MRI can provide similar information on bone erosions and synovitis as expensive high-field MRI units [4]. If low-field scanners can replace high-field scanners in clinical studies, the costs of making such studies would be reduced significantly.

The cartilage in OA patients degenerates by losing thickness and integrity, and typical relevant quantitative measures of the cartilage status are volume and thickness maps. When finding such measures the segmentation of the cartilage is a crucial step. Many segmentation methods rely heavily on expert user interaction, but having experts to perform manual slice-by-slice delineation of the cartilage is too time consuming for routine clinical use and is inclined to inter-

Y. Liu, T. Jiang, and C. Zhang (Eds.): CVBIA 2005, LNCS 3765, pp. 230–239, 2005.

and intra-user variability. In order to find a cost-effective and precise cartilage segmentation, methods that are partly or fully automated are being developed. The main challenges in cartilage segmentation are the thin structure of the cartilage and the low contrast, both between the cartilage and surrounding soft tissues and between different cartilage compartments.

1.1 Related Work by Others

Several groups have developed semi-automated/automated methods for cartilage segmentation. Lynch et al. [5] combine user interaction with active contours, and Solloway et al. [6] use active shape models for slice-by-slice cartilage segmentation. 2D methods has limited continuation between slices and since they have to be converted into a 3D segmentation when finding for example thickness maps, it is advantageous to perform segmentation in 3D directly.

Among the 3D techniques that have been developed, Grau et al. [7] have a segmentation method that is based on a watershed approach. Pakin et al. [8] have developed a region growing scheme that is followed by a two-class clustering for automatic segmentation. Warfield et al. [9] presents a semi-automatic segmentation method that iterates between a classification step and a template registration step, which is shown to a lower variability compared to repeated manual segmentations.

1.2 Overview of Our Work

The 3D segmentation techniques described in section 1.1 all require some amount of manual interaction except for the method of Pakin et al. [8], and the methods are evaluated only on small data sets. Neither Grau et al. nor Pakin et al. evaluate their methods on scans from OA patients. In this paper, we present a segmentation method that combines a tibial cartilage vs. rest and a femoral cartilage vs. rest approximate kNN classifier with a rejection threshold for the background class for the segmentation of tibial and femoral medial cartilage. Our method is evaluated on a large data set containing both healthy and osteoarthritic knees. We show that by introducing the rejection threshold, two binary classifiers are sufficient for our three-class classification task. OA is more often observed in the medial compartments [10], therefore we focus on medial cartilage in this work.

Besides comparing our method to state-of-the-art cartilage segmentation methods, we do a comparison between the combination of binary classifiers and previous work where the cartilage is segmented using a hierarchical approach, combining one two-class and one three-class kNN classifier [11]. We also compare our results to a direct three-class classifier. Features are selected by forward selection followed by backward selection, and we consider the importance of of a suitable criterion function in the feature selection for the classifier performance.

2   Methods

2.1   Image Acquisition

An Esaote C-Span low-field 0.18 T scanner dedicated to imaging of extremities acquires Turbo 3D T1 scans (40° flip angle, T_R 50 ms, T_E 16 ms). The scans are made through the sagittal plane and have four different voxel sizes, $(0.7031/0.7813/0.8594/0.9375) \times 0.7031 \times 0.7031 mm^3$. After automatically removing boundaries that contain no information, the scan size is $104 \times 170 \times 170$ voxels.

The scans have been manually segmented on a slice-by-slice basis by a radiologist. A scan slice with the tibial and femoral medial cartilage manually segmented is shown in Figure 1. We use 111 scans of both left and right knees,

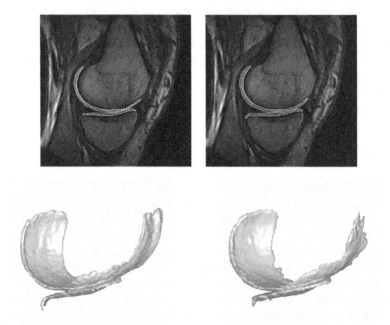

Fig. 1. The segmentation of tibial and femoral medial cartilage. Top row shows one slice (170x170 pixels) and the bottom row are the 3D visualizations. Manual segmentations are to the left and automatic segmentations to the right. The sensitivity, specificity and DSC of our automatic segmentation are 88.68%, 99.88% and 0.812 for this scan.

the right knees are reflected about the center in the sagittal plane in order to treat all scans analogously. The test subjects are both males and females, aged between 22 and 79 years, and diagnosed as having a Kellgren and Lawrence Index [12] between 0 and 3. There are 98 scans of healthy knees (KL index $\leq$ 1) and 13 of osteoarthritic knees (KL index > 1).

2.2   Cartilage Classification

We implement our classifier in an Approximate Nearest Neighbor (ANN) framework developed by Mount and colleagues [13]. The ANN classifier is in principle a kNN-classifier, but allows for faster computations if an error is tolerated. The ANN search algorithm returns k points such that the ratio of the distance between the ith reported point ($1 \leq i \leq k$) and the true ith nearest neighbor is at most $1 + \epsilon$. Given a set S of n data points in R^d, the k nearest neighbors of a point in S can be computed in $O((c_{d,\epsilon} + kd)\log n)$ time, where $c_{d,\epsilon} = d[1 + 6d/\epsilon]^d$, thus the computational complexity increases exponentially with the dimensions. One difficulty in classification tasks is the tradeoff between computational complexity and accuracy. After experimenting with different values we set $\epsilon = 2$ and $k = 100$ for a reasonable such tradeoff.

There are three classes we wish to separate, tibial medial cartilage, femoral medial cartilage and background. We combine one binary classifier trained to separate tibial cartilage from the rest and one trained to separate femoral cartilage from the rest with a rejection threshold, described in section 2.6.

2.3   Features

We here introduce a set of candidate features, and in section 2.4 we describe our feature selection scheme. We are interested in features that describe the geometry of the object in question, and therefore have the 3-jet as candidate features since they can describe all local 3D geometric features up to third order [14]. All derivatives are achieved by the convolution with Gaussian derivatives, defined as $I_{i_1,\dots,i_n} = I * D_{i_1,\dots,i_n}G(\sigma)$, where G is a Gaussian, D the differential operator and σ is the scale. All features are examined on three scales, ($0.65mm$, $1.1mm$ and $2.5mm$), to cover the range of different cartilage thicknesses. The x-, y and z axes are defined as the sagittal-, coronal- and axial axes. The eigenvalues and the eigenvectors of the Hessian and the structure tensor are also candidate features. The Hessian,

$$H(\sigma) = \begin{pmatrix} I_{xx} & I_{xy} & I_{xz} \\ I_{yx} & I_{yy} & I_{yz} \\ I_{zx} & I_{zy} & I_{zz} \end{pmatrix},$$

describes local curvature and is among other things used for locating vessels, and the structure tensor,

$$ST(\sigma_{out}, \sigma) = G(\sigma_{out}) * \begin{pmatrix} I_x I_x & I_x I_y & I_x I_z \\ I_y I_x & I_y I_y & I_y I_z \\ I_z I_x & I_z I_y & I_z I_z \end{pmatrix},$$

examines the local gradient distribution. We would also like to examine some third order properties and therefore evaluate the third order tensor, in Einstein annotation $L_{www} = I_{ijk}I_iI_jI_k/(I_iI_i)^{3/2}$, in the gradient direction as candidate features. Besides these features related to the geometry, we also include the location in the image and the intensity as candidate features, because these are features that are highly relevant for a radiologist when visually inspecting the images. The intensities smoothed on the three scales are also candidate features.

2.4   Training of the Classifier

Feature selection can not only reduce computational time and complexity, it can also provide better classification accuracy due to the curse of dimensionality. The features of the classifiers are selected by sequential forward selection followed by sequential backward selection. In the forward selection we start with an empty feature set and expand the search space by adding one feature at the time according to the outcome of a criterion function. The backward selection starts with the features found by the sequential forward selection and iteratively excludes the least significant feature according to the criterion function. All features are examined in every iteration, which means that the same feature can be selected several times.

For the two-class classifier we forward propagate until there are 60 features in the feature set and we back propagate until there are 39 features left in the set. As criterion function for the two-class classifiers we use the area under the ROC curve (AUC). The ROC curve is determined by varying the threshold for the classifier and plot the ratio of false positives against the ratio of true positives. A perfect classifier has an $AUC = 1$ and a random performance yields $AUC = 0.5$. In the two-class classification case, the AUC is a well established criterion function. However, this criterion function is not easily extendable to N-class classification tasks where $N > 2$. Mossman [15] has developed ROC analysis for multi-class classification by varying the class sensitivities as decision thresholds to form 3D surfaces. For three-class classification there are 6 such surfaces, and the volumes under the surfaces (VUS) are the performance metrics, similar to the AUC in 2D. A perfect classifier has $VUS = 1$ and chance performance yields $VUS = 0.17$. However the sensitivities does not provide a complete description of the operator performance because it ignores the $N^2 - N$ misclassification probabilities. Edwards et al. [16] has generalized ROC analysis for multi-class classification tasks into what they call the hypervolume under the ROC hypersurface, a performance metric that take all misclassification probabilities into account. However they conclude that the hypervolume may not be a useful performance metric when $N > 2$. For the three-class classifier, we take the average of the six Mossman's VUS's as the criterion function. We forward propagate until there are 75 features in the set, and then back propagate until there remains 54 features. The direct three-class classifier has less features than two binary classifiers together, but we do not include more features because as described in section 2.2 the computational complexity increases exponentially with the dimensionality.

We use 25 scans for the training of the classifier, the same 25 scans are used in the feature selection, threshold selection and for the training data set for the final classifier.

2.5   Selected Features

We train one tibial cartilage (ω_{tm}) vs. rest, one femoral cartilage (ω_{fm}) vs. rest and one background (ω_b) vs. rest classifier. In addition we train a classifier that directly separates the three classes. The selected features for the different

Table 1. The features selected for the different classifiers. The number corresponds to the significance with 1 as the most significant feature. $ST(\sigma_{out}, \sigma)$ and $H(\sigma)$ stands for the eigenvalues if nothing else is stated.

Feature/classifier	ω_{tm}	ω_{fm}	ω_b	Direct 3-class
I_x, I_y, I_z $\sigma = 0.65$	5		9	9
I_x, I_y, I_z $\sigma = 1.1$	7	3	13	14
I_x, I_y, I_z $\sigma = 2.5$	4	4	4	1
Position	1	1	1	2
Intensity				4
Intensity smoothed	2	5	2	5
$H(0.65mm)$		8		
$H(1.1mm)$	8	10,11	6	13, 14, 15
$H(2.5mm)$	10	9,13	5	8
$ST(1.1mm, 0.65mm)$		2*		16*
$ST(2.5mm, 0.65mm)$	11, 12, 13	12	10, 11, 12	
$ST(2.5mm, 1.1mm)$				7
I_{xxx} all scales				6
I_{zzz} all scales	6	6		
I_{xxz} all scales				11
I_{xx} all scales				3
I_{yy} all scales	9		7	17,18
I_{zz} all scales	3	7	3	
I_{xy} all scales			8	12
I_{yz} all scales				10

* eigenvector corresponding to largest eigenvalue

classifiers are presented in Table 1. The position, the intensity smoothed on the three scales and the first order derivatives on $\sigma = 2.5mm$ are highly ranked by all classifiers. The structure tensor and the Hessian are repeatedly selected by all classifiers, but the direct three-class classifier has selected features from the 3-jet more frequently than the others.

2.6   Setting a Threshold for the Classifier

The outcome of an ω_i vs. rest classifier can be seen as the posterior probabilities that, for all the voxels in the image, a voxel j with feature vector $\mathbf{u}_{i,j}$ belongs to class ω_i. We denote it $P(\omega_i|\mathbf{u}_{i,j})$ or $P_{i,j}$ for short. In one-versus-all classification, which is commonly used for multi-class classification [17], one builds ω_i vs. rest classifiers for $i = 1, \ldots N$ and perform a winner-takes-all vote between them, assigning j to the class ω_i with the highest posterior probability. In the scans, roughly 0.2% of the voxels belong to tibial cartilage and 0.5% to the femoral cartilage, making the background the by far largest class. Our approach is similar to one-versus all, but due to the dominance of the background class we replace the background vs. rest classifier by a rejection threshold, which states that a the posterior probability should be higher than a threshold T before it can be assigned to a cartilage class. The decision rule is:

236   J. Folkesson et al.

$$j \in \begin{cases} \omega_{tm}, & P_{tm,j} > P_{fm,j} \text{ and } P_{tm,j} > T; \\ \omega_{fm}, & P_{fm,j} > P_{tm,j} \text{ and } P_{fm,j} > T; \\ \omega_b & \text{otherwise.} \end{cases}$$

Using the features found from feature selection, the 25 training scans are leave-one-out evaluated. The results of varying the threshold for the tibial cartilage vs. rest and femoral cartilage vs. rest classifiers are seen in Figure 2. The Dice similarity coefficient (DSC) is considered a useful statistical measure for studying accuracy in image segmentation [18]. It measures the spatial volume overlap between two segmentations A and B and is defined as $DSC(A, B) = \frac{2 \times |A \cap B|}{|A| + |B|}$. The rejection threshold is set to 0.98, because as demonstrated in Figure 2, the maximum DSC occurs then.

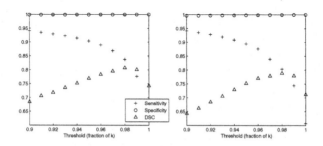

Fig. 2. The results of varying the threshold in leave-one-out evaluation of the training set. The tibial vs. rest classifier performance is demonstrated to the left, and the femoral vs. rest classifier to the right.

3   Results

We classify the scans according to the decision rule in section 2.6, and the largest connected component is selected as the segmentation. The sensitivity, specificity and DSC are calculated using manual segmentations by a radiologist as gold standard. The results are displayed in Table 2 and are visualized in Figures 1 and 3. The results of our method is distinctly higher than those of the fully automatic method of Pakin et al [8]. The sensitivity and DSC of our method is not as high as that of Grau et al. [7], but we have evaluated our method on far more scans, including osteoarthritic knees, and without manual interaction.

In Table 2 we also compare the results of our segmentation method to the results we obtained using a hierarchical approach [11], where the the voxels are first roughly partitioned into cartilage/non-cartilage using a two-class classifier, then a three-class classifier partitions the voxels that are classified as cartilage in the first round into tibial cartilage, femoral cartilage and background. The classifiers are trained similar to what is described in this paper. The threshold is not optimized for maximal DSC, however the average DSC does not exceed 0.802 for any threshold. The test set in [11] contains 2% osteoarthritic knees compared

Table 2. The results of our combined binary classifier method (denoted 'This work') compared to two state-of-the-art methods, the hierarchical method in [11] and a direct three-class classifier, evaluated with comparisons to manual segmentations.

Method	This work	Pakin	Grau	Hierarchical	Direct 3-class
Sensitivity	84.17%	66.22%	90.03%	90.01	81.25%
Specificity	99.89%	99.56%	99.87%	99.80%	99.85%
DSC	0.811	Unavailable	0.895	0.795	0.768
Test set	86	1	7	46	86
Manual labor	0	0	5-10 min	0	0

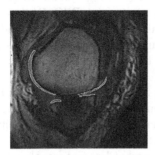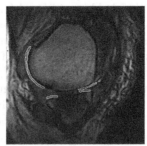

Fig. 3. The segmentation of an osteoarthritic knee, diagnosed as having KL index 3, in a slice where the cartilage is degraded. To the left is a gold standard segmentation and to the right our automatic segmentation. The sensitivity, specificity and DSC of the automatic segmentation are 86.12%.

to 8% in this work. The direct three-class classifier performs distinctly worse than the hierarchical classifier and our combined binary classifier method.

The radiologist re-segmented the tibial medial cartilage in 31 scans in order to determine intra-rater variability for the gold standard segmentations. The average DSC between the two manual segmentations is 0.857, which explains the fairly low values of the DSC in our evaluation since we cannot expect our method to resemble the expert better than the expert itself. The corresponding DSC of the automatic segmentation versus expert for the tibial cartilage of the 31 scans is 0.823. Ideally, several trained experts should segment every scan several times and a more robust gold standard could then be determined using STAPLE [19], but with our large amount of data it is too labor intensive.

We believe that the ω_b vs. rest classifier could add little more information to our final class decisions. Still, we examine its effect by temporarily including it in the decision rules, making them:

$$j \in \begin{cases} \omega_{tm}, & P_{tm,j} > P_{fm,j} \text{ and } P_{tm,j} > P_{b,j} \text{ and } P_{tm,j} > T; \\ \omega_{fm}, & P_{fm,j} > P_{tm,j} \text{ and } P_{fm,j} > P_{b,j} \text{ and } P_{fm,j} > T; \\ \omega_b & \text{otherwise.} \end{cases}$$

The average sensitivity, specificity and DSC using this rule remained exactly the same as for the two binary classifiers with rejection threshold. Using a pure one-versus-all approach without the threshold T yielded a large number of false positives for the cartilage classes an has an average sensitivity, specificity and DSC of 98.5%, 98.9% and 0.48.

4   Discussion

Our segmentation method combines two binary kNN classifiers trained to distinguish tibial cartilage respectively femoral cartilage from the rest of the image and incorporates a rejection threshold for allowing a voxel to be classified as cartilage. The threshold is optimized for maximizing DSC. We have shown that this classifier can replace a one-versus-all classifier without degrading the performance. This means that the background vs. rest classification is unnecessary, which saves approximately one third of the computational time compared to a one-versus-all approach.

In the feature selection, the criterion function determines what features that will be included in the classifier, and thus has a major impact on the classifier performance. The kNN classifier is inherently a multi-class classifier, but still the combination of binary classifiers yields better results than the hierarchical approach even though the former has somewhat less features than the latter. We believe this to be related to the fact that a good generalization to multi-class classification of the AUC in the two-class case is yet to be discovered.

We have demonstrated a cartilage segmentation algorithm that compared to state-of-the-art methods outperforms the to our knowledge only fully automatic method, and has a performance comparable to a semi-automatic method.

References

1. Felson, D.T., Lawrence, R.C., Hochberg, M.C., McAlindon, T., Dieppe, P.A., Minor, M.A., Blair, S.N., Berman, B.M., Fries, J.F., Weinberger, M., Lorig, K.R., Jacobs, J.J., Goldberg, V.: Osteoarthritis: New insights, part 2: Treatment approaches. Annals of Internal Medicine **133** (2000) 726–737
2. Graichen, H., Eisenhart-Rothe, R., Vogl, T., Englmeier, K.H., Eckstein, F.: Quantitative assessment of cartilage status in osteoarthritis by quantitative magnetic resonance imaging. Arthritis and Rheumatism **50** (2004) 811–816
3. Pessis, E., Drape, J.L., Ravaud, P., Chevrot, A., Ayral, M.D.X.: Assessment of progression in knee osteoarthritis: results of a 1 year study comparing arthroscopy and mri. Osteoarthritis and Cartilage **11** (2003) 361–369
4. Ejbjerg, B., Narvestad, E., adn H.S. Thomsen, S.J., Ostergaard, M.: Optimised, low cost, low field dedicated extremity mri is highly specific and sensitive for synovitis and bone erosions in rheumatoid arthritis wrist and finger joints: a comparison with conventional high-field mri and radiography. Annals of the Rheumatic Diseases **13** (2005)
5. Lynch, J.A., Zaim, S., Zhao, J., Stork, A., Peterfy, C.G., Genant, H.K.: Cartilage segmentation of 3d mri scans of the osteoarthritic knee combining user knowledge and active contours. Volume 3979., SPIE (2000) 925–935

6. Solloway, S., Hutchinson, C., Vaterton, J., Taylor, C.: The use of active shape models for making thickness measurements of articular cartilage from mr images. Magnetic Resonance in Medicine **37** (1997) 943–952
7. Grau, V., Mewes, A., Alcañiz, M., Kikinis, R., Warfield, S.: Improved watershed transform for medical image segmentation using prior information. IEEE Transactions on Medical Imaging **23** (2004)
8. Pakin, S.K., Tamez-Pena, J.G., Totterman, S., J.Parker, K.: Segmentation, surface extraction and thickness computation of articular cartilage. Volume 4684., SPIE (2002) 155–166
9. Warfield, S.K., Kaus, M., Jolesz, F.A., Kikinis, R.: Adaptive, template moderated, spatially varying statistical classification. Medical Image Analysis (2000) 43–55
10. Dunn, T., Lu, Y., Jin, H., Ries, M., Majumdar, S.: T2 relaxation time of cartilage at mr imaging: comparison with severity of knee osteoarthritis. Radiology **232** (2004) 592–598
11. Folkesson, J., Dam, E., Olsen, O.F., Pettersen, P., Christiansen, C.: Automatic segmentation of the articular cartilage in knee mri using a hierarchical multi-class classification scheme, to appear in MICCAI (2005)
12. Kellgren, J., Lawrence, J.: Radiological assessment of osteo-arthrosis. Annals of the Rheumatic Diseases **16** (1957)
13. Arya, S., Mount, D.M., Netanyahu, N.S., Silverman, R., Wu, A.Y.: An optimal algorithm for approximate nearest neighbor searching in fixed dimensions. Journal of the ACM **45** (1998) 891–923
14. Florack, L.: The Syntactical Structure of Scalar Images. PhD thesis, University of Utrecht (1993)
15. Mossman, D.: Three-way rocs. Med. Decis. Making **19** (1999) 78–79
16. Edwards, D.C., Metz, C.E., Nishikawa, R.M.: The hypervolume under the roc hypersurface of near-guessing and near-perfect observers in n-class classification tasks. IEEE Transactions on Medical Imaging **24** (2005) 293–299
17. Yeang, C.H., Ramaswamy, S., Tamayo, P., Mukherjee, S., Rifkin, R.M., Angelo, M., Reich, M., Lander, E., Mesirov, J., Golub, T.: Molecular classification of multiple tumor types. Bioinformatics **1** (2001)
18. Zou, K.H., Warfield, S.K., Bharatha, A., Tempany, C.M., Kaus, M.R., Haker, S.J., III, W.M.W., Jolesz, F.A., Kikinis, R.: Statistical validation of image segmentation quality based on a spatial overlap index. Acad Radiol **11** (2004) 178–189
19. Warfield, S.K., Zou, K.H., Wells, W.M.: Simultaneous truth and performance level estimation (staple): An algorithm for the validation of image segmentation. **23** (2004)

Computer-Aided Diagnosis (CAD) for Cervical Cancer Screening and Diagnosis: A New System Design in Medical Image Processing

Wenjing Li[1], Viara Van Raad[1], Jia Gu[1], Ulf Hansson[1],
Johan Hakansson[1], Holger Lange[1], and Daron Ferris[2]

[1] STI Medical Systems, Honolulu, HI, 96813, USA
{wli, vraad, jgu, uhansson, jhakansson, holger}@sti-hawaii.com
[2] Medical College of Georgia, Augusta, GA, 30912, USA
dferris@mail.mcg.edu

Abstract. Uterine cervical cancer is the second most common cancer among women worldwide. Physicians visually inspect the cervix for certain distinctly abnormal morphologic features that indicate precursor lesions and invasive cancer. We introduce our vision of a Computer-Aided-Diagnosis (CAD) system for cervical cancer screening and diagnosis and provide the details of our system design and development process. The proposed CAD system is a complex multi-sensor, multi-data and multi-feature image analysis system. The feature set used in our CAD systems includes the same visual features used by physician and could be extended to new features introduced by new instrument technologies, like fluorescence spectroscopy. Preliminary results of our research on detecting the three most important features: blood vessel structures, acetowhite regions and lesion margins are shown.

1 Introduction

Uterine cervical cancer is the second most common cancer in women worldwide, with nearly 500,000 new cases and over 270,000 deaths annually. Invasive disease is preceded by pre-malignant Cervical Intraepithelial Neoplasia (CIN). If it can be detected early and treated adequately, cervical cancer can be prevented [1].

Colposcopy is the primary diagnostic method used in the US to diagnose CIN and cancer, following an abnormal cytological screening (Papanicolaou smear). The purpose of a colposcopic examination is to identify and rank the severity of lesions, so that biopsies representing the highest-grade abnormality can be taken, if necessary. A colposcopic examination involves a systematic visual evaluation of the lower genital tract (cervix, vulva and vagina), with special emphasis on the subjective appearance of metaplastic epithelium comprising the transformation zone on the cervix (Fig.1(a)). For this purpose a colposcope (Fig.1 (b)) is used. A colposcope is a low powered binocular microscope with a built in white light source and objective lens attached to a support mechanism. During the exam, a 3-5% acetic acid solution is applied to the cervix, causing abnormal and metaplastic epithelia to turn white. Cervical cancer precursor lesions and invasive cancer exhibit certain distinctly abnormal morphologic

Y. Liu, T. Jiang, and C. Zhang (Eds.): CVBIA 2005, LNCS 3765, pp. 240–250, 2005.

features that can be identified by colposcopic examination. Lesion characteristics such as margin shape, color or opacity, blood vessel caliber, intercapillary spacing and distribution, and contour are considered by physicians (colposcopists) to derive a clinical diagnosis. These colposcopic signs, when considered aggregately, determine the severity of the neoplasia and discriminate abnormal findings from similarly appearing, anatomically normal variants. Various colposcopic indices, based on grading lesion characteristics, provide clinicians structured approaches to predicting histologic findings. However, due to the subjective nature of the examination, the accuracy of colposcopy is highly dependent upon colposcopist experience and expertise.

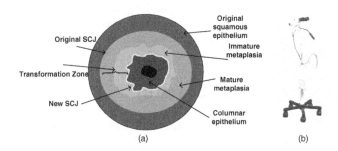

Fig. 1. (a) A schematic presentation of a cervix, (b) A colposcope

Digital imaging is revolutionizing the medical imaging field and enabling sophisticated computer programs to assist the physicians with Computer-Aided-Diagnosis (CAD). Clinicians and academia have suggested and shown proof of concept to use automated image analysis of cervical imagery for cervical cancer screening and diagnosis. A computer system was readily able to discriminate CIN3 from normal epithelium and immature metaplasia [2]. Since intercapillary distances increase proportionally with disease severity, these tiny distances can be automatically measured by computer to predict the specific level of cervical neoplasia [3].

Various image processing algorithms have been developed to detect different colposcopic features. Van Raad used active contour models at multiple scales to detect the transformation zone [4]. Yang et al. applied deterministic annealing technique to detect the acetowhite epithelium regions [5]. Gordon and his coworkers, applied Gaussian Mixture model to segment three tissue types (original squamous, columnar, and acetowhite epithelium) using color and texture information [6]. Ji et al [7] presented a generalized texture analysis algorithm for classifying the vascular patterns from colposcopic images. Balas [8] and Orfanoudaki et al. [9] analyzed the temporal decay of the acetic acid whitening effect by measuring the intensity profile over time. Furthermore, several approaches for tissue classification have been developed: a simple colposcopic lesion contour classification method by artificial neural network [10], a rule-based medical decision support system for detecting different stages of cervical cancer using the signs and symptoms from physical examination [11], the classification of cervical tissue based on spectral data using multi-layered perceptrons and Radial Basis Function (RBF) networks [12]. These various examples support the feasibility of automated image analysis to detect cervical neoplasia.

Based on experience gained in developing Hyperspectral Diagnostic Imaging (HSDI^{TM}), fluorescence and reflectance spectroscopy imaging technology for cervical cancer, we transformed our strategy for cervical cancer detection to include a versatile CAD system, capable of incorporating many features (including spectroscopy). The system is called ColpoCAD^{TM}. The heart of ColpoCAD^{TM} is a complex multi-sensor, multi-data and multi-feature image analysis system. A functional description of the envisioned ColpoCAD^{TM} system with the system design and development process of the image analysis system is discussed in this paper. We also include preliminary results of our research for detecting and extracting the three most important cervical neoplasia pathological features: blood vessel structure, acetowhite and lesion margin. As this is a new and complex field in medical image processing, various computer vision and image processing techniques are involved. This paper establishes the framework and the foundation for collaboration and discussion between industry, academia, and medical practitioners.

2   Computer-Aided Diagnosis(CAD)

ColpoCAD^{TM} includes all functions that are related to colposcopy and that can be provided by a computer, from automation of the clinical workflow to automated patient diagnosis and treatment recommendation. It is a software program that may run on various processing platforms such as computers, DSP/FPGA processing boards, embedded systems, etc., and that interfaces to a cervical data acquisition system such as a digital/video/optical Colposcope with digital/film-based camera. We start with a functional description of the envisioned CAD system for colposcopy. Next, the core of the CAD system, a modular and open system design for the image analysis system is presented. We also introduce the development process that effectively manages the complexity of developing such a system.

Table 1. Functional Description of ColpoCAD^{TM} System
High-resolution still images from the examination are displayed on a high-resolution monitor.
Live video of the examination can be viewed and replayed.
Images and video can be enhanced by glint removal, green filter, etc.
Diagnostic features, such as acetowhite regions, vessel structure, lesion margins, acetowhite decay, and contour can be automatically displayed.
Feature measurements can be provided to the physician on demand.
Automated lesion detection and tissue diagnosis can be shown to the physician.
Suggested biopsy sites can be indicated.
Reference images of similar lesions and their characteristics can be brought up from a reference database and shown to the physician for comparison.

2.1   Functional Description

The capabilities of ColpoCAD^{TM} originate from a technology-driven vision which captures all feasible CAD system functionality. A system description of a "technology-based" CAD system for colposcopy is summarized in Table 1. The CAD system architecture is flexible, so that a range of products (screening device, colposcopy adjunct, etc.) can be based on this framework. We note that the current ColpoCAD system design provides automated image analysis for the examination of the ectocervix only, and currently excluding the examination of the vulva, vagina, and endocervical canal. These aspects of the colposcopic examination will need to be provided by Colposcopy, until addressed by ColpoCAD. The envisioned functions of the CAD system are comprised of the following components: (1) Image enhancement, (2) Feature extraction, (3) Reference database, and (4) Diagnosis and directed biopsies.

Image Enhancement

A "digital colposcope" can provide numerous image enhancements, including:

- Green filter to accentuate vasculature.
- Mapping the color-space of one colposcope to that of another can provide the same image appearance, to normalize differences due to receiver and light source variation.
- General image enhancements, like contrast, brightness, zoom, sharpening, etc.
- Glare removal to provide information in the image regions that are normally destroyed by glare. Since colposcopists use glare patterns to assess the contour of the lesions (3D topology), glare-free images should only be provided in addition to images with glare. Glare can be removed by designing the acquisition system with cross-polarization or by software.
- 3D topology-based illumination normalization to lighten dark regions on the periphery of the cervix. 3D reconstruction of the cervix can compensate for the differences in illumination due to the 3D topology of the cervix.

Feature Extraction

A colposcopist uses various features to assess the cervix. Those features can be automatically extracted from the cervical data and shown to the colposcopist to help the assessment. A core feature set includes the visual features used by colposcopists during a colposcopic examination. This feature set can be extended to include new features introduced by novel instrument technologies, like fluorescence and impedance, and any other plausible feature that can be extracted from the cervical data. Colposcopic features include (1) Anatomic, (2) Epithelial acetowhitening, (3) Blood vessel structure, (4) Lesion margin sharpness and shape (5) Contour, (6) Lugol's iodine staining.

Image enhancement can be provided to emphasize specific features in the imagery, in particular colposcopic features. These individual features can be classified in terms of their significance to the tissue diagnosis: normal, low-grade, high-grade and cancer. The extracted and classified features can be presented to the colposcopist individually or combined as an overlay on an image of the cervix (preferable a universal reference image - typically a color image after acetic acid application), similar to the colposcopic impression annotation.

Reference Database

A colposcopic diagnosis can be assisted by providing matching examples of reference lesions/cervixes including their diagnosis. The key is to be able to characterize all lesions by their feature parameters (i.e. a quantitative expression of qualitative characteristics, such as the "straightness" of a border, or "whiteness" of an acetowhite lesion). A reference database can be built from cervical data sets for which the diagnosis and the feature parameters of all lesions are available. The ground truth for the diagnosis can be determined by expert colposcopists and pathologists. The feature parameters can be determined by expert colposcopists and pathologists as well or automatically calculated by feature extraction algorithms. The search keys of the reference database are the feature parameters.

Diagnosis and Directed Biopsies
ColpoCAD-based Tissue diagnosis provides the colposcopist with the automated detection, localization and classification (in terms of severity: normal, low-grade, high-grade or cancer) of all lesions on the cervix. Note that not one feature alone can provide reliable tissue diagnosis. All available features, starting with the obvious visual ones used by colposcopists, and adding those from new instrument technologies should be integrated into one system to optimize performance. Automated assessment of the adequacy of the examination (visualization of the entire transformation zone) should also be provided, as this affects patient management options. One important goal of colposcopy is to direct where biopsies should be taken. Based on the feature extraction and tissue diagnosis, the CAD system determines the minimum number of biopsies needed, identifies where these sites are located and displays their locations. Ultimately, the final goal is that the patient diagnosis can be derived directly from the computer's analysis, once clinical studies demonstrate equivalent or better performance compared to standard colposcopy and pathology.

2.2 ColpoCAD™ System Design

The image analysis system design is driven by the following objectives:

- To build the core system on visual features used by colposcopists;
- To fuse all available data in order to optimize performance;
- To provide the flexibility to work on data sets from different instruments;
- To provide architecture that enables systematic evolution of CAD system for colposcopy.

The system takes color calibrated data of the cervical examination as input and provides as output the detected features and their classification, the tissue diagnosis for all locations on the cervix and an assessment of the examination adequacy. Calibration parameters, demographic parameters, patient history and a system sensitivity parameter are used as the parameters of the system. The system architecture is open, modular, and feature-based. The architecture identifies three basic processing layers: (1) data registration, (2) feature extraction and (3) classification. In the data registration layer, all calibrated exam data is spatially registered to a selected reference image, such that all extracted features can be fused in the classification layer and data can be exchanged among feature extraction modules. The feature extraction layer is divided into distinct modules by evaluating distinct anatomical and physiological phenomena for each module. Each feature extraction module can use any of the registered data sources for processing. The classification layer consists of the tissue diagnosis module that provides the classification of each individual feature and combines

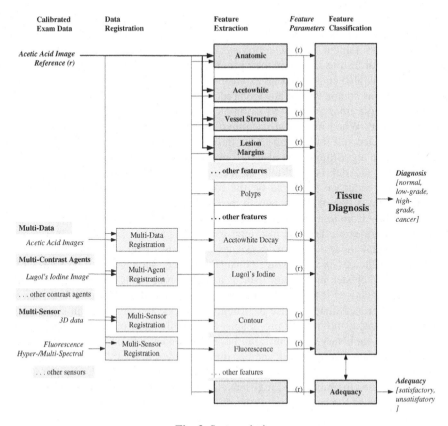

Fig. 2. System design

the outputs of all feature extraction modules in order to determine the tissue diagnosis for all locations on the cervix, and the determination of the adequacy of the exam. The exam adequacy determination is based on its own specific feature extraction modules and/or the feature parameters from other feature extraction modules.

Fig. 2 illustrates our proposed system configuration. The core system (highlighted in gray) consists of the extraction of the anatomic features and the three most important colposcopic features: acetowhite, vessel structure, and lesion margins; the determination of the adequacy of the exam, and the tissue diagnosis. It uses only one RGB image as input, therefore, by definition, this should be the reference image and no data registration is required. The reference image should be taken at the moment in time after application of 5% acetic acid when the acetowhite effect is still visible and the blood vessels can be seen again (blood vessels may be difficult to observe immediately after the application of acetic acid). This is a compromise for the acetowhite and vessel structure feature extraction modules. When more images are available after application of acetic acid, the acetowhite and vessel structure feature extraction modules should use the most appropriate image as their input to optimize the performance. The temporal decay of acetowhitening requires a series of images after application of acetic acid to be assessed. A colposcopist uses the glare pattern associated with surface relief, stereoscopic view and the movement of the colposcope to assess the 3D contour feature. For the digital colposcopy system, we use 3D reconstruction of the cervix for its assessment. The 3D topology of the cervix can also be used for precise measurements of lesions to follow their progression over multiple exams. The Lugol's iodine feature is also considered an extension of the core system when images using Lugol's iodine as contrast agent are acquired.

When multiple images are used as input, all images need to be registered to the reference image. When images are acquired at different times, the registration algorithms need to account for the soft-tissue movement as well as patient and instrument movement. The algorithms must also accommodate common "contaminants" such as blood, mucus and debris. Multiple intra-examination data registration of an acetowhite decay sequence seems to be the fundamental registration problem, as the reference image is one of the images in the sequence, and the acetowhite effect only changes slightly from image to image. However, it is a more challenging task to register not only intra-exam data, but also inter-exam data, to the pixel level when images are taken several months apart to detect lesion changes over time. In this case, the appearance of the cervix can change considerably over such a long time frame. One approach is to register inter-exam data at a higher processing level, such as at the level of the diagnosed lesions. The image registration with different contrast agents against the reference image is also a difficult task. Due to the physician's manipulation and instrument movement, the images after application of contrast agents, like Lugol's iodine, look very different from the images taken with no contrast agent. The multi-sensor data registration task can be simplified by acquiring the data from different sensors close to the moment when the reference image is taken. We previously described a means to embed (and register) a reflectance image in fluorescence hyperspectral data, when the acquisition of the reflectance and fluorescence data cannot be interleaved [13].

2.3 ColpoCAD^{TM} Algorithm Development Process

The performance of image processing algorithms depends highly on the quality of the available data sets. Unfortunately, existing cervical image databases share many shortcomings, including: glare, no camera calibration, no color calibration, only one image in a patient data set, limited or no pathology ground truth for the entire cervix including all different tissue classes, and no ground truth for feature annotations. For the development of a multi-data, multi-contrast agents, multi-sensors fusion system, complete data sets per patient are required. Data sets from patients receiving Loop Electrosurgical Excision Procedure (LEEP) provide a rich distribution and variety of all tissue classes and different colposcopic findings, which are suitable for the development process. One reason for the paucity of high quality standardized imaging data, and an impediment to develop CAD systems for colposcopy is that standard colposcopic examinations involve visual inspection of the cervix using an optical colposcope, and images of the cervix are not routinely taken. Furthermore, digital colposcopy, a technology that could eventually ameliorate this problem is still in its infancy.

Another critical component of the CAD system development is the definition of the feature parameters. The variation in feature parameters is related to disease severity.

In the case of colposcopic features, the parameters need to be defined and refined in collaboration with expert colposcopists. A systematic, iterative approach for defining and refining the feature parameters is made possible by defining the feature parameters at a level where it is meaningful to the colposcopist and by providing ground truth annotations for those defined feature parameters. The definition of the feature parameters is a difficult exercise because colposcopists typically define colposcopic findings in qualitative terms, rather than quantitative terms that a computer can understand. Colposcopic indices or assessment systems, such as those published by Reid [14] and Rubin and Barbo [15], have been defined by colposcopists in an attempt to formalize colposcopy. These assessment systems use qualitative terms to describe the observable phenomena of the colposcopic features and classify them by their implied severity. For our purposes, equivalent quantitative feature parameters need to be defined.

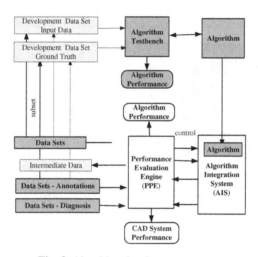

Fig. 3. Algorithm development process

We have defined a set of parameters for the colposcopic features that are assessed by colposcopists. We have also acquired extensive multi-data, multi-contrast-agent and multi-sensor high-quality calibrated data set. This extensive data resource will facilitate the development of the CAD system. We have also developed an Algorithm Integration System (AIS) and an automated Performance Evaluation Engine (PEE). An illustration of our algorithm development process using the AIS and PEE is shown in Fig. 3. The AIS allows outputting of all intermediate data calculated by every algorithm in the system. The PEE controls the AIS and evaluates each algorithm against its "ground truth" annotations and determines the overall performance of the system by providing a Receiver Operator Characteristic (ROC) curve. The AIS also provides data selection, algorithm selection and parameters variation to evaluate different system configurations. This platform enables the CAD system development effort to focus on developing and refining the image processing algorithms.

3 Preliminary Results

We have prototyped a few image processing algorithms for glare removal, anatomical feature detection, acetowhite region detection, and blood vessel mosaic and punctation structure detection for the technology using a RGB image data set from 111 human subjects participating in a clinical study of our HSDI^{TM} instrument [16].

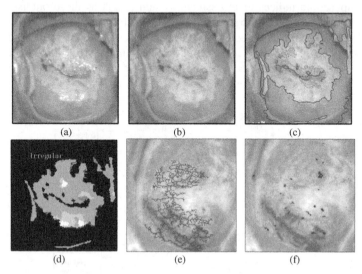

Fig. 4. Preliminary results. (a) Original Image, (b) Glint Removal, (c) Segmentation Results for Cervix Region (black contour), Acetowhite (Blue), Columnar Region(Green contour), and Os (Green Region), (d) Multi-level acetowhite Regions and its irregular contour (e) Mosaic vessels, (f) Punctation vessels

Glare in the cervical images need to be removed when using an instrument that does not provide cross-polarized imagery. An example of our glare removal algorithm [17] is shown in Fig. 4 (b). Colposcopists assess the color of the acetowhite regions. Because the ealier HSDI data set was not color calibrated, we prototyped the detection of multi-level acetowhite regions on the basis of different intensity levels, rather than color information [18]. The resulting defined acetowhite regions also serve as an input for lesion margin analysis. The detection of acetowhite regions requires the knowledge of cervical anatomic features, like the cervix, columnar region and the os, to guide and adapt the processing. Examples of the anatomic feature detection and acetowhite region detection algorithms are shown in Fig. 4 (c) and (d). One lesion margin characteristic assessed by colposcopists is the smoothness of the lesion margin. We developed an algorithm prototype to classify every location of a lesion margin to be either smooth or irregular as show in Fig. 4(d). We have also developed algorithm prototypes to detect mosaic and punctation vessel patterns. Examples are shown as Fig. 4 (e) and (f).

4 Future Work

ColpoCAD™ is a new system in medical imaging that presents great opportunities to apply existing state-of-the-art technologies to a new application. It is based on the development of a complex image analysis system, that in order to achieve the highest possible performance, require the collaboration of experts in a wide variety of disciplines, like image registration, mathematic morphology, machine learning, 3D reconstruction, human factors, and databases, etc.. Recognizing the complexity and the importance of such a system, we have introduced a novel concept for the research and development of this image processing system, by extending our in-house research and development to an "industry guided open academic research collaboration". Our goal is to improve women's health care by providing cost-effective CAD-based systems for cervical cancer screening and diagnosis. A CAD system for colposcopy, a "machine colposcopist expert", has the potential to revolutionize cervical cancer screening and diagnosis worldwide.

References

1. D. Ferris, etc. Modern Colposcopy, Textbook and Atlas, 2nd Edition (2002).
2. E.D. Dickman etc. Identification of cervical neoplasia using a simulation of human vision, Journal of Lower Genital Tract Disease, Vol.5, No.3 (2001) 144-152.
3. M.S. Mikhail etc. Computerized measurement of intercapillary distance using image analysis in women with cervical intraepithelial neoplasia: correlation with severity. Obstet. Gynocol. Vol.95 (2000), 52-3.
4. V.Van Raad, Active contour models-A multiscale implementation for anatomical feature delineation in cervical images. Proc. of ICIP (2004) 557-560.
5. S. Yang etc. A multispectral digital cervigram™ analyzer in the wavelet domain for early detection of cervical cancer. Proc. of SPIE on Medical Imaging, Vol.5370 (2004) 1833-1844.
6. S. Gordon etc. Image segmentation of uterine cervix images for indexing in PACS. Proc of the 17th IEEE Symposium on Computer based Medical Systems (2004).
7. Q. Ji etc. Texture Analysis for classification of cervix lesions. IEEE Trans. on Medical Imaging, Vol.19, No.11, (2000), 1144-1149.
8. C. Balas, A novel optical imaging method for the early detection, quantitative grading and mapping of cancerous and precancerous lesions of cervix, IEEE Trans. on Biomedical Engineering, Vol.48, No.1, (2001), 96-104.
9. I.M. Orfanoudaki, etc. A clinical study of optical biopsy of the uterine cervix using a multispectral imaging system, Gynecologic Oncology Vol.96, (2005) 119-131.
10. I. Claude et. Contour features for colposcopic iamge classification by artificial neural networks, Proc. of ICPR (2002), 771-774.
11. P. Mitra etc. Staging of cervical cancer with soft computing, IEEE Trans. on Biomedical Imaging, Vol.47, No. 7, (2000), 934-940.
12. K. Tumer etc. Ensembles of radial basis function networks for spectroscopic detection of cervical precancer, IEEE Trans. on Biomedical Engineering, Vol.45, No.8, (1998).
13. H. Lange etc. Reflectance and fluorescence hyperspectral elastic image registration, Proc. of SPIE on Medical Imaging, Vol.5370, (2004).

14. R. Reid etc. Genital warts and cervical cancer. VII. An improved colposcopic index for differentiating benign papillomaviral infections from high-grade cervical intraepithelial neoplasia. Am. J. Obstet. Gynecol Vol.153, No.6, (1984) 611-8.
15. M.M. Rubin and D.M. Barbo. Ch.9a: Rubin and Barbo Colposcopic Assessment system. Colposcopy: Principles and practice. W.B. Saunders Company (2002) 187-195.
16. U. Gustafsson etc. Fluorescence and reflectance monitoring of human cervical tissue in vivo: a case study, Proc. of SPIE on Photonics West Biomedical Optics, Vol.4959, (2003).
17. H. Lange, Automatic glare removal in reflectance imagery of the uterine cervix, Proc. of SPIE on Medical Imaging. Vol.5747, (2005).
18. H. Lange, Automatic detection of multi-level Acetowhite regions in RGB color images of the uterine cervix, Proc. of SPIE on Medical Imaging, Vol.5747, (2005).

Constrained Surface Evolutions for Prostate and Bladder Segmentation in CT Images

Mikael Rousson[1], Ali Khamene[1], Mamadou Diallo[1],
Juan Carlos Celi[2], and Frank Sauer[1]

[1] Imaging and Visulization Dept.,
Siemens Corporate Research,
755 College Rd East, Princeton NJ 08540 USA
[2] Oncology Care Systems,
Siemens Medical Solutions,
Hans-Bunte-Str. 10, 69123, Heidelberg Germany

Abstract. We propose a Bayesian formulation for coupled surface evolutions and apply it to the segmentation of the prostate and the bladder in CT images. This is of great interest to the radiotherapy treatment process, where an accurate contouring of the prostate and its neighboring organs is needed. A purely data based approach fails, because the prostate boundary is only partially visible. To resolve this issue, we define a Bayesian framework to impose a shape constraint on the prostate, while coupling its extraction with that of the bladder. Constraining the segmentation process makes the extraction of both organs' shapes more stable and more accurate. We present some qualitative and quantitative results on a few data sets, validating the performance of the approach.

1 Introduction

Accurate contouring of the gross target volume GTV and critical organs is a fundamental prerequisite for successful treatment of cancer by radiotherapy. In adaptive radiotherapy, the treatment plan is further optimized according to the location and the shape of anatomical structure during the treatment sessions. Successful implementation of adaptive radiotherapy calls for development of a fast, accurate and robust method for automatic contouring of GTV and critical organs. This task is specifically more challenging in the case of the prostate cancer. The main reason is first, there is almost no intensity gradient at the bladder-prostate interface. Second, the bladder and rectum fillings change from one treatment session to another and that causes variation in both shape and appearance. Third, the shape of the prostate changes mainly due to boundary conditions, which are set (due to pressure) from bladder and rectum fillings.

The introduction of prior shape knowledge is often vital in medical image segmentation due to the problems outlined above [2,7,6,11,3,10,5]. In [6], authors use both shape and appearance models for prostate and rectum. In [5] authors propose a shape representation and modeling scheme that is used during both the learning and the segmentation stage. The proposed approach in this paper is

Y. Liu, T. Jiang, and C. Zhang (Eds.): CVBIA 2005, LNCS 3765, pp. 251–260, 2005.

focused on segmenting the bladder and prostate only. We have pursued another method for the rectum segmentation and the details of that is not the focus of this paper. The main differentiator of this approach from the other ones is the fact that we do not try to enforce the shape constraints on the bladder. The main reason is to increase the versatility and applicability of the method on larger number of datasets. The argument here is that the bladder filling dictates the shape of the bladder; therefore the shape is not statistically coherent to be used for building shape models and the consequent model based segmentation. However, the shape of the prostates across large patient population show statistical coherency. Therefore, we present a coupled segmentation framework with a non-overlapping constraint, where the shape prior, depending on the availability, can be applied on any of the shapes. Related works proposed to couple two level set propagations [9,11]. However, in the proposed approach, we formulate the coupling in a Bayesian inference framework. This drives to the coupled surface evolutions, where no overlap is possible.

The rest of the paper is organized as follows. In Section 2, we introduce the main contribution of the paper: a Bayesian inference to couple the extraction of two structures. Section 3 presents a probabilistic integration of prior shape knowledge. Then, these two formulations are combined for the special case of joint prostate and bladder segmentation in Section 4. In 5th and last section, we present qualitative and quantitative validations.

2   A Bayesian Inference for Coupled Level Set Segmentations

The level set representation [8] permits to describe and deform a surface without introducing any specific parameterization and/or a topological prior. Let $\Omega \in \mathbb{R}^3$ be the image domain, it represents a surface $\mathcal{S} \in \Omega$ by the zero crossing of an higher dimensional function ϕ, usually defined as a signed distance function:

$$\phi(x) = \begin{cases} 0, & \text{if } x \in \mathcal{S}, \\ +\mathcal{D}(x, \mathcal{S}), & \text{if } x \text{ is inside } \mathcal{S}, \\ -\mathcal{D}(x, \mathcal{S}), & \text{if } x \text{ is outside } \mathcal{S}. \end{cases} \quad (1)$$

where $\mathcal{D}(x, \mathcal{S})$ is minimum Euclidean distance between the location x and the surface. This representation permits to express geometric properties of the surface like its curvature and normal vector at given location, area, volume, etc... It is then possible to formulate segmentation criteria and advance the evolutions in the level set framework.

In our particular problem, we need to extract several structures from a single image. Rather than segmenting each one separately, we propose a Bayesian framework where the most probable segmentation of all objects is jointly estimated. We consider the extraction of two structures represented by two level set functions ϕ_1 and ϕ_2. The optimal segmentations of a given image I is obtained by maximizing the joint posterior distribution $p(\phi_1, \phi_2|I)$. Using the Bayesian theorem we have:

$$p(\phi_1, \phi_2|I) \propto p(I|\phi_1, \phi_2)\, p(\phi_1, \phi_2) \qquad (2)$$

The first term is the conditional probability of an image I and will be defined later using intensity properties of each structure. The second term is the joint probability of the two surfaces. We use the latter term to impose a non-overlapping constraint between the surfaces. Posteriori probability is often optimized by minimizing its negative logarithm. This gives the following energy functional for minimization process:

$$E(\phi_1, \phi_2) = \underbrace{-\log p(I|\phi_1, \phi_2)}_{E_{\text{data}}} \underbrace{-\log p(\phi_1, \phi_2)}_{E_{\text{coupling}}} \qquad (3)$$

A gradient descent approach with respect to each level set is employed for the minimization. The gradients of each level set can be computed as follows:

$$\begin{cases} \dfrac{\partial \phi_1}{\partial t} = -\dfrac{\partial E_{\text{data}}}{\partial \phi_1} - \dfrac{\partial E_{\text{coupling}}}{\partial \phi_1} \\[3mm] \dfrac{\partial \phi_2}{\partial t} = -\dfrac{\partial E_{\text{data}}}{\partial \phi_2} - \dfrac{\partial E_{\text{coupling}}}{\partial \phi_2} \end{cases} \qquad (4)$$

2.1   Non-overlapping Constraint

In this section, we define the joint probability $p(\phi_1, \phi_2)$ which serves as the coupling constraint between the surfaces. For this purpose, we make the assumptions that the level set values are spatially independent and that $\phi_{1,x}$ (the value of ϕ_1 at the position x) and $\phi_{2,y}$ are independent for $x \neq y$. These two assumptions give:

$$p(\phi_1, \phi_2) = \prod_{x \in \Omega} \prod_{y \in \Omega} p(\phi_{1,x}, \phi_{2,y}) \propto \prod_{x \in \Omega} p(\phi_{1,x}, \phi_{2,x}) \qquad (5)$$

Let H_ϵ be a regularized version of the Heaviside function defined as:

$$H_\epsilon(\phi) = \begin{cases} 1, & \phi > \epsilon \\ 0, & \phi < -\epsilon \\ \dfrac{1}{2}\left(1 + \dfrac{\phi}{\epsilon} + \dfrac{1}{\pi}\sin\left(\dfrac{\pi\phi}{\epsilon}\right)\right), & |\phi| < \epsilon. \end{cases}$$

The non-overlapping constraint can then be introduced by adding a penalty, when the voxels are inside both structures, i.e. when $H_\epsilon(\phi_1)$ and $H_\epsilon(\phi_2)$ are equal to one:

$$p(\phi_{1,x}, \phi_{2,x}) \propto \exp\left(-\alpha H_\epsilon(\phi_{1,x}) H_\epsilon(\phi_{2,x})\right) \qquad (6)$$

where α is a weight controlling the importance of this term. We will see later, in the application section, that it can be set once for all. The corresponding term in the energy is:

$$E_{\text{coupling}}(\phi_1, \phi_2) = \alpha \int_\Omega H_\epsilon(\phi_{1,x}) H_\epsilon(\phi_{2,x})\, dx \qquad (7)$$

2.2   Image Term

Following recent works [1,9], we define the image term using region-based intensity models. Given the overlapping constraint, the level set functions ϕ_1 and ϕ_2 define three sub-regions of the image domain: $\Omega_1 = \{x, \phi_1(x) > 0 \text{ and } \phi_2(x) < 0\}\}$ and $\Omega_2 = \{x, \phi_2(x) > 0 \text{ and } \phi_1(x) < 0\}\}$, the parts inside each structure and $\Omega_b = \{x, \phi_1(x) > 0 \text{ and } \phi_2(x) > 0\}$, the remaining part of the image. Assuming intensity values to be independent, the data term is defined from the prior intensity distributions $\{p_1, p_2, p_b\}$ for each region $\{\Omega_1, \Omega_2, \Omega_b\}$:

$$p\left(I|\phi_1, \phi_2\right) = \prod_{x \in \Omega_1} p_1\left(I(x)\right) \prod_{x \in \Omega_2} p_2\left(I(x)\right) \prod_{x \in \Omega_b} p_b\left(I(x)\right) \tag{8}$$

If a training set is available, these probability density functions can be learned with a Parzen density estimate on the histogram of the corresponding regions. In section 4, we will use an alternative approach, which considers user inputs. We can write the corresponding data term, which depends only on the level set functions:

$$
\begin{aligned}
E_{data}(\phi_1, \phi_2) = &- \int_{\Omega} H_\epsilon(\phi_{1,x})(1 - H_\epsilon(\phi_{2,x})) \log p_1(I(x))\, dx \\
&- \int_{\Omega} H_\epsilon(\phi_{2,x})(1 - H_\epsilon(\phi_{1,x})) \log p_2(I(x))\, dx \\
&- \int_{\Omega} (1 - H_\epsilon(\phi_{2,x}))(1 - H_\epsilon(\phi_{1,x})) \log p_b(I(x))\, dx
\end{aligned} \tag{9}
$$

2.3   Energy Minimization

The calculus of the variations of the global energy (3) with respect to ϕ_1 and ϕ_2 drives a coupled evolution of the level sets:

$$
\begin{cases}
\dfrac{\partial \phi_1}{\partial t} = \delta(\phi_1) \left((1 - H_\epsilon(\phi_2)) \log \dfrac{p_b(I(x))}{p_1(I(x))} - \alpha H_\epsilon(\phi_2) \right) \\[3mm]
\dfrac{\partial \phi_2}{\partial t} = \delta(\phi_2) \left((1 - H_\epsilon(\phi_1)) \log \dfrac{p_b(I(x))}{p_2(I(x))} - \alpha H_\epsilon(\phi_1) \right)
\end{cases} \tag{10}
$$

One can see that the data speed becomes null as soon as the surfaces overlap each other and therefore, the non-overlapping constraint will be the only one to act.

3   Shape Constrained Segmentation

As mentioned in the introduction, the image data may not be sufficient to extract the structure of interest; therefore prior knowledge has to be introduced. When the structure's shape remain similar from one image to another, a shape model can be built from training samples. Several types of shape models have been proposed in the literature [2,7,6,11,3,10,5]. Such models can be used to constrain the extraction of similar structures in other images. A straightforward approach is to estimate the instance from the modeled family that fits the best to the observed image [11,5,4]. This assumes the shape model to be generic enough to describe accurately the new structure. To add more flexibility, one can impose the segmentation not to belong to the shape model but to in limited range defined by a given distance [10,3]. This allows to capture small image-specific details that can not be captured in a global model. In the following, we present a general Bayesian formulation of this shape constrained segmentation.

For the sake of simplicity, we consider the segmentation of a single object represented by ϕ. Assuming a set of training shapes $\{\phi^1, \dots, \phi^N\}$ available, the optimal segmentation is obtained by maximizing:

$$
\begin{aligned}
p\left(\phi | I, \{\phi^1, \dots, \phi^N\}\right) &\propto p\left(I, \{\phi^1, \dots, \phi^N\} | \phi\right) p\left(\phi\right) \\
&\propto p\left(I | \phi\right) p(\phi) p\left(\{\phi^1, \dots, \phi^N\} | \phi\right) p\left(\phi\right) \\
&\propto p\left(I | \phi\right) p(\phi) p\left(\phi | \{\phi^1, \dots, \phi^N\}\right) p\left(\{\phi^1, \dots, \phi^N\}\right) \\
&\propto p\left(I | \phi\right) p(\phi) p\left(\phi | \{\phi^1, \dots, \phi^N\}\right)
\end{aligned}
\tag{11}
$$

The independence between I and $\{\phi^1, \dots, \phi^N\}$ is used to obtain the second line, and $p\left(\{\phi^1, \dots, \phi^N\}\right) = 1$ gives the final expression. The corresponding maximum a posteriori can be obtained by minimizing the following energy function:

$$
E(\phi) = \underbrace{- \log p\left(I | \phi\right)}_{E_{\text{data}}} \underbrace{- \log p\left(\phi\right)}_{E_{\text{regul}}} \underbrace{- \log p\left(\phi | \{\phi^1, \dots, \phi^N\}\right)}_{E_{\text{shape}}}
\tag{12}
$$

The first term integrates image data and can be defined according to section 2.2. The second one can be used to introduce a priori regularity of the segmentation. The last one introduces the shape constraint learned from the training samples. Following [7,11,10], this last term is built from a principal component analysis of the aligned training level sets. An example of such modeling on the prostate is shown in Figure 1. The most important modes of variation are selected to form a subspace of all possible shapes. The evolving level set can then be constrained inside this subspace [11,4] or it can be attracted to it [7,10] by defining the probability of a new instance as:

$$
p\left(\phi | \{\phi^1, \dots, \phi^N\}\right) \propto \exp\left(-d^2(\phi, Proj_{\mathcal{M}}(\phi))\right)
\tag{13}
$$

where $d^2(,)$ is the squared distance between two level set functions and $Proj_{\mathcal{M}}(\phi)$ is the projection of ϕ into the modeled shape subspace $\mathcal{M}$. More details can be found in [7,11,10].

In the next section, we combine this shape constrained formulation with the coupled level set Bayesian inference presented in section 2 for the joint segmentation of the prostate and the bladder.

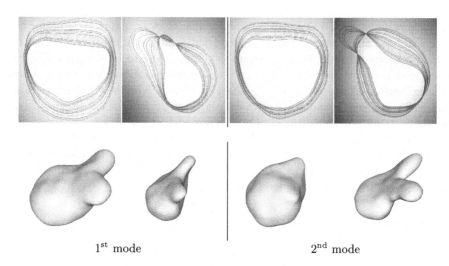

Fig. 1. Prostate shape model- Top: shape variations in 2D views, Bottom: generated shapes

4   Application to the Joint Segmentation of the Prostate and the Bladder

The main difficulty in segmenting the prostate and bladder is the prostate-bladder interface and the lack of reliability on the data on the lower part of the prostate (see Figure 2). There seems to be a notable intensity gradient around the bladder except from the side that is neighboring prostate. Besides, there seems to be a good statistically coherency among the shapes of the prostates from a patient population. However, the statistical coherency does not hold for the bladder shape, since the shape is dictated by the filling that can be unpredictable. Based on these arguments, we consider a model-based approach for the extraction of the prostate only. A coupled segmentation approach with a non-overlapping constraint resolves the ambiguity on the interface. To summarize, we design an approach that jointly segment the prostate and the bladder by including a coupling between the organs and a shape model of the prostate. The framework developed in the last two sections allows us to express this in a probabilistic way. Let ϕ_1 be the level set representing the prostate boundary and ϕ_2, the bladder one. Given N training shapes of the prostate $\{\phi_1^1, \ldots, \phi_2^N\}$, the posterior density probability of these segmentations is:

$$p\left(\phi_1, \phi_2 | I, \{\phi_1^1, \ldots, \phi_2^N\}\right) = \frac{p\left(I, \{\phi_1^1, \ldots, \phi_2^N\} | \phi_1, \phi_2\right) p\left(\phi_1, \phi_2\right)}{p(I, \{\phi_1^1, \ldots, \phi_2^N\})} \qquad (14)$$

Since the image and the training contours are not correlated, we have:

$$p\left(\phi_1, \phi_2 | I, \{\phi_1^1, \ldots, \phi_2^N\}\right) \propto p\left(I | \phi_1, \phi_2\right) p\left(\phi_1, \phi_2\right) p\left(\phi_1 | \{\phi_1^1, \ldots, \phi_2^N\}\right) \qquad (15)$$

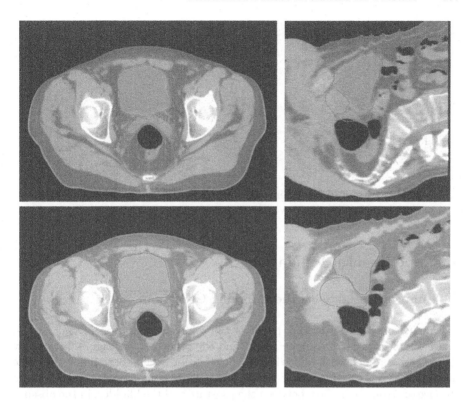

Fig. 2. Prostate and bladder segmentation without (top) and with (bottom) coupling

Each factor of this relation have been described in Section 2 and 3. Hence, the optimal solution of our problem should minimize the following energy:

$$E(\phi_1, \phi_2) = E_{\text{data}}(\phi_1, \phi_2) + E_{\text{coupling}}(\phi_1, \phi_2) + E_{\text{shape}}(\phi_1) \qquad (16)$$

The first two terms have been described in equation (9) and (7). Only the shape energy need some clarification. In our implementation, a two step approach has been chosen. In a first time, we follow [11,4] by constraining the prostate level set in the subspace obtained from the training shapes. Then, we add more flexibility to the surface by considering the constraint presented in equation (13).

For initialization, the user clicks inside each organ. ϕ_1 and ϕ_2 are then initialized as small spheres centered on these two points. They also serve to define the intensity models of the organs by considering a Parzen density estimate of the histogram inside each sphere and outside voxels are used for the background. Using the user input to define intensity distributions of the organs has proved to be reliable. The intensity of each organ being relatively constant, its mean value can be actually guessed with a good confidence and the approach does not show a big sensitivity to user inputs.

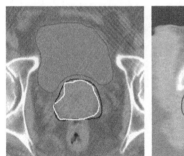 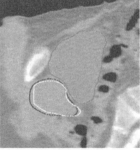 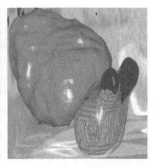

Fig. 3. Prostate and bladder segmentation - Red: bladder segmentation, Black: prostate segmentation, White: ground truth prostate

5   Experimental Validations

5.1   Improvements with the Coupling Constraint

The main contribution of this paper is the joint segmentation of two organs, where one incorporates a shape model and the other not. In Figure 2, we show the results obtained with and without coupling. In both experiments, the same shape model was considered for the prostate (with seminal vesicles). Given the absence of strong boundary between the prostate and the bladder, in the absence of coupling, the bladder leaks inside the prostate and the prostate is shifted toward the bladder. Segmenting both organs at the same time with coupling constraint solve this problem. Related works were able to obtain correct results for the prostate without this coupling but the coupling make it a lot more robust to the initialization and to the image quality. Moreover, imposing a shape model to the bladder is definitely not appropriate given its large variations intra- and inter-patient, and so, the coupling is mandatory to extract this organ.

5.2   Validation on a Large Dataset

To assess the quality of our results, we use several quantitative measures similar to the ones introduced in [6]:

- ρ_d, the probability of detection, calculated as the fraction of the ground truth volume that overlap with the estimated organ volume. This probability should be close to 1 for a good segmentation.
- ρ_{fd}, the probability of false detection, calculated as the fraction of the estimated organ that lies outside the ground truth organ. This value should be close to 0 for a good segmentation.
- c_d, the centroid distance, calculated as the norm of the vector connecting the centroids of the ground truth and estimated organs. The centroid of each

organ is calculated using the following formula assuming the organ is made up of a collection of N triangular faces with vertices (a_i, b_i, c_i) :

$$c = \frac{\sum_{i=0}^{N-1} A_i R_i}{\sum_{i=0}^{N-1} A_i} \qquad (17)$$

where R_i is the average of the vertices of the ith face and A_i is twice the area of the ith face: $R_i = (a_i + b_i + c_i)/2$ and $A_i = \|(b_i - a_i) \otimes (c_i - a_i)\|$.

- s_d, the surface distance, calculated as the median distance between the surfaces of the ground truth and estimated organs. To compute the median distance, we generated a distance function using the ground truth volume.

In Figure 4, we show the measures obtained for the prostate segmentation on 16 images (4 patients with 4 images each) for which the manual segmentation was available. These images are $512 \times 512 \times 100$ pixels with a spacing of $1\text{mm} \times 1\text{mm} \times 3\text{mm}$. To conduct these test, we used a leave-one-out strategy, i.e. the shape of considered image was not use in the shape model. The model was built from all the other images and is so an inter-patient model. We obtained an average accuracy between 4 and 5 mm, i.e., between one and two voxels. The percentage of well-classified was around 82%. The average processing time on a PC with the process of 2.2 GHz is about 12 seconds.

Patient	ρ_d	ρ_{fd}	c_d (mm)	s_d (mm)
1	0.93	0.20	3.5	4.1
2	0.82	0.12	5.8	4.2
3	0.88	0.16	5.2	4.0
4	0.93	0.19	4.0	3.9
5	0.84	0.20	5.5	4.0
6	0.85	0.22	5.9	3.7
7	0.89	0.20	3.4	2.9
8	0.84	0.28	3.1	4.5
9	0.80	0.35	8.7	4.9
10	0.88	0.27	8.0	4.3
11	0.67	0.19	4.8	3.7
12	0.84	0.35	8.6	6.7
13	0.73	0.20	7.7	5.4
14	0.83	0.09	2.3	3.1
15	0.84	0.19	4.0	4.0
16	0.85	0.15	3.2	3.7
Average	0.84	0.21	5.2	4.2

Fig. 4. Quantitative validation of the prostate segmentation - From left to right: probability of detection, probability of false detection, centroid distance and average surface distance

6 Conclusion

We have proposed a new Bayesian framework to segment jointly several structures. We developed a probabilistic approach that integrates a coupling between the surfaces and prior shape knowledge. This general formulation has been adapted to the important problem of prostate segmentation for radiotherapy. By coupling the extraction of the prostate and bladder, we were able to constrain the problem and make it well-posed. Qualitative and quantitative results were presented to validate the performance of the proposed approach. Future works will consist of the joint extraction of all three organs including the rectum.

References

1. T. Chan and L. Vese. Active contours without edges. *IEEE Transactions on Image Processing*, 10(2):266–277, February 2001.
2. T. Cootes, C. Taylor, D. Cooper, and J. Graham. Active shape models-their training and application. *Computer Vision and Image Understanding*, 61(1):38–59, 1995.
3. D. Cremers, S. J. Osher, , and S. Soatto. Kernel density estimation and intrinsic alignment for knowledge-driven segmentation: Teaching level sets to walk. *Pattern Recognition*, 3175:36–44, 2004.
4. D. Cremers and M. Rousson. Efficient kernel density estimation of shape and intensity priors for level set segmentation. In *MICCAI*, October 2005.
5. E.B. Dam, P.T. Fletcher, S. Pizer, G. Tracton, and J. Rosenman. Prostate shape modeling based on principal geodesic analysis bootstrapping. In *MICCAI*, volume 2217 of *LNCS*, pages 1008–1016, September 2004.
6. D. Freedman, R.J. Radke, T. Zhang, Y. Jeong, D.M. Lovelock, and G.T. Chen. Model-based segmentation of medical imagery by matching distributions. *IEEE Trans Med Imaging*, 24(3):281–292, March 2005.
7. M. Leventon, E. Grimson, and O. Faugeras. Statistical Shape Influence in Geodesic Active Contours. In *Proceedings of the International Conference on Computer Vision and Pattern Recognition*, pages 316–323, Hilton Head Island, South Carolina, June 2000.
8. S. Osher and J. Sethian. Fronts propagating with curvature dependent speed: algorithms based on the Hamilton–Jacobi formulation. *J. of Comp. Phys.*, 79:12–49, 1988.
9. N. Paragios and R. Deriche. Geodesic active regions: a new paradigm to deal with frame partition problems in computer vision. *Journal of Visual Communication and Image Representation, Special Issue on Partial Differential Equations in Image Processing, Computer Vision and Computer Graphics*, 13(1/2):249–268, march/june 2002.
10. M. Rousson, N. Paragios, and R. Deriche. Implicit active shape models for 3d segmentation in mr imaging. In *MICCAI*. Springer-Verlag, September 2004.
11. A. Tsai, W. Wells, C. Tempany, E. Grimson, and A. Willsky. Mutual information in coupled multi-shape model for medical image segmentation. *Medical Image Analysis*, 8(4):429–445, December 2004.

Curvilinear Structure Based Mammographic Registration

Lionel C.C. Wai and Michael Brady

Medical Vision Laboratory, Robotics Research Group, University of Oxford,
Parks Road,Oxford OX1 3PJ, United Kingdom.
{lwai,jmb}@robots.ox.ac.uk

Abstract. Mammographic registration is a challenging problem due in part to the intrinsic complexity of mammographic images, and partly because of the substantial differences that exist between two mammograms that are to be matched. In this paper, we propose a registration algorithm for mammograms which incorporates junctions of Curvilinear structures (CLS) as internal landmarks. CLS depict connective tissue, blood vessels, and milk ducts. These are detected by an algorithm based on the monogenic signal and afforced by a CLS physical model. The junctions are extracted using a local energy (LE)-based method, which utilises the orientation information provided by the monogenic signal. Results using such junctions as internal landmarks in registration are presented and compared with conventional approaches using boundary landmarks, in order to highlight the potential of anatomical based feature extraction in medical image analysis. We demonstrate how computer vision techniques such as phase congruency (PC), local energy (LE) and multi-resolution can be applied in linear (1-D) and junction (2-D) detection as well as their application to medical image registration problems.

1 Introduction

Because mammograms are so variable anatomically, and because there is wide variation in image formation, radiologists often have considerable difficulty in detecting and diagnosing disease from a single image. For this reason, they are trained to compare mammograms: two different views of the same breast, left vs right same view, and especially to detect significant changes in the "same" view at two different times. For this reason, temporal mammogram registration has increasingly recognized as a key component of computer-aided detection (CAD) in mammography, though to date (unlike microcalcification detection) no commercial systems are available. The challenge of reliably matching temporal mammogram pairs is the reason the word "same" above is in quotation marks: there are likely to be very different imaging parameters, compounded by a slightly different compression of the breast, so that the two images can appear quite dissimilar. Often, a striking dissimilarity concerns the CLS which depict connective tissue, blood vessels, and milk ducts, and whose appearance is quite sensitive to breast compression. For this reason, several algorithms either work entirely from the breast boundary, ignoring internal landmarks, or attempt to remove the CLS in a preprocessing step [1-5]. van

Y. Liu, T. Jiang, and C. Zhang (Eds.): CVBIA 2005, LNCS 3765, pp. 261–270, 2005.
© Springer-Verlag Berlin Heidelberg 2005

Engeland et al analyzed the use of primary structures such as nipple, center of mass and pectoral muscle as landmarks. [4] Also, numerous studies have proposed the use of one-dimensional features as internal landmarks. Among them are the pseudo-linear structures proposed by Vujovic [5] and the nonlinear filter suggested by Zweiggler [6].

Marias [3] demonstrates that whereas aligning the boundaries of two mammograms provides a good basis for registration, it is necessary to augment this with landmarks internal to the breasts. They suggest detecting small features such as microcalcifications, though their presence is not guaranteed. This paper starts from the observation that while the appearance of the CLS are sensitive to compression, in practice, the difference in compression is of the order of 0.5cm [17], and so major CLS structures often do appear in both images. If a CLS junction appears in both images, as it often does, then it should be used as a landmark: removing all the CLS in a preprocessing step is overly defeatist! Though the segmentation of the CLS has been presented in [7], it will be overviewed in this paper for completeness.

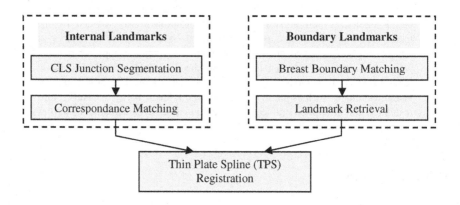

Fig. 1. Schematic of the CLS based registration framework

2   CLS Physics

Anatomically, CLS are composed of structures including blood vessels, milk ducts and connective stroma, and they project as ridge-like features on a mammogram. The dimensions of such structures range from 1800 microns to 5 microns in width. For a digital mammogram with a resolution of 50 microns per pixel, the detectable range lies between 1800 microns to 180 microns [8]. In mass and calcification segmentation, the CLS are considered as noise. On the other hand, as we will show, the CLS can be a reliable feature for registration. Thus the segmentation of the CLS is important both in noise removal and landmark selection.

The CLS junctions satisfy the invariance requirement for temporal pairs of mammograms. A possible factor that might in principle cause changes in the CLS network is the angiogenesis [9] that typically accompanies cancer development. However, arteries and veins are less sensitive to the Vascular Endothelium Growth

Factor (VEGF) than the microvessels or capillaries, and the latter (micron scale) are generally invisible in mammograms.

3 Segmentation of CLS Junctions as Internal Landmarks

The segmentation of the CLS is inevitably multi-resolution. This is because of the variation in the widths of vascular structures and the need for noise suppression. To implement this, the image is firstly processed by a set of Difference of Gaussian (DoG) band-pass filters to form the scale-space. The phase of the image can be obtained from three quadrature filters, by convolving these (approximately bandpass) scale-space images f with the Riesz Transform pair of filters h_1, h_2, to form the monogenic signal [10]:

$$f_M(x_1, x_2) = (f(x_1, x_2), (h_1 * f)(x_1, x_2), (h_2 * f)(x_1, x_2)) \tag{1}$$

in which f is the DoG filtered images and the h_1 and h_2 are the Riesz transform, defined more naturally in the Fourier domain by:

$$H_1(u_1, u_2) = i \frac{u_1}{\sqrt{u_1^2 + u_2^2}} \text{ and } H_2(u_1, u_2) = i \frac{u_2}{\sqrt{u_1^2 + u_2^2}}. \tag{2}$$

The vector-valued filter, the monogenic signal, gives a substantially more robust phase estimation for two dimensional images than is provided by a set of steerable filters in several orientations [11].

Given the monogenic signal images, the problem becomes how to localize the ridges of the CLS in order to extract the "skeleton" (and junctions). The phase congruency (PC) approach is adopted detect such features [12]. PC is a measure of the phase similarity of the Fourier components of a point. The phase congruency of a point with spatial coordinate given by x can be defined as follows:

$$PC(x) = \underset{\theta \in (0, 2\pi)}{Max} \frac{\int_{-\infty}^{\infty} a_\omega \cos(\omega x + \phi_\omega - \theta) d\omega}{\int_{-\infty}^{\infty} a_\omega d\omega}. \tag{3}$$

Based on the idea of ridge detection, which rests on the support of monogenic signal and phase congruency, the degree of scale span of the multiresolution filters is determined based on tuning on a set of CLS with certain widths and cross-section profiles on the image. The model based tuning provides a performance enhancement for higher-level applications. For example, if the CLS are to be identified are then removed, the CLS width range should be as wide as possible. On the other hand, if CLS segmentation is for registration, only salient and large vessels are needed so that the CLS detector should be biased towards CLS at higher scales. Thus the CLS model can improve the specificity and selectivity of the detector for different applications.

The model we use is adopted from Cerneaz[8], who introduced a two medium modelthat estimates the CLS intensity profile on a x-ray film. The CLS are assumed

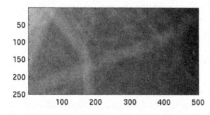
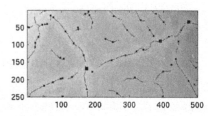

Fig. 2. Sample outputs of the CLS and junction detector. The CLS junction selection is based on neighborhood orientation information and local energy (LE). The large markers are the final junctions, while the smaller ones are rejected candidates (i.e. number of branches <= 2).

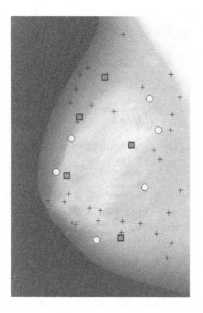
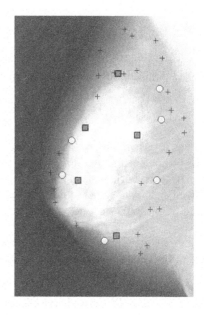

Fig. 3. This figure shows a set of CLS junctions on a pair of temporal mammograms (Mediolateral Oblique (MLO) – right breast) and the final pairs of corresponding landmarks. Round dots denotes the final corresponding pairs, crosses being the rejected CLS junctions. The squares are corresponding pairs of saliency points extracted using the Kadir/Brady algorithm (start scale 150; end scale 120) [18]. The star near the nipple of the left mammogram is the only rejected saliency point. (Please refer to Part 6: Results and Discussion)

to have an elliptic cross section when the breast is compressed during screening. Based on this relationship, the pixel intensity profile on a digitised image can be modeled.

As CLS are typically low contrast and since poor signal-to-noise can badly affect the performance of the CLS detector, local energy (LE) thresholding is used [13] to suppress undesirable responses. LE is related to phase congruency (in discrete terms):

$$LE(x) = PC(x)\sum_n A_n, \tag{4}$$

where A_n is the amplitude of the nth bandpass filter. A typical output of our CLS (junction) detector is shown in Fig. 2.

Apart from noise removal, local energy is also used to segment CLS junctions. First, the algorithm detects those pixels which have a *local maxima* of LE, based on the notion that the convergence, or intersection, of ridges will result in a point with higher LE. In the second step, these candidate points (points with local maxima) are then searched through a neighbourhood of radius r, where $r=kLE(x)$ to find any CLS (branches) that point towards that candidate point, by comparing the orientation of the CLS and the vector pointing to the branch from the junction point. The orientation information is computed from the monogenic signal. A junction is detected if the number of branches is more than 2.

With the junction extracted, the algorithm then matches up the corresponding junctions based on a joint measure of the LE and the Euclidean distance difference between the junction points. A sample output is demonstrated in Fig. 3.

4 Boundary Landmarks Segmentation and Matching

In addition to landmark registration, we improve both the boundary landmark generation and matching method relative to a previous approach in our Laboratory [3]. To generate boundary landmarks, the breast boundary is first segmented using a phase-based approach in the same multi-resolution framework as the CLS detection [14] and the points extracted are parameterized using a cubic spline. Thus a regularised curvature can be retrieved from the spline function. For the boundary matching process, instead of directly deducing the curvature from the spline, we estimate it in a multi-resolution framework: we compute the curvature $\kappa(t,s)$, in which t is the spline parameter and s is the scale, that is, curvature scale-space (CSS) [15]. Then matching between breast boundaries can be implemented as a rigid registration/correlation problem between two CSS maps. The result is an output of the scaling and the shift of the boundary curve of the source image being warped to the target image.

Compared with the approach of Marias, who use a model to find out three extremum (nipple, rib and axilla) of boundary curvature (which can only be feasible on a certain type of breasts), our approach is more reliable because it can accommodate almost all types of breast boundaries without enforcing a specific model to it. Also, in our approach, the number of boundary landmarks can be easily partitioned to ensure a better mapping between temporal mammograms. It also provides a potential way of robust registration implementation if there is a rigid registration pipeline available.

An example of the boundary landmarks generated and matched between temporal pairs and some of the registration result is shown in Fig. 4.

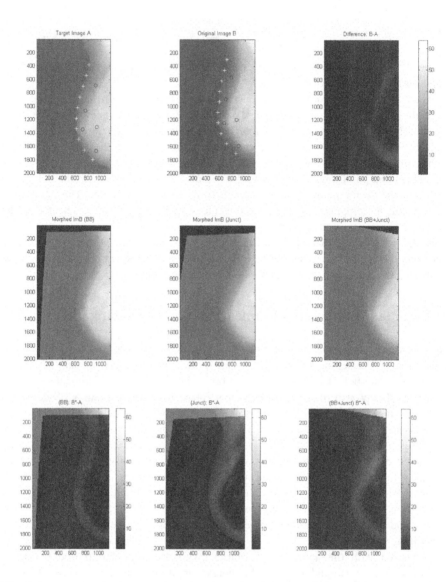

Fig. 4. An example of temporal pair registration using Thin Plate Spline (TPS) [16]. The upper row shows the temporal pairs. (The crosses are the location of boundary landmarks). The original difference image is showed top right. The middle row is the warped moving images and the bottom row shows the difference measure. Just using boundary landmarks improves the registration near the boundary; but does not improve the structural difference within the parenchyma. One can observe a 'white band' present in every difference image after registration. This is the due to the intensity difference which can be traced back to the difference in tube voltage and the compression force of the breast between the screening. (which can be partly reduced by transforming the image into SMF format [17])

5 Registration Method

After the landmarks are detected and correspondences are established, the warp is generated using the paired landmark point sets. In this study, we use Thin Plate Splines (TPS) [16] as the warp function of the registration of the source to target image, defined as in the following equation:

$$f(x,y) = a_1 + a_2 \cdot x + a_3 \cdot y + \sum_{i=1}^{n} w_i \cdot U\left(\left|L_F(i) - (x,y)\right|\right) \cdot \tag{5}$$

In this equation, $f(x,y)$ is the warp function, $L_F(i)$ is the ith landmark in the fixed (source) image and w_i is the landmark weighting coefficient. U is the biharmonic function $U(r) = -r^2 \log r^2$. In the MATLAB Spline Toolbox implementation, the coefficients are optimized by a weighted measure of the position error and the bending energy of the warp:

$$pE_f + (1-p)I_f \tag{6}$$

where

$$E_f = \sum_n \left| L_M - f(L_F) \right|^2 \tag{7}$$

and

$$I_f = \iint_{\mathbb{R}^2} \left(\frac{\partial^2 f}{\partial x^2}\right)^2 + 2 \cdot \left(\frac{\partial^2 f}{\partial x \partial y}\right)^2 + \left(\frac{\partial^2 f}{\partial y^2}\right)^2 dx dy \cdot \tag{8}$$

In our implementation and all the experimental results presented in this paper, $p=0.7$. The Thin Plate Spline is a robust and commonly-used warping function used in non-rigid registration. It has the advantage of being efficient for local deformations. Inititutively speaking, the warping of thin plate spline resembles the warping of one x-ray film towards another.

After generating the TPS function with the landmarks from two images, the second (moving) image is warped toward the fixed image by using the TPS. This is done in practice by inversely warping the coordinate frame of the fixed image towards that of the moving image. After that, the intensity of each pixel in the warped image is determined by regularization. In our implementation we use linear interpolation as the regulariser.

6 Results and Discussion

Demonstrations of the proposed registration framework are presented in Fig. 3-5. As seen in Fig. 3, the landmark matching framework has been successful in matching pairs of landmarks, and that there are sufficiently many internal landmarks. However, some pairs of junctions that are candidates to be matched are currently missed in our approach, which is based on the measure of LE and Euclidean distance. A better measure could be developed to obtain higher yield of internal landmarks.

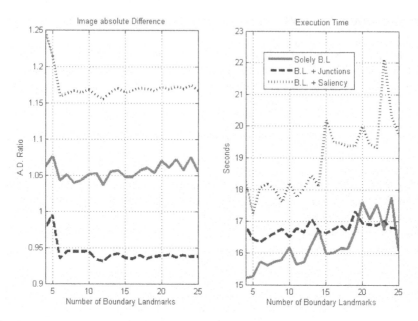

Fig. 5. Registration using solely Boundary Landmarks (B.L.) versus Boundary Landmarks with Junctions or Saliency Point as internal landmarks. The temporal pair being registered is shown in Fig. 3. We vary the number of boundary landmarks used but the number of internal landmarks is constant (i.e. 6 pairs of internal landmarks for the B.L. + Junctions case and 5 pairs for the B.L. + Saliency case.) On the Left shows the image absolute difference (A.D.) Ratio of the breast area, in which the image difference before registration is 1. On the right shows the execution speed of thin plate spline (TPS), which has a positive relationship to the complexity of warping.

One can observe the functional difference between boundary landmarks and internal landmarks in Fig. 4. The boundary landmarks improve the shape correspondence between breasts whereas the junction landmarks strengthen the structural correspondence of tissue. From the temporal registration example presented, use of the internal landmarks improves the registration by highlighting the contrast between different tissue (like the thickness of the upper part of the breast in Fig. 4).

Another comparison is shown in Fig. 5, in which we compare the relationship between registration with internal (junction) landmarks and the registration without internal landmarks. We also investigate whether the numbers of boundary landmarks affect the registration performance. When performing registration without internal landmarks, using 8-12 boundary landmarks gives the best registration performance. The performance gain decreases with more boundary landmarks because of over-fitting. When internal landmarks are incorporated in the registration, the absolute difference is far lower than using solely boundary landmarks. The difference measure also shows a lesser variation, in other words a higher confidence level. We also compared our algorithm with Marias's approach of using saliency points as internal landmarks for registration. It is found that using saliency points, like CLS junctions, can enhance the reliability of image difference measure. However, in terms of the image difference measure, the CLS junctions prove to be a better choice of internal landmarks than saliency.

Similar results are obtained in the execution time as well. For registration with both boundary landmarks (B.L.) and junctions, execution time is more stable than using boundary landmarks solely, whereas the execution speed increases in the solely B.L. case and B.L with saliency as landmarks. As the execution speed implies the complexity of warping, the result indicates that the higher discrepancies exist between the position expressed by boundary and that by saliency landmarks. These results demonstrates the important role of CLS junctions in ensuring registration performance and implementation reliability.

7 Conclusions

A landmark-based registration framework of mammograms has been presented in this paper. We have demonstrated how various ideas in computer vision may be applied for feature detection and registration of medical images, including multi-resolution (scale-space) analysis, phase congruency, local energy and monogenic signal. Through proposing new methods in both boundary matching and landmark (control-point) identification, we have demonstrated improvements to current methods [3]. We also provide further evidence on the significance of including internal landmarks in mammographic registration.

Compared with previous mammographic registration approaches, our approach incorporates the notion of multi-resolution into both the framework of boundary and internal landmark detection. The advantages of multi-resolution analysis have been shown with higher stability and accuracy in feature detection, and this enhances the registration performance as a result. However, the speed of multi-resolution is the prominent challenge that needs to be addressed in our future work.

Acknowledgements. Lionel Check-Chiu Wai would like to thank for the support from the Croucher Foundation, Hong Kong. Michael Brady acknowledges support from EPSRC for the IRC in Medical Images and Signals (MIAS), and for the eDiamond project.

References

1. M. Y. Sallam, K. W. Bowyer, "Registration and difference analysis of corresponding mammogram images", *Medical Image Analysis*, vol. 3, iss 2, pp. 103-118, 1999.
2. R. Marti, R. Zwiggelaar, C. Rubin, "Automatic registration of mammograms based on linear structures", in *Information Processing in Medical Imaging (IPMI 2001)*, pp. 162-168, LNCS 2082, Springer-Verlag, 2001.
3. K. Marias, C. Behrenbruch, S. Parbhoo, A. Seifalian, M. Brady, " A Registration Framework for the Comparison of Mammogram Sequences", *IEEE Transactions on Medical Imaging,* Vol. 24, No. 6, pp. 782-790, 2005.

4. S. van Engeland, P. Snoeren, J. Hendriks and N. Karssemeijer, "A Comparison of Methods for Mammogram Registration", *IEEE Transactions on Medical Imaging,* vol. 22, No. 11, pp. 1436-1444, 2003.
5. N. Vujovic, "Establishing the correspondence between control points in pairs of mammographic images," *IEEE Transactions on Image Processing,* vol. 6, no. 10, pp. 1388-1399, 1997.
6. R. Zwiggelaar, T. Parr, C. Taylor, "Finding orientated line patterns in digital mammographic images", in *Proceedings 7th British Machine Vision Conference,* pp. 715-724, 1996.
7. L. C. C. Wai, M. Mellor, M. J. Brady, "A multi-resolution CLS detection algorithm for mammographic image analysis", *7th International Conference on Medical Image Computer and Computer Assisted Intervention (MICCAI),* vol. 2., pp. 865-872, 2004.
8. N. Cerneaz, "Model-based analysis of mammograms", DPhil Thesis, University of Oxford, 1994 (see also Chapter 11 of Highnam and Brady q.v.)
9. N. Weidner, J.P. Semple, W.R. Welch, J. Folkman, "Tumor angiogenesis and metastasis-correlation in invasive breast carcinoma", *New England Journal of Medicine,* vol. 324, No. 1, pp. 1-8, 1991.
10. M. Felsberg, G. Sommer, "A new extension of linear signal processing for estimating local properties and detecting features", in *Proceedings of DAGM Symposium,* Spinger-Verlag, pp. 195-202, 2002.
11. V. U. B. Schenk, M. Brady, "Finding CLS using multiresolution oriented local energy feature detection," in *Proceedings 6th International Workshop on Digital Mammography (IWDM 2002),* June 2002.
12. P. Kovesi, "Image features from phase congruency", *Videre: A Journal of Computer Vision Research,* Vol.1, No.3, 1999.
13. V. U. B. Schenk, "Visual identification of fine surface incisions", DPhil Thesis, University of Oxford, 2001.
14. C.E. Tromans, M. J. Brady and R. Warren, "Breast Boundary Segmentation and its use in Breast Density Estimation", *Proceedings of the International Workshop on Digital Mammography (IWDM 2004),* E. Pisano (ed.) to appear, 2005.
15. F. Mokhtarian and A. K. Mackworth, "A Theory of Multi-Scale, Curvature-Based Shape Representation for Planar Curves," *IEEE Trans. Pattern Analysis and Machine Intelligence,* vol. 14, no. 8, pp. 789-805, 1992.
16. F. L. Bookstein, "Principal Warps: Thin-Plate Splines and the Decomposition of Deformations", *IEEE Trans. Pattern Analysis and Machine Intelligence,* vol. 11, No. 6, 1989.
17. R. Highnam, M. Brady, *Mammographic Image Analysis,* Kluwer Academic, 1999.
18. T. Kadir, M. Brady, "Scale Saliency and Image Description", *International Journal of Computer Vision,* vol. 45, No.2, pp. 82-105, 2001.

Deformable Registration for Generating Dissection Image of an Intestine from Annular Image Sequence

Suchit Pongnumkul, Ryusuke Sagawa,
Tomio Echigo, and Yasushi Yagi

The Institute of Scientific and Industrial Research, Osaka University,
8-1 Mihogaoka, Ibaraki, Osaka, 567-0047, Japan
{p-suchit, sagawa, echigo, yagi}@am.sanken.osaka-u.ac.jp

Abstract. Examination inside an intestine by an endoscope is difficult and time consuming, because the whole image of the intestine cannot be taken at one time due to the limited field of view. Thus, it is necessary to generate a dissection image, which can be obtained by extending the image of an intestine. We acquire an annular image sequence with an omnidirectional or wide-angle camera, and then generate the dissection image by mosaicing the image sequence. Though usual mosaicing techniques transform an image by perspective or affine transformations, these are not suitable for our situation because the target object is a generalized cylinder and the camera motion is unknown a priori. Therefore, we propose a novel approach for image registration that deforms images by a two-dimensional-polynomial function which parameters are estimated from optical flow. We evaluated our method by registering annular image sequences and we successfully generated dissection images, as presented in this paper.

1 Introduction

Examining a patient's intestine using an endoscope is difficult and time consuming, because the field of view of a camera is restricted and the doctor can only look at a small part of the intestine at a time. It would be desirable for an easy-to-understand view to be available for medical doctors. This is especially important when a lot of data is involved, for example, when a doctor compares patients among those who have similar symptom.

The most easy-to-understand way for an examination is to operate and cut open the intestine for a view of the whole intestine, but it is impossible for many reasons. The generation of images, which look like cut-and-expanded intestine, is required. Thus by using this representation a doctor can examine the wide area of an intestine at a glance without performing an operation. Videos that are taken by an endoscope can be used to generate such images by utilizing an adapted video mosaicing technique.

A number of methods have been explored and proposed in the video mosaicing literature. S. Peleg and J. Herman [9] developed a panoramic mosaicing method using manifold projection. Szeliski [13] developed an image-based video mosaicing method using 8-DOF projective image transformation parameters between pairs of input images. His

Y. Liu, T. Jiang, and C. Zhang (Eds.): CVBIA 2005, LNCS 3765, pp. 271–280, 2005.
© Springer-Verlag Berlin Heidelberg 2005

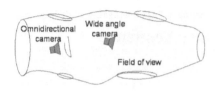

Fig. 1. Omnidirectional and wide-angle cameras inside an intestine

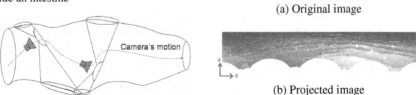

(a) Original image

(b) Projected image

Fig. 2. The camera motion is unknown a priori when examining inside an intestine **Fig. 3.** An image of intestine's model taken by endoscope

method can be used when a target is a plane (planar image mosaicing) or the optical centers of images are approximately fixed throughout the video capture (panorama image mosaicing). Swaminathan and Nayar [12] developed a non-metric method for calibrating wide-angle lenses and polycameras, seeking the distortion parameters that would map the image curves to straight lines. But the method does not apply in our objective because of the lack of straight lines in an intestine.

On the other hand, a number of non-rigid body registration methods have been proposed in the field of medical image, for example, free-form deformation(FFD) [3], global transformation using affine transformation and local transformation controlled by FFD model based linear singular blending(LSB) B-spline [14], finite element method (FEM) [6]. These methods work well only if the motion between two images is small.

As mentioned earlier, existing methods make use of the knowledge of camera position or rigid-object shapes. However, the shape of intestine is non-rigid and an endoscopic image sequence contains large motions. Moreover, the trajectory of the camera takes a meandering path as shown in Fig. 2, since the shape of the tube is not a simple cylinder. Therefore, a new image registration approach is required. In this paper, we propose a novel method to generate a dissection image of an intestine from an image sequence, where the dissection image look like the image obtained by cutting the intestine lengthwise and opening out its inside. And we also propose a novel deformable registration method for non-rigid object using the multiple variable polynomial functions (two-dimensional-polynomial functions) which parameters are estimated from optical flow.

The examination of an intestine by an endoscope can be considered as capturing a sequence of images of the inside of a generalized cylinder (in this paper called a "tube object") using a camera. Each image in the sequence captures a part of the tube, and combining them will yield an image of the whole tube. We acquire an image sequence of a tube using an omnidirectional or a wide-angle camera. These cameras have a large field of view as shown in Fig. 1. Thus, they obtain the image of the inside wall of a tube object. Fig. 3(a) shows an image captured by an endoscope; from this image, we utilize the annular area and apply an appropriate formula to obtain a stripe of a dissection image, as shown in Fig. 3(b). After we obtain a sequence of parts of the dissection images, we need to register and mosaic them to form a full dissection image of the intestine. In this paper, our method accomplishes the deformable registration of images by fitting a two-dimensional-polynomial function, which restricted by shape of a generalized cylinder.

This paper is organized as follows. Section 2 gives an overview of our approach. Section 3 explains our deformable registration. Section 4 presents our experimental results. Finally section 5 summarizes our findings.

2   Generating a Dissection Image

In our approach, we take the annular images with a 360 degree view camera with no information about the camera's motion; however, we assume that the camera's motion is continuous, and the characteristic of the observed target is a smooth tube. Our approach to mosaic the annular image sequence is a feature-based approach with steps as shown below:

1. Detect optical flows
2. Project input image into panoramic image
3. Register the projected image
4. Mosaic the registered image

We detect the optical flows from our input image sequence, and then project the input image into panoramic image. After that, we use the detected optical flow in our image registration. Finally, we mosaic the transformed image into mosaicing image.

2.1   Computing Optical Flows and Estimating the Pose of the Camera

We compute optical flows by extracting and tracking feature points. Our method is based on the KLT feature tracker [8] and the feature points are detected using [11]. Fig. 4 shows an example of the result of computing optical flows. Each feature point is detected at the point where the texture changes steeply and the black lines depict the vectors of optical flows.

After computing optical flows, we estimate the pose of the camera using optical flows. The purpose is to reject the outliers of optical flows and cancel the rotation of the camera before projecting the input image into a panoramic image coordinate. Our method first estimates the epipolar geometry using 7 point matches [15] or 8 point matches [7]. Next, we refine the solution by reprojecting the feature points using the estimated parameters [10]. Since our method accomplishes a robust estimation with a RANSAC approach [5], we can reject false optical flows as outliers.

Because the deformation of an input image, which is caused by the rotation of the camera does not change according to the distance from the camera, an image without deformation can be created by applying the inverse rotation to the input image. On the other hand, the deformation by the translation of the camera cannot be easily restored because it depends on the distance from the camera to the object viewed. We explain the solution to this issue in section 3.

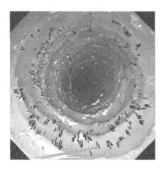

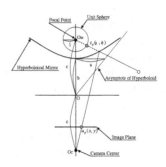

Fig. 4. Detected optical flow (black lines)   **Fig. 5.** Projection model of a hyper-omnidirectional camera

2.2 Projection into Spherical Coordinates

The next step is to project an annular image into spherical coordinates. If we use cylindrical coordinates, the mapping function can diverge when the direction of the camera changes. Thus, we use spherical coordinates. There are several ways to capture the annular image, using an omnidirectional or a wide-angle camera. In this section, we explain the method to generate a panoramic image in a spherical coordinate from the image of a hyper-omnidirectional camera [4]. Even if we use a different type of camera, we can generalize the image into spherical coordinate, which make the computation is similar.

Figure 5 shows the projection model of a hyper-omnidirectional camera system. Every ray point to the focal point of the hyperboloidal mirror through a point $S_p(\theta, \phi)$ on the spherical coordinates of the mirror. It reflects to the camera center through a point $u_p(x, y)$ in the annular image coordinates. Thus, we can project the annular image taken by a hyper-omnidirectional camera into a unit sphere by the following computation:

$$\beta = \arctan\left(\frac{-\left((b^2 + c^2)\sin(\phi \cdot \pi/n_h - \pi/2) - 2bc\right)}{-\left((b^2 - c^2)\cos(\phi \cdot \pi/n_h - \pi/2)\right)}\right)$$

$$r = f \tan\left(\frac{\pi}{2} - \beta\right)$$

$$x = c_x + r \cos\left(2\theta\frac{\pi}{n_w}\right) \tag{1}$$

$$y = c_y + r \sin\left(2\theta\frac{\pi}{n_w}\right)$$

where n_w and n_h are the width and height, respectively, of a projected image, a, b and c are the parameters of the hyperboloidal mirror, and (c_x, c_y) is the center of the annular image. From these equations, we can project each pixel (x, y) of an annular image into a point (θ, ϕ) of the spherical coordinates. A sample of a captured annular image is shown in Fig 3(a), and Fig 3(b) shows the image after projecting.

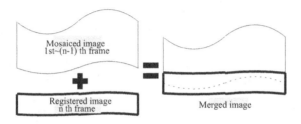

Fig. 6. Image mosaicing

2.3   Image Registration

The third step is image registration that determines the spatial transformation, which maps points from one image to corresponding points on the second image, and transforms the image from the determined map. Since our target object is a tube object, a perspective or affine transformation is not suitable. Therefore, we propose deformable registration by fitting a two dimensional polynomial function. The detail is described in section 3.

2.4   Image Mosaicing

After image registration, the remaining operation is to merge the registration results into the mosaic image. As Fig 6 shows the idea of merging a registered image from the n-th frame on the left side of the figure into a mosaic image, which is created by mosaicing from the first to the (n-1)-th images. We simply mosaic the registered images by overwriting the new registered image on the mosaic image to make a new mosaic image.

3   Deformable Image Registration by Polynomial Transformation

Most image mosaicing techniques transform images by perspective or affine transformations for registration. However, these transformations only work for images of stationary planar objects taken with a perspective camera. Since our images are annular images taken by omnidirectionally with a wide-angle camera, and the target is a tube object, these methods do not work. Therefore, we propose a novel approach for image registration that deforms images by fitting two-dimensional-polynomial functions.

3.1   Model of Optical Flow

If we separate the motion vector to the components along the θ-axis and the ϕ-axis, we can define the model of optical flows depending on θ and ϕ position of the optical flows; because the object and the motion of the camera are constrained to a smooth tube and continuous motion, respectively.

Motions Along θ-axis. Because the input image is an annular image sequence taken from an omnidirectional or wide-angle camera, the motion vectors have periodicity

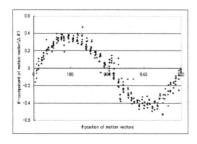 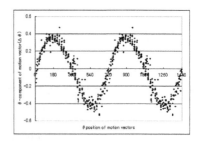

Fig. 7. Detected optical flow (black lines)   **Fig. 8.** Projection model of a hyper-omnidirectional camera

along the θ-axis after projecting into a spherical coordinate. Because our target object is a smooth tube, the θ-component of the motion vectors has 2 extrema as shown in Fig 7, which shows the θ-component of motion vectors that are detected from an input annular image sequence

When fitting this data into a polynomial function, since the data has periodicity along θ-axis and is extracted from an annular image sequence, we use 2 cycles of the data, as shown in Fig 8, to approximate the periodicity by a polynomial function. Thus, the number of extrema is 4. If we use a polynomial function for fitting, the degree must be at least 5.

If the object is a real cylinder and the camera moves minutely at the center of the object along the θ-axis, the θ-component of the motion vectors becomes a sine function $\Delta\theta = \sin(\theta)$, where $\Delta\theta$ is the θ-component of a motion vector and θ is the position of the optical flow. Even in other cases, for example, when the camera is not at the center of the tube or where the tube is not a perfect cylinder, the function between θ and $\Delta\theta$ is similar to a sine function. Therefore, when we fit a polynomial function to the data, the degree of the function is sufficient if we can fit the polynomial function to a sine function. We empirically find that a 10-degree polynomial function is sufficient for fitting the objects that we operate on in this paper with the function.

Motion Along ϕ-axis. The ϕ-component of the motion vectors, depend on the motion along the ϕ-axis. Fig 9 shows the situation where the camera moves along the ϕ-axis.

If the distance between the camera origin O and the wall of tube is r and the camera moves rC along the ϕ-axis, where C is an arbitrary constant, the positions of a feature point satisfies

$$C = \tan(\phi) - \tan(\phi') \tag{2}$$

where ϕ and ϕ' are the ϕ-positions of a feature point before and after the motion, respectively. After algebraic manipulation, Eq. 2 becomes

$$\tan(\Delta\phi) = \frac{2C(\cos(2\phi) - 1)}{C\sin(2\phi) - 2} \tag{3}$$

where $\Delta\phi = \phi' - \phi$. Fig 10 shows the function of Eq.3 where $-\pi/2 \le \phi \le \pi/2$ and $C = \pi/180$. Since it has only an extremum, we can estimate this function by fitting a second degree polynomial function.

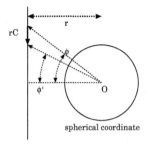

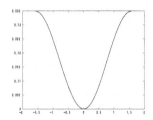

Fig. 9. Detected optical flow (black lines)   **Fig. 10.** Projection model of a hyper-omnidirectional camera

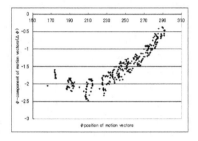

Fig. 11. Relation between ϕ position(ϕ) and ϕ-component($\Delta\phi$) of motion vectors

Fig 11 shows the ϕ-components of optical flows that are detected from an annular image sequence captured by an omnidirectional camera. As described above, the function has an extremum. Thus, it can be approximated by a second degree polynomial function. When we use a wide-angle camera, it cannot observe the lateral and backward directions, in which ϕ is around or less than zero. Since the distribution of the ϕ-components of optical flows are almost linear in such cases, we use a first degree polynomial function for fitting.

3.2 Polynomial Transformation

From the model of optical flows described above, we approximate the distribution of optical flows by a polynomial functions. By putting them together, we model the distribution of optical flows by two-dimensional-polynomial functions as follows:

$$\theta_{new} = \sum_{i=0}^{n}\sum_{j=0}^{m} C_{i,j}^{[\theta]}\theta^i\phi^j \tag{4}$$

$$\phi_{new} = \sum_{i=0}^{n}\sum_{j=0}^{m} C_{i,j}^{[\phi]}\theta^i\phi^j \tag{5}$$

where θ and ϕ are the position of a feature point before the motion, θ_{new} and ϕ_{new} are those after the motion, and $C_{ij}^{[\theta]}$ and $C_{ij}^{[\phi]}$ are the coefficients of the polynomial function.

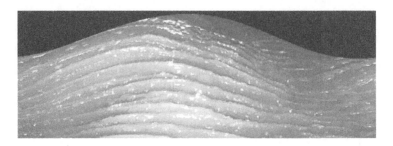

Fig. 12. Generated dissection image of an intestine model

By substituting the position of a feature point for θ, ϕ, θ_{new} and ϕ_{new}, we obtain two linear equations of $C_{ij}^{[\theta]}$ and $C_{ij}^{[\phi]}$. If the degree of θ and ϕ in Eq. (3) is N and M, the number of coefficients is $2NM$. Thus, if we have more than NM feature points, we can determine the coefficients. Since the system becomes linear equations that consist of $2NM$ variables, we estimate the coefficients by a least square method.

If we fit the data to polynomial functions with $2NM$ variables; that is, we model the shape of the object and the camera motion by the polynomial functions with $2NM$ variables. Though the degree of freedom of the shape is quite reduced, we can efficiently model a tube object to create the dissection image.

4   Experiments

To test our method, we set up an experiment using an endoscope and a model of an intestine. The endoscope has a wide-angle camera, with an image angle of approximately 140 degrees (diagonal). Fig 3 shows the input image and the projection into spherical coordinates. Fig 12 shows the mosaicing result from 150 images. Though the object is not a perfect cylinder and the motion is not straight and not at a constant speed, our method successfully generated a mosaicing image.

Next, to evaluate the error of our proposed method, we used the annular image sequence of a checker-pipe (shown in Fig 13) acquired by the hyper-omnidirectional camera. The camera moved along a meandering path. The size of the input image was 640 × 480 pixels and the size of the panoramic image of spherical coordinates was 720 × 360 pixels. We computed our deformable registration on a PC with a Pentium4 3.2GHz processor. The computational time for the two images was 680 msec for fitting 750 data and 0.11 msec to transform one pixel. We compared our method with a simple method that transform images only by translation along the θ and ϕ axes. Table 1 shows the roots of mean square (RMS) errors for both methods, which are computed from the differences of the positions of feature points after registration. We used a 5-degree polynomial for θ, and a 2-degree polynomial for ϕ, that is the minimum requirement as shown in 3.1. Our method successfully reduced the errors.

Fig 14 shows one part of the mosaicing results after registration. Fig 14(a) is registered by translation, and Fig 14(b) is the same part registered by our deformable registration. These results were generated from 250 images. Though the shape of the target

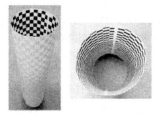

Fig. 13. Used target object

Table 1. Comparison of root of the mean square of the size of the optical flow after transformation

registration	RMS
translation	1.265132995
our approach	0.612701392

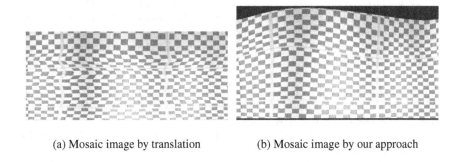

(a) Mosaic image by translation   (b) Mosaic image by our approach

Fig. 14. Comparison of the Results

object is a simple cylinder, the mosaicing result was distorted because of the meandering camera motion. On the other hand, the distortion in the results of the deformable registration was reduced from that done by only translation.

5   Conclusion

This paper described a novel method to generate a dissection image of the inside of an intestine. While examinations inside a tube object are difficult and time consuming due to the limited field of view, our method provides an easy-to-understand view for inspecting an intestine. Since a perspective or affine transformation is not suitable for registration of annular images, we proposed a deformable registration by fitting a two dimensional polynomial function. The proposed method successfully creates a dissection image of a generalized cylinder with arbitrary camera motion. Even if the object moves and deforms during observation, it is possible for our method to mosaic images.

As future work, since residual error exists after polynomial fitting, we will apply other deformable registration techniques that have more degrees of freedom, for example, a FEM-based method [1,2] to the imaging problem.

References

1. L. Cohen and I. Cohen. Finite-element methods for active contour models and balloons for 2-d and 3-d images. *PAMI*, 15(11):1131–1147, November 1993.
2. T. F. Cootes, G. J. Edwards, and C. J. Taylor. Active appearance models. *Lecture Notes in Computer Science*, 1407:484–498, 1998.
3. R. D, S. LI, H. C, H. DL, L. MO, and H. DJ. Nonrigid registration using free-form deformations: application to breast mr images. *IEEE Transactions on Medical Imaging*, 18(8):712–721, 1999.
4. K. Daniilidis and C. Geyer. Omnidirectional vision: Theory and algorithms. In *ICPR*, pages 1089–1096, 2000.
5. M. Fischler and R. Bolles. Random sampling consensus: a paradigm for model fitting with application to image analysis and automated cartography. *Commun. Assoc. Comp. Mach.*, 24(6):381–395, 1981.
6. J. Gee and D. Haynor. Numerical methods for high dimensional warps, 1998.
7. R. Hartley. In defense of the eight-point algorithm. *IEEE Transactions on Pattern Analysis and Machine Intelligence*, 19(6):580–593, 1997.
8. B. Lucas and T. Kanade. An iterative image registration technique with an application to stereo vision. In *Proc. International Joint Conference on Artificial Intelligence*, pages 674–679, 1981.
9. S. Peleg and J. Herman. Panoramic mosaics by manifold projection, 1997.
10. M. Pollefeys. *Self-calibration and metric 3D reconstruction from uncalibrated image sequences*. PhD thesis, ESAT-PSI, K.U.Leuven, 1999.
11. J. Shi and C. Tomasi. Good features to track. In *Proc. IEEE Conference on Computer Vision and Pattern Recognition*, pages 593–600, 1994.
12. R. Swaminathan and S. K. Nayar. Nonmetric calibration of wide-angle lenses and polycameras. *IEEE Transactions on Pattern Analysis and Machine Intelligence*, 22(10):1172–1178, 2000.
13. R. Szeliski. Image mosaicing for tele-reality applications. In *WACV94*, pages 44–53, 1994.
14. S. Tang and T. Jiang. Nonrigid registration of medical image by linear singular blending techniques. *Pattern Recogn. Lett.*, 25(4):399–405, 2004.
15. Z. Zhang. Determining the epipolar geometry and its uncertainty: A review. *International Journal of Computer Vision*, 27(2):161 – 195, 1998.

Distance-Intensity for Image Registration

Rui Gan and Albert C. S. Chung

Lo Kwee-Seong Medical Image Analysis Laboratory,
Department of Computer Science,
The Hong Kong University of Science and Technology, Hong Kong
{raygan, achung}@cs.ust.hk

Abstract. In this paper, a novel one-element voxel attribute, namely *distance-intensity* (DI), is defined for associating spatial information with image intensity for registration tasks. For each voxel in an image, the DI feature encodes spatial information at a global level, and is about the distance of the voxel to its closest object boundary, together with the original intensity information. Without the help of image segmentations, the computation of the DI map is carried out by applying a Poisson process on a vector field that combines both gradient and *distance-gradient*. Mutual information (MI) is adopted as a similarity measure on the DI feature space. A multi-resolution registration method is then used for aligning multi-modal images. Experimental results show that, as compared with the conventional MI-based method, the proposed method has longer capture ranges at different image resolutions. This leads to more robust registrations. Randomized registration experiments on clinical 3D CT, MR-T1 and MR-T2 datasets demonstrate that the new method gives higher success rates than the traditional MI-based method.

1 Introduction

General promising results have shown that mutual information (MI) as a voxel intensity-based similarity measure is well-suited for multi-modal image registration [1,2]. However, it has been suggested that the conventional MI-based registration can result in misalignment for some cases [3,4] and then room for improvement exists. The standard MI measure only takes intensity information into account. Therefore, a known disadvantage is the lack of concern on any spatial information (neither local nor global) which may be present in individual images to be registered [5,6]. As a simple illustration, a random perturbation of image points identically on both images results in unchanged MI value as that of the original images.

Several researchers have proposed adaptations of the standard MI-based registration framework to incorporate spatial information. Pluim et al. [4] multiplies the conventional MI measure with an external local gradient term to ensure the alignment of locations of tissue transitions. The probing results indicated that the registration function of the combined measure is smoother than that of the standard MI measure. But this approach does not directly extend the MI based similarity measure. Butz et al. [7] applies MI to edge measure (e.g., gradient

Y. Liu, T. Jiang, and C. Zhang (Eds.): CVBIA 2005, LNCS 3765, pp. 281–290, 2005.

magnitude) space to align object surfaces. However, MI based on edge measure is sensitive to the sparseness of joint edge feature histograms. This may increase the difficulty of the optimization procedure. Moreover, Rueckert et al. [6] exploits higher-order MI for 4D joint histograms which are built on the co-occurrence of intensity pairs of adjacent points. This method was shown to be robust to local intensity variation. However, only one neighbor is considered at a time in this approach and plenty of spatial information which may be present globally or within large neighborhood system has been ignored.

In this paper, a novel one-element voxel attribute, namely *distance-intensity* (DI), is defined to incorporate spatial information with intensity for registration tasks. The DI feature encodes globally defined spatial information for each voxel. This is about the distance of the voxel to its closest object boundary, together with original intensity information. Without the help of image segmentations, the computation of DI map is carried out by applying a Poisson process on a vector field that combines both gradient and *distance-gradient*. Then, mutual information is exploited as a similarity measure on the DI feature space. To increase computational efficiency and robustness of the proposed method, the registration procedure is a multi-resolution iterative process.

Based on the results on clinical 3D CT, MR-T1 and MR-T2 image volumes, it is experimentally shown that the proposed method has relatively longer capture ranges[1] than the traditional MI-based method at different image resolutions. This can obviously make the multi-resolution image registration more robust. Moreover, the results of around 400 randomized registration experiments reveal that our method gives higher success registration rates than the conventional MI-based method.

2   Distance-Intensity Attribute

2.1   Definition

In our proposed registration approach, a novel one-element attribute, namely *distance-intensity* (DI), is assigned to each voxel in an image. Within individual images, the DI feature is designed for consolidating spatial information at a global level with intensity. In other words, the DI feature depends not only on image intensity, but also on the distance of a voxel to its closest object boundary.

Given an image $I(\mathbf{v})$ over domain Ω, where $\mathbf{v} = (x, y, z)$ denotes voxel position, we define a distance-intensity (DI) map, $DI(\mathbf{v})$, of the image as

$$DI(\mathbf{v}) = I(\mathbf{v}) + \Big(I(\mathbf{v}) - I\big(\mathbf{v} + \mathbf{d}(\mathbf{v})\big) \Big) \log_D |\mathbf{d}(\mathbf{v})|, \qquad (1)$$

where $\mathbf{d}(\mathbf{v})$ is the vector from $\mathbf{v}$ to the closest boundary voxel of other objects[2] and $D = \max_{\mathbf{v}} |\mathbf{d}(\mathbf{v})|$. Here the function $\log_D(\cdot)$ limits the influence of $\mathbf{d}(\mathbf{v})$.

---

[1] Capture range represents the range of alignments from which a registration algorithm can converge to the correct maximum.

[2] This implies that two voxels $\mathbf{v}$ and $\mathbf{v} + \mathbf{d}(\mathbf{v})$ belong to different objects.

Following this definition, when a voxel is at or near object boundary, the DI value approximates its original intensity value. Thus, structure transitions remain unchanged. On the other hand, when voxel position moves from boundaries towards interiors of homogenous regions (either background regions or anatomical structures), the DI value smoothly and gradually varies. With this property, the DI map of homogenous regions can provide global and detailed spatial information about the distance of a voxel to its closest object boundary, as well as intensity information. A graphical illustration for these properties will be presented in Section 2.3.

2.2   Computation

It is noted that there is no available object segmentation (or boundary) in our registration process, i.e., $\mathbf{d}(\mathbf{v})$ is not derivable. However, we found that the gradient of DI map can be robustly estimated. Consequently, an accurate and smooth solution of the DI map can be computed by applying a Poisson process on a vector field. The estimated solution approximates the gradient of DI map.

The gradient of DI map, $\nabla DI(\mathbf{v})$, is given as follows,

$$\nabla DI(\mathbf{v}) = \nabla I(\mathbf{v}) + \left(I(\mathbf{v}) - I(\mathbf{v} + \mathbf{d}(\mathbf{v}))\right) \frac{\nabla|\mathbf{d}(\mathbf{v})|}{|\mathbf{d}(\mathbf{v})|\log D}$$
$$+ \left(\nabla I(\mathbf{v}) - \nabla I(\mathbf{v} + \mathbf{d}(\mathbf{v})) \cdot \frac{\partial(\mathbf{v} + \mathbf{d}(\mathbf{v}))}{\partial \mathbf{v}}\right) \log_D |\mathbf{d}(\mathbf{v})|, \qquad (2)$$

where $\frac{\partial(\mathbf{v}+\mathbf{d}(\mathbf{v}))}{\partial \mathbf{v}}$ is the Jacobian matrix. Note that as compared with the first two terms in Eq. 2, the third term provides little influence: If $\mathbf{v}$ is inside homogenous regions, $\nabla I(\mathbf{v})$ and $\nabla I(\mathbf{v} + \mathbf{d}(\mathbf{v}))$ tend to zero; otherwise, when $\mathbf{v}$ is at or close to boundary, $\log_D |\mathbf{d}(\mathbf{v})|$ is tiny and inclines to zero. Therefore, we have

$$\nabla DI(\mathbf{v}) \approx \nabla I(\mathbf{v}) + \left(I(\mathbf{v}) - I(\mathbf{v} + \mathbf{d}(\mathbf{v}))\right) \frac{\nabla|\mathbf{d}(\mathbf{v})|}{|\mathbf{d}(\mathbf{v})|\log D}. \qquad (3)$$

This represents a weighted combination of gradient and *distance-gradient*.

Distance-Gradient: The distance-gradient operator (∇_d) on two different voxels ($\mathbf{v}_1$ and $\mathbf{v}_2$) is defined as

$$\nabla_d I(\mathbf{v}_1, \mathbf{v}_2) = \left(I(\mathbf{v}_1) - I(\mathbf{v}_2)\right) \frac{\mathbf{v}_1 - \mathbf{v}_2}{|\mathbf{v}_1 - \mathbf{v}_2|^2}. \qquad (4)$$

With this definition, the second term in Eq. 3 becomes $\frac{1}{\log D} \nabla_d I(\mathbf{v}, \mathbf{v} + \mathbf{d}(\mathbf{v}))$ by the fact that $\nabla|\mathbf{d}(\mathbf{v})| = \frac{\mathbf{d}(\mathbf{v})}{|\mathbf{d}(\mathbf{v})|}$ almost everywhere. Moveover, we make the following hypothesis, which is often satisfied in practice,

$$|\nabla_d I(\mathbf{v}, \mathbf{v} + \mathbf{d}(\mathbf{v}))| = \max_{\mathbf{v}' \in \Omega} |\nabla_d I(\mathbf{v}, \mathbf{v}')|. \qquad (5)$$

Consequently, Eq. 3 becomes

$$\nabla DI(\mathbf{v}) \approx \mathbf{F}(\mathbf{v}) = \nabla I(\mathbf{v}) + \frac{1}{\log D} \nabla_d I(\mathbf{v}, \hat{\mathbf{v}}),$$

$$\text{with} \quad \hat{\mathbf{v}} = \arg \max_{\mathbf{v}' \in \Omega} |\nabla_d I(\mathbf{v}, \mathbf{v}')|. \tag{6}$$

Poisson Process: Following Eq. 6, the vector field $\mathbf{F}(\mathbf{v})$ approximates $\nabla DI(\mathbf{v})$. In order to compute the DI map, one may use a direct integral approach on $\mathbf{F}(\mathbf{v})$. However, we have observed that it is unstable for real applications due to the insufficient capability of handling noise. The noise is cumulated and may result in a quite noticeable error. Therefore, we propose to minimize the following energy functional to derive an optimal solution of DI map, $\widehat{DI}(\mathbf{v})$,

$$\iiint_{\mathbf{v} \in \Omega} |\nabla \widehat{DI}(\mathbf{v}(x,y,z)) - \mathbf{F}(\mathbf{v}(x,y,z))|^2 dx dy dz. \tag{7}$$

$\widehat{DI}(\mathbf{v})$ can be obtained by solving a Poisson equation [8], $\nabla^2 \widehat{DI} = \nabla \cdot \mathbf{F}$, where $\nabla^2 = (\frac{\partial^2}{\partial x^2} + \frac{\partial^2}{\partial y^2} + \frac{\partial^2}{\partial z^2})$ and $\nabla \cdot$ are Laplacian and divergence operators respectively. Obtaining the unique solution of Poisson equation is a well studied problem. In our work, Neumann boundary conditions are exploited. Then, the gradient descent flow minimizing the total energy is given by

$$\widehat{DI}_t(\mathbf{v}(x,y,z)) = \nabla^2 \widehat{DI}(\mathbf{v}(x,y,z)) - \nabla \cdot \mathbf{F}(\mathbf{v}(x,y,z)). \tag{8}$$

2.3   Graphical Illustration

As a detailed description, we computed the DI map of a clinical CT image volume obtained from the Retrospective Image Registration Evaluation (RIRE) project[3]. A slice from the volume is shown in Fig. 1a, while Fig. 1c presents the corresponding slice from the DI map. (Note that values from individual images are re-scaled to $[0, 1]$ for a fair comparison.) It is observed that, for those voxels at or near object boundaries, their DI values approximate the original intensity values. This implies that structure transitions remain unchanged. Meanwhile, when voxel position moves from boundaries towards interiors of homogenous regions (either background regions or anatomical structures), the DI value smoothly and gradually varies. However, due to the limitation of image quality, such smooth changes may not be clearly displayed in Fig. 1c.

Furthermore, Figs. 1b and 1d respectively present the value profiles of the same line (marked as red dashed lines) in Figs. 1a and 1c. As suggested by Fig. 1d, the value variation from boundaries towards homogenous regions is smooth and gradual. It is worth noting that, although there is little intensity change at

---

[3] The images and the standard transformation(s) were provided as part of the project, Retrospective Image Registration Evaluation, National Institutes of Health, Project Number 8R01EB002124-03, Principal Investigator, J. Michael Fitzpatrick, Vanderbilt University, Nashville, TN.

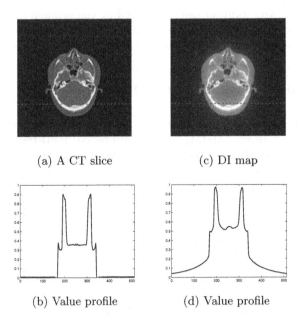

(a) A CT slice   (c) DI map

(b) Value profile   (d) Value profile

Fig. 1. (a) and (c) are slices respectively selected from a clinical CT image volume and its corresponding DI map. (b) and (d) are value profiles of lines in (a) and (c), which are marked as red dashed lines.

the middle of the line in Fig. 1b, a small and smooth saddle can be found in Fig. 1d located at the corresponding position. The raised white boundary slightly below the line cause this saddle. It is because, as discussed above, the DI feature encodes spatial information at a global level.

3   Mutual Information (MI) Based Image Registration

As we have discussed above, the DI feature encodes spatial information at a global level together with original intensity information. We adopt it as voxel attribute for registration tasks. Mutual information (MI) [9] is then exploited as a similarity measure to measure the degree of dependence of the DI feature space. Given a geometric transformation, the 2D joint DI distribution can be approximated by either Parzen windowing or histogramming [10]. Histogramming is employed in this paper because the approach is computationally efficient. The trilinear partial volume distribution interpolation [1] is exploited to update the joint histogram for non-grid alignment.

To accelerate the registration process and ensure the robustness of the proposed method, we exploit a multi-resolution approach based on the Gaussian Pyramid representation [2]. Rough estimates can be found using downsampled images and treated as starting values for optimization at higher resolutions. Then the fine-tuning of the solution can be derived at the original image resolution. In this paper, the MI value at each resolution is maximized via the Powell's direction set method in multidimensions [11].

4   Experimental Results and Discussions

To evaluate the MI similarity measure on the novel distance-intensity attribute (hereafter referred to as **MI-DI**) and the proposed multi-resolution registration method, we have performed experiments on different image modalities: CT, rectified MR-T1 (T1-rec), and rectified MR-T2 (T2-rec). The traditional MI similarity measure on intensity (hereafter referred to as **MI-I**) [1,2] has also been applied for comparison.

4.1   Comparisons on Capture Range

CT – T1 (3D – 3D) Registration. Three pairs of clinical CT (around $512 \times 512 \times 30$ voxels and $0.65 \times 0.65 \times 4$ mm^3) and T1-rec ($256 \times 256 \times 26$ voxels and around $1.26 \times 1.26 \times 4.1$ mm^3) image volumes – datasets #1, #2 and #3 – were obtained from RIRE. Note that all image pairs used in our experiments (CT, T1-rec and T2-rec) were first registered by the conventional multi-resolution MI based registration method and were then examined by an experienced consultant radiologist to ensure that the final alignments are correct and acceptable. This procedure was employed for a better presentation of the probing results and also for further facilitating the experiments that will be described in Section 4.2.

Figs. 2a and 2d respectively plot the translational probes for registering the low resolution (Level 3) testing image pairs from three datasets for MI-I and MI-DI. At the original image resolution (Level 0), Figs. 2b and 2e plot the translational probes and Figs. 2c and 2f plot the rotational probes based on MI-I and MI-DI respectively. As observed in Figs. 2a and 2b, for the translational probes of MI-I at different image resolutions, it would occur obvious local maxima when the misalignment of two images is relatively large. On the contrary, Figs. 2d and 2e suggest that the shape of the probing curves based on MI-DI is improved and the capture ranges of MI-DI can be relative longer than those of MI-I. This is because, with the proposed distance-intensity attribute, regions with homogenous intensities (including anatomical structures and background regions) can provide varying information related to the distance of a voxel to its closest object boundary. Therefore, when the misalignment increases, the MI-DI values would keep decreasing. With this finding, it would be expected that the optimization procedure for registration will be benefited and the registration robustness can be increased. On the other hand, for the rotational probes, the capture ranges of MI-I and MI-DI are comparable (see Figs. 2c and 2f).

T1 – T2 (3D – 3D) Registration. Three pairs of clinical T1-rec and T2-rec image volumes – datasets #4, #5 and #6 – obtained from RIRE were used for

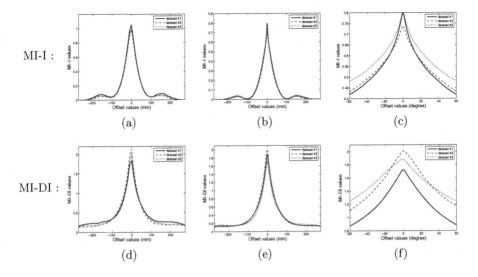

MI-I :

(a)   (b)   (c)

MI-DI :

(d)   (e)   (f)

Fig. 2. Probing curves for 3D – 3D registration on three CT and T1-rec datasets (#1, #2 and #3). Translational probes for registering the low resolution (Level 3) image pairs: (a) MI-I and (d) MI-DI. Translational probes for registering the original resolution (Level 0) image pairs: (b) MI-I and (e) MI-DI. Rotational probes for registering the original resolution image pairs: (c) MI-I and (f) MI-DI.

the experiments. The results of translational probes are shown in Figs. 3a (MI-I) and 3d (MI-DI) for the low resolution (Level 3) registration and in Figs. 3b (MI-I) and 3e (MI-DI) for the original resolution (Level 0) registration. Figs. 3c and 3f respectively plot the rotational probes based on MI-I and MI-DI for the original resolution (Level 0). Similar results of the capture ranges are obtained as compared with CT – T1 registrations.

4.2   Performance Comparisons on Registration Robustness

A series of randomized experiments have been designed to study the registration robustness of the proposed MI-DI based method and the conventional MI-I based method. The testing image pairs were datasets #1 (CT – T1) and #6 (T1 – T2). The experiments took 100 tests on each testing image pair for either method. At each trial, the pre-obtained ground truth registration (see Section 4.1) was perturbed by 6 uniformly distributed random offsets for all translational and rotational axes. The perturbed registration was then treated as the starting alignment. The random offsets for X and Y axes were drawn between [-150, 150]mm, while those for Z axis and each rotational axis were respectively drawn between [-70, 70]mm and [-20, 20] degrees. (Note that for either testing dataset the same set of randomized starting alignments was used for both methods for a fair comparison.)

MI-I :

MI-DI :

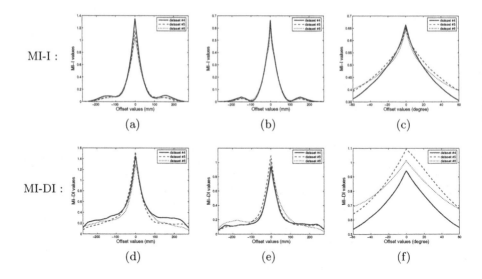

(a)   (b)   (c)

(d)   (e)   (f)

Fig. 3. Probing curves for 3D – 3D registration on 3 T1-rec and T2-rec datasets (#4, #5 and #6). Translational probes for registering the low resolution (Level 3) image pairs: (a) MI-I and (d) MI-DI. Translational probes for registering the original resolution (Level 0) image pairs: (b) MI-I and (e) MI-DI. Rotational probes for registering the original resolution image pairs: (c) MI-I and (f) MI-DI.

To evaluate each derived registration with respect to the ground truth registration, the translational error (which was the root-sum-square of the differences for three translational axes) and the rotational error (which was the real part of a quaternion) were computed. In our experiments, the threshold vector for assessing registration success was set to $(2mm, 2°)$, because registration errors below $2mm$ and $2°$ are generally acceptable by experienced clinicians [12,13].

The success rates of the MI-I based method and the MI-DI based method for datasets #1 and #6 are listed in Table 1. It is suggested that the MI-DI based method (Column **MI-DI**) has higher success rates as compared with the MI-I based method (Column **MI-I**) for both datasets. Based on these experiments, we also observed that the majority of failed cases for the MI-DI based method had about $180°$ misalignment for one rotational axis, while registration errors for other axes were quite small. (It is meant that, after registration, the brain in

Table 1. The success rates with the MI-I based method and the MI-DI based method for datasets #1(CT – T1) and #6 (T1 – T2)

Testing	Success rate	
dataset	MI-I	MI-DI
#1 (CT – T1)	66%	80%
#6 (T1 – T2)	68%	85%

the floating image was inverted along a rotational axis.) Oppositely, for the MI-I based method, most of the failed cases had large translational and rotational misalignments simultaneously. This observation somehow implies that, along the translational axes, the capture ranges of MI-DI are longer than those of MI-I.

5 Conclusion

To conclude, this paper has designed a new one-element voxel attribute, namely distance-intensity (DI), for registration tasks. In an image at a global level, for each voxel, the DI feature encodes spatial information about the distance of the voxel to its closest object boundary, as well as the original intensity information.

The DI map of an image can be computed without image segmentations. To compute the DI map, we have demonstrated how to apply a Poisson process on a vector field combining both gradient and distance-gradient. Then, mutual information (MI) has been adopted as a similarity measure on the DI attribute space and a multi-resolution registration method has been proposed for aligning multi-modal images.

The experimental results on clinical 3D CT, MR-T1 and MR-T2 datasets have indicated that the proposed method has relatively longer capture ranges than the conventional MI-based method at different image resolutions. Moreover, a series of randomized experiments on precisely registered clinical image pairs have demonstrated that the success rates of our method are higher than those of the conventional MI-based method.

Acknowledgements

The authors would like to acknowledge the support from the Hong Kong Research Grants Council (HK RGC) under grant (HKUST6155/03E).

References

1. Maes, F., Collignon, A., et al.: Multimodality Image Registration by Maximization of Mutual Information. IEEE Trans. Med. Img. **16** (1997) 187–198
2. Wells, W., Viola, P., et al.: Multi-Modal Volume Registration by Maximization of Mutual Information. Medical Image Analysis **1** (1996) 35–51
3. Penney, G., Weese, J., et al.: A Comparison of Similarity Measures for Use in 2D-3D Medical Image Registration. IEEE Trans. Med. Img. **17** (1998) 586–595
4. Pluim, J., et al.: Image Registration by Maximization of Combined Mutual Information and Gradient Information. IEEE Trans. Med. Img. **19** (2000) 809–814
5. Pluim, J., Maintz, J., Viergever, M.: Mutual-Information-Based Registration of Medical Images: A Survey. IEEE Trans. Med. Img. **22** (2003) 986–1004
6. Rueckert, D., Clarkson, M., et al.: Non-rigid registration using higher-order mutual information. In: Proc. SPIE, Medical Imaging: Image Processing. Volume 3979. (2000) 438–447
7. Butz, T., Thiran, J.P.: Affine registration with feature space mutual information. In: MICCAI. (2001) 549–556

8. Zwillinger, D.: Handbook of Differential Equations, 3rd ed. Boston, MA: Academic Press (1997)
9. Cover, T., et al.: Elements of Information Theory. John Wiley & Sons, Inc. (1991)
10. Bishop, C.: Neural Networks for Pattern Recognition. Oxford U. Press (1995)
11. Press, W., Teukolsky, S., et al.: Numerical Recipes in C, 2nd Edition. Cambridge University Press (1992)
12. Hajnal, J.V., et al.: Medical Image Registration. CRC Press LLC (2001)
13. Zhu, Y., Cochoff, S.: Likelihood Maximization Approach to Image Registration. IEEE Trans. Image Processing **11** (2002) 1417–1426

Efficient Population Registration of 3D Data

Lilla Zöllei[1], Erik Learned-Miller[2], Eric Grimson[1], and William Wells[1,3]

[1] Computer Science and Artificial Intelligence Lab, MIT
[2] Dept. of Computer Science, University of Massachusetts, Amherst
[3] Radiology Department, Brigham and Women's Hospital

Abstract. We present a population registration framework that acts on large collections or *populations* of data volumes. The data alignment procedure runs in a simultaneous fashion, with every member of the population approaching the *central tendency* of the collection at the same time. Such a mechanism eliminates the need for selecting a particular reference frame *a priori*, resulting in a non-biased estimate of a digital atlas. Our algorithm adopts an affine *congealing* framework with an information theoretic objective function and is optimized via a gradient-based stochastic approximation process embedded in a multi-resolution setting. We present experimental results on both synthetic and real images.

1 Introduction and Motivation

The registration of two data sets is the problem of identifying a geometric transformation which maps the coordinate system of one to that of another or, more generally, establishing a homology among the input images when the number of input images to be aligned is more than two. In this scenario, it is not one, but a group of transformations that needs to be identified in order to put all the inputs into correspondence. We are particularly motivated by the *population* registration problem, which includes the registration of collections of images or volumes, where the number of inputs is greater than twenty or potentially much greater.

Depending on the nature of the images to be processed, we distinguish between mono- and multi-modal registration tasks. In the former, the inputs are acquired by the same, and in the latter case by different, types of imaging devices. A registration problem that lies between these two categories is the so-called template-to-subject registration which involves the alignment of an image or a set of images with a template constructed independently from the current alignment. (The template, as explained below, can be one member of the input image set or a probabilistic representation of prior knowledge about the imaged object.) In computer vision, template-registration tasks are common when there is some prior information about the standard characteristics of the input and / or when one wishes to compare a current sample of a group to previously processed ones. The results can then be further studied to carry out statistical inference on shape, population characteristics or on abnormal variability. They could also be used as a pre-processing step for segmentation studies.

Y. Liu, T. Jiang, and C. Zhang (Eds.): CVBIA 2005, LNCS 3765, pp. 291–301, 2005.

In the medical domain the same task has become increasingly important and is referred to as atlas-to-subject registration. Its prevalence can be explained by the accessibility of rapidly growing image databases and faster computers that allow for population studies and various data mining tasks. We were initially inspired by the availability of such data volumes; thus our examples are all from the medical domain. Note, however, that the algorithm formulation is very general and it is not restricted to only medical input data sets.

In this work, we demonstrate a new unbiased and computationally efficient framework for aligning populations of 3D medical images for the purpose of digital (anatomical) atlas construction. We believe that defining a robust inter-subject registration technology that enables the comparison of large numbers of images will allow us to build better structural atlases, and to further analyze inter-subject differences.

2   Background and Previous Work

Several approaches exist that propose the alignment of multiple data sets into the same coordinate frame. Besides the details of the registration algorithm applied, there is a significant difference in how each method interprets the common coordinate frame (or template). For some specific applications, the desired template is already established. The input volumes then do not need to be managed as a set, they can be aligned with the reference frame individually. This approach is advantageous when single input volumes need to be compared to the template. If, however, the input volumes are to be treated (simultaneously) as a group, other mechanisms are required.

For the rest of the applications, the digital template is not available, so that too has to be generated along with the aligning transformations. In the medical community, recently, there have been several approaches proposed [3,6,12,11,14]. One group of algorithms selects a standard coordinate frame (for example, based upon certain anatomical structures) and requires the algorithm to position all the inputs into that frame. The mean of the so-aligned images is then computed. Such methods have been performed, for instance, with the usage of the Talairach anatomical coordinate system [1,13]. A major disadvantage of these methods is that the images need to be pre-processed in order to have the matching landmarks reliably identified in them. That is a time-consuming and potentially error-prone procedure.

Other approaches select one of the current data volumes to be the common reference frame [3]. After all the other volumes are aligned to this, their *mean* is computed. The problem here is the introduction of bias into the procedure by claiming that one sample volume can represent the standard reference. Even if the procedure is re-run several times or the selection of the particular reference frame is carried out in a more careful manner, we cannot always ensure a non-biased implementation of this process. In the case of anomalies present in the input, the registration results could be significantly distorted.

Instead, there is growing interest in generating *mean models* as a *by-product* of a larger-scale registration process. That formulation eliminates the introduction of a bias into the registration framework by simultaneously evolving the data sets towards a common reference. According to one approach, the "mean" is initially defined and the images are aligned to that reference image [14]. The process is iterated until the optimal alignment is found. Another approach follows that same scheme, but it performs non-rigid alignment of 2D scans using a minimum description length criterion [12]. Because of memory limitations, these algorithms can currently handle only a limited number (< 10) of input volumes. We note that algorithms in this subgroup are closely related to a maximum likelihood framework where each voxel distribution is represented by a Gaussian with a mean equal to the voxel mean and a fixed variance. When using our framework - congealing - though, each voxel has a separate, individually optimized non-parametric distribution. Since the distribution of tissues at a particular voxel is usually highly non-Gaussian, it would seem that our framework is more appropriate.

Another approach within this same category defines the image set registration problem by the generalization of a one-to-one alignment framework [10]. The authors estimate the joint density function of all the inputs and construct a maximum likelihood-type similarity metric. For computational ease the input images are pre-segmented into a handful of anatomical classes. A drawback of this approach is that that it requires the construction of a joint density function whose size grows exponentially with the number of input images. While the amount of data available only grows linearly, the number of samples required for a good density estimation grows exponentially.

3   Our Method

We are interested in formulating the problem as an analogy to an inter-subject image set alignment task. We use a technique called *congealing* as a basis of our framework. This approach was first introduced in the machine learning and computer vision literature, offering a solution to the hand-written digit recognition problem [8,9]. There, a model of the *central tendency* of binary input images was recovered and used for classification purposes.

The objective function proposed in the congealing framework is the total voxel-wise entropy of the input image volumes. The entropies are computed at each coordinate location and then these quantities are added together. This formulation thus models distributions of each voxel *conditioned on spatial location* rather than treating each position as equivalent. This is in contrast with the popular mutual information or joint entropy methods for alignment where entropy is measured *within* an image and the voxel distribution is assumed to be *i.i.d.*([7,10,15]). The sum of voxel-wise entropies is approximately equivalent to finding the maximum likelihood latent image in the population [8], and using it as an alignment criterion results in a low total entropy joint image. This outcome represents the underlying shape of the imaged objects and its residual variation.

Warfield et al. have already applied a preliminary version of the congealing approach to the problem of fusing MRI scans of 22 pre-term infants and producing an atlas of the developing white matter [14]. In that implementation, the intra-cranial cavity (ICC) of all the input volumes was pre-segmented to allow for binary congealing, and one member of the population was also set to be stationary (resulting in a biased result). A nine parameter affine transformation was identified for all the inputs. (A model created by this method on adult brain scans is referred to as *control model* in Section 5 and is shown in Fig. 4 (b).)

Our contribution to the congealing framework lies in its adaptation to a population of grayscale-valued 3D data volumes without introducing any bias and a computationally efficient implementation via a stochastic gradient-based optimization procedure in a multi-resolution framework.

3.1 The Objective Function

As mentioned already, our congealing framework adopts the sum of voxel-wise entropies as a joint alignment criterion. The main intuition behind using such an objective function is that, when in proper alignment, intensity values at corresponding coordinate locations from all the inputs form a low entropy distribution. That statement holds even if the intensity values are not identical. Hence noise or bias fields, and what is more, corresponding multi-modal inputs can also be accommodated. An entropy-based objective function is also appropriate to handle data sets whose intensities form multi-modal distributions. That property is of great benefit when the population consists of (sufficient number of representatives of) data volumes with widely varying intensity profiles. For example, the tissue intensities at a particular voxel location in the cortex would likely include some white matter voxels, some gray matter voxels, and a small percentage of other tissue types. The distribution of brightness values in such a distribution is frequently multi-modal.

If we denote the collection of m input volumes as $\mathcal{I} := \{I_1, I_2, ..., I_m\}$, then our goal is to identify the set of m transformations, $\mathcal{T} := \{T_1, T_2, ..., T_m\}$ (one transformation associated with each volume), such that the objective function f of total voxel-wise entropies is minimized. The objective function is then:

$$f(\mathcal{I}, \mathcal{T}) = f(T_1(I_1), ..., T_m(I_m)) = \sum_{i=1}^{N} H(\mathcal{I}(\mathcal{T}(\mathbf{x_i}))),$$

where $\mathbf{x_i} \in \mathcal{R}^3$ indicates a particular coordinate location in the data coordinate system, H is the Shannon entropy and N is the total number of voxel locations in the data coordinate system. This measure actually forms an upper bound on the true entropy of the image distribution. By minimizing this upper bound, we approximate the minimum of the true entropy [8].

In the current implementation we use 12-parameter affine transformations. Our convention orders the transformation components as the rotation, scaling and shearing followed by the displacement. Accordingly, $\forall j \; T_j(\mathbf{x_i}) = (D_j +$

$Sh_j S_j(R_j(\mathbf{x_i})))$, where D_j is the displacement, R_j is the rotation, S_j is the anisotropic scaling and Sh_j is the shearing component of transformation T_j.

As both the size and number of our expected image volumes are large, memory allocation and computational speed are both of serious concern. Consequently, we apply a stochastic sampling framework and the EMMA[1]-style entropy estimator in our framework [15]. Instead of considering all the locations in the data coordinate space, we propose a random selection of them. Then an approximation of the total sum of voxel-wise entropies is computed for a particular alignment configuration. We write the modified objective function (approximating expectation with sample average) as:

$$f(\mathcal{I}, \mathcal{T}) = -\frac{1}{m}\sum_{i=1}^{M}\sum_{j=1}^{m}\log p(I_j(T_j(\mathbf{x_i}))),$$

where M now indicates the number of randomly selected sample points. Note, that the samples in this reduced set of coordinate locations are not fixed but re-generated at each iteration of the algorithm. As the experiments show, this modification enabled us to significantly reduce the overall number of voxel locations considered in our computations.

3.2 The Optimization

In the original framework of the congealing algorithm, a coordinate descent optimization was used to guide the minimization of the objective function. As this technique is not computationally efficient for our purposes, we have implemented an iterated stochastic gradient-based update mechanism (similar to that of [15]) that significantly reduces the processing time.

3.3 Transformation Normalization

We have a normalization step included at the end of each iteration, where we compose each transformation estimate by the inverse of the mean transformation matrices. This update is necessary as it ensures that the average movement of points at corresponding coordinate locations is zero, thus preventing the images from drifting out of the field of view.[2]

3.4 The Multi-resolution Framework

It is widely known in the registration literature that optimization functions can easily become trapped in local minima. Although congealing already mitigates

---

[1] The name EMMA refers to "Empirical entropy manipulation and analysis"
[2] This normalization criterion is different from the one presented in [8], where the normalization aimed to maintain a zero mean displacement estimate and a mean transformation matrix of determinant 1.

some problems of local minima [8], we also constructed a multi-resolution registration framework. This implementation starts the processing of the data sets at a down-sampled and smoothed level and then refines the results during the higher resolution iterations. Not only does this framework improve the optimization, it also boosts computation speed and memory usage efficiency. The number of hierarchy levels is mostly dependent on the quality and the original size of the input images. For the experiments presented in this work, it was sufficient to use a maximum of three levels of hierarchy.

4   Medical MRI Experiments

We ran experiments on three different populations of MRI acquisitions. The first set consisted of 22 baby brain volumes. Each brain volume was 176 by 186 by 110 voxels, with each voxel measuring 1.0 by 1.0 by 2.0 millimeters in size. The second and third data sets consisted of 28 and 127 adult brain volumes. These volumes were 256 by 256 by 124 voxels, with each voxel measuring 0.9375 by 0.9375 by 1.5 millimeters. Due to page limitations, we will demonstrate the results only on the third set of the images. We believe that this is the first report of simultaneous registration run on such a large collection of input volumes.

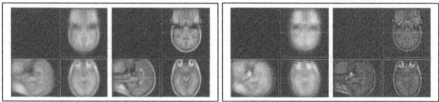

(a) Data set of 127 MRI volumes   (b) Synthetic data set of 40 MRI volumes

Fig. 1. Orthogonal slices of the mean volume of the samples before and after alignment: (a)adult brain data set of 127 MRI volumes (b) synthetic data set of 40 MRI volumes.

The experiments on the 127 medical scans were executed on three different resolution levels (where the volumes were (32 by 32 by 31), (64 by 64 by 62) and (128 by 128 by 124) voxels). The largest offset was obtained on the lowest level and then refinement was computed on the higher hierarchy levels. In our experiments we only had to select between 800 - 1500 samples, which constitutes just .05-2.5% of the total voxels, and no more than 250 iterations were necessary. The total running time for the experiment was approximately six hours.

The results of the experiments are displayed in Fig. 1 (a). This figure portrays three orthogonal slices of the mean volumes computed before and after the experiments. As a qualitative measure, we can establish that following the population alignment, the data volumes properly line up and the mean volumes have clean and sharp boundaries.

5 Validation

Validating our results and verifying our alignment is a complex task. In this section we provide both qualitative and preliminary quantitative results.

Visually we can confirm that the mean volumes computed after the congealing process have much sharper boundaries than prior to alignment (see Fig. 1 and Fig. 4 (c)). This is an indirect indicator of how good an agreement has been achieved. Looking at the central slices extracted from all the input volumes after the congealing process (see Fig. 2 (b) and 3 (b)) also suggests that the algorithm has managed to find a good quality alignment.

We also provide a quantitative analysis obtained from running our algorithm both on a synthetic image population and from comparing one of our adult brain models to an already existing one.

5.1 Synthetic Example

As a control study, we selected one particular medical MRI volume from a group of adult brain acquisitions and created a database of transformed volumes by

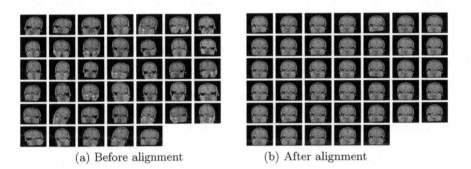

(a) Before alignment   (b) After alignment

Fig. 2. Synthetic data set of 40 MRI volumes. Central slices of the input images (a) before and (b) after the population alignment.

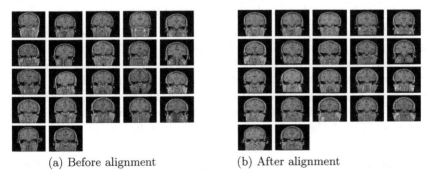

(a) Before alignment   (b) After alignment

Fig. 3. The adult brain data set of 22 MRI volumes used to make our atlas. Central slices of the input images (a) before and (b) after the population alignment.

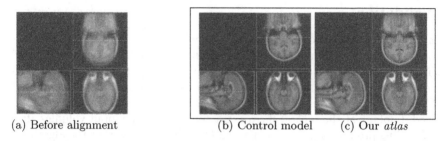

(a) Before alignment   (b) Control model   (c) Our *atlas*

Fig. 4. 3D views of the mean volume created from the adult brain data population of 22 images: (a) before population alignment (b) the control model and (c) the model estimate of our algorithm

applying affine transformations to it. The magnitude of these transformations varied between $+/-10$ degrees for rotation, $+/-10$ mm for displacement, between $[.85, 1.15]$ factors for scaling and between $+/-.1$ factors of shearing. At the onset of the algorithm, 40 volumes were randomly generated as inputs. All the input volumes were 124 by 256 by 256 voxels, with each voxel measuring .9375 by .9375 by 1.5 mm. The twelve parameters of the affine transformations were recovered after running our algorithm on two levels of the hierarchy. The number of samples used was .05% of the total number of voxels and fewer than 400 iterations were necessary to achieve convergence. The total running time was 2964 seconds. The results of these experiments can be seen in Fig. 1 (b) and 2 (b). The former illustrates the mean volumes computed before and after the congealing process, while the latter displays the central slices of each of the input volumes before and after the alignment. For the initially selected adult brain scan, we had access to the segmentation of two sub-cortical structures, the left and right thalamus (LT and RT). After the congealing alignment was executed, we applied the resulting transformations to these segmentations and then computed an overlap measure on the so-aligned binary images. The measure of our choice was $f_{\text{overlap}}(A_1, A_2) = \frac{|A_1 \cap A_2|}{min(|A_1|,|A_2|)}$ (A_i indicating binary variables), which can be easily generalized to higher number of inputs.

The overlap scores indicate great improvement, they increased from 0 to .745 and to .75 in the case of LT and RT, respectively. These numbers might seem a bit low, but as the overlap metric we use is quite conservative, we further interpret these results. For the left thalamus, .745 means that all 40 input segmentations agreed 74.5% of the time and 34 inputs are sufficient to reach an 89% score. Similarly, for the right thalamus, .75 means that all 40 inputs agreed 75% of the time, and 35 inputs are sufficient to reach a 90% score.

Several factors may influence the magnitude in a decrease of this score. First, when computing the intersection, even single misaligned voxels can significantly reduce the metric value. Second, transforming the binary structures introduces quite a high variation in the size of these relatively small anatomical structures:

the standard deviation of the structure sizes (after the transformations have been applied with nearest neighbor interpolation) was 149 voxels.[3]

We also analyzed the transformations resulting from the congealing process. Computing exact error measurements (even when knowing the ground truth offsetting transformations) is difficult as the transformations recovered by our alignment process are able to recover the inverse of the offsetting transformations only up to a common term. Therefore, we recovered both a dispersion and a bias term of the resulting errors across all the input volumes via an analysis similar to the consistency measures introduced in [4]. Our dispersion scores (indicating accuracy) were in the range $[0.05, 0.15]$ and the bias terms (indicating the magnitude of the common term) in the $[0, 2]$ voxel range.

5.2   Atlas Comparison

As an additional experiment, we also compared one of our resulting atlases to a previously generated template. More specifically, we ran our algorithm on 22 adult brain volumes (with the same parameters as indicated in Section 5.1) and compared that to a *control model* whose generation is explained in details [14]. Qualitatively, we first assess the success of the congealing algorithm (Fig.3) and then we compare the atlases in Fig.4 (b) and (c) and establish that they are highly similar. (Note the 3D view of the mean volume in the original setup is demonstrated in Fig. 4 (a)).

For a quantitative analysis, we used the same segmentation-overlap study as in the case of the synthetic experiments. In the case of LT, our overlap measure was .474027 vs .428483 of the *control model* and in the case of RT we obtained .439664 vs .496284. Our performance thus is comparable to that of the atlas.

These overlap measures are even lower than in Section 5.1. That is because in this experiment we process inter-subject scans and the normal variability in their differences can only be explained to a certain extent by affine transformations. Currently we are implementing a viscous fluid-based non-rigid warp [2] to add to our multi-resolution framework. Such a dense deformation model should be able to eliminate some of the remaining local disagreements in our alignment results.

6   Summary and Conclusions

In this paper, we introduced a new population registration framework. Without any pre-processing step, we used a congealing-type alignment method to efficiently put a large collection of data volumes into correspondence. The algorithm builds on an information theoretic objective function and currently uses fully parameterized affine transformations. We introduced an approximate stochastic sampling framework which allowed us to process only a small number of samples

---

[3] We indeed experimented with other interpolation methods, which resulted in lower standard deviations, but as the minimum component size was also increased in this manner, the end result did not change significantly from the one that we report here.

from the inputs. The optimization is implemented in a stochastic gradient-based optimization framework that enables a substantial increase in speed.

Acknowledgment

This work has been supported by NIH 5 P41 RR13218 and NIH Roadmap for Medical Research, Grant U54 EB005149 as a member of the National Alliance for Medical Image Computing (NAMIC). Information on the National Centers for Biomedical Computing can be obtained from http://nihroadmap.nih.gov/ bioinformatics.

References

1. D. Collins. 3D Model-Based Segmentation of Individual Brain Structures from Magnetic Resonance Imaging Data. PhD thesis, McGill University, Montreal, Canada, 1994.
2. E. DAgostino, F. Maes, D. Vandermeulen, and S. P. A viscous fluid model for multimodal non-rigid image registration using mutual information. Medical Image Analysis, 7:565575, 2003.
3. A. Guimond, J. Meunier, and T. J.-P. Average brain models: A convergence study. Technical Report 3731, INRIA, July 1999.
4. H. Johnson and G. E. Christensen. Consistent landmark and intensity-based image registration. IEEE Transactions on Medical Imaging, 21(5):450461, May 2002.
5. S. Joshi, B. Davis, M. Jomier, and G. Gerig. Unbiased diffeomorphic atlas construction for computational anatomy. NeuroImage, September 2004.
6. P. Lorenzen, B. Davis, and G. Gerig. Multi-class posterior atlas formation via unbiased kullback-leibler template estimation. In LNCS, volume 3216, pages 95 102, September 2004.
7. F. Maes, A. Collignon, D. Vandermeulen, G. Marchal, and P. Suetens. Multimodality image registration by maximization of mutual information. IEEE Transactions on Medical Imaging, 16(2):187198, 1997.
8. E. Miller. Learning from One Example in Machine Vision by Sharing Probability Densities. PhD thesis, Massachusetts Institute of Technology, February 2002.
9. E. Miller, N. Matsakis, and P. Viola. Learning from one example through shared densities on transforms. In IEEE Conference on Computer Vision and Pattern Recognition, volume 1, pages 464471, 2000.
10. C. Studholme and V. Cardenas. A template-free approach to volumetric spatial normalization of brain anatomy. Pattern Recognition Letters, 25(10):11911202, July 2004.
11. P. Thompson, R. Woods, M. Mega, and A. Toga. Mathematical/computational challenges in creating deformable and probabilistic atlases of the human brain. In Human Brain Mapping, volume 9 (2), pages 8192, February 2000.
12. C. Twining and C. Marsland, S. Taylor. Groupwise non-rigid registration: The minimum description length approach. In Proceedings of BMVC, 2004.
13. D. Van Essen, H. Drury, S. Joshi, and M. Miller. Functional and structural mapping of human cerebral cortex: Solutions are in the surfaces. In National Academy of Sciences, volume 95, pages 788795, 1998.

14. S. Warfield, J. Rexilius, P. Huppi, T. Inder, E. Miller, W. Wells, G. Zientara, F. Jolesz, and R. Kikinis. A binary entropy measure to assess nonrigid registration algorithms. In Fourth International Conference on Medical Image Computing and Computer-Assisted Intervention (MICCAI), Lecture Notes in Computer Science, pages 266274. Springer, October 2001.
15. W. Wells, P. Viola, H. Atsumi, S. Nakajima, and R. Kikinis. Multi-modal volume registration by maximization of mutual information. In Medical Image Analysis, volume 1, pages 3552, 1996.

Efficient Symbolic Signatures for Classifying Craniosynostosis Skull Deformities

H. Jill Lin[1], Salvador Ruiz-Correa[1,2], Raymond W. Sze[1,2],
Michael L. Cunningham[1,2], Matthew L. Speltz[1], Anne V. Hing[2],
and Linda G. Shapiro[1]

[1] University of Washington, Seattle, WA, USA
[2] Children's Hospital and Regional Medical Center, Seattle, WA, USA

Abstract. Craniosynostosis is a serious and common pediatric disease caused by the premature fusion of the sutures of the skull. Early fusion results in severe deformities in skull shape due to the restriction of bone growth perpendicular to the fused suture and compensatory growth in unfused skull plates. Calvarial (skull) abnormalities are frequently associated with severe impaired central nervous system functions due to brain abnormalities, increased intra-cranial pressure and abnormal build-up of cerebrospinal fluid. In this work, we develop a novel approach to efficiently classify skull deformities caused by metopic and sagittal synostoses using our newly introduced symbolic shape descriptors. We demonstrate the efficacy of our methodology in a series of large-scale classification experiments that compare the performance of our symbolic-signature-based approach to those of traditional numeric descriptors that are frequently used in clinical research. We also demonstrate an application of our symbolic descriptors in shape-based retrieval of skull morphologies.

1   Introduction

Craniosynostosis, the premature fusion of the fibrous skull joints or sutures, is a common condition of childhood, affecting 1 in 2500 individuals. As an infant's brain grows, open sutures allow the skull to develop normally. The early closure of one or more sutures results in abnormal head shapes due to the restriction of osseous growth perpendicular to the closed sutures and compensative growth of unaffected calvarial plates. Sagittal synostosis is the most common form of isolated suture synostosis with an incidence of approximately 1 in 5000 [8]. Early closure of the sagittal suture results in scaphocephaly, denoting a long narrow skull often associated with prominent ridges along the prematurely ossified sagittal suture (Fig. 1b). Metopic synostosis is less common than sagittal synostosis, affecting 1 in 15,000 individuals [8]. The premature fusion of the metopic suture produces trigonocephaly, denoting a triangular shaped head (Fig. 1c).

The diagnosis of craniosynostosis is typically made on the basis of clinical judgments, with CT imaging to confirm the clinician's impression. Although quantitative measures of head shape are not often used for clinical diagnosis,

Y. Liu, T. Jiang, and C. Zhang (Eds.): CVBIA 2005, LNCS 3765, pp. 302–313, 2005.

research has been conducted to compare the timing [12] and outcomes of serious surgical procedures that involve the complete reconstruction of the skull (Fig. 1b and c), sometimes in combination with cranial molding techniques [4] [5] [12].

Recent advances in multi-detector computed tomography (CT) technology enable unprecedented accuracy in the detection of fused skull sutures. However, image interpretation remains largely confined to subjective description. Most imaging studies in patients with craniosynostosis emphasize qualitative shape features and relegate quantitative assessments to the measurement of a ratio or an angle between anthropometric landmarks, therefore disregarding the broad range of shape variations that are of fundamental interest in understanding the pathogenesis and clinical course of affected patients.

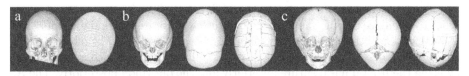

Fig. 1. Frontal and top views of a) a normal skull, b) a patient affected with sagittal synotosis, and c) a patient affected with metopic synostosis. Post-surgical reconstructions are also shown.

Attempts to classify craniosynostosis malformations by combining morphometric techniques [2][9] and likelihood-based or dissimilarity-based classification methods have been published in [9], with high cross-validation error rates (32-40% average for sagittal synostosis and 18-27% average for metopic synostosis), likely due to the limited sampling of skull anatomy. More recently, alternative numeric shape descriptors have been proposed to predict sagittal synostosis with high true positive (TP) and true negative (TN) classification rates [15] [16] [17].

In this paper, we develop a novel methodology to accurately and efficiently predict sagittal and metopic synostosis diagnosis using off-the-shelf support vector machines and our newly introduced *symbolic shape descriptors* [10]. Our approach utilizes a *folding* technique proposed in [7] to significantly reduce the computational complexity at classification time as compared to that of the algorithm described in [10]. Furthermore, we utilize bootstrap [3] and cross-validation techniques for model selection [19] to show that our efficient algorithm does not compromise classification accuracy, and outperforms numeric descriptors that are traditionally used in clinical settings. Finally, we suggest that our proposed technique to quantify synostotic phenotypes will be important for future studies to determine correlations with surgical planning, long term outcome measurements, deficits in neurocognition and potential genetic and environmental causes.

The task we want to approach can be formally described as follows. We are given a random sample of M skull shapes labeled as sagittal (1), metopic (2) and normal (3), respectively. Using the skull shape information, we wish to construct a set of symbolic shape descriptors and a classification function in order to accurately and efficiently predict the label of a new skull shape.

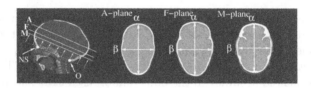

Fig. 2. The scaphocephaly severity indices SSI-A, SSI-F and SSI-M are computed as the head width to head length ratio β/α as measured on CT bone slices that are defined by internal anatomical landmarks on cerebral ventricles

2   Source of Images

Our shape descriptors are extracted from CT image slices from skull imaging. In order to standardize our computations, we use a calibrated lateral view of a 3-D reconstruction of the skull to select three CT slice planes defined by internal brain landmarks. These planes are parallel to the skull base plane, which is determined by using the frontal nasal suture anteriorly and the opisthion posteriorly. The A, F and M planes are shown in Figure 2. The A-plane is at the top of the lateral ventricle, the F-plane is at the Foramina of Munro, and the M-plane is at the level of the maximal dimension of the fourth ventricle. Using standard image segmentation and spline interpolation techniques [6], it is possible to extract the oriented outline from a CT bone image at the level of any of the planes defined above (Fig. 3a). The points of an oriented outline (such as point P in Fig. 3b) have a direction defined by their corresponding tangent vectors.

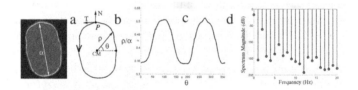

Fig. 3. a) Bone CT slice at the level of the A-plane. b) Oriented outline counter with clockwise direction; c) same outline represented in polar coordinates (ρ, θ); and d) 21 components of the corresponding cranial spectrum. Key: α (maximum outline length), T (tangent vector), N (normal vector), and (CM) center of mass.

3   Numeric Shape Descriptors

Numeric shape descriptors can range from a single number per planar slice to a large matrix of numbers. In our previous work, we proposed three descriptors of increasing complexity. The *scaphocephaly severity indices* (SSIs) [17] describe skulls with numbers representing ratios. These ratios are the head width to length, β/α, computed at the three planes defined above and are denoted by

SSI-A, SSI-F, and SSI-M, respectively (Fig. 2). Note that the ratio β/α measures the deviation of a skull outline shape from a perfect circle ($\beta/\alpha = 1$). The *cranial spectrum* (CS) [16] describes a skull shape with the magnitude of the Fourier series coefficients of a periodic function. This function is derived from a normalized oriented outline by using polar coordinates with origin at the center of mass of the outline (Fig. 3b). This representation encompasses shape information that cannot be captured by the SSI ratios, and is closely related to traditional DFT-based descriptors [13]. We use the first $R = 50$ coefficients of the spectrum in our experiments.

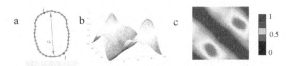

Fig. 4. a) Oriented contour represented as a sequence of N evenly spaced points. b) Cranial image. c) Top view of cranial image with normalized distance scale.

The *Cranial Image* (CI) [15] descriptor is a matrix representation of pairwise normalized square distances computed for all the vertices of an oriented outline that has been discretized into N evenly spaced vertices. Let D be a symmetric matrix with elements $D_{ij} = d_{ij}/\alpha$, for $i, j = 1 \cdots, N$, where d_{ij} is the Euclidean distance between vertices i and j, α is the maximum length of the contour (Fig. 4a), and N is a number between 100 and 500. Since the outline is oriented, the vertices can be sequentially ordered up to the selection of the first vertex. As a consequence, the matrix D is defined up to a periodic shift along the main diagonal. The CI of an oriented outline is defined as an equivalence class of distance matrices parametrized by a set of operators Θ_n that permutes the rows and columns of D to produce the aforementioned shift; more precisely, CI= $D(\Theta_n)$, $n = 1, \cdots, N$. The definition of CI can be extended to incorporate an arbitrary number of oriented outlines by computing inter and intra-oriented outline distances for each of the vertices of all of the outlines representing a

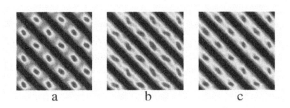

Fig. 5. Cranial images for a patient diagnosed with a) sagittal synostosis, b) metopic synostosis, and c) normal head shape. Cranial images were constructed using three consecutive oriented outlines at the levels of the A-plane, F-plane and M-plane

skull. For example, the vertices of outlines at the A, F, and M planes could be arranged from 1 to N, from $N + 1$ to $2N$, and from $2N + 1$ to $3N$, respectively (Fig. 5).

4   Symbolic Shape Descriptors

Symbolic shape descriptors (SSDs) were developed in [10] to overcome the computational complexity of cranial image descriptors. More specifically, the worst case complexity of a ν-SVM classification function that uses cranial images is $O(ML^3N^3)$, where M is the number of skulls in the training set, L is the number of oriented outlines used to represent a skull, and N is the number of vertices per outline. Such complexity limits the practical use of CIs in applications where several outlines are required to represent a 3-D skull shape.

The goal of symbolic shape descriptors is to encode global geometric properties that differentiate our shape classes (sagittal, metopic and normal) by probabilistic modeling of their local geometric properties. This paradigm can produce a compact representation of 3-D shape that improves the classification performance of numeric descriptors and reduces the computational complexity of the classification function to $O(MP)$ with $P \ll L^3N^3$. However, the *standard* SSD algorithm in [10] requires the computation of $(M+1)V + (M+1)P + P$ parameters for every test skull shape, where V is the vocabulary in the training set(to be defined below) and where the typical values of M, V and P are 100, 5×10^3, and 20, respectively. To overcome this issue, we adapt the *folding* technique described in [7], which only requires the computation of P parameters for every new skull shape. The training and testing steps of our *efficient* SSD algorithm are described below.

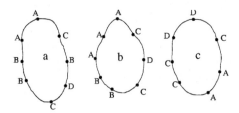

Fig. 6. Symbolic labels are assigned to the vertices of the oriented outlines by applying k-means clustering to their numeric attributes. Oriented outlines of a) sagittal, b) metopic and c) normal head shapes, respectively, taken at the level of the A-plane.

Training Algorithm. The input of the efficient SSD learning algorithm is a set of skull shapes $\mathcal{S} = \{S_1, \cdots, S_M\}$. Each shape is represented by L oriented outlines, and each outline is discretized into N evenly spaced vertices. For the sake of simplicity, we assume that $L = 1$. The training algorithm is as follows:

1. For each shape S_j in $\mathcal{S}$ and each vertex v_i of S_j, compute the vector of distances from all other vertices of S_j to v_i. This vector is the same as the i-th row of the CI matrix descriptor (Fig. 5).
2. Cluster these vectors by k-means clustering with user-selected k and assign each cluster a symbolic label. Each vertex receives the label of its cluster.
3. Compute a *bag of words* (*BOW*) representation of the skull outlines in $\mathcal{S}$. More specifically, the symbols associated with the vertices of an oriented outline are used to construct strings of symbols or words. The word size is fixed at some integer $1 \leq W \leq N$. For instance, when $W = 3$, each word contains three symbols. A *BOW* representation for the outline in Figure 7a is the unordered set $s=\{'CAA','AAB','ABB','BBC','BCD', 'CDB','DBC','BCA'\}$.
4. Compute a $M \times V$ co-occurrence matrix of counts $[n(s_i, w_j)]_{ij}$ for the training set where $n(s_i, w_j)$ denotes the number of times the word w_j occurs in the *BOW* s_i associated with the skull outline S_i.
5. Apply *probabilistic latent semantic analysis* (PLSA) to the co-occurrence matrix of the training set [7]. PLSA is a latent variable model which associates an unobserved class variable $z_k \in z_1, \ldots, z_P$ with each observation, and an observation being the occurrence of a word in a particular *BOW*. The PLSA (also called aspect model) is formally defined as $P(s_i, w_j) = P(s_i) \sum_{k=1}^{P} P(w_j|z_k)P(z_k|s_i)$, where $P(s_i, w_j)$ denotes the probability that a word occurrence will be observed in a particular *BOW* s_i, $P(w_j|z_k)$ denotes the class-conditional probability of observing the word w_j given the aspect z_k, and $P(z_k|s_i)$ denotes a *BOW*-specific probability distribution over the latent variable space. The equation above can be conveniently parametrized as $P(s_i, w_j) = \sum_{k=1}^{P} P(z_k)P(w_j|z_k)P(s_i|z_k)$, which is symmetric in both entities, *BOW* and words, and where $P(s_i|z_k)$ denotes the class-conditional probability of a specified *BOW* conditioned on the unobservable class variable z_k.
6. Use the class-conditional probabilities $P(s|z)$ estimated in the previous step to construct the symbolic shape descriptors for the outlines in $\mathcal{S}$. More specifically, for each outline S_i in the training set, form its corresponding *symbolic shape descriptor* as the P-dimensional vector $[P(s_i|z_1), \cdots, P(s_i|z_P)]$.
7. Use cross-validation on the training set of symbolic shape descriptors computed in the previous step for selecting the model of a ν-SVM classification function.

The outputs of the training algorithm are the k-means cluster centers, the set of words in the training set (vocabulary), the $P(w|z)$ parameters of the PLSA model, and a ν-SVM classification function for the symbolic shape descriptors.

An intuitive interpretation for the aspect model can be obtained by observing that the conditional distributions $P(w_j|s_i)$ are convex combinations of the P class conditionals or *aspects* $P(w_j|z_k)$. Loosely speaking, the modeling goal is to identify conditional probability mass functions $P(w_j|z_k)$ such that the *BOW*-specific word distributions are as faithfully as possible approximated by convex combinations of the aspects [7]. In our context, words encode local geometric properties of the outline shapes; therefore, the global geometric properties of the outlines in S are modeled as convex combinations of local *geometric aspects*. This means that $BOWs$ that have similar co-occurrence word distributions can be represented by similar geometric aspects. In fact, the PLSA model tends to cluster BOW-word pairs [7]. The parameters of the PLSA model can be estimated using the standard Expectation Maximization algorithm [1]. For the sake of space, the reader is invited to consult [7] for a comprehensive description of the PLSA model and its implementation details.

Testing Algorithm. The inputs are a new skull shape S_{new}, the k-means cluster centers, the vocabulary of the training set, the $P(w|z)$ parameters of the PLSA model, and a ν-SVM classification function.

1. Use the k-means cluster centers and a nearest neighbor rule to assign symbolic labels to the vertices of the test skull outline S_{new}.
2. Compute the occurrence vector corresponding to the test skull S_{new} using the vocabulary of the training set.
3. Use the class-conditional probabilities $P(w|z)$ estimated from the training set to compute $P(s_{new}|z)$ for the test skull S_{new}, and form the symbolic shape descriptor $[P(s_{new}|z_1), \cdots, P(s_{new}|z_P)]$. Note that the $P(w|z)$ parameters are kept fixed (not updated at each M-step) for estimation of $P(s_{new}|z)$. In doing so, $P(s_{new}|z)$ maximizes the likelihood of the skull shape S_{new} with respect to the previously trained $P(w|z)$ parameters.
4. Use the classification function and the symbolic shape descriptor computed in the previous step to predict the label of S_{new}.

The output of the efficient SSD algorithm is the label of S_{new}.

4.1 ν-SVMs and Model Selection

We use ν-SVMs with a Gaussian kernel $k(x, x') = \exp(-d(x, x')^2/\sigma^2)$ to measure similarities between shape descriptors (SSIs, cranial spectrum, and symbolic shape descriptors), where the function d is the Euclidean distance, and σ is the *width* parameter of the kernel. The worst case computational complexity for this kernel is $O(Mr)$, where r is the dimension of the x vectors. We use the kernel $k_\Theta(D, D') = \max_n \ k(D(\Theta_n), D')$ to measure the similarity between cranial images. We select the width σ of the kernel (and the k, W and P parameters of the symbolic shape descriptors) by minimizing the *leave-one-out error* (LOOE) estimate of the expected classification error [18]. We bound the variance of our statistical estimators (LOOE and confusion matrices) by computing *bootstrap* confidence intervals [3].

5   Experimental Results

Our sample population consists of 60 CT head scans from children with sagittal synostosis, 13 head scans diagnosed with metopic synostosis and 41 scans of

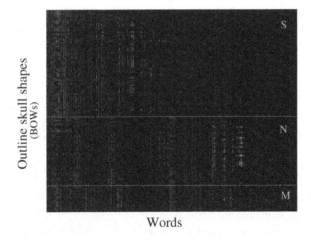

Fig. 7. Co-occurrence matrix of word counts (displayed as a color image) corresponding to the skull shapes in our sample population. Each skull shape is represented using three outline shapes ($L = 3$) at the level of the A, F and M planes. Key: Sagittal (S), Normal (N) and Metopic (M).

age-matched controls with normal head shapes. Computed tomography data are acquired with a multi-detector system that produces isotropic 3-D images with 0.5 mm resolution. Three-dimensional reconstructions of each patient's skull are generated with a high performance workstation (Figs. 1 and 2).

5.1 *BOW* Representation

We compute co-occurrence matrices of counts for the *BOW* representation of the skull outlines in our population sample. Our data reveal that this symbolic representation encodes distinctive shape information that can be used to differentiate sagittal, metopic and normal skull shapes. This can be seen in Fig. 7, which shows as a color image of a co-occurrence matrix for skull shapes represented by three oriented outlines at the A, F and M levels ($L = 3$, $k = 150$ and $W = 5$). It is clear from the figure that the distributions of word frequencies for each of the classes differ significantly. Our data also show that for both $W > 5$ and $k > 250$ the co-occurrence matrix becomes too sparse and word count estimates become unreliable. Values $k < 30$ do not allow us to discriminate between skull shape classes.

5.2 Classification Results

Table 1 shows the classification performance for the SSI, CS, CI and standard SSD descriptors computed separately for the three oriented outlines ($N=200$, $R=50$, $L=1$, $k=150$ and $W=3$). Standard SSD descriptors computed from single

Table 1. Classification confusion matrices for SSIs, CS, CI and standard SSD descriptors computed for individual oriented outlines OA, OF and OM. Outlines were generated at the A, F and M planes, respectively. Key: Sagittal (S), Metopic (M) and Normal (N).

		SSI			CS			CI			SSD		
		S	M	N	S	M	N	S	M	N	S	M	N
	S	0.98	0.00	0.05	0.98	0.00	0.04	1.00	0.00	0.05	1.00	0.00	0.07
OA	M	0.00	0.85	0.54	0.00	0.62	0.07	0.00	0.31	0.00	0.00	0.77	0.12
	N	0.02	0.15	0.41	0.02	0.38	0.88	0.00	0.69	0.95	0.23	0.80	0.88
	S	0.93	0.00	0.00	0.98	0.00	0.00	0.95	0.00	0.05	1.00	0.00	0.07
OF	M	0.00	0.85	0.51	0.00	0.93	0.07	0.00	0.92	0.05	0.00	0.92	0.05
	N	0.07	0.15	0.49	0.02	0.07	0.93	0.05	0.08	0.90	0.00	0.08	0.88
	S	0.88	0.00	0.20	0.90	0.00	0.10	0.91	0.08	0.12	0.97	0.00	0.10
OM	M	0.00	0.76	0.51	0.00	0.85	0.00	0.02	0.85	0.02	0.00	0.85	0.00
	N	0.12	0.23	0.29	0.10	0.15	0.90	0.07	0.07	0.85	0.03	0.15	0.90

Table 2. Classification confusion matrix and $p = 0.05$ confidence intervals for standard SSD computed using all three oriented outlines associated with the A-plane, F-plane and M-plane levels. Key: Symbolic shape descriptors (SSD), Saggital (S), Metopic (M) and Normal (N).

Standard SSD Algorithm

	S	M	N
S	**1.00 [0.99,1.00]**	0.00[0.00, 0.01]	0.07 [0.05, 0.09]
M	0.00 [0.00 0.01]	**1.00 [0.98, 1.00]**	0.00 [0.00, 0.02]
N	0.00 [0.00 0.01]	0.00 [0.00 0.08]	**0.93 [0.90 0.96]**

Table 3. Classification confusion matrix and $p = 0.05$ confidence intervals for efficient SSD computed using all three oriented outlines associated with the A-plane, F-plane and M-plane levels. Key: Symbolic shape descriptors (SSD), Saggital (S), Metopic (M) and Normal (N).

Efficient SSD Algorithm

	S	M	N
S	**1.00 [0.99,1.00]**	0.00[0.00, 0.01]	0.07 [0.05, 0.09]
M	0.00 [0.00 0.01]	**1.00 [0.94, 1.00]**	0.00 [0.00, 0.02]
N	0.00 [0.00 0.01]	0.00 [0.00 0.06]	**0.93 [0.89 0.97]**

outlines perform better than SSIs and have comparable performance to those of CS and CI descriptors.

Table 2 shows the results for standard SSDs computed from all three outlines ($L=3$). Table 3 shows the related results for efficient SSDs. These results are superior than those on single slices alone. Although the performance of effi-

$$z_1 \qquad z_4 \qquad z_{12} \qquad z_{13} \qquad z_{14}$$

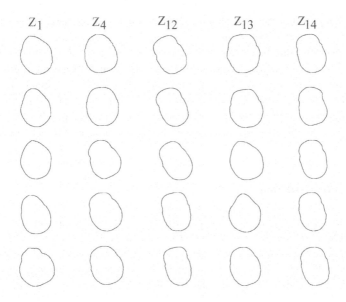

Fig. 8. Skull shapes are ranked based on the computed $P(s|z)$. Shapes in aspect z_1 belong to metopic, in aspect z_4 belong to normal, and aspect z_{12} and z_{14} belong to sagittal. Aspect z_{13} includes a mix of metopic and normal skull shapes.

cient SSDs and standard SSDs are comparable, the standard SSDs requires the computation of $(M+1)V+(M+1)P+P$ parameters ($\sim 10^5$), while the efficient SSDs only requires the calculation of P parameters ($M{=}113$, $V{=}5 \times 10^3$ and $P{=}15$).

5.3 Shape-Based Skull Ranking

The five skull shapes with the highest $P(s_i|z_k)$ for $z = 1, 4, 12, 13, 14$ are shown in Fig. 8. Note that the top ranked shapes for aspects z_{12} and z_{14} represent shape features only evident in sagittal synostosis, while aspect z_1 encodes features only observed in the metopic class. Aspect z_4 encodes features that are only evident in the class of normal shapes. Also note that the sagittal skulls in column z_{12} have flatter and wider tops in contrast to the sagittal skulls in column z_{14}. These observations suggest that SSD descriptors could be used to stratify skull shapes in different subcategories. This kind of aspect-based shape ranking can be potentially used to develop automatic retrieval applications of skull morphologies.

6   Conclusions

This paper presents an improved and efficient approach to the symbolic shape descriptors proposed in [10]. This method is compared with our previous work on numeric shape descriptors and standard SSDs for accurate prediction of sagittal and metopic diagnoses. We show that the symbolic shape descriptors computed from three oriented outlines outperform all of the numeric shape descriptors. We also show that efficient SSDs have equal classification performance to standard SSDs. Because the computational complexity of the efficient SSD approach is further reduced from that of the standard SSD method, efficient SSD is the preferred algorithm that can be potentially used to represent 3-D skull shape of large data sets without significant increase in the complexity at classification time.

Acknowledgements

This work is supported in part by The Laurel Foundation Center for Craniofacial Research, The Marsha Solan-Glazer Craniofacial Endowment, The Biomedical and Health Informatics Training Grant (T15 LM07442), and a grant from NICDR R01-DE-13813. The authors gratefully acknowledge the suggestions made by Daniel Gatica-Perez regarding the use of PLSA in our application.

References

1. Dempster, A.P., Laird, N.M., Rubin, D.B.: Maximum likelihood from incomplete data via the EM algorithm. J. Royal Statist, Soc. B, **39** (1977)
2. Dryden I., Mardia K. V.: Statistical Shape Analysis. New York: John Wiley and Sons(1998)
3. Efron, B.: The Jackknife, the Bootstrap, and Other Resampling Plans. Society for Industrial and Applied Mathematics (1982)
4. Fata, J.J., Turner, M.S.: The reversal exchange technique of total calvarial reconstruction for sagittal synostosis. Plast. Reconst. Surg. **107** (2001) 1637–1646
5. Guimaras-Ferreira, J., Gewalli, F., David, L., Olsson, R., Freide, H., Lauritzen, C.G.K.: Spring-mediated cranioplasty compared with the modified pi-plasty for sagittal synostosis. Scand. J. Plast. Surg. Hand Surg. **37** (2003) 209–215
6. Haralick, R.M., Shapiro, L.G.: Computer and Robot Vision. Addison-Wesley (1992)
7. Hofmann, T.: Unsupervised learning by Probabilistic Latent Semantic Analysis. Machine Learning **42** (2001) 177–196
8. Lajeunie, E., Le Merrer, M., Marchac, C., Renier, D.: Genetic study of scaphocepaly. Am. J. Med. Gene. **62** (1996) 282-285
9. Lale, S.R., Richtsmeier, J.T.: An invariant approach to statistical analysis of shape. Chapman and Hall/CRC (2001).
10. Lin, H.J., Ruiz-Correa, S., Shapiro, L.G., Hing, A.V., Cunningham, M.L., Speltz, M.L., Sze, R.W.: Symbolic shape descriptors for classifying craniosynostosis deformations from skull imaging. In press, Proceedings of the IEEE Conference on Engineering in Medicine and Biology Society (2005).
11. Lynch, M., Walsh, B.: genetic and analysis of quantitative trait. Sinauer Associates (1998)
12. Panchal, J., Marsh, J.L., Park, T.S., Hauffman, B., Pilgram, T., Huang, S.H.: Sagittal craniosynostosis outcome assessment for two methods of timing and interventions. Plast. Reconstr. Surg. **103** (1999) 1574–1579

13. Rao, C.: Geometry of circular vectors and pattern recognition of shape of a boundary. Proc. Nat. Acad. Aci. **95** (2002) 12783
14. Ruiz-Correa, S., Shapiro, L.G., Meilă, M.: A new paradigm for recognizing 3-D object shapes from range data. IEEE International Conference on Computer Vision bf 2 (2003) 1126–1133
15. Ruiz-Correa, S., Sze, R.W., Lin, H.J., Shapiro, L.G., Speltz, M.L., Cunningham, M.L.: Classifying craniosynostosis deformations by skull shape imaging. In press, Proceedings of the IEEE Conference on Computer-Based Medical Systems (2005)
16. Ruiz-Correa, S., Sze, R.W., Starr, J.R., Hing, A.V., Lin, H.J., Cunningham, M.L.: A Fourier-based approach for quantifying sagittal synostosis head shape. American Cleft Palate-Craniofacial Association Meeting (2005)
17. Ruiz-Correa, S., Sze, R.W., Starr, J.R., Lin, H.J., Speltz, M.L., Cunningham, M.L., Hing, A.V.: New scaphocephalyseverity indices of sagittal craniosynostosis: A comparative study with cranial index quantifications. Submitted to the American Cleft Palate-Craniofacial Association Journal (2005)
18. Scholköpf, B., Smola, A.J.: Learning with Kernels. Cambridge University Press (2002)
19. Vapnik V.V.: Statistical Learning Theory. John Wiley and Sons (1998)

Elastic Interaction Models for Active Contours and Surfaces

Albert C.S. Chung[1], Yang Xiang[2], Jian Ye[2], and W.K. Law[1]

[1] Lo Kwee-Seong Medical Image Analysis Laboratory,
Department of Computer Science,
The Hong Kong University of Science and Technology, Hong Kong
[2] Department of Mathematics,
The Hong Kong University of Science and Technology, Hong Kong

Abstract. In this paper, we propose a new framework for active contour and surface models. Based on the concepts of the elastic interaction between line defects in solids, this framework defines an image-based speed field for contour evolution. Different from other level set based frameworks, the speed field is global and defined everywhere in the whole space. It can offer a long-range attractive interaction between object boundary and evolving contour. The new framework is general because it can be easily extended to higher dimension. Using the Fast Fourier Transforms, we also introduce an efficient algorithm for finding the values of the image-based speed field. Some experiments on synthetic and clinical images are shown to indicate the properties of our model.

1 Introduction

Extracting a surface from medical data is clinically an important step because the extracted boundary surface can provide essential ssvisual and quantitative information about the shape and size of the biological objects, e.g. brains and vessels.

Active contour models have widely been used for image segmentation and surface extraction. The classical snakes approach evolves and finds object boundary based on forces derived from the internal energy of the contour and local image gradient [4].

If the moving contour is not close enough to the target object, the capture range of the contour can be limited. Then, an additional constant balloon force was introduced along the contour normal direction to accelerate the contour motion and increase the capture range [1].

To offer more flexibility in handling multiple objects and their topological changes, the level set framework [6,5] was used to model the moving contour. The dynamic equation is given as

$$\frac{\partial \phi}{\partial t} = g(\nabla I) \left(\nabla \cdot \left(\frac{\nabla \phi}{|\nabla \phi|} \right) + \nu \right) |\nabla \phi|, \tag{1}$$

where $\phi(x, y)$ is the level set function whose zero level set represents the contour. All terms before $|\nabla \phi|$ gives the speed of the embedded contour along its normal

Y. Liu, T. Jiang, and C. Zhang (Eds.): CVBIA 2005, LNCS 3765, pp. 314–323, 2005.
© Springer-Verlag Berlin Heidelberg 2005

direction. The first term $\nabla \cdot \left(\frac{\nabla \phi}{|\nabla \phi|} \right)$ smooths and shortens the contour based on contour curvature. The second term ν is the constant balloon force making the contour expand or shrink depending on its sign. The gradient function $g(\nabla I)$ gives very small value at the boundary and makes the speed of the moving contour small. As such, the evolving contour will stop on the object boundary. However, without the constant balloon force, the capture range can be short and the contour cannot reach the narrow concave regions of the object boundary. This is because the effect of ∇I, defined by $g(\nabla I)$ in Eq. 1, is localized near the boundary. While with the balloon force, there is a limitation that the balloon force cannot make some parts of contour shrink while other parts of the contour expand. Therefore, the initial contour must be placed entirely outside or inside the object to be detected.

In this paper, inspired by the elastic interaction between line defects in solids, we propose an active contour method offering a long-range attractive interaction between two contours (object boundary and evolving contour). We shall define a long-range attraction generated by the object boundary and acting on the evolving contour for solving the segmentation problem. The speed field due to this interaction is calculated efficiently using the Fast Fourier Transforms, and is defined everywhere in the space. No force extension is needed, as it is commonly needed in the conventional level set based active contour methods. We also use the level set framework to handle the topological changes during the contour evolution. This framework is general and can be applied to the N-dimensional segmentation problems. It is experimentally shown that the method can be effective in detecting elongated and tubular structures, e.g. brain vessels.

2 Method

2.1 2D Segmentation Based on Elastic Interaction

The main goal of this section is to define a speed field v for encouraging attractive interaction between object boundary and moving contour during the contour evolution. The level set framework is employed to represent the moving contours in 2D and surfaces in 3D [6]. Let ϕ be the level set function. The evolution equation is given as $\frac{\partial \phi}{\partial t} = v|\nabla \phi|$, where v represents a speed field, in which the values of speed are well defined in the whole space.

We now define the speed field v of a two dimensional moving contour. As shown in Fig. 1, the (blue) contour $\gamma(s)$ represents the object boundary and another (red) contour represents the moving contour. At any point $\mathbf{P}$ on the moving contour, the speed is derived based on the elastic interaction between line defects in solids [2] and our previous work [10]. The speed field v is defined as

$$v = - \int_{\gamma(s)} \frac{\mathbf{r} \cdot \mathbf{n}}{r^3} ds, \tag{2}$$

where $\mathbf{r}$ is a vector between point $\mathbf{P}$ and a point on $\gamma(s)$, $r = |\mathbf{r}|$ denotes the Euclidean distance between these two points, and $\mathbf{n}$ represents the normal di-

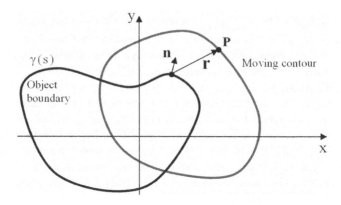

Fig. 1. Elastic interaction between object boundary (blue) and moving contour (red)

rection. Under this definition, the speed inside the object boundary and outside the object boundary are different in sign.

We describe how the speed function defined above can be used for image segmentation problem. Let an image be $I(x, y)$ located in the $z = 0$ plane, where $(x, y) \in \Omega$ and Ω denotes the image domain. The speed field is set to depend on the intensity values in the image by replacing the normal direction $\mathbf{n}$ in Eq. 2 by the image gradient ∇I. However, the image-based speed function is singular on the contour $\gamma(s)$. The singularities can then be smeared out if the normal direction $\mathbf{n}$ is replaced with the gradient of the smoothed image $\nabla(G_\sigma * I)$, where G_σ represents a Gaussian smoothing filter with standard deviation σ. Therefore, the image-based speed field v is given as

$$v = -\int_\Omega \frac{\mathbf{r} \cdot \nabla(G_\sigma * I)}{r^3} dx dy, \tag{3}$$

where Ω denotes the image domain and $(x, y) \in \Omega$.

Another important property of the speed field v is that it is a long range speed field generated by the object boundary, and there is no need to place the initial contour entirely inside or outside the object. Thus the moving contour can "see" the far away boundary by the interaction between object boundary and evolving contour boundary. Also, the sign of the speed depends on the direction of the contour and the object boundary, so that the contour is not necessarily to be placed entirely inside or near the object boundary. The direction of the object boundary $\mathbf{t}$ is defined as

$$\mathbf{t} = \frac{1}{|\nabla(G_\sigma * I)|} \left(\frac{\partial(G_\sigma * I)}{\partial y}, -\frac{\partial(G_\sigma * I)}{\partial x}, 0 \right). \tag{4}$$

For instance, if an object has a stronger intensity than the background, the direction of the object boundary is counterclockwise; and is clockwise vice versa. The direction of the moving contour, i.e. the zero level contour of the level set function $\phi(x, y)$, can also be defined similarly, with $G_\sigma * I$ replaced by ϕ in Eq. 4. The level set function is chosen such that the moving contour has an opposite direction with respect to the object boundary. As a result, the moving contour is attracted to the object boundary under the speed field v.

In the above definition of speed function, the image noise also generates a speed field for the moving curve, resulting in spurious contours. The speed generated by the noise is relatively small as compared with that by the object boundary. We remove this contribution of the noise by adding the interaction within the moving contour, so that the relative weak interaction between the noise and the moving contour can be overcome. The speed field v is now defined as

$$v = -\int_\Omega \frac{\mathbf{r} \cdot \nabla(G_\sigma * I + wH(\phi))}{r^3} dx dy, \tag{5}$$

where w is an adjustable coefficient and H is the Heaviside function, which is defined as

$$H(\phi) = \begin{cases} 0 & \text{if } \phi \le -\epsilon, \\ \frac{1}{2}(\sin(\frac{\pi\phi}{2\epsilon}) + 1) & \text{if } -\epsilon < \phi < \epsilon, \\ 1 & \text{if } \phi \ge \epsilon, \end{cases} \tag{6}$$

where ϵ is a small constant.

The values of the speed field v can be solved efficiently using the Fast Fourier Transform (FFT) algorithm. It is well known that in three dimensional space, $-1/4\pi r$ is the solution of the Poisson equation,

$$-\triangle \frac{1}{4\pi r} = \delta, \tag{7}$$

where δ is the three dimensional Dirac delta function. Performing the Fourier transformations on both sides of the above equation, we can get

$$\widehat{\frac{1}{r}} = \frac{1}{m^2 + n^2 + l^2} \cdot \frac{1}{2\pi^2}, \tag{8}$$

where m, n, and l are frequencies in the Fourier space. Thus

$$\widehat{\nabla \frac{1}{r}} = \frac{(im, in, il)}{m^2 + n^2 + l^2} \cdot \frac{1}{2\pi^2}. \tag{9}$$

In order to perform the FFT algorithm to get the values of speed (Eq. 5), we have to change our formulation from two dimensional space to three dimensional space. To achieve this goal, we multiply a factor $\delta(z)$, where $\delta(z)$ is one-dimensional Dirac delta-function. Therefore, Eq. 5 can be re-written as

$$v = -\int_z \int_\Omega \frac{\mathbf{r}}{r^3} \cdot (\nabla(G_\sigma * I(x, y) + wH(\phi)(x, y)), 0)\delta(z) dx dy dz. \tag{10}$$

Let the Fourier coefficients of the function $G_\sigma * I + wH(\phi)$ be $\{d_{mn}\}$. The Fourier coefficients of the function $(\nabla(G_\sigma * I(x, y) + wH(\phi)(x, y)), 0)$ are then

$\{(imd_{mn}, ind_{mn}, 0)\}$. Performing the Fourier transformation on both sides of Eq. 10, based on Eq. 9, we get

$$\hat{v} = \frac{(im, in, il)}{m^2 + n^2 + l^2} \cdot \frac{1}{2\pi^2} \cdot (imd_{mn}, ind_{mn}, 0) \cdot \frac{1}{2\pi} \cdot (2\pi)^2,$$
$$= -\frac{1}{\pi} \cdot \frac{m^2 + n^2}{m^2 + n^2 + l^2} d_{mn}. \tag{11}$$

Finally, we have

$$v(x, y) = -\int_{-\infty}^{\infty} \sum_{m,n} \frac{1}{\pi} \frac{m^2 + n^2}{m^2 + n^2 + l^2} d_{mn} e^{imx} e^{iny} dl, \tag{12}$$

$$= -\sum_{m,n} \frac{\sqrt{m^2 + n^2}}{2} \cdot d_{mn} e^{imx} e^{iny}. \tag{13}$$

To obtain a smooth moving contour, we can introduce a small curvature term associated with a small weight μ. Now, the evolution equation is given as

$$\frac{\partial \phi}{\partial t} = \left(\mu \nabla \cdot \left(\frac{\nabla \phi}{|\nabla \phi|} \right) + v \right) |\nabla \phi|. \tag{14}$$

2.2   Extension to 3D Segmentation Problem

Similarly, we define our three dimensional speed field v as

$$v = -\int_S \frac{\mathbf{r} \cdot \mathbf{n}}{r^4} dA, \tag{15}$$

where S represents the object boundary in 3D. By replacing the normal direction $\mathbf{n}$ by the gradient of the smoothed image $\nabla(G_\sigma * I)$, the value of speed v is now relying on the image intensity values in an image volume $I(x, y, z)$, where $(x, y, z) \in \Omega$ and Ω denotes the image domain. In order to perform FFT algorithm to solve the image-based speed function, we have to change the formulation to 4D space. The speed function is re-written as

$$v = -\int_w \int_\Omega \frac{\mathbf{r}}{r^4} \cdot (\nabla(G_\sigma * I(x, y, z) + wH(\phi)(x, y, z)), 0)\delta(w)dxdydzdw, \tag{16}$$

where $\delta(w)$ is the one-dimensional Dirac delta-function. Let the Fourier coefficients of the function $G_\sigma * I + wH(\phi)$ be $\{d_{mnl}\}$. Similarly to 2D problem described in the previous section, performing FFT on both sides of Eq. 16 and following by taking the inverse FFT, we get

$$v(x, y, z) = -\sum_{m,n,l} \frac{\sqrt{m^2 + n^2 + l^2}}{8} \cdot d_{mnl} e^{imx} e^{iny} e^{ilz}, \tag{17}$$

where m, n, and l are frequencies in the Fourier space.

2.3   Numerical Implementation

For the numerical implementation of Eq.(14), we use central difference for the curvature term, Godunov's scheme [7] combined with fifth order WENO derivative [3] for the term $v|\nabla\phi|$, and the forward Euler method in time. Re-initialization for ϕ is used to reduce the numerical errors [9]. The initial zero level contour of ϕ is set to be the zero crossing of the speed field generated by the image only, i.e. $\phi = v/|v|$, where v is calculated using $w = 0$. This gives an initial contour very close to the object boundary, so that the object boundary can then be found and the noise be removed efficiently after short-time evolution.

3   Results

The proposed method has been applied to synthetic images and four sets of 3D Rotational Angiographic (RA) images. We have also implemented the gradient vector flow (GVF) method [12,11,8]. Since the results using these GVF methods [12,11,8] are similar in the comparisons, all results are obtained using the modified GVF method with the balloon force [8].

3.1   Synthetic Images

In this section, all results were obtained using a numerical mesh with the size of 128×128 pixels. The width and length were equal to 2 units. The pixel width was $dx = dy = 2/128$.

Fig. 2 shows the results on an image with multiple objects, which have different intensity and topology, but without noise. Given that the intensity values range between 0(white) and 1(black), the intensity values of the four objects were 3/9, 4/9, 5/9 and 6/9 (see Fig. 2(a)). As shown in the figure, the image has thin features such as convex (bottom left) and concave (top right) regions. The parameters of our method were set as follows: $\sigma = 0.8$ (Eq. 5), $w = 0.35$ (Eq. 5), $\epsilon = dx$ (Eq. 6)and $\mu = 0.002$ (Eq. 14). Our method found the object boundaries accurately (see Fig. 2(b)). In fact, for this image without noise, the zero level contour of the speed field v gives the object boundary directly. In this case, no evolution is needed. Fig. 2(c) shows that the speed field is globally defined and can have long influence on the moving contour.

The bottom row of Fig. 2 shows the results obtained using the GVF method with adaptive bidirectional balloon force. Unlike our method, this method needs extension of force (velocity) field based on the diffusion of gradient information. The parameters were set as follows: $\mu = 0.02$, $\sigma_E = 2dx$, $\beta = 0.002$ and $\epsilon = 0.1$ (see [8] for definitions of the parameters). We set a circle as the initial contour (see Fig. 2(d)). As shown in Fig. 2(e), not all parts of the contour were attracted to the correct boundaries of the objects (see the bottom left object in Fig. 2(e)). Fig. 2(f) shows the corresponding force field of the GVF method. From the figure, it is observed that, at the middle between two adjacent objects, the contour cannot move further. This is because the extended velocity is perpendicular to the normal direction of the zero level set.

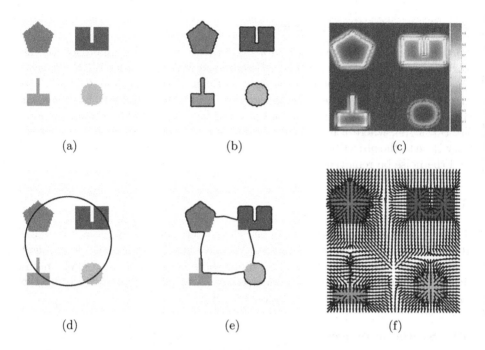

(a)   (b)   (c)

(d)   (e)   (f)

Fig. 2. (a) An input image with multiple objects, (b) results obtained using our method, (c) speed field v of our method (Note that $log_2(|v| + 1)$ is shown for better visualization.), (d) initial contour for GVF method, (e) results obtained using the GVF method and (f) GVF force field

Our method has been applied to the same image (see Fig. 2(a)) but with different levels of noise. The SD of the background noise $\sigma_B = 0.0621$ was obtained from the real 3D-RA images, which will be described in the next section.

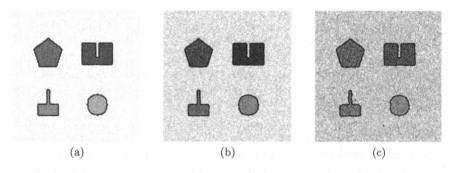

(a)   (b)   (c)

Fig. 3. Synthetic images with different levels of noise: (a) $0.5\sigma_B$, (b) σ_B and (c) $2\sigma_B$. Intensity values range between 0(white) and 1(black) in the images.

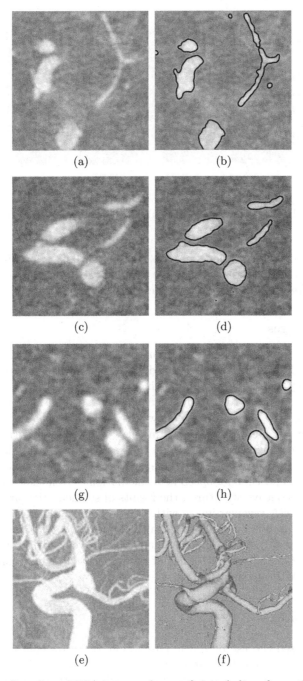

Fig. 4. Image slices from 3DRA image volumes. Original slices for patients 1 (Fig.a), 2 (Fig.c) and 3 (Fig.e). Results obtained using our method for patients 1 (Fig.b), 2 (Fig.d) and 3 (Fig.f). Fig.g and Fig.h show the MIP image and the corresponding 3D view of the result obtained using our method.

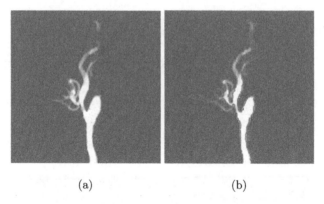

(a)   (b)

Fig. 5. (Fig.a) DSA vascular image. (Fig.b) The corresponding segmentation result.

The errors of segmentation were 0%, 0.06% and 0.63% for Figs. 3(a), 3(b) and 3(c) respectively. It shows that the proposed method can give reasonable segmentation results when noise level increases.

3.2 Real Images

We have applied our 3D segmentation method on four 3D-RA clinical datasets acquired by a Philips Integris Imager medical system at the Department of Diagnostic Radiology and Organ Imaging, Prince of Wales Hospital, Hong Kong. The data volume was around $100 \times 100 \times 100$ voxels with a voxel size of $0.75 \times 0.75 \times 0.75\text{mm}^3$. Figs. 4(a), 4(c) and 4(e) show three selected image slices. Contours obtained using our method are shown in Figs. 4(b), 4(d) and 4(f) respectively (note that the contours are lying inside the vascular regions). The initial contours were obtained directly using the speed field, and then evolved using the level set method and FFT for speed field calculation. Given that the vasculature has convex and concave structures, the results of segmentation are satisfactory. Fig. 5 shows a DSA vascular image with thin and elongated structures, and the intensity values are low (weak linkage) in the upper half of the image. As shown in the figure (Fig. 5b), our method can help capture weak edges connected along the strong edges. A 3D surface of one of the segmented image volumes and the corresponding MIP are shown in Figs. 4(g) and 4(h).

4 Conclusion

We have proposed the use of elastic interaction for active contour and surface models. Our method has been applied to the synthetic and real image volumes for image segmentation. The experimental results show that, for images without noise (e.g. synthetic images), the zero level set of the speed function can give contour very near to the target object boundary. For images with noise (e.g. real images), the initial contour can be efficiently computed and then object details can be detected via contour evolution using the Fast Fourier Transform (FFT) algorithm. It is experimentally shown that our method can be effective in detecting elongated and tubular structures, e.g. brain vessels in 3DRA or DSA.

References

1. L.D. Cohen. On active contour models and balloons. *Computer Vision and Graphic Image Processiong Conference*, 53(2):211–331, 1991.
2. J.P. Hirth and J. Lothe. *Theory of Dislocations, 2nd edition*. John Wiley & Sons, Inc., New York, 1982.
3. G.S. Jiang and D. Peng. Weighted ENO schemes for Hamilton-Jacobi equations. *SIAM Journal on Scientific Computing*, 21(6):2126–2143, 2000.
4. M. Kass, A. Witkin, and D. Terzopoulos. Snakes: Active contour models. *International Journal of Computer Vision*, 1(4):321–331, 1988.
5. R. Malladi, J.A. Sethian, and B.C. Vemuri. Shape modeling with front propagation: A level set approach. *IEEE Transactions on Pattern Analysis and Machine Intelligence*, 17(2):158–175, 1995.
6. S. Osher and J.A. Sethian. Fronts propagating with curvature-dependent speed: algorithms based on Hamilton-Jacobi formulations. *Journal of Computational Physics*, 79:12–49, 88.
7. S. Osher and C.W. Shu. High-order essentially nonoscillatory schemes for Hamilton-Jacobi equations. *SIAM Journal of Numerical Analysis*, 28(4):907–922, 1991.
8. N. Paragios, O. Mellina-Gottardo, and V. Ramesh. Gradient vector flow fast geometric active contours. *IEEE Transactions on Pattern Analysis and Machine Intelligence*, 26(3):402–407, 2004.
9. D. Peng, B. Merriman, S. Osher, H.K. Zhao, and M. Kang. A PDE-based fast local level set method. *Journal of Computational Physics*, 155(2):410–438, 1999.
10. Y. Xiang, A.C.S. Chung, and J. Ye. A New Active Contour Method based on Elastic Interaction. *IEEE International Conference on Computer Vision and Pattern Recognition*, 1:452–457, 2005.
11. C. Xu and J.L. Prince. Generalized gradient vector flow external forces for active contours. *Signal Processing*, 71(2):131–139, 1998.
12. C. Xu and J.L. Prince. Snakes, shapes, and gradient vector flow. *IEEE Transaction on Image Processing*, 7(3):359–369, 1998.

Estimating Diameters of Pulmonary Nodules with Competition-Diffusion and Robust Ellipsoid Fit

Toshiro Kubota[1] and Kazunori Okada[2]

[1] CAD Solutions, Siemens Medical Solutions
[2] Real-Time Vision & Modeling department, Siemens Corporate Research

Abstract. We propose a new technique to extract a pulmonary nodule from helical thoracic CT scans and estimate its diameter. The technique is based on a novel segmentation, or label-assignment, framework called competition-diffusion (CD), combined with robust ellipsoid fitting (EF). The competition force defined by replicator equations draws one dominant label at each voxel, and the diffusion force encourages spatial coherence in the segmentation map. CD is used to reliably extract foreground structures, and nodule like objects are further separated from attached structures using EF. Using ground-truth measured manually over 1300 nodules taken from more than 240 CT volumes, the performance of the proposed approach is evaluated in comparison with two other techniques: Local Density Maximum algorithm and the original EF. The results show that our approach provides the most accurate size estimates.

1 Introduction

Measuring the size of pulmonary nodules from X-ray computed tomography (CT) data is an important practice for diagnosis and progression analysis of lung cancer. The nodule size often plays an important role in choosing a proper patient care, and is also an effective feature to separate true nodules from nodule-like spurious findings. Typically, the size is represented by the diameter of the nodule. In clinical practice, it is conventional to use the 2D diameter-based estimation because the manual reading can be done readily by scanning through a CT volume slice by slice. Automating this task for computer-aided diagnosis (CAD) is, however, a difficult problem due to intensity variations, partial volume effects, attachment to other structures, and noise [1,2,3,4,5,6]. Although a truly 3D based volume estimate may give more accurate information for diagnosis and prognosis, we anticipate the trend of the 2D approach will continue for foreseeable future.

A CT-based screening protocol specified by the International Early Lung Cancer Action Program (I-ELCAP) details how the diameter of pulmonary nodules should be measured and how the measurements should be used for determining the patient management. According to the protocol, the result of an initial

Y. Liu, T. Jiang, and C. Zhang (Eds.): CVBIA 2005, LNCS 3765, pp. 324–334, 2005.

CT screening of lung is considered positive if at least one solid or part-solid nodule with 5.0mm or more in diameter or at least one non-solid nodule with 8.0mm or more in diameter is found [7]. Although these 5mm and 8mm thresholds are likely to become smaller as more accurate screening becomes possible with high resolution multi-detector helical CT (MDCT), the importance of nodule size in cancer diagnosis will stay unchanged.

Despite an existing large body of works, nodule segmentation is still an active open problem. More accurate and efficient algorithms will be extremely useful for detection and diagnosis of lung cancer. We consider the segmentation problem in a semi-automated setting where a rough location of a potential nodule is known. There are many candidate detection algorithms that can be used to fully automate our system, in particular as a part of a CAD system. Therefore, our semi-automated treatment does not lessen the importance of the problem and the usefulness of our algorithm.

Recently, a semi-automated size estimation algorithm using a robust Gaussian ellipsoid fitting (EF) was proposed by [8]. Given a marker positioned near a nodule, the algorithm computes the location, orientation and radii of an ellipsoid by fitting a Gaussian-based model to the intensity variation nearby the marker. It employs scale-space mean-shift and a robust scale estimator to find the solution. The volume and diameter of the nodule can be estimated from the ellipsoid. Their work verified the estimation accuracy using a large clinical database [8]. However, the technique tends to be inaccurate in the diameter measurement for small nodules due mainly to the small sample size problem.

The main contribution of this work is a new diameter estimation technique that improves the accuracy and the speed of the original EF. The proposed technique is based on a combination of EF and a technique using *competition-diffusion* segmentation (CD) [9]. The competition-diffusion is a class of reaction-diffusion systems that employ a competitive learning mechanism ([10,11]) as the system's reaction term. To our knowledge, this work is the first attempt to apply CD to medical image segmentation problems. It also differs fundamentally from other well-known reaction-diffusion-based segmentation solutions [12,13]. Our experimental results indicate that CD is highly effective and fast in segmenting solitary nodules, but is not applicable to non-solitary ones. On the other hand, EF is stable and applicable to both solitary and non-solitary nodules, but inaccurate for small solitary ones. Thus, our idea is to apply CD to solitary nodules and EF to non-solitary ones. We use the CD segmentation to determine if the nodule is solitary or non-solitary.

The paper is organized as follows. In Section 2, three segmentation algorithms, CD, EF and Local Density Maximum (LDM) [14], are described. They are compared against the proposed hybrid approach in our experiments. Section 3 describes a diameter estimation technique using the segmentation results. Section 4 introduces the proposed hybrid method (HB). Section 5 shows our experimental results. Section 6 gives summary and concluding remarks.

2   Segmentation

2.1   Competition-Diffusion System

Formulation. The goal of the present system is to assign to each location a class label from a set of n classes. We first assign each location a state vector $\boldsymbol{x} \in S^n$, where $S^n = \{(x_1, x_2, ..., x_n)|x_i \geq 0, \sum_i x_i = 1\}$ is called n simplex. Each component in the state vector gives a normalized fitness of the particular class. The closer the state value is to *1*, the more fitting the location is to the class. Initially, the class assignment is ambiguous and contaminated with noise in the observation. We then use the competition-diffusion system to filter out the noise and bring one dominant value in the state vector representation at each location. The final segmentation is obtained by assigning the dominant class to each location. The diffusion process brings good spatial coherence to the segmentation map, and the competition process selects the most fitted label and prevents the diffusion process from oversmoothing the state vector representation.

Associated with $\boldsymbol{x}$ is a spatial coordinate vector $\boldsymbol{r} \in \Gamma$ where Γ is some manifold in 3-dimension. Let Φ be the space of functions, $\Gamma \to S^n$, and we consider the following initial value problem.

$$\dot{\boldsymbol{x}}(\boldsymbol{r}, t) = \begin{pmatrix} \dot{x}_1(\boldsymbol{r}, t) \\ \dot{x}_2(\boldsymbol{r}, t) \\ \vdots \\ \dot{x}_n(\boldsymbol{r}, t) \end{pmatrix} = \begin{pmatrix} g_1(\boldsymbol{x}(\boldsymbol{r}, t)) \\ g_2(\boldsymbol{x}(\boldsymbol{r}, t)) \\ \vdots \\ g_n(\boldsymbol{x}(\boldsymbol{r}, t)) \end{pmatrix} + \mu \begin{pmatrix} H(\boldsymbol{x}(\boldsymbol{r}, t)) \\ H(\boldsymbol{x}(\boldsymbol{r}, t)) \\ \vdots \\ H(\boldsymbol{x}(\boldsymbol{r}, t)) \end{pmatrix} \tag{1}$$

$$\boldsymbol{x}(\boldsymbol{r}, 0) = \boldsymbol{x}_0 \in \Phi \tag{2}$$

where $\dot{x}$ is the time derivative of x, the first term in the right hand side is a competition term, the second term is a diffusion term, and μ is a positive number that balances the competition term and the diffusion term. We call g_i a component-wise inhibition operator $(g_i : S^n \to [0, 1])$ and $\boldsymbol{g} = [g_1, g_2, ..., g_n]^T$ a competition operator $(G : S^n \to S^n)$. H is a general form of a linear diffusion operator. Our motivation is to encourage spatial homogeneity in the segmentation with the diffusion term and to bring a dominant class at each pixel with the competition term.

We consider a component wise inhibition operator of the following form:

$$g_i(\boldsymbol{x}) = x_i \left(f_i(\boldsymbol{x}) - \bar{f}(\boldsymbol{x}) \right) \tag{3}$$

where f_i is a fitness function of the ith class, and

$$\bar{f}(\boldsymbol{x}) = \sum_i x_i f_i(\boldsymbol{x}) \tag{4}$$

is the average fitness. Equation (3) is often called a replicator equation and has been used to model ecological progression among multiple species. With a suitable choice of the fitness functions, the population of the species reaches an equilibrium state where the multiple species coexist. On the other hand, by choosing another set of fitness functions, we can derive a state where only one species survives or dominates. In our state space representation, it corresponds to the state where $x_i = 1$ and $x_j = 0$, $\forall j \neq i$. We call this a *mutually exclusive state*. We call the state *internal* when $x_i > 0$ $\forall i$. For our segmentation problem, we want to derive a state vector representation at each location with one dominant component. We call the state *dominant* when there exists a class whose state value is strictly the largest. The dominant state may not necessarily be a mutually exclusive one as the diffusion force prevents it from reaching the state at the boundary between different classes.

Let us first list properties of the above initial value problem. Their proof can be found in [15].

- If $\boldsymbol{x}(0) \in \Phi$, then $\boldsymbol{x}(t) \in \Phi$, $\forall t > 0$.
- If f_i is Lipschitz continuous, then the initial value problem of (1) has a unique solution.
- A mutually exclusive state is a stable fixed point if at the fixed point $f_i > f_{j \neq i}$ and $f_i > 0$ where i is the dominant class.
- An internal fixed point is unstable when the fitness function is linear, symmetric and positive definite.

When we use linear fitness function, then the Lipschitz condition is satisfied. The condition of the third item is satisfied if the diagonal elements of the fitness matrix are positive and larger than any of the off-diagonal elements in their respective columns. Thus, to draw a unique solution with a dominant class at every location, we use a linear fitness function with a fitness matrix of $\boldsymbol{M}$ that is symmetric, positive, and $M_{ii} > M_{ij}$ $\forall i$. The fitness function is

$$f_i(\boldsymbol{x}) = (\boldsymbol{M}\boldsymbol{x})_i \tag{5}$$

with $(\boldsymbol{v})_i$ being the ith component of a vector $\boldsymbol{v}$. The solution gives a dominant class at each location except in degenerate cases when $\boldsymbol{x}(\boldsymbol{r})$ reaches a configuration that is constant everywhere and is also a fixed point at every $\boldsymbol{r}$.

Nodule Segmentation. We use CD to extract nodules, vessels, and other bright foreground structures. For solitary nodules, this step extracts them reliably. For non-solitary nodules, we further apply the robust Gaussian ellipsoid fit to separate nodules from the attached structures.

For nodule segmentation, we provide two classes: background (class 1) and foreground (class 2) that includes nodules, vessels, and other pulmonary structures. Hence $n = 2$. An important design issue for applying CD to a particular segmentation task is the initialization of $\boldsymbol{x}$ ($\boldsymbol{x}_0$ in (1)). we choose the following formula for segmenting pulmonary nodules.

$$x_2(\boldsymbol{r}) = e^{-2(1-\min(1, I(\boldsymbol{r})/1000))^2} \tag{6}$$

$$x_1(\boldsymbol{r}) = 1 - x_1(\boldsymbol{r}) \tag{7}$$

where $I(\boldsymbol{r})$ denotes the CT value of the input volume at $\boldsymbol{r}$, and 1000 is near the upper CT value of non-calcified pulmonary nodules. Hence for voxels with $I \geq$

1000, $x_2 = 1$ and $x_0 = 0$. For voxels with $I < 1000$, x_2 decreases monotonically as I deviates from 1000 while x_1 increases. x_2 takes the minimum value of e^{-2} when $I = 0$. Another design issue is the fitness matrix. We use a 2 by 2 identity matrix which satisfies the above condition for assuring dominant states.

It is convenient to have different time steps for the competition term and the diffusion term in (1). This is equivalent to having spatially variant μ in (1). We use $0.5\bar{f}$ for the time step of the competition term and 0.5 for the diffusion term. Using a linear isotropic diffusion, (1) can be discretized as

$$x_i(\boldsymbol{r}, n+1) = 0.5 \frac{x_i(\boldsymbol{r}, n) f_i(\boldsymbol{x}(\boldsymbol{r}, n))}{\bar{f}(\boldsymbol{x}(\boldsymbol{r}, n))} + 0.5 \bar{x}_i(\boldsymbol{r}, n) \qquad (8)$$

where $\bar{x}$ is the average value of the six-neighbors. For our experiments, we repeat the iteration for four times, with which one class emerges as a dominant one over the other at each voxel.

2.2   Robust Gaussian Ellipsoid Fit

This technique robustly fits a 3D anisotropic Gaussian function to the nodule's intensity distribution in a multiscale fashion, given a marker positioned near a target nodule. An ellipsoid that approximates the nodule's boundary is derived as a specific iso-level or equal-probability contour of the fitted Gaussian. Various nodule size features (e.g., maximum diameter, volume, sphericity) are computed analytically from radii of the ellipsoid. The multiscale analysis is given by i) performing a robust mean shift-based Gaussian model fitting for each of Gaussian scale space images constructed over a set of discrete analysis scales, and ii) find the most stable estimate among the multiscale model estimates by minimizing a form of Jensen Shannon divergence used as a stability criterion. The solution is efficient because the mean shift formulation removes the explicit construction of the Gaussian scale space that are computationally expensive.

At each scale, the nodule center location as Gaussian mean is estimated by the convergence of the scale space mean shift procedures. In the neighborhood of this estimated mean, local data analysis is performed by the mean shift procedures initialized at a set of neighboring points. The anisotropic tumor spread as Gaussian covariance is estimated by a constrained least-squares solution of a linear system constructed with the convergent mean shift vectors. Using information only from the convergent vectors facilitates the robustness, removing outlier samples from the above estimation framework. Due to this, the solution is effective for segmenting wall- or vessel-attached cases. In our experiment, we followed the parameter settings recommended in [8]. The scale space is conceived with 18 analysis scales with 0.25 interval $(0.5^2, .., 4.75^2)$. And 35% 3D confidence ellipsoid is used for deriving an equal-probability contour from the fitted Gaussian. This confidence threshold was determined experimentally.

2.3   Local Distribution Maximum

The technique applies thresholding at multiple levels followed by connected component analysis on each thresholded volume. It then searches for objects and their *plateaus* in the multiple thresholded volumes. The search starts from the volume with the highest threshold value and moves to ones with lower threshold values sequentially. A new object is found when a connected component has no overlaps to components in the previous volume. An object becomes a plateau when the ratio between the volume of the object and the volume of its bounding box suddenly decreases by more than some fraction (say η) or the object merges with another plateau. Important parameters of the method are the threshold values and η. In our experiment, we set $\eta = 1/30$ following the recommendation in [14] and set 12 threshold levels between 0 and 1100 with an increment of 100.

3   Diameter Estimation

According to the I-ELCAP protocol [7], "the diameter of a nodule is estimated as the average length and width where length is measured on a single CT image that shows the maximum length; and width is defined as the longest perpendicular to the length." Typically, the CT image is selected along the axial direction, due mainly to high-resolution and isotropic nature of the axial view. We follow closely with the protocol to estimate the diameter from the segmentation.

For LDM and CD, the diameter of a nodule is estimated as follows. After the segmentation and connected component analysis, the component that is closest to the marker is selected as the target nodule. In most cases, the marker is contained within the component, but in some cases, it lies on the background due to inaccurate marker positioning. Next, the component is analyzed slice by slice in the axial view. For each axial slice, 2-dimensional connected component analysis is performed, an ellipse is fitted to each component, and the geometrical mean of the axes is recorded for each ellipse. Among all 2-dimensional connected components, we select the one with the maximum geometrical mean for diameter measurement. The diameter is then estimated as the average width and height of the bounding box enclosing the selected component. Use of the geometrical mean instead of an arithmetic mean gives a slightly better agreement with the ground-truth.

For EF, the diameter is estimated as follows. First, an ellipsoid directly derived from the estimated covariance is projected on the axial plane, and then the radii of the ellipse on the projection plane is computed. The diameter is estimated as the arithmetic mean of the radii times the scaling constant of 1.6416, corresponding to the 35% confidence limit.

4   Hybrid Method

When a nodule is attached to another structure, CD will segment both of them together and result in a large over-estimated volume. This segmented volume usually stretches out to the boundary of the bounding volume (21x21x21 in our experiments). This observation leads to a simple test for the nodule type. If the segmentation volume touches one of six boundaries of the bounding volume, it is considered non-solitary. Otherwise, it is considered solitary. We can also compute the ratio between the segmentation volume and the volume of the bounding box enclosing the segmentation to check if the segmentation has a reasonably spherical shape. In our experiments, we only used the boundary check to determine if the nodule is solitary.

By using this solitary/non-solitary check of a nodule with CD segmentation, we implement a hybrid approach to the diameter estimation problem. For each given marker, a sub-volume of 21x21x21 voxels is extracted. CD segmentation is then applied to the volume, followed by the boundary check. If the boundary check indicates the nodule to be solitary, we apply the diameter estimation by the CD segmentation. Otherwise, we apply EF on the sub-volume and estimate the diameter. This hybrid approach is denoted by HB in the rest of the paper.

5   Experiments

In this section, we evaluate the performance of HB in comparison to EF, LDM and CD. We use 1349 nodules taken from over 240 CT volumes for the evaluation. Certified radiologists placed markers by eye-appraisal, resulting in at least one marker for each nodule. A 21x21x21 bounding volume is used as an input. The ground-truth diameter for each nodule is measured by human experts (both radiologists and scientists in the medical imaging field) following the IELCAP protocol.

First, we qualitatively evaluate the segmentation results of EF, LDM and CD. Figures 5(a)-(l) show some illustrative examples of segmentation results and their diameter estimates. In each figure, the left, middle and right images are the result's axial slices for EF, LDM and CD, respectively. The location of the slice is at the center of the ellipsoid computed by EF. The EF results are displayed by an ellipse (conic) on the cutting plane with the original data superimposed. The first number at the top-left corner is the ground-truth and the second number is the EF's estimate. The numbers in the LDM and CD results are the respective estimates.

As stated in Section 1, EF has difficulties in processing small nodules. This is observed in Figures 5(g)-(h). EF can also segment a part of the surrounding background as a nodule, leading to an over-estimation of the diameter as shown in Figure 5(h). A problem associated with LDM is its sensitivity to the pre-determined threshold levels, which are typically set by a fixed increment. The segmentation of an object becomes inaccurate when the intensity distribution of the object has an overlap with the distribution of its plateau. This can be observed in Figures 5(i)-(j). The degree and the frequency of the problem can be reduced by increasing the number of threshold levels, but at the cost of increasing the computational load. CD is effective in estimating the diameter of solitary nodules. However, the technique is not applicable to nodules attached to other structures such as the lung wall as seen in Figures 5(k)-(l).

Next, the estimation accuracy is quantitatively evaluated with the ground-truth. According to the CD-based boundary test, there are 614 solitary and 735 non-solitary nodules in the data set. We first evaluate the performance of EF,

LDM and CD separately for the two types of nodules. The squared difference between the estimates and the corresponding ground-truth is used as error metric. Figures 2-3 show the results for solitary and non-solitary cases, respectively.

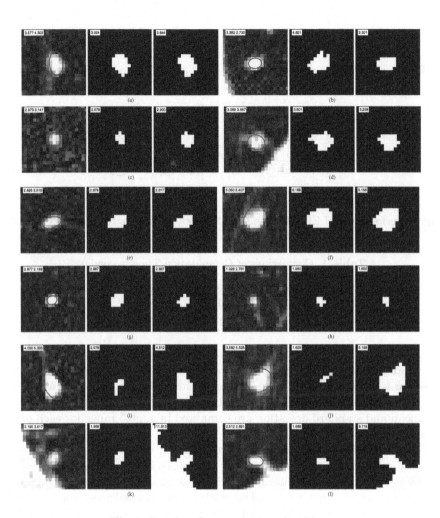

Fig. 1. Results of segmentation algorithms

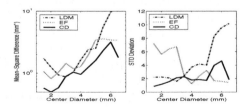

Fig. 2. Estimation performance of EF, LDM and CD for solitary nodules

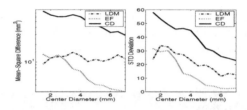

Fig. 3. Estimation performance of EF, LDM and CD for non-solitary nodules

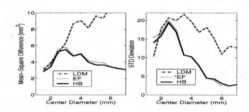

Fig. 4. Performance of EF, LDM and HB for both solitary and non-solitary nodules

Table 1. Comparison of Computation Time (seconds)

Method	EF	LDM	CD	HB
mean	1.26	0.269	0.0510	0.651
std	0.25	0.18	0.014	0.7

The mean is shown in log scale to improve the visibility of the plots while the deviation is shown in linear scale. The error statistics are computed as a function of the diameter sampled discretely between 1 and 7 with a 0.5mm interval. The mean and standard deviation are computed in a ±0.5 range for each of the center diameter.

For solitary nodules, the error tends to positively correlate with the diameter. Thus the squared difference error can be normalized by the corresponding center diameter for better interpretation. CD is more accurate than EF and LDM across all sizes except at 3mm where LDM with 0.2913 normalized-error is slightly better than CD with 0.2972 normalized-error. For non-solitary nodules, CD is the least accurate and EF is the most accurate one. For EF and CD, the error tends to negatively correlate with the diameter while it stays around $2.5mm^2$ for LDM. The large error by CD is due to the over-segmentation problem.

Next, the performance of HB is evaluated using both nodule types together. Figure 4 shows the mean and the standard deviation of the squared difference errors in linear scale for EF, LDM and HB using the same diameter ranges as in Figures 2-3. HB constantly gives a smaller error than other methods in all sizes. This is not a surprising result; HB analyzes the solitary and non-solitary nodules by CD and EF whose accuracy in their respective categories has been verified above. Table 1 summarizes the computational efficiency of each estimation technique computed as the mean and standard deviation over 1349 nodules. The results indicate that CD is computationally most efficient while EF is most expensive. HB is about 50% faster than EF.

6 Conclusion

We introduced a new pulmonary nodule size/diameter estimation technique that combined robust Gaussian ellipsoid fit (EF) and competition-diffusion segmentation (CD). The technique first uses CD to separate foreground structures from the background, and applies EF if necessary to separate a nodule from attachment. If the nodule is solitary, the CD step alone is sufficient. A simple test on the CD segmentation accurately separates solitary and non-solitary cases.

Our experiments show that this hybrid method outperforms EF, CD and Local Density Maximum. For solitary nodules (see Figure 2), the mean-square difference error between the estimates and the ground-truth is 1.19 mm^2 with EF and 0.73 mm^2 with CD: a 35% reduction. The hybrid method is also twice as fast as EF.

References

1. van Ginneken, B., ter Harr Romeny, B.M., Viergever, M.A.: Computer-aided diagnosis in chest radiography: A survey. IEEE TMI **20** (2001) 1228–1241
2. Reeves, A.P., Kostis, W.J.: Computer-aided diagnosis of small pulmonary nodules. Seminars in Ultrasound, CT, and MRI **21** (2000) 116–128
3. Ko, J.P., Naidich, D.P.: Computer-aided diagnosis and the evaluation of lung disease. J. Thorac Imaging **19** (2004) 136–155
4. Armato, S., et al.: Computerized detection of pulmonary nodules on CT scans. RadioGraphics **19** (1999) 1303–1311
5. Fan, L., Novak, C., Qian, J., Kohl, G., Naidich, D.: Automatic detection of lung nodules from multi-slice low-dose CT images. In: SPIE Med. Imag. (2001)
6. Lee, Y., et al.: Automated detection of pulmonary nodules in helical CT images based on an improved template-matching technique. IEEE TMI **20** (2001) 595–604
7. Henschke, C.I., et al.: CT screening for lung cancer: Frequency and significance of part-solid and nonsolid nodules. Am. J. Roentgen. **178** (2002) 1053–1057
8. Okada, K., Comaniciu, D., Krishnan, A.: Robust anisotropic Gaussian fitting for volumetric characterization of pulmonary nodules in multislice CT. IEEE TMI **24** (2005) 409– 423
9. Kubota, T., Espinal, F.: Reaction-diffusion systems for hypothesis propagation. In: ICPR00. (2000) Vol III: 547–550
10. Pelillo, M.: The dynamics of nonlinear relaxation labeling processes. Journal of Mathematical Imaging and Vision **7** (1997) 309–323
11. Carpenter, G.A., Grossberg, S.: A massively parallel architecture for a self-organizing neural pattern recognition machine. Computer Vision, Graphics, and Image Processing **37** (1987) 54–115
12. Tek, H., Kimia, B.: Volumetric segmentation of medical images by three-dimensional bubbles. CVIU **64** (1997) 246–258

13. Zhu, S., Mumford, D.: Prior learning and gibbs reaction-diffusion. PAMI **19** (1997) 1236–1250
14. Zhao, B., Gamsu, G., Ginsberg, M.S., Jiang, L., Schwartz, L.H.: Automatic detection of small lung nodules on CT utilizing a local density maximum algorithm. Journal of Applied Clinical Medical Physics **4** (2003) 248–260
15. Kubota, T., Okada, K.: Competition-diffusion and its properties. Technical report, Siemens Medical Solutions USA, CAD Solutions (2005)

Fast 3D Brain Segmentation Using Dual-Front Active Contours with Optional User-Interaction

Hua Li[1,2], Anthony Yezzi[1], and Laurent D. Cohen[3]

[1] School of ECE, Georgia Institute of Technology, Atlanta, GA, USA
[2] Dept. of Elect. & Info. Eng., Huazhong Univ. of Sci. & Tech., Wuhan, P.R. China
[3] CEREMADE, UMR 7534 University Paris-Dauphine, 75775 Paris Cedex France
hua.li@ece.gatech.edu

Abstract. Important attributes of 3D brain segmentation algorithms include robustness, accuracy, computational efficiency, and facilitation of user interaction, yet few algorithms incorporate all of these traits. Manual segmentation is highly accurate but tedious and laborious. Most automatic techniques, while less demanding on the user, are much less accurate. It would be useful to employ a fast automatic segmentation procedure to do most of the work but still allow an expert user to interactively guide the segmentation to ensure an accurate final result.

We propose a novel 3D brain cortex segmentation procedure utilizing dual-front active contours, which minimize image-based energies in a manner that yields more global minimizers compared to standard active contours. The resulting scheme is not only more robust but much faster and allows the user to guide the final segmentation through simple mouse clicks which add extra seed points. Due to the global nature of the evolution model, single mouse clicks yield corrections to the segmentation that extend far beyond their initial locations, thus minimizing the user effort. Results on 15 simulated and 20 real 3D brain images demonstrate the robustness, accuracy, and speed of our scheme compared with other methods.

1 Introduction

Three dimensional image segmentation is an important problem in medical image analysis. Determining the location of the cortical surface of the human brain from MRI imagery is often the first step in brain visualization and analysis. Due to the geometric complexity of the brain cortex, manual slice by slice segmentation is quite difficult and time consuming. Thus, many automatic segmentation methods have been proposed which eliminate or nearly eliminate user interaction.

The active contour model has been widely applied in medical imaging, which was introduced in [1] as the "snakes" and is an energy minimization method. Malladi and Sethian [2] showed the initial contributions on 3D segmentation of medical images, after that, numerous contributions [3,4,5,6,7,8] have been made on the segmentation of complex brain cortical surfaces.

These methods used the active contour model as the final step for the cortex segmentation, applied geometric and anatomical constraints and/or utilized

Y. Liu, T. Jiang, and C. Zhang (Eds.): CVBIA 2005, LNCS 3765, pp. 335–345, 2005.

significant pre-processing of the data to obtain desirable final segmentations. Furthermore, curve evolution process in these methods are very time-consuming.

Some other methods were also proposed for brain segmentation, such as fuzzy set methods [9,10], Bayesian Methods [11], Markov random field methods [12,13,14], expectation-maximization (EM) algorithm [15] and so on. These methods were aimed at segmenting the brain tissues automatically, and limiting the user interaction to choosing the parameters of the automatic process, setting initial surfaces for surface evolution, or restricting regions to be processed. It is usually impossible or very difficult and unintuitive for experts to guide the segmentation process with their professional knowledge for improving the accuracy of the final result. In our opinion, methods that allow simple and intuitive user interaction (while minimizing the need for such interaction as much as possible) are more useful than totally automatic methods given the importance of high accuracy and detail in cortical segmentation.

In this paper, we propose a novel 3D brain cortex segmentation scheme based on dual-front active contours which are faster and yield more global image-based energy minimizers compared to other active contours models. This scheme also adapts easily to user interaction, making it very convenient for experts to guide the segmentation process by adding useful seed points with simple mouse clicks. This scheme is very fast and the total computation time is less than 20 seconds. Experimental results on 15 simulated and 20 real 3D brain images demonstrate the robustness of the result, the high reconstruction accuracy, and the low computational cost compared with other methods.

2   Cortex Segmentation by Dual-Front Active Contours

2.1   3D Brain Cortex Segmentation with Flexible User-Interaction

The basic idea of dual-front active contour model is proposed by the authors in [16] for detecting the object boundaries. Using this model, the segmentation objective is achieved by iteratively dilating the initial curve to form a narrow region and then finding the new closest potential weighted minimal partition curve inside by dual front evolution.

Due to the complex and convoluted nature of the cortex and the partial volume effects of MRI imaging, the segmentation of cortex must be considered in three dimensions. Here we propose the 3D brain cortex segmentation scheme based on the dual-front active contours. This scheme is simple, fast, and accurate with flexible user-interaction. In Fig 1, we show an overall diagram of this scheme. And we will give the details about choosing the active region and the potentials in the following subsection.

2.2   Active Region and Potentials Decision By Histogram Analysis

The original dual front active contours use morphological dilation to form the narrow active region from an initial curve. In fact, this is just one way to obtain

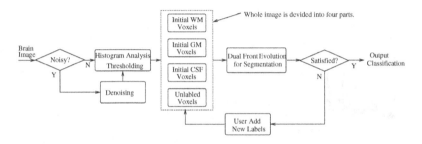

Fig. 1. Overall diagram of 3D brain cortex segmentation process

the active region, we may use some other methods to define the active regions for a given segmentation, or class of images. And for the 3D brain tissue segmentation, the morphological dilatation is not a good solution because of the complex and convoluted structure of cortex. It is possible that the labels of some tiny and convoluted parts may be changed during dilation, and this will affect the result's accuracy.

In this subsection, we give a simple way to decide the active region by analyzing the histogram of the MRI normal brain image. The Fig. 2 shows the histogram analysis of the three tissues in brain: CSF, GM, and WM. Panel (a) is the histogram of a sample 3D MRI elderly brain image. There are three peaks and two bottoms in the histogram. These three peaks approximate to the average mean value of the three tissues. In fact, the neighborhoods of these two bottoms correspond to the voxels located around the boundary of different tissues. Because of the partial volume effect, it is hard to separate these voxels just by simple thresholding. We treat these voxels as unlabeled voxels, and use dual-front evolution to separate them.

As shown in the Panel (b) of Fig. 2, by setting different thresholds, the whole 3D image may be divided into GM seeds, WM seeds, CSF seeds, background points, and unlabeled voxels which are the voxels within the two regions R_1 and R_2 around these two bottoms. Background points are ignored for the computation. For the image with high noise level, we will smooth it first, then calculate the histogram and divide it.

Now, for the potentials for different labeled curves, we use region-based information for guiding the fronts' evolution. We calculate the mean values u_{CSF}, u_{GM} and u_{WM}, the variance values σ^2_{CSF}, σ^2_{GM} and σ^2_{WM}, of the three different kind of voxels with different labels l_{CSF}, l_{GM} and l_{WM}. Then the propagation potentials for the labeled points (x, y) are decided by

$$\widetilde{P}_l(x,y) = w_1 \cdot \exp(-\frac{|\overline{I}(x,y) - u_l|^2}{2\sigma_l^2}) + w_2 \quad \text{if} L(x,y) = l(l_{CSF}, l_{GM}, l_{WM}), \quad (1)$$

where $\overline{I}(x, y)$ is the average value of the image intensity in a window of size 3×3 centered at the examined point.

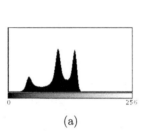
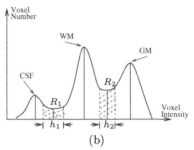

(a)   (b)

Fig. 2. The active region location is decided by the histogram analysis and thresholding of the 3D MRI brain image. (a): the histogram of a sample 3D MRI brain image; (b): the center of R_1 is the bottom between the peaks of CSF and WM, the center of R_2 is the bottom between the peaks of CSF and WM. h_1 and h_2 decide the size of R_1 and R_2.

3 Experimental Results

In this section, we show validations of our approach on various 3D simulated and real MRI brain image data sets. We use $T1$-weighted images for our test because they provide the best gray/white contrast and are commonly used for neuroanatomical analysis. All the experimental results shown in this section are obtained from 3D volume process directly.

To evaluate the efficiency of our method for every tissue type T (GM, WM, and CSF), four probability measures are defined by equation

$$TP = \frac{N_B \cap N_R}{N_R}, FN = \frac{N_R - N_B \cap N_R}{N_R}, FP = \frac{N_B - N_B \cap N_R}{N_R}, OM = \frac{TP}{1 + FP}, \quad (2)$$

where N_R is the number of reference ground truth voxels of tissue T. N_B is the number of voxels detected by our algorithm as the voxels of tissue T.

3.1 Validation on Simulated MR Brain Data

In Fig. 3, we present the results of the segmented WM tissues for five different slices of one 3D simulated brain image provided by BrainWeb [17]. We use the potentials defined by Eq. 1 with $\omega_1 = 1$ and $\omega_2 = 0.1$. The size of R_1, h_1, is equal to 20, the size of R_2, h_2, is equal to 10 (see the Fig. 2).

In Table 1, we also give the comparison of the GM segmentation results on the same 3D simulated image of our scheme and other three methods, the fuzzy C-means method [18] implemented by ourselves, the Hidden Markov Method [12] provided by the website of FMRIB Software Library(http://www.fmrib.ox.ac.uk/fsl/), and the coupled surface algorithm reported in [7].

In Fig. 4, the 3D models of segmented GM and WM surfaces from our method, and the ground truth data are also shown. From these segmentation results and comparison results, we can see that our scheme performs better than

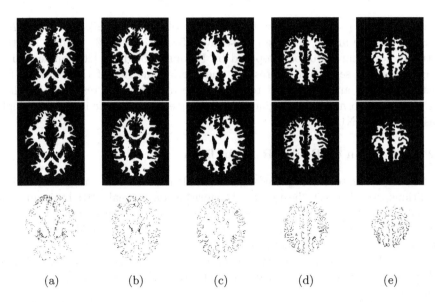

(a)   (b)   (c)   (d)   (e)

Fig. 3. Comparison of the segmentation results from our method with the ground truth data of five slices of one 3D simulated brain image provided by BrainWeb [17], which is $T1$ modality, $1mm$ slice thickness, 3% noise level, 20% INU. And the image size is $181 \times 217 \times 181$.

The top row presents the segmentation results obtained from our method; the middle row shows the ground truth data provided by BrainWeb database; the bottom row shows the difference between the segmentation results from our method and the ground truth data. These five columns correspond to five slices of the test 3D image.

Table 1. Comparison of the gray matter segmentation results of our method with some other methods on one 3D simulated brain image, which is the same one as that in Fig. 3

Rate	Fuzzy C-means Method	Hidden Markov Method	Coupled Surface Algorithm	Dual-Front Active Contours
TP (%)	87.3	92.3	92.8	93.3
FN (%)	12.7	7.7	7.2	6.7
FP (%)	23.2	5.7	6.0	5.6
Overlap Metric	0.708	0.873	0.875	0.883
Time (s)	373	500	3600	15

the other three methods in the accuracy of result and the computational efficiency.

We also test our method on 15 3D simulated brain images provided by Brain-Web [17,19], which are $T1$ modality, $1mm$ slice thickness, different noise levels 1%, 3%, 5%, 7%, and 9%, and different INU settings 0%, 20%, and 40%. All images are the same size of $181 \times 217 \times 181$. We still use the potentials defined by Eq. 1 with $\omega_1 = 1$ and $\omega_2 = 0.1$. The size of R_1, h_1, is 20, the size of R_2, h_2 is 10. For the image with high noise levels 5%, 7%, and 9%, we first use the isotropic nonlinear diffusion proposed by Perona and Malik [20] for denoising images. For the segmentation results, the overlap metrics of three tissues for these 15 images are from 0.747 to 0.944. The measurement results show that our scheme performs well in segmenting the cortex even for the image with high noise level and INU setting.

3.2 Validation on Real MR Brain Data

To further evaluate our segmentation method under a wide range of imaging conditions, we also test the proposed algorithm on 20 real MRI brain images and compare the segmentation results with the manual segmentation by experts and some other segmentation methods. The 20 normal MR brain data sets and their manual segmentations were provided by the Center for Morphometric Analysis at Massachusetts General Hospital and are available at ISBR website http://www.cma.mgh.harvard.edu/ibsr/.

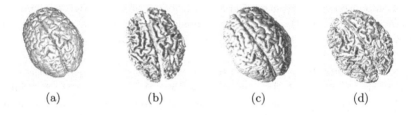

(a)   (b)   (c)   (d)

Fig. 4. Comparison of the 3D models of the GM and WM surfaces from our method and from the ground truth data. The test image is the same one as that in Fig. 3. (a) and (b) are the 3D models of the GM and WM surfaces obtained from our method; (c) and (d) are the 3D models of the GM and WM surfaces from the ground truth.

Fig. 5 shows the overlap metric, the average overlap metric of the CSF, GM and WM segmentation results on 20 normal brains, from the manual method, various automatic segmentation results provided by ISBR, the hidden Markov method [12] provided by the website of FMRIB Software Library (http://www.fmrib.ox.ac.uk/fsl/), and our proposed scheme. For the segmentation of these real brain images, we still use the potentials defined by Eq. 1 with $\omega_1 = 1$ and $\omega_2 = 0.1$. The size of R_1, h_1, is 20, the size of R_2, h_2, is 10. For these 20 brain images, the histograms are not as that shown in Fig. 2, we need to choose the two bottoms manually. So how to decide the two bottoms automatically need further research.

In this comparison with other segmentation methods, except for the methods provided by ISBR [21], we also compare our method with the other three recently proposed methods, the Bayesian method proposed in [11] (MPM-MAP); the couple-surface algorithm [7] (ZENG), and the hidden Markov method [12]

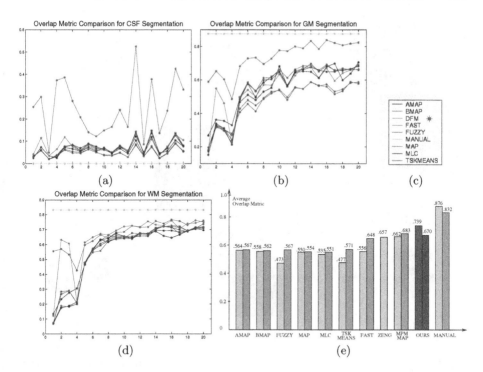

Fig. 5. The overlap metric of the CSF, GM, and WM segmentation results on 20 normal real brain images from various segmentation methods. The results of some automatic segmentation methods provided by ISBR. AMAP: adaptive MAP; BMAP: biased MAP; FUZZY: fuzzy c-means; MAP: Maximum Aposteriori Probability; MLC: Maximum-Likelihood; TSKMEANS: tree-structure k-means; FAST: Hidden Markov method [12]; MPM-MAP: the Bayesian method proposed in [11]; ZENG: the couple-surface algorithm [7]; DFM: our scheme.

(FAST). But with the rapid development of the medical image processing technology, it is impossible to compare all the related methods and test our methods on all the real brain images. This study is just the initial step of our research work on brain image analysis. We will still work on it, and improve the model's robustness and the segmentation's accuracy.

3.3 Simple and Useful User Interaction

The above two subsections show the segmentation result of our scheme with automatic thresholding only. Furthermore, our scheme is very convenient for users to add simple seed points just by mouse clicks to improve the segmentation accuracy dramatically. Fig. 6 gives an example of this nice property.

In Fig. 6, the first row shows one slice of the test 3D image (Panel (a)) which is the same as that in Fig. 3, the ground truth data of the WM tissue (Panel (b))

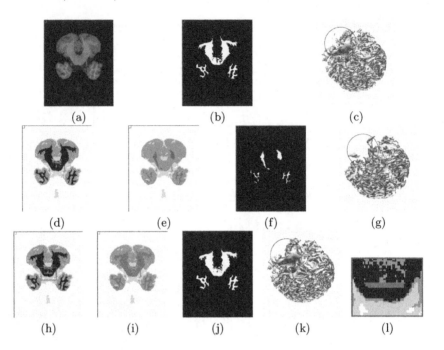

Fig. 6. The simple user interaction can improve the segmentation accuracy dramatically. The blue line in figure (l) is the zoom-in of the user added seed points in figure(h). The difference of the segmentation result from the automatic thresholding (fig.(g)), the automatic thresholding with manual correction (fig.(k)), and the ground truth (fig.(c)) are shown in the red circles of figure (c), (g), and (k).

in this slice, and the corresponding 3D model of the WM tissue (Panel (c)). The second row shows the segmentation result based on one automatic thresholding. When setting the active region according to the Fig. 2, if the region R_2 is shifted to high intensity region, and the size of R_2 is large, we get the different active region between WM and GM tissue. The black voxels in Panel (d) present the unlabeled voxels after setting this threshold, and the different labeled voxels (shown in the figures with different colors) present different tissues' seed points. After segmentation, the WM tissue is shown in Panel (e), the 3D model of segmented WM is shown in Panel (g). Here we can see, if automatic thresholding cannot provide enough WM seed points, the segmented WM tissue is incorrect. In this case, the third row shows the segmentation result after user interaction. As shown in Panel (h), the user interaction is just several mouse clicks within seconds to add some new seed points manually only on one slice, then we run the dual-front evolution again to segment GM and WM. The segmented boundary of GM/WM is shown in Panel (i), the extracted WM tissue and the corresponding 3D model are shown in Panel (j) and Panel (k). The figures show that the accuracy of the result after user interaction is much better than that just based on automatic thresholding. This sample shows that our method allow the simple user-interaction, we will still research on the efficiency of the user-interaction.

3.4   Computational Time

Another nice property of our methods is the high computational efficiency. We test our method on 15 simulated 3D MR brain images and 20 real normal 3D MR brain images. The average total computation time is around 20 seconds, in which the average computational time for the histogram analysis is around 5 seconds and the average computational time for dual front evolution is around 15 seconds, on the 2.5 GHz Pentium4 PC processor.

We downloaded the software of the Hidden Markovian method from the website of FMRIB Software Library (http://www.fmrib.ox.ac.uk/fsl/), and implemented the fuzzy C-means method [18] for the comparison with our method. On the same computer, the average computational time of Hidden Markovian method for the same test images used in our method is around 550 seconds, the average computational time of the fuzzy C-means method for the same images is around 450 seconds. The comparison shows that our method is much faster then these two methods. The average overlap metric for gray matter and white matter segmentation of these two methods are 0.473 and 0.567 from fuzzy C-means methods, 0.556 and 0.648 from Hidden Markov method, which are lower than that of 0.739 and 0.670 from our method.

Although the average overlap metric for white matter segmentation of the Bayesian method proposed in [11] on the same 20 real brain data sets is 0.683 (shown in Fig. 5), a little higher than that of 0.670 from our method, they reported that the computational time is around 280 seconds which is much slower than our methods.

Because many active contour model based methods always combined with some pre-processing methods such as fuzzy C-means, Bayesian segmentation, and etc. The active contour model is just implemented as the final step to yield the final cortical surface, it is hard for us to give an exact comparison. Here, we give the brief discussion about the computational time of some active contour model based methods.

Xu's method [6] combined the adaptive fuzzy C-means algorithm [9], they reported that the computational time for the final deformable surface algorithm is about 3 hours. As for the coupled surface method proposed by Zeng [7], it was reported that for a 3D image of the whole brain with the voxel size of $1.2 \times 1.2 \times 1.2mm^3$, their algorithm runs in about $1h$ on a SGI Inigo2 machine with a 195MHz R10000 processor for the implementation of skull stripping, cortex segmentation and measurement simultaneously. They also reported that the average overlap metric for gray matter segmentation on the same 20 normal brain images provided by ISBR is 0.657, which is lower than that of our method, 0.739. Goldenberg [8] also adopted the coupled surfaces principle and used the fast geodesic active contour approach to improve the computational time for cortex segmentation. They reported that the computational time of their method is about 2.5 mins for a $192 \times 250 \times 170$ MR image of the whole brain on a Pentium3 PC. But they did not give the quantitative analysis of the segmentation results.

4   Conclusions and Future Work

In this paper, we propose a novel scheme for 3D brain cortex segmentation based on dual-front active contours. The cortex segmentation results from the synthetic and real MR brain images, and the computation time compared with other methods demonstrate the high reconstruction accuracy, the low computational cost and the minimum user interaction of this scheme. In the future, our research work will focus on the following aspects.

First, our dual-front active contour model is very fast, and easy to be implemented, it is flexible to combine with other methods as the post-processing method and improve the segmentation accuracy further. We will work on the combination of the current model with some powerful INU bias compensation methods and smooth methods to improve the model's robustness.

Second, in this paper, we just use the region-based information to guide the curve evolution because the interfaces among difference tissues is not clear (because of the partial volume effect). We are also working on proposing some better local operators, and combine them with the region-based information in the potentials to improve the accuracy of the segmentation result further.

Third, our model can be generalized to multi-spectral data, which is very common in MR imaging. In this case, the voxel intensities are assume to be vectors instead of scalars, and how to design the potentials, and the thresholds need further investigation.

Fourth, we are working on finding the better methods to choose active region automatically for improving the method's generality.

This dual front active contour model provides a novel, simple idea for 3D brain tissue segmentation, and also has strong potential applications in other medical image analysis domains, where a volumetric layer is the study of interest. Examples include the left ventricular (LV) myocardium of the heart and the boundary of the liver.

References

1. Kass, M., Witkin, A., Terzopoulos, D.: Snakes: Active contour models. International Journal of Computer Vision 1 (1988) 321–332
2. Malladi, R., Sethian, J.: A geometric approach to segmentation and analysis of 3d medical images. In: Processings of Mathematical Methods in Biomedical Image Analysis, MMBIA'96. (1996)
3. Davatzikos, C., Bryan, R.: Using a deformable surface model to obtain a shape representation of the cortex. IEEE Trans. on Medical Imaging 15 (1996) 785–795
4. Teo, P., Sapiro, G., Wandell, B.: Creating connected representations of cortical gray matter for functional mri visualization. IEEE Trans. on Medical Imaging 16 (1997) 852–863

5. Dale, A., Fischl, B., Sereno, M.: Cortical surface-based analysis. NeuroImage **9** (1999) 179–194
6. Xu, C., Pham, D., Rettmann, M., Yu, D., Prince, J.: Reconstruction of the human cerebral cortex from magnetic resonance images. IEEE Trans. on Medical Imaging **18** (1999) 467–480
7. Zeng, X., Staib, L., Schultz, R., Duncan, J.: Segmentation and measurement of the cortex from 3D MR images using coupled surfaces propagation. IEEE Transactions on Medical Imaging **18** (1999) 100–111
8. Goldenberg, R., Kimmel, R., Rivlin, E., Rudzsky, M.: Cortex segmentation: A fast variational geometric approach. IEEE Trans. on Medical Imaging **21** (2002) 1544–1551
9. Pham, D., Prince, J.: Adaptive fuzzy segmentation of magnetic resonance images. IEEE Trans. on Medical Imaging **18** (1999) 737–752
10. Liew, A., Yan, H.: An adaptive spatial fuzzy clustering algorithm for 3d mr image segmentation. IEEE Trans. on Medical Imaging **22** (2003) 1063–1075
11. Marroquin, J., Vemuri, B., et al.: An accurate and efficient bayesian method for automatic segmentation of brain mri. IEE Trans. on Medical Imaging **21** (2002) 934–945
12. Zhang, Y., Brady, M., Smith, S.: Segmentation of brain mr images through a hidden markov random field model and the expectation maximization algorithm. IEEE Trans. on Medical Imaging **20** (2001) 45–57
13. Ruan, S., Moretti, B., Fadili, J., Bloyet, D.: Fuzzy markovian segmentation in application of magnetic resonance images. Computer Vision and Image Understanding **85** (2002) 54–69
14. Leemput, K.V., Maes, F., Vandermeulen, D., Suetens, P.: Automated model-based tissue classification of mr images of the brain. IEEE Trans. on Medical Imaging **18** (1999) 897–908
15. Kapur, T., Grimson, W., et al.: Segmentation of brain tissue from magnetic resonance images. Medical Image Analysis **1** (1996) 109–127
16. Li, H., Elmoataz, A., Fadili, J., Ruan, S.: Dual front evolution model and its application in medical imaging. In: MICCAI2004. Volume 3216., Rennes/Saint-Malo, France (2004) 103–110
17. BrainWeb: Mcconnell brain imaging center, montreal neurological institute. (http://www.bic.mni.mcgill.ca/brainweb/)
18. Bezdek, J.: Pattern Recognition with Fuzzy Objective Functions Algorithms. Plenum (1981)
19. Cocosco, C., Kollokian, V., Kwan, R., Evans, A.: Brainweb: Online interface to a 3D MRI simulated brain database. NeuroImage **5** (1997) S425
20. Perona, P., Malik, J.: Scale-space and edge detection using anisotropic diffusion. IEEE Trans. on PAMI **12** (1990) 629–639
21. Filipek, P., Richelme, C., Kennedy, D., Caviness, V.: The young adult human brain: an mri-based morphometric analysis. Cerebral Cortex **4** (1994) 344–360

Improved Motion Correction of fMRI Time-Series Corrupted with Major Head Movement Using Extended Motion-Corrected Independent Component Analysis

Rui Liao[1], Martin Mckeown[2], and Jeffrey Krolik[3]

[1] Siemens Corporate Research, Inc., 755 College Rd East, Princeton, NJ 08540, USA
[2] University of British Columbia, Vancouver, British Columbia, V6T 2B5, Canada
[3] Pratt School of Engineering, Duke University, Durham, NC 27708, USA

Abstract. An extension of previously-described Motion-Corrected Independent Component Analysis (MCICA) for improved correction of significant patient head motion in fMRI data is proposed. For fMRI time-points corrupted with relatively large motion, i.e. on the order of half a voxel, only partial images subject to minimal interpolation artifact are initially used in MCICA, allowing for an accurate estimation of the activation weights of the underlying ICA components. The remaining voxels that are irretrievably corrupted with gross motion in the motion-corrupted time-points are treated as missing data, so the final component maps of the ICA components are estimated from an optimally motionless reference ensemble. Interpolation artifact therefore is minimized in the final registered image, which can be mathematically expressed as a weighted combination of the extended reference ensemble. Experiments demonstrate that the proposed method was robust to the presence of simulated activation and the number of reference images used. While the previous version of MCICA already achieved noticeably decreased registration error than SPM and AIR, the proposed method further reduced the error by thirty percent when correcting simulated gross movements applied on real fMRI time-points. With a real fMRI time-series acquired during a motor-task, further increased mutual information and more clustered activation in the primary and supplementary motor areas were observed.

1 Introduction

A typical fMRI experimental session requires subjects to lay motionless during tens of minutes. Even cooperative subjects with head constraints may show both slow and unpredictable abrupt displacements of a millimeter or more. For very young, old, or ill subjects, the displacement could be significantly larger, i.e. several millimeters. Head motion can result in large signal changes that can be difficult to differentiate from changes due to true brain activation. When motion corresponds to the underlying task, misinterpretation of what signal changes are due to motion and what are due to changes in brain activation is a serious challenge [1].

We have recently proposed a novel method, named Motion-Corrected Independent Component Analysis (MCICA), for retrospective motion correction of fMRI time-

Y. Liu, T. Jiang, and C. Zhang (Eds.): CVBIA 2005, LNCS 3765, pp. 346–355, 2005.

series [2]. In contrast with the conventional registration approaches, MCICA has the advantage of incorporating multiple reference images in a practical manner for alignment purpose, which allows for brain activations present in an fMRI time-series to be implicitly modeled and hence will not interfere with motion estimation. Experiments demonstrated that compared to the LS-based similarity metric implemented in SPM and AIR, two widely-used registration packages [3] [4], MCICA was more robust to the addition of simulated activation and did not lead to detection of false activations after correction of simulated task-correlated motion. With actual fMRI data the time course of the derived continually task-related ICA component became more correlated with the underlying behavioral task after preprocessing with MCICA, and the associated activation map was more clustered in the expected area without spurious activation at the brain edge [6].

In MCICA, the final registered image is achieved by taking data-adaptive linear combinations of basis images, instead of using a non-adaptive general-purpose resampling kernel, which minimizes interpolation artifacts and provides potentially nonrigid-body motion correction [2]. To generate the basis images, a dense search in the limited range of the possible translation/rotation needed is performed. Although interpolation error is present in each basis image, it can be compensated to some degree by an optimal linear operator, i.e. the data-adaptive filter estimated by MCICA. It was demonstrated that for real fMRI data corrupted with artificial motion, the final registered image obtained by MCICA achieved higher fidelity to the original image, compared to the images obtained by SPM, AIR, or Cubic interpolation even with the perfectly known motion-compensation parameters (i.e. the inverse of the artificially applied rigid-body motion) [2].

Nevertheless, for images corrupted with relatively large motion, i.e., on the order of half a voxel, it has been observed that the interpolation artifact at the brain edge in the rotated/shifted basis images is too large to be sufficiently compensated by a linear combination of the basis images. Fig. 1 compares the errors in the intensity values caused by cubic interpolation with the known motion-compensation parameters (Fig. 1.a) and that produced by the Least-Mean-Square (LMS) combination of the rotated/shifted basis images (Fig. 1.b), for a real fMRI volume that was corrupted by an artificial 3D movement of mean discrepancy of 0.65 voxels when integrated over the brain. The registration error for each voxel is represented by the brightness (intensity) in the image. It can be seen that the error at the brain edge for the LMS solution using the rotated/shifted basis images is relatively high, although it becomes smaller (dimmer) than that caused by cubic interpolation.

In this paper, we suggest an extension of MCICA algorithm for improved compensation of relatively large motion effect in fMRI data. Specifically, for a time-point containing grossly corrupted data, some severely motion-affected voxels may be treated as missing data. Time courses of the underlying ICA components are estimated using only suitable subsets of voxels that are likely to be helpful for motion estimation, and corresponding component maps are estimated using extended optimally motionless reference ensemble. In essence, the final registered image is reconstructed as a weighted summation of the extended reference ensemble, instead of a weighted summation of the rotated/shifted basis images. Fig. 1.c displays the errors obtained by the LMS combination of the extended reference ensemble, which is clearly lower than that achieved for the LMS solution using the rotate/shifted basis images (Fig. 1.b). The summation of the extended reference ensemble using the weights estimated by the proposed method achieves comparable result (Fig. 1.d).

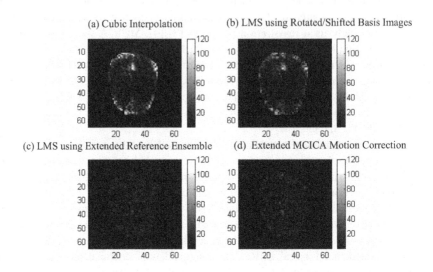

Fig. 1. Comparison of errors of cubic interpolation (a), LMS linear combination of rotated/shifted basis images (b), LMS linear combination of extended reference ensemble (c) and extended MCICA for large motion correction (d), for an image corrupted with motion of mean discrepancy of 0.65 voxels when integrated over the whole brain

2   Extended Motion-Corrected Independent Component Analysis

When ICA model $\mathbf{X} = \mathbf{AS}$ is applied to fMRI data analysis, the data matrix $\mathbf{X}$ (time-by-voxel) is formed by concatenating all voxel values in a volume acquired at a single time-point as a row vector, and then concatenating all such row vectors for the whole time-series along the column direction. It is assumed that the observed fMRI data are the linear sum of the contributions from several spatially independent processes. The component maps of the independent processes are collected as rows in the component map matrix $\mathbf{S}$ (component-by-voxel), and the corresponding activation courses are collected as columns in the time course matrix $\mathbf{A}$ (time-by-component). The objective of ICA is to determine the unmixing matrix $\mathbf{W}$, to achieve the time course estimation $\tilde{\mathbf{A}} = \mathbf{W}^{-1}$, and the component map estimation $\tilde{\mathbf{S}} = \mathbf{WX}$. With the Infomax algorithm [5], $\mathbf{W}$ is estimated by maximizing $H[\mathbf{Y}]$ where $H[\cdot]$ denotes the Shannon (joint) entropy of a random vector of which each row of $\mathbf{Y}$ is viewed as an independent realization, and $\mathbf{Y}$ is a nonlinear transformation of $\mathbf{X}$:

$$\mathbf{Y} = g\left(\tilde{\mathbf{S}}\right) = g(\mathbf{WX}) \tag{1}$$

For fMRI signals with super-Gaussian distributions, the nonlinear transfer function is typically chosen to be the logistic function $g(\tilde{s}) = \dfrac{1}{1+e^{-\tilde{s}}}$. It can be shown that,

$$H[\mathbf{Y}] = H[\mathbf{X}] + E\{\log|J|\} \qquad (2)$$

where $E\{\cdot\}$ denotes statistical expectation and $|J|$ is the absolute value of the determinant of the Jacobian matrix of the transformation from $\mathbf{X}$ to $\mathbf{Y}$.

The core idea of the MCICA algorithm is based on the observation that motion effects within fMRI data will result in an increase in $H[\mathbf{X}]$ and a decrease in $H[\mathbf{Y}]$ in Eq.(2) [2]. The entropy difference, $E\{\log|J|\}$, therefore can be used as the objective function to be maximized for motion mitigation of fMRI data. For an fMRI time-series, an appropriate number of optimally motionless time-points are selected as the reference ensemble (typically consisting of ten time-points in our applications). Each time-point in the time-series is then brought into alignment with the reference ensemble one by one. Specifically, in order to align one time-point denoted by the column-vector $\mathbf{x}_1$ (transpose of a given row in the data matrix $\mathbf{X}$), the proposed objective function, $E\{\log|J|\}$, is maximized for the following matrix with respect to the data-adaptive filter $\mathbf{p}$:

$$\mathbf{X}^r = \begin{bmatrix} \mathbf{R}^T\mathbf{p} & \mathbf{x}_2 & \cdots & \mathbf{x}_q \end{bmatrix}^T \qquad (3)$$

Here the column-vector $\mathbf{x}_i$ ($i = 2, \cdots, q$) represents the time-points that act as the 'reference ensemble', and $\mathbf{R}$ is the basis image matrix whose rows collect different translations and/or rotations of the time-point to be registered, $\mathbf{x}_1$, after gross alignment using the principal axes of activation method. Therefore in the previously-described MCICA algorithm in [2], the final registered image for the time-point $\mathbf{x}_1$ is obtained as $\mathbf{R}^T\mathbf{p}$, which is a linear sum of the rotated/shifted basis images weighted by the estimated data-adaptive filter $\mathbf{p}$.

In this paper we propose an extension of MCICA algorithm by exploiting the property that under the ICA model each voxel in the image is assumed to be independent. In particular, we can choose voxels that are likely to be helpful for motion estimation and discard other less suitable voxels. For images corrupted with large motion, we propose choosing voxels in a ring torus configuration as voxels near the center of mass will be largely unaffected by pure rotations, and the voxels at the brain edge may be affected by significant interpolation errors in the rotated/shifted basis images. This submatrix, $\mathbf{X}^r_{ICA}$, that contains the voxels in the ring torus region, is used in MCICA for an accurate estimation of the data-adaptive filter $\mathbf{p}$, the time course matrix $\mathbf{A} = \mathbf{W}^{-1}$, and the partial component maps for the ring torus region $\mathbf{S}^r_{ICA} = \mathbf{W}\mathbf{X}^r_{ICA}$.

We notice that it is not appropriate to apply the estimated data-adaptive filter $\mathbf{p}$ to all voxels in the volume to calculate the complete registered image because, as shown in Fig. 1.b, a linear summation of the rotated/shifted basis images is not sufficient to recover the voxels at the brain edge. Nevertheless, the time course matrix $\mathbf{A}$ obtained from the voxels in the ring torus region is common to all voxels. In another words, we have obtained the enhancement/suppression weights for the ICA components contributing to the time-point to be registered. We can thereby obtain the complete registered image as the linear combination of the complete component map $\mathbf{S}^r$ weighted by the estimated enhancement/suppression weights contained in $\mathbf{A}$. The only problem left is to calculate the complete component map matrix $\mathbf{S}^r$.

The complete component map matrix $\mathbf{S}^r$ can be estimated by running Infomax ICA directly on a motionless data matrix $\hat{\mathbf{X}}$, named 'extended reference ensemble', which is formed by replacing the time-point to be registered (the first time point in our simplified example in this paper) in the data matrix $\mathbf{X}^r$ with an extra image free of motion. However, in order to directly apply the previously estimated enhancement/suppression weights, that is, to calculate the complete registered image as the corresponding row of the matrix product $\mathbf{AS}^r$, the calculated component map $\mathbf{S}^r$ should have proper order and variance, or in another words, should contain $\mathbf{S}^r_{ICA}$ as a submatrix. Unfortunately, there is indeterminacy inherent in the ICA model in the variance and the order of the estimated components. Moreover, ICA is not a deterministic algorithm, which means it generates a little bit different outputs for different runs. Therefore, in our experiment, we directly estimate the unmixing matrix $\hat{\mathbf{W}}$ for $\hat{\mathbf{X}}$ by minimizing $\left\| \hat{\mathbf{W}}\hat{\mathbf{X}}_{ICA} - \mathbf{S}^r_{ICA} \right\|$ with the solution:

$$\hat{\mathbf{W}} = \mathbf{S}^r_{ICA}\hat{\mathbf{X}}^T_{ICA}(\hat{\mathbf{X}}_{ICA}\hat{\mathbf{X}}^T_{ICA})^{-1} \tag{4}$$

where $\hat{\mathbf{X}}_{ICA}$ is the submatrix containing the same indexes of columns (the voxels in the ring torus region) from $\hat{\mathbf{X}}$ as $\mathbf{X}^r_{ICA}$ from $\mathbf{X}^r$. The complete component map $\mathbf{S}^r$ is then obtained as:

$$\mathbf{S}^r = \hat{\mathbf{W}}\hat{\mathbf{X}} \tag{5}$$

whose corresponding submatrix optimally approximates $\mathbf{S}^r_{ICA}$ in the sense of least mean square error. Since the estimated ICA components are a linear transformation of the extended reference ensemble, the final registered image, which is obtained as the corresponding row (the first row in our simplified example in this paper) of the matrix product $\mathbf{AS}^r = \mathbf{A}\hat{\mathbf{W}}\hat{\mathbf{X}}$, is essentially a linear combination of the images in the extended reference ensemble $\hat{\mathbf{X}}$, with the weights as the corresponding row in the matrix product $\mathbf{A}\hat{\mathbf{W}}$.

3   Experiments

The performance of the extended MCICA algorithm was quantitatively evaluated on both surrogate data and real fMRI time-series, and was compared with that of SPM and AIR.

a) MCICA: To generate the basis images in $\mathbf{R}$, we first estimated any large motion by aligning the centroid and principal axes of activation of the image to be registered to that of the mean image of the reference ensemble. The preprocessed image was then rotated about its centroid using all combinations of the rotation angles of [-2, -1, 0, 1, 2] degrees in three dimensions. Two translated versions were then generated for each of the rotated images by random three-dimensional translations within [-0.25 0.25] voxels. Voxels within two voxels' distance of the automatically detected brain edge using thresholding and/or within five voxels' distance of the center of mass were excluded when estimating the data-adaptive filter $\mathbf{p}$ in MCICA.

b) LS-SPM: The standard realignment algorithm in SPM2 was used. The default option of 4th-degree B-spline interpolation was used for resampling.

c) LS-AIR: A second implementation of the least-square approach in AIR 5.05 was used. The recommended option of Chirp-Z interpolation was chosen for resampling and the recommended six-parameter rigid-body model for intra-subject image registration was used.

In the first experiment, the robustness of the proposed extended MCICA algorithm to the number of reference images used was explored. A simulated data set $\mathbf{X}$ was formed by left-multiplying a component map matrix $\mathbf{S}$ mimicking $n=9$ brain activations, with a time course matrix $\mathbf{A}$ consisting of sinusoids corrupted with noise. A simulated brain image with high contrast at the artificial 'brain' edge was then added to each row of $\mathbf{X}$ to mimic the global variance of real fMRI brain images. The first row of $\mathbf{X}$ was moved by a random 3D motion to produce a mean discrepancy of 0.65 voxels when integrated over the whole brain. Different numbers of observations (selected from the 2nd row to the 11th row) in $\mathbf{X}$ were then used as the reference ensemble to register the artificially-moved image in extended MCICA. In SPM and AIR, the original motionless image was used as the reference image to register its artificially-moved version. Fig. 2 demonstrates the mean absolute registration error (MAE, defined as the mean of the absolute intensity differences of voxels in the brain area between the registered image and the known correct image free of motion) versus the number of reference images used. It is clear that the registration error obtained by the extended MCICA algorithm was significantly and consistently lower than that obtained by SPM, AIR, and cubic interpolation with perfectly correct rigid-body transformation. Note that the registration result of the proposed method closely followed the LMS solution using the corresponding extended reference ensemble, suggesting that the weights for the reference ensemble estimated by the extended MCICA algorithm were near-optimal.

The second experiment investigates the influence of activation level (strength) on registration accuracy. We tested five different levels of mean signal increase: 0.64%, 1.28%, 2.56%, 5.12% and 10.25%, which were generated by superimposing the first row in $\mathbf{X}$ with one component map selected from S multiplied by different levels of activation weights. These images were then again corrupted by a random 3D motion of a mean discrepancy of 0.65 voxels and were registered using the extended reference ensemble consisting of 10 observations in $\mathbf{X}$ (i.e. from the 2nd row to the 11th row). To eliminate simulated motion specificities as a potential confound, ten different motion parameters (with fixed translation and rotation amplitudes about the centroid resulting in an average of 0.65 voxels of mean discrepancy across the brain) were generated randomly for each set of experiments, and the results were averaged +over the ten realizations. Fig. 3 demonstrates the mean absolute error (MAE) versus activation level introduced into the image to be registered. It can be seen that the errors for SPM and AIR increased monotonically with increasing activation strength. In contrast, the performance of MCICA was relatively invariant to the increase of activation level.

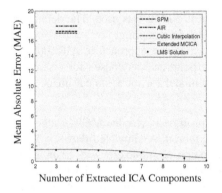

Fig. 2. Registration results of extended MCICA for large motion correction with different numbers of reference images used

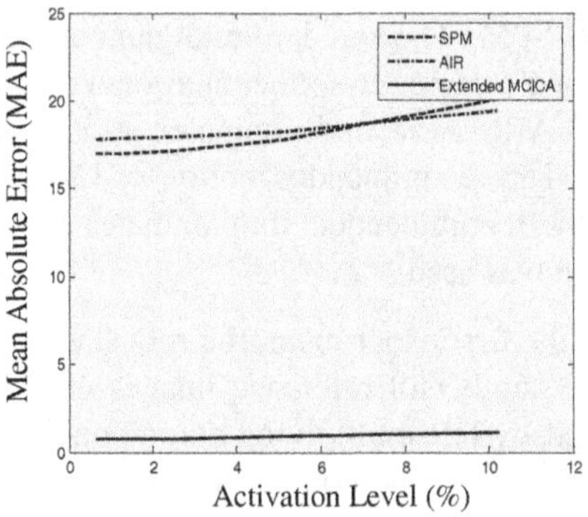

Fig. 3. Influence of activation level of the image to be registered on registration accuracy for motion correction of large motion

Fig. 4 plots the MAE as a function of the amplitude of the artificial movement (in the unit of mean discrepancy over the brain) applied to real fMRI data. Specifically, for a real fMRI time-series, an optimal sub-series consisting of eleven time-points with minimized discrepancy between their centroids and principal axes of activation was selected. One time-point among the selected sub-series was then artificially moved by random 3D motions of different amplitudes. In MCICA, the other ten time-points in the sub-series were used as the extended reference ensemble to register the artificially-moved time-point. In SPM and AIR, the perfect reference image, that is, the original image without the artificial motion applied, was used for registration. The original image was then used as the gold standard to evaluate the registration accuracy. Both the previous version of MCICA (dotted line) and the proposed extended MCICA algorithm (circle line) were used to register the images corrupted by motions of mean discrepancies from 0.02 voxles to 0.7 voxels. The solid line represents the performance of the hybrid MCICA algorithm in which the proposed extended algorithm was utilized for correcting motions with discrepancies larger than 0.32 voxels. Experiments were finally performed on a real fMRI times-series made up of 65 3D images acquired during a simple motor task of both-hand movement. Six time-points in the times-series that were corrupted with relatively large motion (i.e. movement of mean discrepancy large than 0.32 voxels) were motion corrected using the proposed

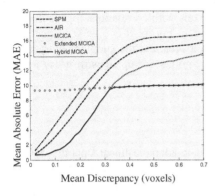

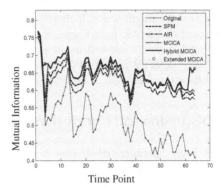

Fig. 4. Registration error versus amplitude of the artificial motion applied to the image to be registered for real fMRI time-series

Fig. 5. Comparison of mutual information between the first time-point and subsequent time-points for the original fMRI data and the four time-series realigned by LS-SPM, LS-AIR, MCICA and Extended MCICA

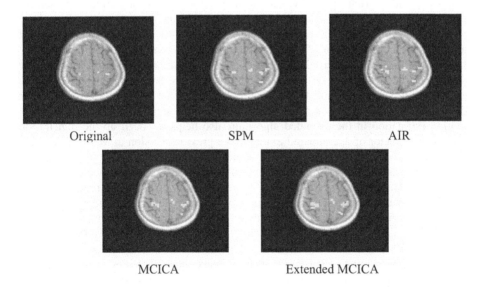

Fig. 6. Comparison of activated areas detected by simple correlation for the original data and the four time-series registered by SPM, AIR, MCICA and extended MCICA

extended MCICA algorithm and are marked by circles in Fig. 5, where the mutual information between the first time-point and all subsequent time-points are plotted. It is obvious that in comparison with SPM, AIR and the previous version of MCICA, the extended algorithm further improved the mutual information between the first-time point and the six time-points corrupted with relatively large motion. In addition, the correlation between the time course of each voxel in the brain and the task-rest behavioral paradigm was calculated, and the voxels with correlations higher than 0.5 were regarded as 'activated' and are highlighted in Fig. 6. It can be seen that more 'activated' voxels clustered in the primary motor area and the supplementary motor area were detected after preprocessing the time-points corrupted with gross motion using the extended MCICA algorithm.

4   Discussion and Conclusions

It has been demonstrated that by designing a data-adaptive linear operator MCICA minimized the spurious artifact introduced by interpolation to the final registered image, and achieved moderate between-slice motion correction [2]. Nevertheless, when patient head motion becomes relatively large, i.e. a significant fraction of a voxel, it is observed that linear combination of the rotated/shifted basis images is not sufficient to compensate for the significant interpolation artifact present at the brain edge in the basis images. Discarding the time-points corrupted with motions on the order of half a voxel, however, may result in an excessive amount of data that must be discarded in aged and patient populations.

In this paper improved compensation of relatively large motion effects in fMRI data using only partial optimal voxels in images for motion estimation is presented. Accurate complete component maps are estimated from the extended 'motionless' reference ensemble, and the final registered image can be mathematically expressed as a weighted combination of the extended reference ensemble. Degradation in the final image due to the interpolation process hence is avoided, which is evidenced by the low registration error in the intensity values at the brain edge, where accurate interpolation is most difficult for any interpolation scheme acting as a low-pass filter due to the sharp intensity variation. In addition, using a smaller number of voxels for motion estimation in the extended algorithm also helps to speed up the registration process by a factor of 2, compared to that in the previous version of MCICA in which all voxels in the brain area were used for motion estimation.

Experiments show that in contrast with SPM and AIR, the proposed method was relatively robust to the level of activation present in the image to be registered. For real fMRI time-point corrupted with relatively large motion (i.e. around half a voxel), the registration error of MCICA in terms of MAE, which was already much smaller than that obtained by SPM and AIR, was further reduced by 30% by the proposed extension. When different numbers of reference images were used to register the artificially-moved image, the performance of the extended algorithm closely followed the LMS curve, which is the optimal solution in terms of least-mean-square error when approximating the original motionless image using a linear summation of the extended reference ensemble. This suggests that the extended MCICA algorithm consistently and reliably converged to the correct solution in the optimization space. Initial promising results, i.e. increased mutual information and more clustered activation maps, were observed for real fMRI time-series of which those time-points corrupted with relatively large motion were registered using the proposed extension.

The proposed method requires that the underlying independent components are sufficiently represented in the regions used for motion estimation so that the comprehensive time course matrix **A** can be estimated. This may be problematic for very focal activations where the activation region is largely treated as missing data. It is further required that the significant underlying components present in the time-point to be registered should be adequately covered in the extended reference ensemble, allowing for an accurate estimation of the complete component maps in $\mathbf{S}^r$. For motion correction of real fMRI time-series, selection of the optimal reference ensemble and the most effective regions for motion estimation may vary among data sets and need further investigation. In addition, automatic method for selecting optimal threshold of motion amplitude above which the proposed extended method is used for registration needs to be devised.

Acknowledgements

The authors are thankful to Chenyang Xu, Frank Sauer and James Williams from Siemens Corporate Research for their support on the continuation of the work.

References

1. Hajnal, J. V., Myers, R., Oatridge, A., Schwieso, J. E., Young, I. R., and Bydder, G. M. : Artifacts due to Stimulus Correlated Motion in Functional Imaging of The Brain. Magnetic Resonance in Medicine 31 (1994) 283-291
2. Liao, R., Krolik, J. L., and McKeown, M. J. : An Information-Theoretic Criterion for Intrasubject Alignment of FMRI Time-Series: Motion Corrected Independent Component Analysis. IEEE Transactions on Medical Imaging 24 (2005) 29 - 44
3. Woods, R. P., Grafton, S. T. Holmes, C. J., Cherry, S. R., and Mazziotta, J. C. : Automate Image Registration: I. General Methods and Intrasubject, Intramodality Validation. Journal of Computer Assisted Tomography 22 (1998) 139-152
4. Friston, K. J., Holmes, A. P., Worsley, K. J., Poline, J. P., Frith, C. D., Frackowiak, R. S. J. : Statistical Parametric Maps in Functional Imaging: A General Linear Approach. Human Brain Mapping 2 (1995) 189-210
5. Bell, A. J., and Sejnowski, T. J. : An Information-Maximization Approach to Blind Separation and Blind Deconvolution. Neural Computation 7 (1995) 1004-1034
6. Liao, R., McKeown, M. J., and Krolik, J. L. : Isolation and Minimization of Effects of Motion on fMRI Data Using Multiple Reference Images. The Second IEEE International Symposium on Biomedical Imaging (2004) 916-919

Local or Global Minima: Flexible Dual-Front Active Contours

Hua Li[1,2] and Anthony Yezzi[1]

[1] School of ECE, Georgia Institute of Technology, Atlanta, GA, USA
[2] Dept. of Elect. & Info. Eng., Huazhong Univ. of Sci. & Tech., Wuhan, China
hua.li@ece.gatech.edu

Abstract. Most variational active contour models are designed to find the "desirable" local minima of data-dependent energy functionals with the hope of avoiding undesirable configurations due to noise or complex image structure. As such, there has been much research into the design of complex region-based energy functionals that are less likely to yield undesirable local minima. Unfortunately, most of these more "robust" region-based energy functionals are applicable to a much narrower class of imagery due to stronger assumptions about the underlying image data. Devising new implementation algorithms for active contours that attempt to capture more global minimizers of already proposed image-based energies would allow us to choose an energy that makes sense for a particular class of energy without concern over its sensitivity to local minima. However, sometimes the completely-global minimum is just as undesirable as a minimum that is too local.

In this paper, we propose a novel, fast and flexible dual front implementation of active contours, motivated by minimal path techniques and utilizing fast sweeping algorithms, which is easily manipulated to yield minima with variable "degrees" of localness and globalness. The ability to gracefully move from capturing minima that are more local (according to the initial placement of the active contour/surface) to minima that are more global makes it much easier to obtain "desirable" minimizers (which often are neither the most local nor the most global). As the examples, we illustrate the 2D and 3D implementations of this dual-front active contour for image segmentation from MRI imagery.

1 Introduction

Since the introduction of snakes [1], active contours have become particularly popular for segmentation applications. Most variational active contour models [2,3,4,5] are designed to find local minima of data-dependent energy functionals with the hope that reasonable initial placement of the active contour will drive it towards a "desirable" local minimum rather than an undesirable configuration that can occur due to the noise or complex image structure.

As such, there has been much research [6,7,8,9,10,11,12] into the design of complex region-based energy functionals that are less likely to yield undesirable local minima when compared to simpler edge-based energy functionals whose sensitivity to noise and texture is significantly worse. Unfortunately,

Y. Liu, T. Jiang, and C. Zhang (Eds.): CVBIA 2005, LNCS 3765, pp. 356–366, 2005.
ⓒ Springer-Verlag Berlin Heidelberg 2005

most of these more "robust" region-based energy functionals are applicable to a much narrower class of imagery compared to typical edge-based energies due to stronger assumptions about the underlying image data.

Devising new implementation algorithms for active contours that attempt to capture more global minimizers of already proposed image-based energies would allow us to choose an energy that makes sense for a particular class of energy without concern over its sensitivity to local minima. The minimal path technique proposed by Cohen et al. [13,14] is one such implementation. It attempts to capture the global minimum of an active contour model's energy between two points. However, for this minimal path technique, the initial points should be located exactly on the boundary to be extracted. Also, a topology-based saddle search routine is needed when they extended this technique to closed curve extraction. And it is not easy to expand to general 3D case [15].

Although many researchers keep their efforts on the design of robust active contour models to find the global minima and avoid the local minma, sometimes the completely global minimum is just as undesirable as a minimum that is too local. In this paper, we propose a novel, fast and flexible dual front implementation of active contours, motivated by minimal path technique and utilizing fast sweeping algorithms. In this model, the segmentation objective is achieved by iteratively dilating the initial curve to form a narrow region and then finding the new closest potential weighted minimal partition curve inside.

This dual-front active contour is easily manipulated to yield minima with variable "degrees" of localness and globalness. The degree of global or local minima can be controlled in a graceful manner by adjusting the width of the dilated narrow region. This ability to gracefully move from capturing minima that are more local (according to the initial placement of the active contour/surface) to minima that are more global makes it much easier to obtain "desirable" minimizers (which often are neither the most local nor the most global). This model guarantees the continuity and smoothness of the evolving curve with the capability to handle topology changes. In addition, it is easy to extend to the 3D case.

2   Dual-Front Active Contours

2.1   Background – The Minimal Path Technique

Given a potential $P > 0$ that takes lower values near desired boundaries, for example, $P = 1/(1 + ||\nabla I||^2)$, the objective of the minimal path method [13,14] is to look for a path (connect the pre-defined two points) along which the integral of $\tilde{P} = P + w$ (w is the constant) is minimal. First, the minimal action map $U_0(p)$ is defined as the minimal energy integrated along a path between the starting point p_0 and any point p, which is

$$U_0(p) = \inf_{A_{p_0,p}} \{E(C)\} = \inf_{A_{p_0,p}} \{\int_\Omega \tilde{P}(C(s))ds\}, \tag{1}$$

where $A_{p_0,p}$ is defined as the set of all paths between p_0 and p. Then, if given the minimal action maps U_0 to p_0 and U_1 to p_1, the minimal path between p_0 and p_1 is exactly the set of points p_g which satisfy

$$U_0(p_g) + U_1(p_g) = \inf_p \{U_0(p) + U_1(p)\}, \tag{2}$$

and this minimal path between p_0 and p_1 is determined by calculating U_0 and U_1 and then sliding back from the saddle point p', which is the first point that two action maps U_0 and U_1 meet each other, on the action map U_0 to p_0 and on the action map U_1 to p_1 according to the gradient descent.

Because the action map U_0 has only one minimum value at the starting point p_0 and increases from the starting point outwards, it can be easily determined by solving the Eikonal Eq. (3) using fast marching algorithm introduced by Sethian et al. [16]. The detailed explanation is shown in [13].

$$||\nabla U_0|| = \widetilde{P} \qquad \text{with} \qquad U_0(p_0) = 0 \tag{3}$$

2.2   Principle of Dual-Front Active Contours

Now we suppose that the image has two regions R_0 and R_1, and we choose one point p_0 inside the region R_0 and another point p_1 inside the region R_1. We still define two minimal action maps $U_0(p)$ and $U_1(p)$ according to the same definition as that in minimal path theory. The potential is also decided by the image features, for example, the potential takes lower values on the boundary of R_0 and R_1.

In the minimal path theory, the points satisfying the Eq. 2 are considered. Contrary to that, we consider the points satisfying the equation $U_0(p) = U_1(p)$. At these points, the level sets of the minimal action map U_0 meets the level sets of the minimal action map U_1. These meeting points form the Voronoi diagram of the image, decompose the whole image into two regions containing the point p_0 and the point p_1 respectively. One region containing the point p_0 is called as region R'_0, and the other region containing the point p_1 is called as region R'_1. All the points in the region R'_0 is closer to p_0 than p_1 in terms of the action map. All the points in the region R'_1 is closer to p_1 than p_0 in terms of the action map. Because the action maps are defined as the potential weighted distance maps, the boundary of regions R'_0 and R'_1 is called as the potential weighted minimal region partition related to the two points p_0 and p_1.

Actually the level sets of the action map U give the evolution of the front. The velocity of the evolving front is decided by the potential. When the evolving front arrives the boundary, the velocity is much lower, and the evolving front almost stops at the boundary. The same situation are for the action maps U_0 and U_1. When choosing the appropriate potentials for calculating the two minimal action maps, it is possible that these two action maps will meet each other at the actual boundary of two regions R_0 and R_1. In other words, we can search the two regions' boundary by calculating the minimal region partition related to the two points inside the two regions respectively.

Without loss of generality, we suppose X be a set of points (for example, a 2D curve or a 3D surface) in the image, U_X is the minimal action with potential $\widetilde{P}_X$ and starting points $\{p, p \in X\}$. Clearly, $U_X = min_{p \in X} U_p$. Then considering two sets $U_{X_i} = min_{p \in X_i} U_p$ and $U_{X_j} = min_{p \in X_j} U_p$, all points satisfying $U_{X_i}(p) = U_{X_j}(p)$ form the boundary of the two regions related to the two point sets X_i and X_j. Because the two action maps are the potential weighted distance maps, this formed boundary is also the potential weighted minimal partition of the regions related to the two point sets X_i and X_j.

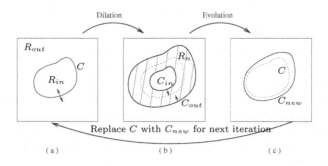

Fig. 1. Iteration process of dual front evolution and dilation. (a): an original contour C separating the region R to regions R_{in} and R_{out}; (b): the curve C is dilated to form the narrow active region R_n; (c): the inner and outer boundaries C_{in} and C_{out} propagate to form the new minimal partition curve C_{new} separating the region R to two regions, and then the curve C is replaced by the curve C_{new} for processing the next iteration.

Therefore, we propose the dual front evolution based on the above analysis to find the potential weighted minimum partition for a defined active region. The evolution principle is shown in Fig. 1. The narrow active region R_n, which is formed by expending the initial curve C, has the inner boundary C_{in} and the outer boundary C_{out}. Then the minimal action maps U_{in} and U_{out} are calculated with different potentials $\widetilde{P}_{in}$ and $\widetilde{P}_{out}$ respectively. When these two action maps meet each other, both evolutions of the level sets of the action maps stop automatically and a minimal partition boundary is formed in region R_n. All points p_g on this minimal partition boundary satisfy the following Eq. (4):

$$\begin{cases} |\nabla U_{in}| = \widetilde{P}_{in} & with \ U_{in}(C_{in}) = 0 \\ |\nabla U_{out}| = \widetilde{P}_{out} & with \ U_{out}(C_{out}) = 0 \\ U_{in}(p_g) = U_{out}(p_g) \end{cases} \qquad (4)$$

The dual front evolution is implemented by labeling the initial curves with different labels, than evolving the labeled curve with different potentials to the unlabeled region until all the points are assigned an unique label. Dual front evolution provides us a method to find the minimal partition curve within a narrow active region. Here this minimal partition is the potential weighted global minima partition only inside the narrow active region, not in the whole image.

Clearly, the degree of this globalness may be changed flexibly according to the size of the narrow active region.

In the dual front evolution, the region-based information and the edge-based information may be unified in the potentials for guiding the curve evolution. The mean values u_{in}, u_{out}, the variance values σ_{in}^2, σ_{out}^2, of the inside region ($R_{in} - R_{in} \cap R_n$) and outside region ($R_{out} - R_{out} \cap R_n$) are calculated. The evolution speeds (or potentials) for the labeled points (x, y) are decided by Eq. (5).

$$\widetilde{P}_{in}(x, y) = w_{in}^r \times f(|I(x, y) - \mu_{in}|, \sigma_{in}^2) + w_{in}^b \times g(\nabla I(x, y)) + w_{in}$$
$$\widetilde{P}_{out}(x, y) = w_{out}^r \times f(|I(x, y) - \mu_{out}|, \sigma_{out}^2) + w_{out}^b \times g(\nabla I(x, y)) + w_{out} \quad (5)$$

where $I(x, y)$ is the value of the image intensity at the examined point. $g(\nabla I(x, y))$ is a function of the image gradient. By choosing different functions f and g, and the different weight for each component of the potentials, this model can be used for different segmentation objectives.

Based on this dual front evolution, we propose the dual-front active contour model. It is an iterative process including dual front evolution and morphological dilation. First, we choose an initial curve, dilate it to form the narrow active region, and use dual-front evolution to find the minimal partition within this active region. Then, we expend the obtained minimal partition curve to form a new narrow active region, and the new potentials for the boundaries of the new active region are also calculated. We repeat this process until the difference between the consecutive obtained minimal partition curves less than the pre-defined threshold.

So, in dual-front active contours, the segmentation objective to find the minima with variable "degrees" globalness in defined region is transferred to find the global minimum partition curve within a narrow active region expanded from the initial contour, and then iteratively replace the current contour with the obtained global minimum partition curve until the final segmentation objective is achieved.

3   The Properties of Dual-Front Active Contours

3.1   Flexible Local or Global Minima

In dual-front active contours, the degree of global or local minima can be controlled in a graceful manner by adjusting the width of the narrow active region for the dual fronts' evolution. This ability to gracefully move from capturing minima that are more local (according to the initial placement of the active contour/surface) to minima that are more global makes this model much easier to obtain "desirable" minimizers (which often are neither the most local nor the most global).

The result of the dual front evolution is the global minimal partition curve inside the active region. So the size and the shape of the narrow active region will affect the final segmentation result. If the size of the active region is small, it possible leads to the problem of local minima because of the local noise. But if the

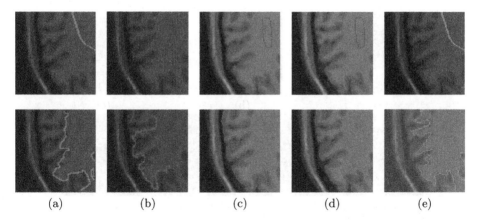

(a)　　　　　(b)　　　　　(c)　　　　　(d)　　　　　(e)

Fig. 2. Comparison of the different segmentation results of the interface of white matter/gray matter from different active contour models with different degrees of local minima and global minima. The gradient information used by panel (a),(b), and (e) is shown in Fig. 3. The top row shows the original image and the initialization for the curve evolution, and the bottom row shows the corresponding edge segmentation results from geodesic active contours (a), the minimal path technique (b), Chan-vese's method (c), Mumford-Shah's method (d) and dual-front active contours (e).

size of the active region is too large, the actual object boundary will be missed. The size of the active region should be selected based on the shape and the size of the detected object, the image quality and the background information, and so on.

In dual-front active contours, we provide very flexible method to define the active region. In fact, the active region is a kind of restricted searching space. The restricted space can be formed by choosing the automatic thresholding, calculating the distance map, using the length of the initial contour's normal, performing the morphological dilation and so on. All these methods can be used for defining the active region. Normally, we use the morphological dilation to obtain the narrow active region because the size of the active region can be controlled easily by adjusting the size of the structure element and the dilation times for the requirement from a given segmentation, or class of images.

The size of active region also can be changed during the evolution process. For example, when the initial curve is far from the object, we may first use the wider active region to expend the searching scale for one iteration, speed up the computation time and avoid the effect of the noise. When the curve, which is obtained after a number of iterations, near the object boundary, we may use the narrow active region for refining the accurate boundary. By the way, if the detected object is bigger, we may use wider active region, otherwise, we should use narrower active region.

In Fig. 2, we compare the different edge detection results by two of the edge-based methods, geodesic active contours [2] and the minimal path technique [13],

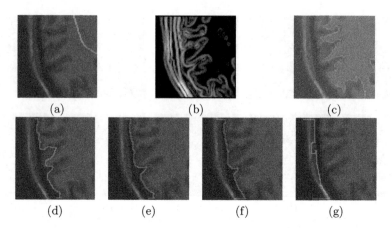

(a)   (b)   (c)

(d)   (e)   (f)   (g)

Fig. 3. By choosing the different size of the narrow active region, the dual-front active contour model achieves different minima.
(a): the original image with the initialization; (b): the corresponding gradient information; (c)-(g): the segmentation result using 5×5, 7×7, 11×11, 15×15, 23×23 pixels circle structuring elements for morphological dilation after 15 iterations.

two of the region-based methods, Chan-Vese's method [8] and Mumford-Shah methods [17], and the dual-front active contours proposed in this paper. This figure is the part of one 2D human brain MRI image, and the segmentation objective is to find the interface of the gray matter and the white matter. We use the above five methods to process this image and obtain the different segmentation result. We can see that, geodesic active contours suffer from undesirable local minima, and the "global minima" found by the minimal path technique is also not exactly what we want, which is effected by the location of the pre-defined two points. Chan-Vese's method and Mumford-Shah's method also found the incorrect global minima. As this figure indicates, our dual-front active contours can control the degree of global or local minima in active contour model, find the correct boundary, and perform better than other methods which find the local minima or global minima.

In Fig. 3, we give another example to demonstrate that, by choosing different narrow active regions with different sizes, the dual-front active contour model achieves different degree's global minima in the whole image. The potential for each point is $\widetilde{P}(x,y) = 1/(|I(x,y) - I_{mean}| + (1 + \nabla I)^2/10) + 0.1$.

3.2   Other Nice Properties

First, the dual front evolution provides the automatic stop criterion in each iteration. The dual front evolution also guarantees the continuity and smoothness of the curve with the capability to handle topology changes. Second, the dual-front active contour model provides automatic stop criterion by comparing the result from consecutive iterations. Third, the dual-front evolution combines the advantages of level-set methods and fast marching methods, avoids the disadvantages of them, and transfers the point-to-point evolution to noncontinuous band-to-band evolution. In this manner, the computational cost is reduced significantly. The detailed information of these properties was shown in [18].

4 Experimental Results

In Fig. 4, we give two other examples to compare the different edge detection results by Chan and Vese's method [8], the Mumford shah algorithm [17], and dual-front active contours. Because Chan's method and Mumford's method are all designed for finding the global minima in the whole image, sometimes, they cannot receive the correct boundary. But for dual-front active contour, the degree of the global minima can be controlled by the size of narrow active region, the model can achieve flexible global degree's minima. In these two examples, the potential for each point is $\widetilde{P}(x, y) = 1/(|I(x, y) - I_{mean}|) + 0.1$.

In Fig. 5, we show that our model can be used for extract the object without clearly gradient information. The panel (a) is a noisy mammogram showing a cyst in the breast, the panel (b) is the corresponding gradient image, the panel (c) shows the middle step of the segmentation process, the panel (d) shows the final segmentation result. In this example, the potential for each point is $\widetilde{P}(x, y) = 1/(|I(x, y) - I_{mean}|) + 0.1$. The structuring element is 5×5 pixels circle for morphological dilation. It is clear from the results that the segmentation of the cyst is refined even with high noise level.

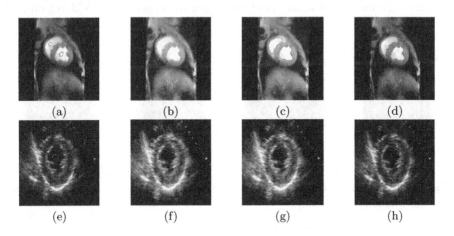

(a)   (b)   (c)   (d)

(e)   (f)   (g)   (h)

Fig. 4. Comparison of different region-based active contours related to the degree of global minima.
(a) and (e): two 2D medical images with the initializations; (b) and (f): the results from Chan-Vese's model suffer from undesirable global minima; (c) and (g): the results from Mumford-Shah model also suffer from the smoothing constraints; (d) and (h): the correct edge extractions from dual-front active contours using 7×7 pixels circle structuring element for morphological dilation.

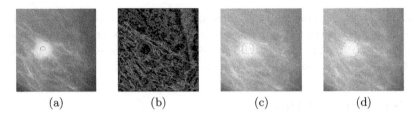

(a)   (b)   (c)   (d)

Fig. 5. The segmentation result on 2D cyst image without gradient informations. The size of the dilation structure element is 5×5 pixels. Panel (a) shows the original image with the initialization. Panel (b) shows the gradient image. Panel (c) shows the middle step of the segmentation process after 5 iterations. Panel (d) shows the segmentation result after 15 iterations.

We also test the dual-front active contours on the simulated MRI 3D brain image data set and extract the interface of gray matter/white matter, as well as applications to specific cortical studies.

Because of the properties of dual-front active contours, the whole segmentation process is considered as a hierarchical decomposition. We assume that the normal brain includes three tissues: GM (gray matter), WM (white matter), and CSF (cerebral spinal fluid). After skull stripping and non-brain tissue removing, we separate the brain region and the background first. Then, we just consider the brain region and use dual-front active contours to segment the brain into CSF and WM+GM two regions. The third step is to restrict the WM+GM region and use dual-front active contours again to separate the WM region and GM region.

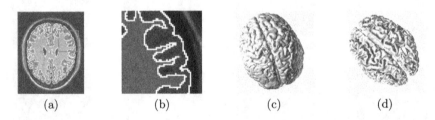

(a)   (b)   (c)   (d)

Fig. 6. The segmented outer and inner cortical surfaces from the MRI brain image with our method

In Fig. 6, we present the segmented outer (CSF-GM interface) and inner (GM-WM interface) cortical surfaces in one slice of the 3D simulated brain image, and a zoom-in of extracted boundaries for this slice. We also show the 3D models of the cortical surfaces. The test image is available from the Brain-Web [19], which is generated from the MS Lesion brain database using the $T1$ modality, $1mm$ slice thickness, 3% noise level and 20% intensity nonuniformity settings. The image size is $181 \times 217 \times 217$. The initialization for the hierarchical segmentation is a sphere centered at $(100, 100, 95)$, and the size is $75 \times 75 \times 150$. The potential for different point is $\tilde{P}(x, y) = 1/(|I(x, y) - I_{mean}|) + 0.1$, and the size of the dilation structure element is $5 \times 5 \times 5$ pixels.

For a 3D brain image ($181 \times 217 \times 217$ voxels in total), Normally, our method requires only 10-20 iterations for segmenting one tissue type (CSF, GM or WM). For each iteration, the computation procedure includes one curve dilation and one dual-front evolution, one iteration last around 15 seconds.

5   Conclusions and Future Work

In this paper, we propose a novel, fast and flexible dual front implementation of active contours, which is easily manipulated to yield minima with variable "degrees" of localness and globalness. This ability to gracefully move from capturing minima that are more local (according to the initial placement of the active contour/surface) to minima that are more global makes it much easier to obtain "desirable" minimizers (which often are neither the most local nor the most global). As the examples, we illustrate the 2D and 3D implementations of this model for object extraction from MRI imagery.

While the underlying principle of the dual front evolution algorithm presented here is based on the authors' earlier work in [18], there are several novelties in the present work which do not appear in the earlier work. Other than the extension to the three dimensions, we have made the very important observation that the dual-front approach may be customed tailored to capture minimizers that are flexible in their degrees of localness and globalness.

As such, we have constructed around this basic building block and algorithm that may be controlled and adapted in ways that other active contour models cannot. This key point, which is not addressed at all in the earlier work [18] greatly extends the usefulness of their model to many important applications in computer vision, especially medical imaging, where user control and interaction is highly desirable.

Furthermore, the 3D algorithm presented in this paper is also quite novel in that is not a mere extension of the 2D algorithm presented in [18]. In fact, the hierarchical decomposition procedure used in our 3D algorithm could also be incorporated to improve even the original 2D algorithm. We believe that this analysis and interpretation of the original algorithm will be of great service to the computer vision community.

References

1. Kass, M., Witkin, A., Terzopoulos, D.: Snakes: Active contour models. International Journal of Computer Vision **1** (1988) 321–332
2. Caselles, V., Kimmel, R., Sapiro, G.: Geodesic active contours. International Journal of Computer Vision **22** (1997) 61–79
3. Yezzi, A., Kichenassamy, S.: A geometric snake model for segmentation of medical imagery. IEEE Trans. on Medical Imaging **16** (1997) 199–209

4. Cohen, L., et al.: On active contour models and balloons. Computer Vision Graphics Image Processing: Image Understanding **53** (1991) 211–218
5. Tek, H., Kimia, B.: Image segmentation by reaction diffusion bubbles. In: Proceedings of International Conference of Computer Vision. (1995) 156–162
6. Zhu, S., Yuille, A.: Region competition: unifying snakes, region growing, and Bayes/MDL for multiband image segmentation. IEEE Trans. on PAMI **18** (1996) 884–900
7. Chakraborty, A., Staib, L., Duncan, J.: Deformable boundary finding in medical images by integrating gradient and region information. IEEE Trans. on Medical Imaging **15** (1996) 859–870
8. Chan, T., Vese, L.: Active contours without edges. IEEE Trans. on Image Processing **10** (2001) 266–277
9. Paragios, N., Deriche, R.: Geodesic active regions: A new framework to deal with frame partition problems in computer vision. Journal of Visual Communication and Image Presentation **13** (2002) 249–268
10. Samson, C., Blanc-Feraud, L., et al.: A level set method for image classification. In: Int. Conf. Scale-Space Theories in Computer Vision. (1999) 306–317
11. Yezzi, A., Tsai, A., Willsky, A.: A statistical approach to image segmentation for bimodal and trimodal imagery. In: Proceedings of ICCV. Volume 2. (1999) 1–5
12. Yezzi, A., Tsai, A., Willsky, A.: A fully global approach to image segmentation via coupled curve evolution equations. Journal of Visual Communication and Image Representation **13** (2002) 195–216
13. Cohen, L., Kimmel, R.: Global minimum for active contour models: A minimal path approach. In: IEEE International Conference on CVPR (CVPR'96). (1996) 666–673
14. Cohen, L.: Multiple contour finding and perceptual grouping using minimal paths. Journal of Mathematical Imaging and Vision **14** (2001) 225–236
15. Ardon, R., Cohen, L.: Fast constrained surface extraction by minimal paths. In: International Conference on Computer Vision-Workshop on VLSM. (2003) 233–244
16. Sethian, J.: Fast marching methods. SIAM Review **41** (1999)
17. Mumford, D., Shah, J.: Optimal approximation by piecewise smooth functions and associated variational problems. Commun. Pure Appl. Math. **42** (1989) 577–685
18. Li, H., Elmoataz, A., Fadili, J., Ruan, S.: Dual front evolution model and its application in medical imaging. In: MICCAI2004. Volume 3216., Rennes/Saint-Malo, France (2004) 103–110
19. Cocosco, C., Kollokian, V., Kwan, R., Evans, A.: Brainweb: Online interface to a 3D MRI simulated brain database. NeuroImage **5** (1997) S425

Locally Switching Between Cost Functions in Iterative Non-rigid Registration

William Mullally[1], Margrit Betke[1], Carissa Bellardine[2], and Kenneth Lutchen[2]

[1] Computer Science Department, Boston University
[2] Department of Biomedical Engineering, Boston University,
Boston, MA 02215, USA

Abstract. In non-rigid image registration problems, it can be difficult to construct a single cost function that adequately captures concepts of similarity for multiple structures, for example when one structure changes in density while another structure does not. We propose a method that locally switches between cost functions at each iteration of the registration process. This allows more specific similarity criteria to be embedded in the registration process and prevents costs from being applied to structures for which they are inappropriate. We tested our method by registering chest computed tomography (CT) scans containing a healthy lung to scans of the same lung afflicted with acute respiratory distress syndrome (ARDS). We evaluated our method both visually and with the use of landmarks and show improvement over existing methodology.

1 Introduction

Registration methods are increasingly in demand by medical practitioners to accurately model the transformations they observe in their image data [1]-[4]. The problem of registering lung images has recently gained notice [5]-[9] largely due to an interest in supporting lung cancer diagnosis. Accurate registration of lung anatomy, however, remains an open problem, especially in the presence of pervasive pathology where normal structures have changed drastically in appearance as when the lung is afflicted with emphysema or acute respiratory distress syndrome (ARDS). In this work, we present a method for registering a chest CT containing a healthy lung to a chest CT of the same lung afflicted with ARDS and present a general framework to solve non-rigid registration problems in which the intensity values of corresponding structures do not change in the same way for all structures in the images.

ARDS is a disease that involves severe flooding and collapse of the lung, thereby making it difficult to breathe and maintain adequate gas exchange. ARDS has a high mortality rate (32% – 45%) [10]. Mechanical ventilation is often a required therapy in order to maintain the necessary O_2 and CO_2 levels of the body. Mechanical ventilation can impose non-physiological forces on the lung that can exacerbate lung injury. Characterizing the heterogeneous nature of the disease and how it is impacted by mechanical ventilation is important for basic survival of these patients [11]. On CT images ARDS is characterized by

Y. Liu, T. Jiang, and C. Zhang (Eds.): CVBIA 2005, LNCS 3765, pp. 367–377, 2005.
© Springer-Verlag Berlin Heidelberg 2005

Before   Case 1   Case 2   Case 3

After

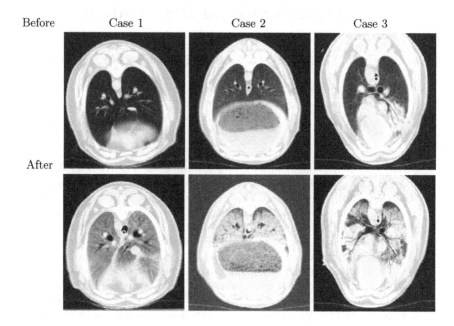

Fig. 1. Axial view of three sheep chests before and after a saline wash of their lungs induced ARDS. A saline wash affected the entire lung of case 1, but did not uniformly affect the lungs of cases 2 and 3 as can be seen from the dark air-filled patches at the top of case 2's lungs and throughout case 3's lungs.

regions within the lung that can be as dense as the tissue surrounding the lung (Fig. 1). Measures on the mechanics of ARDS have been limited to the order of quadrants within the lung [11] rather than the order of the finer anatomical structures visible even in low resolution CT. Non-rigid registration of healthy lung scans to scans of lungs with ARDS can help researchers understand the syndrome and may lead to better treatment options than currently exist. To the best of our knowledge, automatic non-rigid registration approaches have not been applied to this problem.

There are two principle branches of image registration techniques: those guided by image similarity cost functions and those guided by feature detectors. This paper presents a modification to non-rigid registration methods using image-based cost functions. Specifically, we modify the method proposed by Rueckert et al. [12] in which images are aligned by minimizing the "cost" of correspondence between the images by comparing intensity values. In registration problems like this, a similarity function that might be adequate for capturing the spatial deformations of temporally constant density tissue, for example the bony anatomy, might not be sufficient to capture both spatial deformations of structures and temporal changes in tissues density, as in an ARDS inflicted lung. We do not attempt to solve the correspondence problem of lung anatomy imaged before and after the onset of ARDS. Instead, we propose a method to non-rigidly register the tissues surrounding the

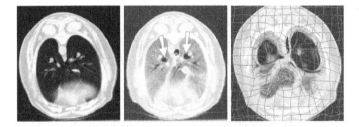

Fig. 2. Axial view of a healthy lung (left) and an ARDS inflicted lung before (middle) and after (right) non-rigid registration using correlation as the only cost to guide registration. The transformation grid is overlaid in the right image. The voxels of the bronchi (indicated by arrows in their original form in the middle image) are inappropriately warped to fill the lung (dark regions in right image). In the iterative registration process, the correlation gradient leads away from correct correspondence within the lung. Correspondence outside the lung is somewhat better.

lung without adversely affecting the topology of the lung. No segmentation is used in our approach. Our approach adaptively changes the character of the cost function at each iteration of the registration process. These changes allow cost functions to be applied only on appropriate anatomy.

2   Methods

We follow the framework proposed by Rueckert et al. [12] in which a multi-level non-rigid registration algorithm is built upon a hierarchical grid of b-splines. Multi-level approaches progress from coarse to fine image resolutions during the process of registration to avoid local minima problems and reduce computation time. A hierarchical b-spline grid controls the transformation T of the source image I_1 into the coordinate system of the target image I_2. The similarity between the two images is evaluated with a cost function of the form:

$$Cost(\theta) = C_{ImageSimilarity}(T(\theta, I_1), I_2) + C_{Regularization}(T(\theta)),$$

where θ designates the positions of the grid points controlling the b-spline. The gradient of this cost function is followed in steps of size μ to find the optimal registration between the two images. The registration process iteratively checks the gradient and modifies the transformation parameters.

The above approach will not work when the cost function does not appropriately embody all the changes that occur between image acquisitions. In Figure 2, for example, correlation was used as the only cost to guide the registration between healthy and ARDS inflicted lungs. The correlation gradient, in effect, pushed the transformation in an anatomically inappropriate direction.

We would like to construct a framework for using cost functions only on the anatomy for which a particular cost function is most appropriate. We can do this by associating each knot θ_i of the b-spline grid for $i = 0, ..., N$, where N is the number of grid control points, with a particular cost function. For $k = 1, ..., K$ cost functions, this takes the form:

$$Cost(\theta_i) = \begin{cases} Cost_1(\theta) & \text{if } f_1(\theta_i, T(\theta, I_1), I_2) > \tau_1 \\ Cost_2(\theta) & \text{if } f_2(\theta_i, T(\theta, I_1), I_2) > \tau_2 \\ \vdots \\ Cost_K(\theta) & \text{otherwise} \end{cases} \tag{1}$$

where f_k are $K - 1$ functions used to decide which cost function to apply by comparing each of them to a threshold τ_k. The cost function association of each control point is decided at each iteration. The algorithm, a modification of Rueckert et al.'s framework that includes our method of cost function selection, is detailed below.

NON-RIGID MULTI-SCALE REGISTRATION ALGORITHM WITH LOCAL COST SWITCHING
Input: Two 3D scans
___
1 **calculate** an initial rigid registration
2 **initialize** the control points $\theta^{(l)}$ and down sample the images to the coarsest resolution, $l = 1$,
3 **repeat**
4   **determine** the cost function $Cost(\theta_i) = Cost_k(\theta)$ to associate with each control point θ_i (Eq. 1)
5   **calculate** $\nabla C = \frac{\partial Cost(\theta_i^{(l)})}{\partial \theta_i^{(l)}}$
6   **for** $\mu = $ max. step size **until** $\mu = $ min. step size
7   **while** $\|\nabla C\| > $ threshold ϵ **or** iteration count $<$ max. iterations **do**
8   **recalculate** the control points $\theta = \theta + \mu \frac{\nabla C}{\|\nabla C\|}$
9   **determine** the cost function $Cost_k(\theta)$ to use at each control point θ_i
10   **recalculate** the gradient vector ∇C
11   **decrease** step size μ
12   **increase** the control point resolution and image resolution l
13 **until** finest level of resolution, $l = L$, is reached
___
Output: θ

We adapted the local cost switching algorithm to the specific application of registering healthy lungs to lungs inflicted with ARDS. We needed to construct cost functions that could appropriately express tissue transformations in this problem. First, we incorporated transformation costs that discourage dramatic bending of the transformation grid and extreme volume changes across the entire image. Secondly, the correspondence of anatomy outside of the lung can be captured by an image-intensity similarity term. We constructed a single cost function incorporating these terms and weighted their contributions to the overall cost using α, β, and γ as follows:

$$Cost() = \alpha \, C_{ImageSimilarity}(T(\theta, I_1), I_2) + \beta \, C_{BendingEnergy}(T(\theta)) + \gamma \, C_{VolumePreservation}(T(\theta)) \tag{2}$$

Specifically, we define $C_{ImageSimilarity}()$ to be the correlation coefficient $\frac{Covariance(I_1, I_2)}{Std.Deviation(I_1) * Std.Deviation(I_2)}$, $C_{BendingEnergy}(T(\theta))$ to be the bending energy

$\frac{1}{V} \int_0^X \int_0^Y \int_0^Z [(\frac{\partial^2 T}{\partial x^2})^2 + (\frac{\partial^2 T}{\partial y^2})^2 + (\frac{\partial^2 T}{\partial z^2})^2 + 2(\frac{\partial^2 T}{\partial xy})^2 + 2(\frac{\partial^2 T}{\partial xz})^2 + 2(\frac{\partial^2 T}{\partial yz})^2] dx dy dz$ of a thin metal plate [12], where X, Y, and Z are the dimensions and V is the volume of the scan, and $C_{VolumePreservation}(T(\theta)) = \int_V |\log(det(Jacobian(T(\theta))))| \, d\theta$ [13].

For the single cost in Eq. 2 to be successful if applied by itself, it must not only relate the anatomy outside the lung which has undergone minimal intensity changes but also the anatomy within the lung which has drastically changed because of the infliction of ARDS. In general, $C_{ImageSimilarity}(T(\theta, I_1), I_2)$ is used to capture such a relationship, but as already shown in Fig. 2, correct anatomic alignment cannot be achieved using the correlation coefficient as the image similarity cost. Moreover, it may not be possible to construct such an image-intensity similarity function that can capture the entire range of anatomical changes seen in comparing scans of healthy lungs to scans of diseased lungs. In such cases where image similarity costs guide registration toward inappropriate solutions, our cost switching framework can be used to allow regions with strong image correlation to non-rigidly align themselves while still correctly deforming regions with weak image similarity. To formulate this, we specify Eq. 1 for two cost functions, $Cost_1$ with an image similarity term and $Cost_2$ without:

$$
\begin{aligned}
Cost_1() &= \alpha \, C_{ImageSimilarity}(T(\theta, I_1), I_2) + \beta \, C_{BendingEnergy}(T(\theta)) \\
&\quad + \gamma \, C_{VolumePreservation}(T(\theta)) \\
Cost_2() &= \beta \, C_{BendingEnergy}(T(\theta)) + \gamma \, C_{VolumePreservation}(T(\theta)),
\end{aligned}
\tag{3}
$$

Because Eq. 1 is applied for $K = 2$, we had to specify one decision function f_1 for Eq. 3. We defined f_1 to be the normalized correlation coefficient with threshold $\tau_1 = 0.5$. This function controls how to switch between the two cost functions at each grid point and differentiates between correlated and uncorrelated image regions. A fixed size patch around the location of each knot point was used as the correlation template. An initial alignment is achieved by performing a rigid registration on high density bony anatomy. The two costs defined in Eq. 3 are assigned in lines 4 and 9 of our cost switching registration algorithm.

It should be noted that with the costs in Eq. 3, we do not expect the anatomy within the injured portions of the lung to achieve perfect alignment. There is no mechanism to draw these regions into correct correspondence except for the bending and volume preservation costs responding to the deformations of surrounding tissues. Tissue outside of these injured regions should achieve good alignment.

3   Experiments

To evaluate our cost switching approach, we used CT scans taken from six sheep (Fig. 1). CT scans were taken both before and after ARDS was induced by treating their lungs with a saline wash. The sheep were placed on ventilators to control the pressure level of air in their lungs. The CT images had resolution $0.71 \times 0.71 \times 10$ mm^3 and captured the entire area of the lung.

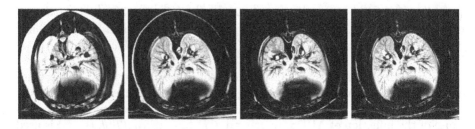

Fig. 3. Absolute difference in intensity values between unregistered scans (left), rigidly registered scans (middle left), single cost non-rigid registration (middle right), and cost switching non-rigid registration (right). The lungs are visible as a result of the density shift induced by the saline wash. Outside of the lungs, the non-rigid approaches improve upon the results of the rigid registration and in this case, our cost switching approach more accurately registered the ribs.

Table 1. Root Mean Squared Error Between Registered Landmarks in the Lung (mm). Rigid and cost switching non-rigid registration driven by non-lung structures result in similar error in lung landmark alignment.

Sheep	Unregistered	Rigid	Single Cost	Cost Switching
1	38.5	15.4	11.9	14.2
2	10.2	7.9	12.1	8.1
3	7.9	6.7	13.3	5.7
4	20.3	8.1	7.2	7.8
5	13.2	9.9	16.8	11.1
6	27.5	9.8	24.2	14.5
Average	19.6	9.6	14.3	10.2

We tested our method by registering images of the same animal imaged at the same pressure level before and after the infliction of ARDS. We validated our registration results both visually and by comparison to ground truth correspondence of landmarks. Figure 3 shows that non-rigid registration approaches reduced the intensity difference between scans for the anatomy outside the lung. As the anatomy outside the lung has not changed in density between imaging, a reduction in the intensity difference reflects a more accurate alignment of anatomy.

Within the lung, since significant density changes have occurred between data acquisitions, density differences are not a useful measure of misalignment. We can, however, evaluate changes in landmark location. The landmarks used consist of branching points of the bronchi and blood vessels within the lung. We used 18-22 landmarks per case. We show the root mean squared error in millimeters between corresponding landmarks in Table 1. We report an average improvement in landmark alignment of 28% by the cost switching approach in comparison to the single cost approach. We report an average degradation in landmark alignment of 6% for the cost switching approach in comparison to the

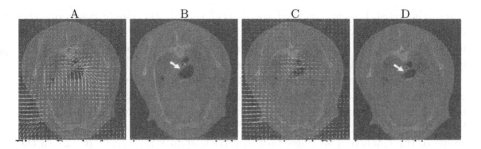

Fig. 4. Results from single cost non-rigid registration (A,B) and cost switching non-rigid registration (C,D) in sheep 1. We show the registered images with an overlay of the local deformation quantities (A,C). Notice the difference in the shape of the trachea (indicated with an arrow). The single cost approach greatly increased the size of the trachea. Our approach stayed closer to physically viable transformation.

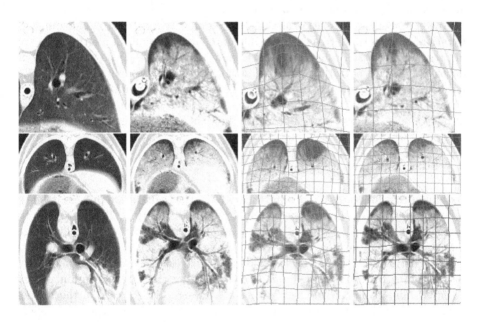

Fig. 5. Axial view of sheep 2 (top) and 3 (middle and bottom). Images are shown with (middle left) and without (left) ARDS before registration. Also shown are the single cost solution (middle right) and our cost switching solution (right) with an overlay of the deformation grid. Notice that the single cost solution expands the dark region at the top of the lung, in the process moving vessel structures away from their corresponding structures. Our approach maintains the character of the rigid transformation within the lung.

rigid approach, where as the single cost approach degraded 49% in comparison to the rigid approach. In all but one case, the cost switching approach maintained the error between landmarks obtained by rigidly registering the scans. In two cases (the most homogeneous of the ARDS scans), the single cost non-rigid approach also maintained the same level of error but in four cases it significantly increased the error, separating the landmarks even more than if the scans had not been registered in three of those cases.

Visual evaluation shows that our cost switching method more accurately registers the ribs than the single cost non-rigid approach (Fig. 3). More significant, however, are the apparent anatomical changes of the trachea, esophagus, and lungs. In Fig. 4 the principal difference between the methods is in the apparent shape of the trachea. The single cost approach greatly increased the size of the trachea. As the only large air filled region in that portion of the body, the trachea was expanded to maximize the correlation with the air filled healthy lungs. Our cost switching approach thus stayed closer to a physically viable transformation. Note that some large deformations were needed to capture changes to the anatomy external to the lung. The single cost approach expanded air filled regions, most notably at the top of the lungs (Fig. 5). Our approach maintained an anatomically appropriate transformations.

Instead of cross-correlation as the image similarity function to guide our registration, other formulations are possible, most notably mutual information. We did test our approach using mutual information and while we do not present in depth results, we note that mutual information drew the anatomy within the lung away from correct correspondence. This performance may indicate that no general purpose similarity function can be defined to represent the density transformation that occurs between a healthy lung and a lung inflicted with ARDS.

4   Discussion and Conclusion

Assigning cost functions at each iteration allows the registration process itself to influence what cost function is used at a particular location. This is similar to several approaches [14,15] for adaptively deciding the impact a particular image point will have in an image registration process. Shen et al. [14] use a hierarchical ordering of "driving voxels" to register images. They propose a similarity measure in a high dimensional space incorporating tissue classification, image intensity, and geometric moment invariants. Using all the voxels in the image, they then find clusters in this space that represent each tissue type. They allow voxels close to the cluster centers to drive registration early in the registration process. They gradually relax the distance they use for determining the driving voxels until all voxel in the image are used. This approach, however, is not appropriate for the application of registering injured lung images in large part because the approach is built upon good segmentation, which has not been reliably demonstrated for injured lungs. Furthermore, Shen et al. eventually apply a single similarity function for all voxels in the images. In the application of injured lung registration, correlation draws some image regions away from correct correspondence, therefore we explicitly deny regions with low correlation from driving the registration process. Moreover, our framework allows for the use of multiple similarity functions, tailored to the requirements of a particular

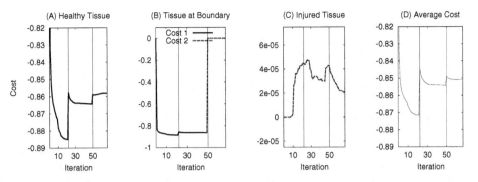

Fig. 6. Typical examples of gradient descent during the registration process at one grid point θ_i for healthy tissue (A), at boundary of healthy and ARDS inflicted tissue (B), within ARDS inflicted tissue (C), and averaged across all transformation grid locations θ (D). Changes in resolution level l occurred at iteration 22 and 50 and are indicated with vertical lines. (A) Outside the lung and within healthy regions of the lung, correlation is strong so $Cost_1$ is used. (B) At the boundary between healthy tissue and injured tissue, correlation can dominate the cost during the low resolution stages of the registration. At the highest resolution, however, strong correlation no longer exists so the registration process automatically switches to $Cost_2$ which does not include correlation costs. (C) Within injured regions of the lung, correlation is weak so $Cost_2$ is used throughout the registration. As the regularizing costs are affected by the movement of neighboring points on the transformation grid, the cost initially increases as other image patches move in response to the gradient of $Cost_1$. The cost begins to decrease once $Cost_1$ no longer drives large movements in other regions of the image. (D) On average, the cost always moves in the direction of a minimum except when the resolution level changes.

application, that can simultaneously drive the registration process on many different image regions of arbitrarily complex description.

Guest et al. [15] propose a reliability measure that can be used on any similarity measure and in any method for computing a registration transformation. The "reliability" of a measure at a particular image point is high if the point matches well to a single point or line in the corresponding image and is low if it matches well to a large region. Our framework can incorporate this measure or any other measure of reliability that is appropriate to a particular application.

We show typical examples of how the cost changed during the registration process in Figure 6. Parameters were set to $\alpha = -1$, $\beta = .001$, and $\gamma = .001$ in Eq. 3. Dues to the low weight given to them, the bending and volume preservation terms did not noticeably impact the solution until the later half of the registration process when the correlation gradient is small. Notice that our algorithm minimizes cost with respect to the transformation parameters and not with respect to the cost function used. The algorithm is not allowed to choose a cost function because it has the lowest value, otherwise, transitions from $Cost_1$ to $Cost_2$ would not occur as seen in Fig. 6 B at iteration 50.

We were limited to using six data sets for a proof of concept test of our approach for registering healthy lungs to diseased lungs. The images came from biomedical study into ARDS where animals were deliberately injured [11]. It is not feasible to obtain a large collection of such images. Our approach may have application to the study of other diseases and injuries to the lung as in pneumonia, asthma, or the effects of near drowning.

Ultimately, to solve the problem of registering CT scans containing healthy lungs to CT scans containing injured lungs, it may be necessary to fuse a feature based approach, perhaps using vessel branching points, to an image similarity approach. Segmentation of these structures, however, is still challenging, especially in the presence of an injury or disease like ARDS. Also, the cost functions used for in our current approach are not directly drawn from biomechanics. The elasticity properties of bones, ligaments, and other tissues should replace the bending energy of thin metal plates and volume preservation costs used here. In addition to formalizing such properties as costs, work remains to apply them to the appropriate anatomy within the registration framework.

In summary, we have presented a novel method for incorporating multiple cost functions into a single registration process. This allows for greater specificity and variation in the definitions of anatomical correspondence used in non-rigid registration problems. We have tested our approach on the difficult problem of registering chest CT scans before and after the infliction of ARDS. By providing a method to register healthy and ARDS inflicted lung scans, we hope to help researchers better understand the syndrome and find new treatment options. Our results demonstrate that being able to selectively apply cost functions on appropriate anatomy does increase the accuracy of the resulting registration.

Acknowledgments

We would like to thank Daniel Rueckert of Imperial College London for providing code which we modified to build our system and Jingbin Wang for discussions. Funding was provided by the National Science Foundation (IIS-0308213, IIS-039009, IIS-0093367, P200A01031, and EIA-0202067).

References

1. H. Lester and S. R. Arridge. A survey of hierarchical non-linear medical image registration. *Pattern Recognition*, 32:129–149, 1999.
2. M. A. Audette, F. P. Ferrie, and T. M. Peters. An algorithmic overview of surface registration techniques for medical imaging. *Med Image Anal*, 4(3):201–217, 2000.
3. Mäkelä Timo, P. Clarysse, O. Sipilä, N. Pauna, Q. C. Pham, T. Katila, and I. E. Magnin. A review of cardiac image registration methods. *IEEE Trans Med Imag*, 21(9):1011–1021, 2002.
4. J. P. W. Pluim, J.B. A. Maintz, and M. A. Viergever. Mutual-information-based registration of medical images: A survey. *IEEE Trans Med Imag*, 22(8):986–1003, August 2003.

5. M. Betke, H. Hong, D. Thomas, C. Prince, and J. P. Ko. Landmark detection in the chest and registration of lung surfaces with an application to nodule registration. *Med Image Anal*, 7(3):265–281, September 2003.
6. V. Boldea, D. Sarrut, and S. Clippe. Lung deformation estimation with non-rigid registration for radiotherapy treatment. In *Medical Image Computing and Computer-Assisted Intervention – MICCAI'03*, pages 770–777. Springer-Verlag, Berlin, 2003.
7. I. Bricault, G. Ferretti, and P. Cinquin. Registration of real and CT-derived virtual bronchoscopic images to assist transbronchial biopsy. *IEEE Trans Med Imag*, 17(5):703–714, 1998.
8. Baojun Li. *The construction of a normative human lung atlas by inter-subject registration and warping of CT images*. PhD thesis, The University of Iowa, 2004.
9. J. N. Yu, F. H. Rahey, H. D. Gage, C. G. Eades B. A. Harkness, C. A. Pelizzari, and J. W. Keyes Jr. Intermodality, retrospective image registration in the thorax. *The Journal of Nuclear Medicine*, 36(12):2333–2338, December 1995.
10. K. F. Udobi, E. Childs, and K. Touijer. Acute respiratory distress syndrome. *American Family Physician*, 67(2):315–322, 2003.
11. C. L. Bellardine, E. P. Ingenito, A. Hoffman, F. Lopez, W. Sandborn, B. Suki, and K. R. Lutchen. Relating heterogeneous mechanics to gas exchange function during mechanical ventilation. *Annls. Biomed. Eng.*, 2005. In press.
12. D. Rueckert, L. I. Sonoda, C. Hayes, D. L. G. Hill, M. O. Leach, and D. J. Hawkes. Nonrigid registration using free-form deformations: Application to breast MR images. *IEEE Trans Med Imag*, 18(8):712–721, August 1999.
13. T. Rohlfing, C. R. Maurer, D. A. Bluemke, and M. A. Jacobs. Volume-preserving nonrigid registration of MR breast images using free-form deformation with an incompressibility constraint. *IEEE Trans Med Imag*, 22(6):730–741, June 2003.
14. D. Shen and C. Davatzikos. Hammer: Hierarchical attribute matching mechanism for elastic registration. *IEEE Trans Med Imag*, 21(11):1421–1439, November 2002.
15. E. Guest, E. Berry, R. A. Baldock, M. Fidrich, and M. A. Smith. Robjust point correspondence applied to two- and three- dimensional image registration. *IEEE Trans Pattern Anal Mach Intell*, 23(2):165–179, February 2001.

Multi-modal Image Registration by Quantitative-Qualitative Measure of Mutual Information (Q-MI)[*]

Hongxia Luan[1], Feihu Qi[1], and Dinggang Shen[2]

[1] Department of Computer Science and Engineering,
Shanghai Jiao Tong University, Shanghai, China 200030
{luan-hx, fhqi}@cs.sjtu.edu.cn
[2] Section of Biomedical Image Analysis, Department of Radiology,
University of Pennsylvania, Philadelphia, PA 19104
dinggang.shen@uphs.upenn.edu

Abstract. This paper presents a novel measure of image similarity, called quantitative-qualitative measure of mutual information (Q-MI), for multi-modal image registration. Conventional information measure, i.e., Shannon's entropy, is a quantitative measure of information, since it only considers probabilities, not utilities of events. Actually, each event has its own utility to the fulfillment of the underlying goal, which can be independent of its probability of occurrence. Therefore, it is important to consider both quantitative and qualitative (i.e., utility) information simultaneously for image registration. To achieve this, salient voxels such as white matter (WM) voxels near to brain cortex will be assigned higher utilities than the WM voxels inside the large WM regions, according to the regional saliency values calculated from scale-space map of brain image. Thus, voxels with higher utilities will contribute more in measuring the mutual information of two images under registration. We use this novel measure of mutual information (Q-MI) for registration of multi-modality brain images, and find that the successful rate of our registration method is much higher than that of conventional mutual information registration method.

1 Introduction

Multi-modality image registration is important to accumulate information from different modality images for diagnosis of diseases, and to align preoperative images with intraoperative images for surgical planning. Mutual information has been suceessfully used as a measure of image similarity for both mono- and multi-modality image registration [1-3]. However, mutual information measurement only considers the matching of intensities, and ignores spatial information in the images. It should be noted that intensity matching not necessarily means anatomical matching. Therefore, it is important to design the registration methods that ensure the anatomical matching.

Spatial information, i.e., relationship of intensities between neighboring voxels, has been widely studied and incorporated into the mutual inforamation based registration

---

[*] This work is supported by NSFC (National Science Foundation of China) 60271033.

Y. Liu, T. Jiang, and C. Zhang (Eds.): CVBIA 2005, LNCS 3765, pp. 378–387, 2005.

procedure. In particular, many methods have been developed to include the image gradients into the registration [4,5]. In [5], the image registration is completed by maximizing both mutual information and matching of gradient maps between two images. Recently, distance map, calculated from grantient map, is proposed for multi-modality image registration [6], in order to make the registration method have larger capture ranges, since gradients are locally defined. On the other hand, the second-order information measures, i.e., the probabilities of co-occurence of intensity pairs within a certain size of image neighbourhood, were introduced into the mutual information based image registration [7]. Also, in order to employ multi-level spatial information simultaneously for image registration, Holden *et al* [8] firstly extracted features such as the luminance, the first and the second order derivatives of the scale space expansion of the image, and then registered two images by maximizing the multi-dimensional mutual information of the corresponding features.

It is important to note that most mutual information based registration methods treat each voxel equally during the registration procedure, regardless of whether some voxels are more useful than others in registration. Actually, different voxels even having same intensity should be treated differently in the registration procedure [9], according to their regional saliency values calculated from the scale-space map [10,11]. For example, WM voxels near to cortex should contribute more than WM voxels inside the large WM regions in measuring the mutual information between two images under registration. In this way, the registration algorithm can focus more on the registration of salient regions.

In this paper, we define a novel measure of image similarity, i.e., quantitative-qualitative measure of mutual information (Q-MI), for robust multimodality image registration. This new measure not only considers the probability of each image intensity, but also considers the utility of each image intensity, during the registration process. Here, we use the saliency value [10] as the utility for voxels in the image. By integrating both probability and utility into the definition of similarity of two images, our method has a much higher successful rate, compared to the conventional mutual information based registration methods, on the images obtained from the BrainWeb [12], indicating the robustness of our method to transformations.

2 Quantitative-Qualitative Measure of Mutual Information (Q-MI)

Before defining quantitative-qualitative measure of mutual information (Q-MI), we will briefly describe the basic concepts of information measure (2.1) and mutual information (2.2). Based on these definitions, we will give our definitions for quantitative-qualitative measure of information (2.3), and for quantitative-qualitative measure of mutual information (2.4).

2.1 Measure of Information

Information measure is a number related to the uncertainty or probability of occurrence of an event or outcome that conveys information [13]. Given a single event E_i with probability of occurrence p_i, the self-information of this event is defined as

$$H(E_i) = -\log p_i \tag{1}$$

The choice of a logarithmic base corresponds to the choice of a unit for measuring information. If the base 2 is used, the resulting units may be called binary digits, or more briefly bits [14]. The average information of a set of n events $E=(E_1, E_2, ..., E_n)$, each with probability of occurrence p_i, is defined as

$$H(E) = H(E_1, ..., E_n) = \sum_{i=1}^{n} p_i(-\log p_i) \tag{2}$$

The above is also called Shannon's entropy [14]. It weights the information per outcome by the probability of that outcome occurring. The Shannon's entropy is a measure of the amount of information required on the average to describe a set of events.

Let $P=(p_1, p_2, ..., p_n)$ be a finite discrete probability distribution of a set of n events $E=(E_1, E_2, ..., E_n)$ on the basis of an experiment whose predicted probability distribution is $Q=(q_1, q_2, ..., q_n)$. Then, a measure of directed divergence, which is called relative information or Kullback-Leibler distance [13], is defined as

$$D(E) = \sum_{i=1}^{n} p_i(\log \frac{p_i}{q_i}) \tag{3}$$

2.2 Measure of Mutual Information

Mutual information is an important concept in information theory and is defined according to relative entropy. Suppose we have two sets of events, $E=(E_1, E_2, ..., E_n)$ with probability distribution $P=(p_1, p_2, ..., p_n)$, and $F=(F_1, F_2, ..., F_m)$ with probability distribution $Q=(q_1, q_2, ..., q_m)$. Mutual information is a measure of the amount of information that the set of events E contains about the set of events F. Thus, mutual information is defined as the relative entropy between the joint distribution and the product distribution as follows,

$$MI(E, F) = \sum_{i=1}^{n} \sum_{j=1}^{m} p(E_i, F_j) \log \frac{p(E_i, F_j)}{p_i q_j} \tag{4}$$

2.3 Quantitative-Qualitative Measure of Information

Shannon's entropy is a quantitative measure of information, since it considers all the events as random abstract events and neglects the particular aspects of those events. From the view of cybernetic system, Belis and Guiasu [15] presented a quantitative-qualitative measure of information in 1968. They thought that the occurrence of an event removes a double uncertainty, i.e., the quantitative one related to its probability of occurrence, and the qualitative one related to its utility for the fulfillment of the goal. The utility of an event is a subjective notion, and it is directly connected to the goal to achieve. Here, we emphasized that the utility of an event is independent of its objective probability of occurrence. For instance, an event of a small probability can have great utility, while an event of a great probability can have small utility.

Let $E=(E_1, E_2, ..., E_n)$ be a finite set of events representing the possible realizations of some experiments. Let $P=(p_1, p_2, ..., p_n)$ be the probabilities of occurrence of those events, and $U=(u_1, u_2, ..., u_n)$ be the utilities of those events. The quantitative-qualitative measure of information is

$$QH(E;U) = \sum_{i=1}^{n} u_i p_i (-\log p_i)$$ (5)

If all utilities are same, equation (5) becomes equation (2), which is Shannon's entropy.

Based on the work of Belis and Guiasu [15], Taneja [16] presented a quantitative-qualitative measure of relative information as follows,

$$QD(E;U) = \sum_{i=1}^{n} u_i p_i \log \frac{p_i}{q_i}$$ (6)

The quantity $u_i \log p_i$ is usually referred as *useful* self-information conveyed by an event with probability of occurrence p_i and utility u_i . Thus, the term $u_i \log(p_i/q_i) = u_i \log p_i - u_i \log q_i$ can be regarded as *useful* information gain in predicting the event E_i. When utilities in equation (6) are ignored, equation (6) becomes equation (3).

2.4 Quantitative-Qualitative Measure of Mutual Information (Q-MI)

As we mentioned above, Shannon's entropy-based mutual information only pays attention to the occurrence of events, and does not consider the particular aspects of events with respect to the goal. In order to consider the particular aspects of events, we define the quantitative-qualitative measure of mutual information (Q-MI) as follows, according to the quantitative-qualitative measure of relative information in equation (6),

$$QMI(E,F;U) = \sum_{i=1}^{n} \sum_{j=1}^{m} u(E_i, F_j) p(E_i, F_j) \log \frac{p(E_i, F_j)}{p_i q_j}$$ (7)

Like definitions given in equations (5) and (6), Q-MI focuses on the *useful* information that one set of events tells about another set of events. When utilities are the same, equation (7) becomes the definition of conventional mutual information.

3   Implementation

This section first describes the method of computing saliency values for each image location and using it as utility for that location. Then, the method of estimating utility for each intensity pair of two images is provided. Finally, the optimization method used in our registration algorithm is briefly described.

3.1 Saliency Measure

Each voxel in the image is unique, and it has its own roles. The only difference between those roles is the amount of significance. For example, the voxels that lie in the region of interest or at the boundary of region of interest are more significant for image analysis and understanding task, compared to the voxels that lie in the background. However, how to characterize each voxel still remains a hot topic in computer vision and pattern recognition fields.

Gradient operator is a simple image detector, able to identify the location of intensity changes. As we indicated in introduction, gradient map has been widely incorporated into the mutual information based registration methods. However, gradient is a local feature, and it is sensitive to noise. On the contrary, saliency measure [10], defined from scale-space map for each voxel in the image, is robust to noise and considers regional information. Accordingly, the saliency definition is adopted here for representing the significance of each voxel, and also the utility of this voxel in image registration.

Saliency measure is defined for each voxel in an image, and it is determined by analyzing entropy in the local regions of different size. For each voxel x, we first calculate the probability distribution of intensity i, $p_i(s,x)$, in a spherical region of radius s, centered at x. Then, we calculate the local entropy $L(s,x)$ from $p_i(s,x)$, as defined below,

$$L(s,x) = -\sum_i p_i(s,x) \log p_i(s,x) \tag{8}$$

The best scale s_x for the region centered at voxel x is selected as the one that maximizes local entropy $L(s,x)$. Since large scale and high local image difference are preferred, the saliency value of voxel x, $A(s_x,x)$, is defined by that maximal local entropy value, weighted by both the best scale s_x and a differential self-similarity measure in the scale space,

$$A(s_x,x) = L(s_x,x) \cdot s_x \cdot \sum_i \left\| \frac{\partial p_i(s,x)}{\partial s} \Big|_{s_x} \right\| \tag{9}$$

By measuring saliency over the whole image, each voxel has a saliency value to represent its significance in the image and also utility in image registration.

3.2 Calculating the Utility of Each Intensity Pair of Two Images

Once the saliency/utility has been defined for each voxel in the two images under registration, we are ready to define the utility for each intensity pair in the two images. Let $I_R(x)$ be the intensity of reference image R at location x, and $I_F(y)$ be the intensity of floating image F at location y. Similarly, let $A_R(x)$ and $A_F(y)$ be the saliency values of voxel x in R and voxel y in F, respectively. Then, the utility of an intensity pair (i,j) can be defined as,

$$u(i, j) = \sum_{\substack{x, y \in \Omega \\ I_R(x)=i, \ I_F(y)=j}} A_R(x) \cdot A_F(y) \qquad (10)$$

where Ω is the overlap region of images R and F. In this paper, we use a *multiplication* operation to combine the saliency values from images R and F. Other combinations of utilities will be tested extensively in future.

3.3 Optimization

The registration problem based on Q-MI can be formulated as an optimization problem. Given a transformation T that maps a floating image F to match with a reference image R, we need to find an optimal transformation T^*,

$$T^* = \arg\max_T QMI(R, T(F); U) \qquad (11)$$

such that our defined Q-MI, i.e., *QMI* in equation (11), is maximized.

Powell's multidimensional set method [17] is used to iteratively search for the maximum value of Q-MI, along each parameter via Brents's method [17]. To increase the robustness and also save the computation time, a multi-resolution framework of registration is performed.

4 Results

A number of experiments have been performed to demonstrate the performance of the proposed Q-MI in multi-modality image registration. The first set of experiments is used to test the performance of our method with respect to noise. The second set of experiments is used to evaluate the robustness of our proposed method. All experiments are performed on PD and T1 MR brain images obtained from Brain Web [12], and 2D slice images are used.

4.1 Visual Demonstration of the Robustness of Our Method to Noises

In this experiment, we evaluate our registration method on 2-dimensional PD and T1 MR brain images. The size of 2D image is 217x181, and the noise level is 1%, 5% and 9%, respectively. PD MR brain image is used as reference image, as displayed in Fig 1a, and T1 MR brain image is used as floating image, as displayed in Fig 1b. Figs 1c and 1d show the color-coded saliency measures for PD and T1 MR brain images, respectively. Since these are the simulation images, the different modality images have been aligned. To visually evaluate the performance of our registration algorithm with respect to different levels of noise, we plot the changes of Q-MI with respect to rotations around z-axis, horizontal shifting and vertical shifting, respectively. Here, parameters R_z, T_x, and T_y denote rotation around z-axis, horizontal shifting, and vertical shifting, respectively.

Figs 2a, 2b and 2c show the results of our Q-MI. It can be clearly observed that the curves of our Q-MI are smooth even in the case of large noise level, indicating the robustness of our method to noise.

4.2 Comparison on Robustness of Registration Methods

For validating the robustness and accuracy of the proposed method, we designed a series of controlled experiments on a pair of brain images with known transformations and noise levels. Similar to the experiments in 4.1, the PD MR brain image is used as the reference image, and the T1 MR brain image is used as the floating image. The floating image is transformed similarly in each of three datasets described below, but additive noises in both reference and floating images are different in the three datasets.

(1) *Test dataset 1*: 1% Gaussian noises were added in both reference and floating images. The floating image is simultaneously rotated and shifted, by a rotation angle uniformly sampled from the range of [-20, 20] degree and the horizontal and vertical shiftings (T_x and T_y) both uniformly sampled from the range of [-40mm, +40mm];

(2) *Test dataset 2*: 5% Gaussian noises were added in both reference and floating images. The floating image is similarly transformed as *Test dataset 1*;

(3) *Test dataset 3*: 9% Gaussian noises were added in both reference and floating images. The floating image is similarly transformed as *Test dataset 1*.

The test datasets 1~3 each generate 1000 randomly transformed images, therefore there are totally 3000 transformed floating images. We applied the registration algorithms, respectively based on conventional mutual information and our Q-MI, to independently register the reference image with each transformed floating image. In order to compare their performances fairly, we used the same optimization technique to perform registrations.

The registration result is regarded as successful if the differences between estimated transformations and ground-truth transformations are less than pre-defined thresholds, i.e., 2 degree for rotation and 2mm for shifting, which is similarly used in [18]. The successful rates of registration based on those two measures are listed in Table 1. Also, for those successful cases of registration, means and standard deviations of rotation errors and shifting errors are calculated, respectively, and listed in Table 2.

Based on Table 1, we can conclude that Q-MI based registration method has a higher success rate than conventional mutual information based method for each test dataset. That is, Q-MI based registration method is more robust, since utility has been incorporated into the mutual information definition. Based on Table 2 that compares registration accuracy for the successful cases, we can observe that the accuracy of Q-MI based registration is comparable to that of conventional mutual information based method.

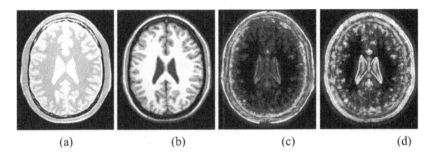

(a)   (b)   (c)   (d)

Fig. 1. The testing MR brain images. (a) PD MR brain image, (b) T1 MR brain image, (c,d) their color-coded saliency measures.

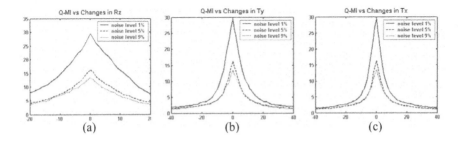

(a)   (b)   (c)

Fig. 2. Changes of Q-MI, with respective to rotations around z-axis R_z (a), horizontal shifting T_x (b), and vertical shifting T_y (c).

Table 1. Successful rates of two registration methods, based on Q-MI and conventional mutual information, respectively, in three datasets

Test Dataset	Successful rate	
	Mutual Information	Q-MI
Dataset 1	60.4%	84.9%
Dataset 2	54.6%	82.4%
Dataset 3	51.0%	76.5%

Table 2. Means and standard deviations of registration errors for the successful cases in three datasets, respectively

Test dataset	Mean and standard deviation					
	Mutual information			Q-MI		
	θ	T_x	T_y	θ	T_x	T_y
Dataset 1	0.03±0.04	0.35±0.53	0.41±0.62	0.13±0.11	0.41±0.59	0.51±0.73
Dataset 2	0.16±0.15	0.39±0.58	0.48±0.67	0.08±0.10	0.47±0.67	0.56±0.78
Dataset 3	0.24±0.24	0.42±0.61	0.50±0.70	0.15±0.17	0.55±0.75	0.58±0.79

5 Conclusion

We have presented a novel measure of image similarity, called quantitative-qualitative measure of mutual information (Q-MI), for registration of multi-modality images. This new measure integrates not only information obtained from the probability of intensity distribution, but also information obtained from the utility of each voxel, defined as value of saliency. This is different from other mutual information registration methods that use spatial information, since spatial information was not used as guidance for the calculation of mutual information. Our experiments on multi-modality MR brain images shows that the successful rate of our method is much higher than that of conventional mutual information based registration method, indicating the robustness of our method. In future, we will test our method extensively on other modality images of brains or other organs. We will also test on 3D images.

References

1. A. Collignon, F. Maes, D. Delaere, D. Vandermeulen, P. Suetens, and G. Marchal, *Automated multi-modality image registration based on information theory*. IPMI, p. 263-274, 1995
2. W.M. Wells, P. Viola, H. Atsumi, S. Nakajima, and R. Kiknis, *Multi-modal volume registration by maximization of mutual information*. Med. Image Anal., 1:35-51, 1996.
3. M. Holden, *et al*, *Voxel similarity measures for 3-D serial MR brain image registration*. IEEE Trans. Med. Imag., 19:94-102, 2000.
4. C.E. Rodriguez-Carranza and M.H. Loew, *A Weighted and Deterministic Entropy Measure for Image Registration Using Mutual Information*. Proceedings of SPIE conference on Image Processing, p.155-166, Feb 1998.
5. J.P.Pluim, J.B. Maintz, and M.A. Viergever, *Image Registration by Maximization of Combined Mutual Information and Gradient Information*. IEEE Trans. Med. Imag., 19:809-814, 2000.
6. R. Gan and A. Chung, *Multi-dimensional Mutual Information Based Robust Image Registration Using Maximum Distance-Gradient-Magnitude*. IPMI'05, 2005.
7. D. Rueckert, M.J. Clarkson, D.L. Hill, and D.J. Hawakes, *Non-rigid registration using higher-order mutual information*. Proceedings of SPIE conference on Image Processing, p.438-447, 2000.
8. M. Holden, L.D. Griffin, N. Saeed, and D.L.G. Hill, *Multi-channel Mutual Information Using Scale Space*. MICCAI, p.797-804, 2004.
9. D. Shen, and C. Davatzikos, *HAMMER: Hierarchical attribute matching mechanism for elastic registration*. IEEE Trans. on Med. Imaging, 21(11):1421-1439, 2002.
10. T. Kadir and M. Brady, *Saliency, Scale and Image Descriptions*. International Journal of Computer Vision, 45:83-105, 2001.
11. X. Huang, Y. Sun, D. Metaxas, F. Sauer, and C. Xu, *Hybrid Image Registration based on Configural Matching of Scale-Invariant Salient Region Features*. Conference on Computer Vision and Pattern Recognition Workshop, June, 2004.
12. D.L. Collins, A.P. Zijdenbos, V. Kollokian, J.G. Sled, N.L. Kabani, C.J. Holmes, and A.C. Evans, *Design and construction of a realistic digital brain phantom*. IEEE Trans. Med. Imag., 17:463-468, 1998.
13. T.M. Cover and J.A. Thomas, *Elements of Information Theory*. New York: Wiley, 1991.

14. C.E. Shannon, *A mathematical theory of communication*. Bell Syst. Tech. J., 27:379-423, 1948.
15. M. Belis and S. Guiasu, *A quantitative-qualitative measure of information in cybernetic systems*. IEEE Trans. Inform. Theory, 14:593-594, 1968.
16. H.C. Taneja and R.K. Tuteja, *Characterization of a quantitative-qualitative measure of relative information*. Inform. Sci., 33:217-222, 1984.
17. W.H. Press, B.P. Flannery, S.A. Teukolsky, and W.T. Vettering, *Numerical Recipes in C*. Cambridge, U.K. : Cambridge Univ. Press, 1992.
18. Y.-M. Zhu and S.M. Cochoff, *Likelihood Maximization Approach to Image registration*. IEEE Trans. on Image Processing, 11(12):1417-1426, 2002.

Multi-scale Vessel Boundary Detection

Hüseyin Tek, Alper Ayvacı, and Dorin Comaniciu

Siemens Corporate Research, Princeton, NJ, USA

Abstract. In this paper, we present a robust and accurate method for the segmentation of cross-sectional boundaries of vessels found in contrast-enhanced images. The proposed algorithm first detects the edges along 1D rays in multiple scales by using mean-shift analysis. Second, edges from different scales are accurately and efficiently combined by using the properties of mean-shift clustering. Third, boundaries of vessel cross-sections are obtained by using local and global perceptual edge grouping and elliptical shape verification. The proposed algorithm is stable to (*i*) the case where the vessel is surrounded by other vessels or other high contrast structures, (*iii*) contrast variations in vessel boundary, and (*iii*) variations in the vessel size and shape. The accuracy of the algorithm is shown on several examples.

1 Introduction

The main goal of the majority of contrast-enhanced (CE) magnetic resonance angiography (MRA) and computed tomography angiography (CTA) is diagnosis and qualitative or quantitative assessment of pathology in the circulatory system. Once the location of the pathology is determined, quantitative measurements can be made on the original 2D slice data or, more commonly, on 2D multi planar reformat (MPR) images produced at user-selected positions and orientations in the volume. In the quantification of stenosis, it is desirable to produce a cross-sectional area/radius profile of a vessel so that one can compare pathological regions to patent (healthy) regions of the same vessel.

Accurate and robust detection of vessel boundaries is often challenging task, Figure 1. Specifically, (*i*) the presence of significant noise levels in CT and MR images often forms strong edges inside vessels. (*ii*) Size of vessels can change drastically along them. (*iii*) The intensity profile of a vessel boundary can be diffused at one side while it can be very shallow on the other sides due to the presence of other vessels or high contrast structures. (*iv*) The presence of vascular pathologies, *e.g.*, calcified plaques, makes the shape of vessel cross-sectional boundary locally deviate from a circular shape. In this paper, we propose a method for detecting vessel boundaries accurately and robustly in the presence of such difficulties.

Previously, Hernandez-Hoyos *et. al.* [7] presented a snake model for segmenting vessel boundaries in the planes orthogonal to the vessel centerline. Wink *et al.* [18] proposed a ray propagation method based on the intensity gradients for the segmentation of vessels and detection of their centerline. Similarly, Tek *et. al.* [16] proposed a segmentation method for the cross-sectional vessel boundaries

Y. Liu, T. Jiang, and C. Zhang (Eds.): CVBIA 2005, LNCS 3765, pp. 388–398, 2005.
© Springer-Verlag Berlin Heidelberg 2005

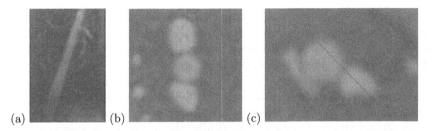

(a)   (b)   (c)

Fig. 1. Detection of vessel boundaries is often a difficult task due to: (a) significant contrast changes along a vessel in MRA. (b) Local deviation from a circular shape. (c) shallow gap edges and diffused edges can be present in the boundary of a vessel.

based on explicit front propagation via ray propagation. However, it is often very difficult to estimate the internal and smoothness parameters to obtain accurate results *robustly*.

In this paper, we propose a new segmentation technique based on multi-scale edge detection, clustering, edge grouping and elliptical shape matching. Specifically, first, edges along a ray are computed in several scales by using mean shift analysis [4]. Second, incorrect edges obtained from multiple scale are eliminated by the mean-shift based clustering algorithm. Third, prominent edges are obtained by selecting edges based on their strengths, and the assumption that vessels are not nested structures. Fourth, smooth and long curve segments are constructed from prominent edges by a local grouping algorithm. Finally, the curve segments that best describes the vessel boundary are determined from the elliptic shape priors. This new algorithm is capable of segmenting vessel boundaries in great detail even in the extreme conditions illustrated in Figure 1. In addition, we propose that 2D cross-sectional vessel boundaries can be successfully used to model 3D vessels very accurately by a centerline tracking algorithm similar to one in [2]. The accuracy and robustness of the 2D cross-sectional boundary detection algorithm is shown on several CTA and MRA data.

1.1   Previous Work

Previously, Tek *et. al.* [16] proposed an approach that is based on explicit front propagation via normal vectors, which then combines smoothness constraints with the mean-shift filtering. Specifically, they considered the curve evolution equation $\partial \mathcal{C}(s,t)/\partial t = S(x,y) \vec{N}$ for the segmentation of vessel boundaries where $\mathcal{C}(s,t)$ is a contour, $S(x,y)$ is the speed of evolving contour and $\vec{N}$ is the vector normal to $\mathcal{C}(s,t)$. In this proposed approach, the contour $\mathcal{C}(s,t)$ is sampled and the evolution of each sample is followed in time by rewriting the curve evolution equation in vector form [16]. The speed of rays, $S(x,y)$ depends on image information and shape priors. They proposed to use $S(x,y) = S_0(x,y) + \beta S_1(x,y)$ where $S_0(x,y)$ measures image discontinuities, $S_1(x,y)$ represents shape priors, and β balances these two terms. In this approach, image discontinuities are detected via *mean-shift analysis* [4] along the rays. Comaniciu and Meer [4] showed that mean-shift analysis, which operates in the joint *spatial-range* domain where the space of the 2-dimensional lattice represents the *spatial* domain and the space of intensity values constitutes the *range* domain, is a powerful method for robustly detecting object boundaries in images.

This algorithm [16] works well in certain applications especially when vessel boundaries are well isolated. However, it is difficult to estimate parameters *i.e.*, spatial, range kernel filter sizes, the amount of smoothness constraints for the robust segmentation of vessels. Specifically, the use of single spatial scale and curvature based smoothness constraints are not enough for accurate results when vessels are not isolated very well. In this paper, we present an approach that robustly handles these difficulties.

2   Multi-scale Edge Detection By Mean Shift Clustering

In this paper, we propose to use the displacement vectors of mean-shift analysis for detecting edges in multiple scales. Unfortunately, the robustness and accuracy of segmentation results heavily depend on the selection of spatial (σ_x) and range (σ_I) scale parameters of mean-shift analysis because vessel boundaries are often in many spatial and range scales. Previously, Comaniciu [3] proposed a statistical technique for the estimation of these parameters directly from images. In this paper, we develop a geometry-based algorithm, which operates solely on the edges of intensity data.

The divergence of displacement vectors corresponds to the edges of structures, Figure 2. In many medical imaging applications, it is often assumed that boundary can be represented by high contrast step edges. However, in reality, diffuse edges, low contrast edges and gap edges occur frequently even in a single cross-sectional vessel boundary, Figure 1. The robust and accurate detection of boundaries in such cases requires edge detection in many scales. However, integration of edge responses from different scales is not an easy task. In this paper, we propose a boundary extraction method which correctly combines the edges obtained from different *spatial* scales of mean-shift filtering along a ray, illustrated step-by-step in Figure 6. It is also possible to apply the filtering in several range scales. However, optimal range kernel size can be obtained directly from the intensity data. Specifically, we experimentally determined that the mean intensity difference between the right and left side of the spatial filters corresponds to the optimal range scales, which is verified in our experiments. In addition, it is assumed that the size of largest diffuse edge is known a priori to set the range of spatial kernels.

There are two main difficulties with obtaining the *correct* edge from multiscale edges: First, multiple erroneous edges often present in the vicinity of the correct edge due to presence of noise in the intensity data. These edges do not corresponds to semantically correct structures, *e.g.* vessel boundary, thus, they should be deleted. Second, there are often several edges along a ray corresponding to the structures of the boundaries. The edge corresponding to the boundary of a vessel can be determined from the geometric properties of the vessels and

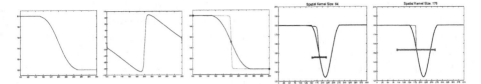

Fig. 2. This figure illustrates the mean-shift filtering of a typical edge. Left: original intensity profile. Middle: Displacement vectors. Divergence of displacement vectors corresponds to the location of the edge. Right: Smoothed intensity and original intensity together.

Fig. 3. Mean-shift based edge detection is depicted on a gap edge. (left) When the correct size mean-shift is applied the correct edge location is obtained. (right) However, larger scale mean-shift moves the edge location to left and lowers the edge strength, E_s.

perceptual edge organization, which is explained in the section. In this section, we describe how to remove incorrect edges along a ray based on *edge confidence* and *edge strength*.

Consider a typical intensity data containing a single edge, Figure 2. While the divergence of displacement vectors defines the location of the edge, the convergence of displacement vectors corresponds to the local mode of intensity, *i.e.* clustering of intensity data. The intensity data can be locally clustered around the edge by mean-shift, if the proper scale, (σ_x) is chosen. We use this fact, *i.e.*, local clustering, to define the *edge confidence* which measures the validity of an edge by checking the presence of local clustering, Figure 2. Specifically, the edge confidence for scale (σ_{xk}) at location i is given by $E_{ci}(\sigma_{xk}) = \frac{\sum_{j=1}^{M} \frac{|I_j^* - I_i|}{|I_c - I_i|}}{M}$ where M is the size of the filter, I_j^* is a smoothed intensity at j, I_c corresponds to the intensity value of the convergence point, *i.e.*, local intensity mode. Observe that this measure is close to one if a local clustering forms around the edge, otherwise, it is close to zero. In this paper, we delete the edges with small confidence (< 0.4) which, for example, forms from applying small-scale mean-shift filtering on diffused edges. While the removal of low confidence edges is important, it cannot solely eliminate all incorrect edges. In fact, several high confidence edges form in the vicinity of a correct edge. To eliminate these incorrect edges, we define *edge strength* as the intensity difference between at edge location and the convergence location. Specifically, the edge strength of an edge location i is given by $E_s(i) = 2|I_i - I_c|$ where I_c is the intensity value of the convergence point. Observe that there are two convergence locations for each divergence location. In ideal conditions, *i.e.*, well isolated step edges, the edge strength does not change based on selection of I_c. However, in real applications, this assumption does not hold and the correct one must be selected. We specifically illustrate this on a gap edge:

Consider a *gap edge*, where the presence of nearby structure alters the intensity profile significantly, Figure 3. The detail analysis of mean-shift filtering points out that the edge location and the edge strength can be accurately computed from *one side* of the filter, Figure 3. Thus, in this paper, we propose the edge strength should be measured from the one side. The correct side is determined from the edge confidences of the sides. Specifically, the side that gives higher edge confidence must be selected for the edge strength. The following observation is then used to eliminate incorrect edges based on their strength and local mode: *An edge is a correct edge if it is not located under the local mode of another edge. If it falls inside the local mode of another edge, it must have higher edge strength.* The local mode of an edge corresponds to the interval between its convergence points. Figure 6a,b illustrates an example.

3   Vessel Boundary Extraction from Multi-scale Edges

In this section, we present an algorithm for selecting the edges that correspond to the cross-sectional boundary of vessels. Specifically, a three-stage algorithm is proposed: prominent edge selection, curve segments from local edge grouping, and curve grouping based on ellipse fitting. The different stages of the proposed algorithm are depicted in detail in Figure 6a-h.

Prominent Edge Selection: In this paper, we propose to use the fact that vessels found CE-MRA/CTA are not embedded inside other bright structures. In other words, they are *locally* surrounded by darker background, *i.e.*, partial nearby bright structures are allowed. This is called *no nested structures* assumption. However, this assumption may not be valid if vessels are fully surrounded by darker appearing plaques, which we have not observed in any data yet. The

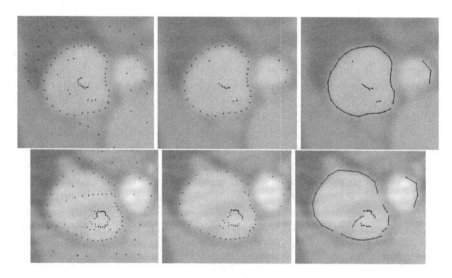

Fig. 4. This figure illustrates the results of prominent edge selection and local edge grouping on two different example. (left) multi-scale edges, (middle) prominent edges, and (right) curve segments after grouping.

prominent edges from multi-scale edges are determined by our *no nested structures* assumption. Geometrically, the first significant edge (strength) encountered during a propagation along the rays from the seed point towards outside often corresponds to the vessel boundary, if there is no significant noise inside the vessels. In other words, an edge is deleted from edge map if there is a much more significant edge present on the right side (outward). Mathematically, the edge E_i is deleted if $E_{si} < k_1 E_{sj}$ where $j > i \geq 0$ or if $k_1 E_{si} < E_{sj}$ where $i > j \geq 0$. k_1 is a parameter which specifies relative strength of edges. In real images, it is not easy to estimate k_1 value that would select edges corresponding to vessel boundaries. Thus, we propose to apply a range of k_1 values to select the prominent edges from multi-scales. In our experiments, all prominent edges are obtained by setting k_1 to $0.1, 0.2, 0.3, 0.5, 0.7, 0.9$ respectively and marking all these prominent edges in a single image. Figure 4 illustrate the proposed algorithm on two real examples. Observe that this algorithm reduces the number of edges significantly while preserving all the important edges.

Curve Segments From Local Edge Grouping: After removing edge elements which are not part of the vessel boundary, the problem of detecting the vessel boundary becomes relatively easy. In this stage, our goal is to organize edge elements into "long smooth curves" via perceptual edge grouping algorithms. Previously, Gestalt psychologists proposed that the human visual system selects those that depict regularities such as good continuation, proximity, symmetry, closure, etc. for the organization of visual data, *e.g.*, [12] These ideas have motivated approaches in computational vision where sets of edge elements which form long smooth curves with few interruptions are grouped together [14,11,6].

The goal of obtaining smooth curve segments in our problem is relatively easy compared to the general edge grouping problem because (1) edge elements are implicitly ordered by rays, (2) very few gaps are present, (3) spurious edges are almost non-existent. Our proposal for grouping edges to obtain curve segments exploits the angle θ_i, and distance (length) L_i between edge elements, Figure 5a. Specifically, edge grouping starts from three edge elements, which forms a smooth curve segment, *i.e.*, small angle θ_i. It then expands in two directions by adding more edge elements based on the neighboring angles which force the curve remain smooth, and the length of neighboring edges which also forces the proximity. When multiple edge elements are "good" candidates for smoothness during the expansion of a curve segment, a branch point forms and new curve segments are initialized from this branch point. This iterative edge grouping terminates when all edge elements are considered for local grouping. This grouping algorithm converts edges to a set of curve segments $\mathcal{C} = \{C_1, ..., C_N\}$. Figure 4 illustrates the results of this local edge grouping algorithm on two examples.

Vessel Boundary From Elliptical Shape Descriptors: After obtaining a set of smooth curve segments from prominent edges, our goal is to select a subset of k curve segments which corresponds to the cross-sectional boundary of vessels. This can be efficiently accomplished by considering all *geometrically possible*

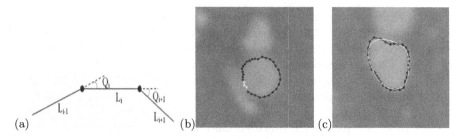

Fig. 5. (a) This figure illustrates the main idea of local grouping. (b) Presence of nearby vessels often remove some of the edges from vessel boundary resulting gaps. The gap between curve segments (black segments) are completed by cubic splines (white curve). (c) Elliptical Fourier Descriptors (white curve) are used for measuring the similarity of curve segments (black) to ellipse with local deformations.

subsets of curve segments and selecting a subset that is most similar to an ellipse. Geometrically possible curve segments correspond to the segments, which form smooth and longer curve segments when they are joined together without breaking them into pieces. Sometimes disjoint curve segments form smooth curves, which then results in gaps between them. In fact, gaps occur often when some parts of vessel boundary do not contain any edge due to the presence of nearby bright structures. For example, when arteries touch veins in MS-325 contrast enhanced MRA, there is no boundary between them, Figure 5b. Similarly, in CTA no boundary between bone and touching vessel may be present due to intensity similarities. In addition, gaps also form in edge grouping stage due to the noise in the vessel boundaries. Thus, we propose that such gaps should be bridged by the best "completion curves" to obtain a closed curve. These completion curves for gaps between curve segments or edge elements are often constructed from circular arcs [17], elastica [10], or Euler-Spiral [8]. In this work, we propose to use cubic splines for computational efficiency. Figure 5b illustrates a smooth completion curve obtained from the cubic spline for a gap between two curve segment.

The curve segments that best represent the cross-sectional boundary of vessel is determined by an elliptical fit measure. Specifically, while the global shapes of vessels resembles an ellipse, it often exhibits local variations from an ellipse due to the presence of nearby vessels. In fact, such local deformations should be preserved for an accurate boundary representation. For this task, we propose to use elliptical Fourier descriptors [15] to obtain the best curve from all the possible sets. Specifically, from given set $\mathcal{C}$, an elliptical fit measure is computed for each geometrically possible subsets of curve segments by elliptical Fourier descriptors. Among them, a subset of curve segments that best fits to an ellipse is selected as the boundary of vessels. Figure 5c illustrates a closed curve constructed from the elliptical Fourier descriptors of a set of curve segments. In our experiment, we used 7 Fourier coefficients since low number of coefficients (< 5) does not capture local deformations of boundary and high number of coefficients (> 10) allows too much local deformation. We experimentally observed

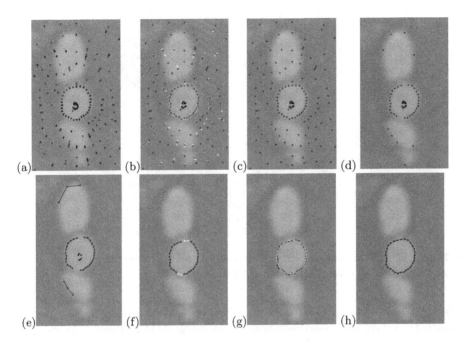

Fig. 6. This figure illustrates the boundary extraction algorithm step by step on a CE-MRA data. White color describes the event taking place at that stage. (a) Multi-scale edges are detected along 1D rays, (b) Incorrect edges (white) are eliminated, (c) Correct edges after deletion of incorrect edges, (d) Prominent edge selection by setting k_1 to $0.1, 0.2, 0.3, 0.5, 0.7, 0.9$, (e) Curve segments obtained from local edge grouping algorithm, (f) Gap completion via cubic spline (white) between curve segments, (g) Elliptic Fourier representation (white) of a curve set, (h) Vessel boundary obtained from an elliptical fit.

that these elliptical descriptors are very accurate in capturing vessel boundaries in great accuracy and robustness.

4   Results and Validations

Figure 6a-h describes the proposed algorithm step by step. The proposed algorithm is applied on several CTA and MRA data sets. Figure 7 illustrates several examples on both CTA and MRA. In all examples, all parameters are constant. Thus, no change in the parameters is needed to obtain accurate results robustly. In addition, the results do not depend on the location of the seed point. The current implementation of our algorithm for a single slice takes 0.15 seconds on Penthium IV 1.8 GHz PC.

The accuracy of results are validated by comparing them against "ground-truth" results created by an expert on 4 patient data sets. Specifically, the 2D cross-sectional vessel boundaries were detected via the proposed algorithm at

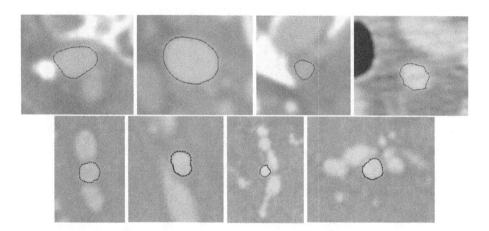

Fig. 7. This figure illustrates the extraction of vessel cross-sectional boundary by the proposed algorithm on several MRA and CTA data

Table 1. This table illustrates the distance differences between computed and expert-constructed vessel cross-sectional boundaries in percentage (%) for 8 different locations. The $(x \pm y); z$ representation describes: x (the average distance difference), y (the standard deviation of this difference) and z (the maximum distance difference between two contours in percentage).

	Patient-1	Patient-2	Patient-3	Patient-4
Contour-1	$(2.98 \pm 1.77);6.93$	$(3.95 \pm 3.02);13.12$	$(7.45 \pm 5.28);21.83$	$(9.82 \pm 5.44);21.71$
Contour-2	$(2.02 \pm 1.28);5.37$	$(3.60 \pm 2.23);11.19$	$(1.69 \pm 0.96);5.01$	$(11.35 \pm 4.00);19.42$
Contour-3	$(2.40 \pm 2.07);9.54$	$(4.29 \pm 3.62);14.82$	$(1.87 \pm 1.37);5.96$	$(13.07 \pm 3.75);19.76$
Contour-4	$(3.36 \pm 2.54);8.78$	$(2.24 \pm 1.40);5.63$	$(2.78 \pm 1.68);6.04$	$(16.72 \pm 5.13);24.76$
Contour-5	$(4.64 \pm 5.03);19.05$	$(3.48 \pm 3.90);13.75$	$(3.73 \pm 3.17);12.69$	$(14.51 \pm 4.85);21.69$
Contour-6	$(3.46 \pm 3.32);15.53$	$(2.58 \pm 2.27);7.07$	$(3.19 \pm 3.03);12.61$	$(13.22 \pm 6.34);25.31$
Contour-7	$(3.19 \pm 4.40);17.99$	$(4.90 \pm 3.40);10.69$	$(3.89 \pm 4.17);14.22$	$(13.25 \pm 3.74);21.49$
Contour-8	$(3.00 \pm 2.56);12.04$	$(4.35 \pm 2.44);10.23$	$(5.80 \pm 4.49);15.58$	$(13.27 \pm 5.45);23.87$

the user selected locations. These results were then compared to the expert generated results in Table 1. We present average error, standard deviation and maximum error between each contour in percentage. Each contour is described by 48 contour points. Let C_i represent a point on the expert-created contour. Similarly, let its corresponding point on the computed contour be represented by $\hat{C}_i$. Since each contour differs in size, percentage errors are used in our validation instead of actual distance in mm. In order to find the percentage difference between two points, we performed a radial comparison using the ratio of the diameter of the user constructed contour to the difference, $|C_i - \hat{C}_i|$. The proposed algorithm performs very well on many data sets. Especially, observe that for the first three data sets mean distance and standard deviations are very

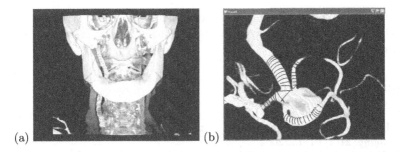

(a)   (b)

Fig. 8. The modeling of vessel is obtained by a simple tracking algorithm which operates on the 2D cross-sectional boundaries of vessels. (a) partial modeling of carotid artery in a CTA is visualized by volume rendering. (b) modeling vessels in the vicinity of a cerebral aneurysm in 3D rotational X-ray angiography.

low. For the Patient-4 the difference is between computed and ground-truth data is relatively high compared to the other data sets. However, the expert is satisfied with the accuracy of the results on Patient-4 because maximum diameter of vessel in that data set was 5 pixels. Thus, maximum error was often less than one pixel.

5   Tracking Vessels

Accurate detection and modeling of vessels is an important task in medical image applications [1,5,19]. Modeling vessels directly from images by the eigenvalue analysis of Hessian matrix has been very popular in vascular image analysis. In these approaches, images are often filtered based on the eigenvalue analysis of Hessian matrix to highlight 3D tubular structures in images. Specifically, a "vesselness measure" is then defined based on the eigenvalue analysis, e.g., [13,9,5]. While the main goal of this paper is the accurate and robust detection of vessel cross-sectional boundary, the 2D cross-sectional vessel boundaries can be successfully used in vessel modeling algorithms. Specifically, we implemented a vessel tracking algorithm that is similar to the one described in [2]. Specifically, direction of vessels are detected by the eigenvalues of Hessian matrix and vessels are tracked by using centerlines and cross-sectional boundaries detected by the current algorithm. Figure 8 illustrates the initial results obtained from this tracking algorithm. It must be observed that while this tracking algorithm cannot segment multiple branches from a single seed, it can be successfully used modeling stenosis and aneurysm very accurately.

6   Conclusion

In this paper, we proposed a method for detecting vessel boundaries accurately and robustly. The proposed algorithm is accurate and stable even where the vessels are surrounded by other vessels or other high contrast structures, contrast variations are present along vessels, and variations in the vessel size and shape are common.

References

1. S. Aylward and E. B. E. Initialization, noise, singularities, and scale in height-ridge traversal for tubular object centerline extraction. *IEEE Trans. on Medical Imaging*, 21(2):61–75, 2002.
2. T. Behrens, K. Rohr, and H. Stiehl. Robust segmentation of tubular structures in 3-d medical images by parametric object detection and tracking. *IEEE Transactions on Systems, Man, and Cybernetics, Part B*, 33(4):554–561, 2003.
3. D. Comaniciu. An algorithm for data-driven bandwidth selection. *IEEE Trans. Pattern Analysis Machine Intell.*, 25(2):281–288, 2003.
4. D. Comaniciu and P. Meer. Mean shift: A robust approach toward feature space analysis. *IEEE Trans. PAMI*, 24(5):603–619, 2002.
5. M. Descoteaux, L. Collins, and K. Siddiqi. Geometric flows for segmenting vasculature in MRI: Theory and validation. In *MICCAI*, 2004.
6. G. Guy and G. Medioni. Inferring global perceptual contours from local features. *IJCV*, 20(1):113–133, 1996.
7. M. Hernandez-Hoyos, A. Anwander, M. Orkisz, J. P. Roux, and I. E. M. P. Doueck. A deformable vessel model with single point initialization for segmentation, quantification and visualization of blood vessesl in 3D MRA. In *MICCAI'00*, 2000.
8. B. B. Kimia, I. Frankel, and A.-M. Popescu. Euler spiral for shape completion. *Int. J. Comput. Vision*, 54(1-3):157–180, 2003.
9. K. Krissian, G. Malandain, N. Ayache, R. Vaillant, and Y. Trousset. Model based multiscale detection of 3d vessels. In *IEEE Conf. CVPR*, pages 722–727, 1998.
10. D. Mumford. Elastica and computer vision. *Algebraic Geometry and Its Applications*, pages 491–506, 1994.
11. P. Parent and S. W. Zucker. Trace inference, curvature consistency and curve detection. *PAMI*, 11(8):823–839, 1989.
12. S. Sarkar and K. Boyer. Perceptual organization using Bayesian networks. In *CVPR*, pages 251–256, 1992.
13. Y. Sato, S. Nakajima, N. Shiraga, H. Atsumi, S. Yoshida, T. Koller, G. Gerig, and R. Kikinis. Three-dimensional multi-scale line filter for segmentation and visualisation of curvilinear structures in medical images. *Med. Image Analysis*, 2(2):143–168, 1998.
14. A. Sha'ashua and S. Ullman. Structural saliency: The detection of globally salient structures using a locally connected network. In *ICCV*, 1988.
15. L. H. Staib and J. S. Duncan. Boundary finding with parametrically deformable models. *PAMI*, 14(2):1061–1075, 1992.
16. H. Tek, D. Comaniciu, and J. Williams. Vessel detection by mean shift based ray propagation. In *Work. on Math. Models in Biomedical Image Analysis*, 2001.
17. S. Ullman. Filling-in the gaps: The shape of subjective contours and a model for their generation. *Biological Cybernetics*, 25:1–6, 1976.
18. O. Wink, W. Niessen, and M. A. Viergever. Fast delination and visualization of vessels in 3-D angiographic images. *IEEE Trans. on Medical Imaging*, 19:337–345, 2000.
19. O. Wink, W. J. Niessen, and M. A. Viergever. Multiscale vessel tracking. *IEEE Trans. on Medical Imaging*, 23(1):130–133, 2004.

Non-rigid Registration for Colorectal Cancer
MR Images

Sarah L. Bond and J. Michael Brady

Wolfson Medical Vision Laboratory, Department of Engineering Science,
University of Oxford, Parks Road, Oxford, OX1 3PJ, UK

Abstract. We are developing a system for patient management in colorectal cancer, in which the need for segmentation and non-rigid registration of pre- and post-therapy images arises. Several methods for non-
rigid registration have been proposed, all of which embody a 'generic'
algorithm to solve registration, largely irrespective both of the kinds of
images and of the application. We have evaluated several of these algorithms for this application and find their performance unsuitable for
aligning pre- and post- therapy colorectal images. This leads us to identify some of the implicit assumptions and fundamental limitations of
these algorithms. None of the currently available algorithms take into
account the issue of scale salience and more importantly, none of the
algorithms "know" enough about colorectal MRI to focus their attention
for registration on those parts of the image that are clinically important.
Based on this analysis, we propose a way in which we can perform registration by mobilizing the knowledge of the particular application, for
example the prior shape knowledge that we have within the colorectal
images as well as knowledge of the large scale non-rigid changes due to
therapy.

1 Introduction

The assessment of computer vision registration techniques presented in this paper arose from our continuing work to develop a system to support patient
management decisions in colorectal cancer. We begin by recalling some of the
salient facts about colorectal cancer and the ways in which its progression is
imaged. Following clinical practice at our site, our work to date has been based
entirely on T2 weighted Magnetic Resonance (MR) images. Then we sketch the
patient management decision we have worked on, evaluating the response to
neo-adjuvant chemo/radiotherapy, which requires the application of image segmentation and registration. To summarize: we established the need for non-rigid
registration, then evaluated a number of prominent research and commercial
methods. We contend that the fundamental problem is that, in their generic
form, the algorithms are not able to mobilize knowledge, whether of anatomy or
of the extensive but (at least qualitatively) predictable physiological responses
following neo-adjuvant chemo/radiotherapy. We show how mobilizing even basic
anatomical knowledge can greatly improve the results of registration.

Y. Liu, T. Jiang, and C. Zhang (Eds.): CVBIA 2005, LNCS 3765, pp. 399–408, 2005.
© Springer-Verlag Berlin Heidelberg 2005

Colorectal cancer is the second most common form of cancer in the western world and kills over 400,000 people each year worldwide. Early and accurate diagnosis is critical in order to assess the risks and determine the best treatment. Increasingly, the results of image analysis are used to determine patient management decisions, for example: whether or not to administer neo-adjuvant chemo/radiotherapy prior to surgery, whether or not there is nodal involvement, and the response of a tumor to such chemo/radiotherapy. We are interested in the local tumor, as seen in the MR data, as this materially affects patient management decisions. More detail about colorectal anatomy and chemo/radiotherapy prior to surgery are presented in Sect. 2.

T2 weighted MR scans are taken before and after the patient has undergone a course of neo-adjuvant chemotherapy or radiotherapy prior to surgery. This enables the consultants to evaluate the effect that the prior treatment has had, and identify the positions of the primary tumor, and any metastatic lymph nodes, that are still present. The tumor and lymph nodes can change dramatically in size and shape as a result of therapy, so their effective comparison pre and post-therapy requires alignment of the images. The best understood, most well-conditioned and predictable registrations assume either a rigid or affine transformation between the pre- and post-therapy images. We have found (Sect. 3.1) that affine registration can align the image positions well based on the rigid features such as the hips and the base of the spine. However, affine does not provide adequate pre- and post-therapy image alignment, largely because of the often substantial, relatively localized changes wrought by therapy.

Recognizing the need for non-rigid registration, we applied a number of well-known research and commercial algorithms. Typical results are presented in Sect. 3.2, and we discuss the poor performance in Sect. 4, asking whether there is something particular about the registration challenge we face or whether there is a more generic issue. We conclude the latter and discuss in Sect. 5 some of the ways in which knowledge of anatomy and physiology might be mobilized to make the performance of these algorithms more reliable, predictable, and accurate.

2   Colorectal Anatomy

We present a very brief introduction to colorectal anatomy in order to enable us to explain the effects of treatment and to frame our discussion of where the non-rigid registration algorithms fail. The main features of interest can be seen in Fig. 1(a). The hips and coccyx are rigid bone structures. The colorectum is where the primary tumor is usually located. The metastatic spread of this tumor into other areas is the key issue in determining patient management. The mesorectum is a layer of fat surrounding the colorectum and contains both lymph nodes and blood vessels. Lymph nodes often contain traces of the tumor as it metastasizes and these structures are therefore also important.

Cancerous tumors cause swelling, primarily in the colorectum and mesorectum. Chemotherapy and radiotherapy are designed primarily to kill cancerous cells in the tumor and in any infected lymph nodes, and to reduce the risk of

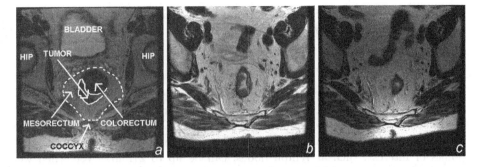

Fig. 1. (a) Anatomy of the region, (b) T2 axial colorectal MR images pre-therapy and (c) post-therapy

metastasis prior to, and during, surgery. Also, they often reduce substantially the swelling in response to the tumor (up to 25%), and this changes both the shape and size of the colorectum and mesorectum.

Neo-adjuvant chemo/radiotherapy is successful, at least to a certain extent, in 50% of cases. Successful (albeit partially successful) response causes the T2-weighted MR signal to reduce in intensity. Any involved lymph nodes are also reduced in size. There is a predictable density change that occurs in the mesorectal fat: it becomes much 'streakier' in appearance in the post-therapy image. The volume of mesorectal fat also decreases, though to varying degrees. The wall of the colorectum often thickens and becomes adematous despite the overall reduction in size. Images corresponding to an equivalent slice from the two pre- and post-therapy data-sets of one of the patients is shown in Fig. 1(b) and (c).

Finally, we note that even in the absence of cancer this area of the body is particularly prone to localized displacement, not least because of bowel and bladder movement. For all of these reasons, the differences between the images pre and post-therapy are most often substantial, to the point where even skilled clinicians have difficulty evaluating patient response to therapy. This motivates the need for image registration to align the anatomy and tumor in the pre- and post-therapy images. The expected changes are substantial, and the descriptions are qualitative, however they do refer to anatomical structures which can be identified [1].

3   Data and Generic Registration Techniques

The pre- and post-therapy images are T2 weighted (TE = 90ms, TR = 3500-5000ms, α = 90 deg, slice thickness = 3mm), axial small field of view, MR images taken at the Radiology Department of the Churchill Hospital, Oxford. The data-sets are 3-D, each consisting of 512 x 512 x 25 voxels of size 0.4mm x 0.4mm x 3mm. Currently, approximately 50 patients per year are treated for colorectal cancer at our site. In the experiments reported in this section, we repeated the application of each of the registration algorithms for a randomly chosen sample comprising nine patients. For each data-set the bias field (an MRI artifact) was removed using a method by Styner et al. [2].

3.1   Affine Registration

For the reasons given in the Introduction, we first implemented affine registration to align the two data-sets. As expected, this gave very poor results, due to the fact that the differences are essentially non-rigid, and due to movement, changes in density, and changes in tumor size. The mean error for manually located points of interest, such as lymph nodes, can be up to 21mm. Even when we placed a larger number of landmarks (17) on the rigid bone structures, and then applied RANSAC [6], a good registration was not achieved, in the sense that the anatomy was not aligned sufficiently for it to be useful to the clinicians. However, affine registration does provide a reasonable global alignment, which can then be used as the first step in non-rigid registration algorithms. This is assumed by several of the non-rigid registration algorithms we experimented with.

3.2   Non-rigid Registration

We have experimented with a representative set of 'generic' research and commercial registration algorithms (and acknowledge gratefully the substantial help that the authors of those algorithms have given us).

Rueckert et al. [3] proposed a registration method using B-splines and mutual information across a uniform grid of control points. This grid is then refined and the procedure is repeated using finer grids until the optimum registration is achieved. The results of a typical application of this algorithm can be seen in Fig.2(a) which shows the warped image computed by the algorithm. Park and Meyer suggested using a mis-match measure [4] in order to determine those areas of the image which seem to be maximally misaligned. They then refine the current grid of control points just in such misaligned areas. Either B-splines or Thin Plate Splines (TPS) can then be placed at these control points in order to perform the registration. A typical set of such control points can be seen in Fig. 2(b). Crum et al. [5] proposed a fluid non-rigid registration algorithm. This was run using normalized mutual information and the difference between the target and the registered source image can be seen in Fig. 2(c). In difference images the mis-registered areas are identified by bright and dark areas, so that a perfectly aligned image would everywhere have the same gray-scale value.

RevealMVS^{TM}, provided to our Laboratory by Mirada Solutions Ltd., as well as ITK (Insight Toolkit www.itk.org) registration methods, were also run on the data. Though its exact form is not made explicit, RevealMVS^{TM} appears to use an algorithm similar to block-matching, whereas ITK uses local affine registration. Typical results of running these algorithms can be seen in the difference images in Fig. 2(d) and (e).

From the results in Fig. 2 it can be seen that the algorithms do not perform well for this application, with small features such as lymph nodes misaligned by up to 30mm in some cases. This is also the case for all the data-sets we

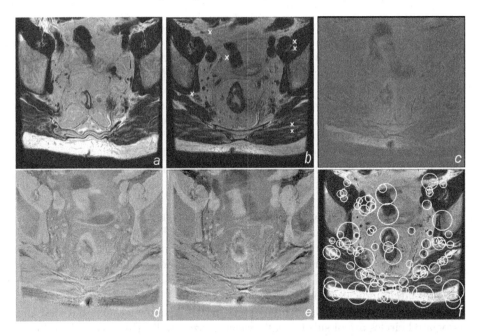

Fig. 2. (a) Result of registration using Rueckert's method. (b) Positions of Control Points found using Park and Meyer's method. Result of registration (difference image) using (c) Crum's method (d) RevealMVS^{TM}, and (e) ITK. (f) Illustration of salience across scale and space.

tested. It seems that the key issue is that the algorithms analyze entropy at a single scale and equate signal complexity with 'interesting features' that drive the registration. However, the area that is of most clinical interest (the mesorectum and colorectum) are the image regions that are the least varying, most bland. The algorithms appear to find, at a coarse scale, points that are locally complex (high entropy) but which are of no clinical interest. These erroneous matches are then largely preserved as the scale of the registration is refined.

4   Need for Scale Saliency

None of the diverse non-rigid registration methods performed well enough to be clinically useful on our pre- and post-therapy data. We contend that there are two main reasons for the observed performance, and that they are quite generic.

The first concerns the saliency, or 'feature-ness', of the images. All of the registration algorithms align the images where there are sufficiently many features, at a certain scale. That is, prior to regularization that propagates local matches, they preferentially align areas of high feature complexity, which is generally equated with high entropy, at the scale of interest. However, Kadir and Brady [7] have demonstrated that scale and saliency are implicitly related, both to each other and to image complexity. That is, features are associated with a particular scale within the image. They show this by considering the entropy of local image regions over a range of scales. They suggest that areas that have a consistently high entropy, that is, if they exist as features over a sufficiently wide range of scales, then they should not in fact be judged salient, since they can not be considered rare, which is the essence of salience. However, if there is a peak at a single scale (or spread over a small range of scales) in the entropies over a particular area then this implies that there is a feature at that position localized to that scale. Kadir and Brady demonstrate that saliency has to be analyzed in terms of scale as well as space. However, all of the non-rigid registration algorithms we experimented with treat the entropy independently at each scale.

Does this matter in practice? To investigate this question, we applied a recent refinement of the algorithm proposed by Kadir and Brady [7] to the colorectal cancer images. We set the algorithm to find the 85 most salient regions across both scale and space (empirically this number produces good results and is insensitive to changes ±5%). A typical result can be seen in Fig. 2(f), where the size of a circle indicates the scale of the feature that has been found. The first thing to note is that the algorithm detects mostly sensible features but that the associated circles are of substantially varying sizes, indicating that it is unlikely that all of the features sought can be detected at a single scale. It should also be noted that the more complex areas of the images, for example the muscle regions in the bottom left and bottom right hand corners of the image, do not yield any salient points. This is because the entropy in these areas is high across the entire range of scales, hence they are not considered salient.

Colorectal images exhibit structure (and complexity) over a wide range of spatial scales, but also have regions that have a high entropy across a range of scales that are, in fact, not salient. Of course, a scale-saliency analysis such as that of Kadir and Brady [7] could be incorporated into non-rigid registration algorithms, though the proper integration of registration of images across a stack of spatial scales is not entirely straightforward.

5   Mobilizing Application-Specific Knowledge in Non-rigid Registration

However, incorporating scale-saliency, though necessary (at least for this task), is not sufficient. We also need the mobilization of appropriate application-specific knowledge that constrains and guides the registration process. In this section, we describe some initial steps toward mobilizing knowledge, hence incorporating segmentation into the registration process. Chen et al. [8] have shown that incorporating segmentation into registration algorithms gives a robust registration and we set out a way in which we can include knowledge of both the anatomy and expected large scale changes into the registration of the pre- and post-therapy data.

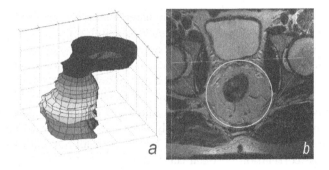

Fig. 3. (a) Segmented colorectum in 3-D, and (b)the constrained region of interest

5.1   Segmentation of the Anatomy

We limit attention to the colorectal and mesorectal regions as this is the area of most clinical interest. The system we have built constructs a local coordinate frame in which the mesorectal region can be reliably and accurately located. We do this by first finding the rigid bone structures (hips and coccyx) which is straightforward given their expected positions, similar sizes, and intensities. We can then use these to locate the colorectum which can be segmented using a Kalman snake, Fig.3(a). From this we can build up a coordinate frame of reference, centered on the colorectum, and defined by the coccyx and hips, which then enables us to "cage" the colorectum, Fig. 3(b). That is, it defines the initial search position of, the scales and size of, the mesorectum, whose boundary is then relatively straightforward to determine. [1] gives more details of the segmentation processes and methods. This anatomical 'map', determining the position of the colorectum and mesorectum, has been shown to accurately locate the anatomical features on all our 9 test data-sets described previously [1]. This 'map' can potentially be extended further to include all the bone regions of the pelvis (not just the hips and coccyx), the bladder and the muscle and fat sections. It has been shown by Christensen et al. [9] that an anatomical atlas can greatly aid registration results in this region of the body due to the large scale deformation that can occur. We are extending this method to combine an automatic fitting of an atlas to the anatomy as both a starting point and constraint for the registration.

5.2   Finding the Deformation Field

We now turn to the issue that therapy causes reduction in tumor size and swelling in the region of the tumor in the colorectum and mesorectum. The warp field for the manually registered pre- and post-therapy images (using landmarks) can be seen in Fig. 4(a). It can be seen that the greatest changes (red) occur in the mesorectal region due to compression. The next stage is to characterize this warp field based on differential invariants, in the manner of Thirion and Calmon [10] and later Rey et al. [11]. Since we can predict the general shape of the deformation field, we can characterize it using the Jacobian of the warp field, and then use this as a regularizer as we seek to match up points of interest. The Jacobian gives a scalar representation of a vector field by characterizing whether a region is shrinking or growing. The actual Jacobian of the warp field, calculated from a manual registration, where the landmarks were known and placed by hand, can be seen in Fig. 4(b). An estimate of this Jacobian found by registering the segmented colorectum, mesorectum and rigid features as described above, can be seen in Fig. 4(c). It can be clearly seen that the general 'shape' of these two Jacobians are similar, and this was the case for all our data-sets, with the minimum cross correlation between the two Jacobians being 0.57.

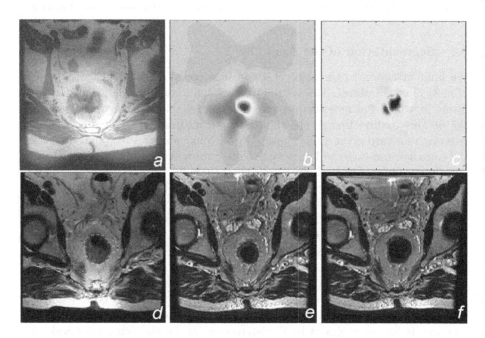

Fig. 4. (a) A visualization of the deformation field, (b) the Jacobian of this deformation field, and (c) the estimated Jacobian using the initial automatic segmentation from the frame of reference. (d)Points of interest on the pre-therapy image, and (e) on the post-therapy image, and (f) the registered post-therapy image.

Points of interest, additional to the automatically segmented rigid bone structures, colorectum and mesorectum, can be placed in and around the colorectal and mesorectal region, as this is where the warping is most likely to occur. These points will mostly include features such such as nodes, vessels etc that are unique to each patient and hence cannot be found using the anatomical 'map'. These features will vary in number between patients, and although they may be few, it is important for the clinical application that they are aligned. The points can be found using the scale salience region detector described previously, constraining the points of interest to within the mesorectum. Points of interest, or features, are found in each image, pre- and post therapy and then corresponding points can then be matched up by minimizing a cost function. This cost function is given by $C = -C_s - \lambda C_r$.

C_s is the cost associated with the similarity based on normalized mutual information between two regions surrounding the points of interest. The size of the surrounding region of interest is taken as the largest scale of the two points being tested, and the area is equivalent to the area of the circles seen in Fig. 2(f). The normalized mutual information is then based on the entropies of these local areas and is given by $(H(A) + H(B))/H(A, B)$ where $H(A)$ and $H(B)$ are the marginal entropies of the two regions A and B for each point, and $H(A, B)$ is the joint entropy of these two regions [12]. C_r is the cost associated with the Jacobian regularizer based on the predicted changes in the data. It is found using the correlation coefficient between the regularizing Jacobian (calculated previously from the registration of the segmented rigid points, colorectum and mesorectum), and the new Jacobian (calculated by incorporating the two possibly corresponding feature points into the warp field). λ is then chosen so as to prevent gross, unlikely warps occurring within the mesorectum. Although the changes can be great, they do occur in a predictable way which is constrained by the initial segmentation of the two images.

Some corresponding points of interest, found from both the initial automatic segmentation and the matching scale-salient regions within the colorectum and mesorectum, can be seen in Figs. 4(d) and 4(e), and the warped image using these landmarks is seen in Fig. 4(f). It can be seen that the colorectum and mesorectum have warped so as to be aligned, without introducing large errors or incorrect matching of regions as occurred using the generic non-rigid algorithms. As well as aligning the large scale anatomical features such as the colorectum, the scale-salient points allow the smaller scale features, that are usually unique to each patient, to also be aligned, providing accurate alignment (within 1mm) of the lymph nodes and vessels in the region of interest. This is a clinically useful result.

6   Conclusions

We have shown that there are fundamental limitations and assumptions imposed on current, generic non-rigid registration algorithms that do not hold for the application of aligning pre- and post-therapy images of colorectal cancer patients. We have then set out a way in which we can mobilize shape knowledge to overcome these limitations and start to develop a robust non-rigid registration framework that makes use of this prior knowledge to perform clinically useful and accurate registrations on colorectal images pre and post-therapy where gross changes have occurred between the two data-sets.

Acknowledgements. The authors would like to thank Dr. Fergus Gleeson, Dr. Helen Bungay and Prof. Neil Mortensen (from the Oxford Radcliffe Hospitals) for providing relevant data and clinical direction. Thanks also to Daniel Rueckert, Hyunjin Park, Charles Meyer, Bill Crum, and Mirada Solutions, Ltd for providing algorithms and software, and finally to the EPSRC for funding.

References

1. Bond, S., Brady, M.: Image Analysis for Patient Management in Colorectal Cancer. To be presented at CARS 05, Berlin, June 2005
2. Styner, M., Brechbuhler, C., Szekely, G., Gerig, G.: Parametric estimate of intensity inhomogeneities applied to MRI. IEEE Trans. Med. Imag. **19** (2000) 153-165
3. Rueckert, D., Sonoda, L.I., Hayes, C., Hill, D.L.G., Leach, M.O., Hawkes, D.J.: Nonrigid Registration Using Free-Form Deformations: Application to Breast MR Images. IEEE Trans. Med. Imag. **18** (1999) 712-721
4. Park, H., Bland, P.H., Brock, K.K., Meyer, C.R.: Adaptive Registration Using Local Information Measures. Med. Imag. Anal. **8** (2004) 465-473
5. Crum, W.R., Hill, D.L.G., Hawkes, D.J.: Information Theoretic Similarity Measures in Non-rigid Registration. IPMI 2003, LNCS **2732** 378-387
6. Fischler, M.A., Bolles, R.C.: Random Sample Consensus: A Paradigm for Model Fitting with Applications to Image Analysis and Automated Cartography. Comm. of the ACM **24** (1981) 381-395
7. Kadir, T., Brady, J.M.: Saliency, Scale and Image Description. Int. J. Comp. Vision **45** (2001) 83-105
8. Chen, X., Brady, M., Lo, J., Moore, N.: Simultaneous Segmentation and Registration of Contrast-Enhanced Breast MRI. IPMI 2005, LNCS
9. Christensen, G., Carlson, B., Chao, K. et al.: Image-based Dose Planning of Intracavity Brachytherapy: Registration of Serial-Imaging Studies Using deformable Anatomic Templates. Int. J. Radiation Oncology Biol. Phys. **51** (2001) 227-243
10. Thirion, J., Calmon, G.: Deformation Analysis to Detect and Quantify Active Lesion in 3D Medical Image Sequences. Research Report 3101. INRIA 1997
11. Rey, D., Subsol, G., Delingette, H., Ayache, N.: Automatic Detection and Segmentation of Evolving Processes in 3D Medical Images: Application to Multiple Sclerosis. IPMI 1999, LNCS **1613** 154-167
12. Studhome, C., Hill, D., Hawkes, D.: An Overlap Invariant Entropy Measureof 3D Medical Image Alignment. Pattern Recognit., **32** (1998) 71-86

Quantizing Calcification in the Lumbar Aorta on 2-D Lateral X-Ray Images

Lars A. Conrad-Hansen[1], Marleen de Bruijne[1], François Lauze[1],
Laszlo B. Tanko[2], and Mads Nielsen[1]

[1] IT University of Copenhagen, Denmark
[2] Center for Clinical and Basic Research, Copenhagen, Denmark

Abstract. In this paper we seek to improve the standard method of assessing the degree of calcification in the lumbar aorta visualized on lateral 2-D X-rays. The semiquantitative method does not take density of calcification within the individual plaques into account and is unable to measure subtle changes in the severity of calcification over time. Both of these parameters would be desirable to access, since they are the keys to assessing important information on the impact of risk factors and candidate drugs aiming at the prevention of atherosclerosis.

Herein we propose to estimate the background of a calcification using inpainting, a technique used in image restoration as well as postprocessing of film, and measure the plaque density as the difference between the background estimation and the original image. Furthermore, we compare total variation inpainting with harmonic inpainting and discuss the potential implications of inpainting for characterizing aortic calcification.

1 Introduction

1.1 What Are We Trying to Achieve?

The ultimate goal is the development of a mass-screening tool, suitable for quantifying the extent of calcification and density of calcific deposits in the lumbar aorta. Although several simple methods have been proposed for the manual semi-quantitative grading of aortic calcification[1,2,3], these methods have limitations especially in terms of capturing small changes in the progression of atherosclerosis. Furthermore, the evaluation may partly depend on the investigator / technician involved, and does not take the changes of the intraluminal expansion or the calcium density of the individual plaques into account.

A mass-screening tool has to deliver reliable and easily reproducible data. Electron-beam computed tomography (EBCT) allows precise quantification of calcium content in the vascular wall and thereby the severity of atherosclerosis [4]. However, this technique is more suitable for clinical research rather than for mass screening purposes, first of all due to high expenses.

A simpler and more easily accessible method is provided by the semi-quantitative grading of aorta calcification visualized by lateral 2-D X-rays of the lumbar section[5,6]. A regrettable limitation of common X-rays though, is that soft tissue, and thus a healthy

Y. Liu, T. Jiang, and C. Zhang (Eds.): CVBIA 2005, LNCS 3765, pp. 409–418, 2005.

aorta, is not visible. Accordingly, inference of the calcification index and its longitudinal changes has to rely solely on the visible calcific deposits in the aorta. To the best of our knowledge there has been no attempt so far as to establishing a computer-based system for quantifying the severity of aorta calcification in an automated fashion.

Essential elements of establishing an automated mass-screening tool are the automated localzation of the lumbar aorta [7], the automated recognition of calcified deposits, and a new method for quantifying the severity of calcification in the plaques. In the present study, we adopted different inpainting methods (total variation and harmonic) - techniques used in image restoration as well as postprocessing of films - to estimate the background of a calcified area. Taking the difference between the estimated background and the actual calcification is expected to provide a measurement of plaque density. These inpainting methods were compared to a simple averaging scheme.

1.2   Semi-quantitative Assessment of Calcified Deposits Using Radiography

The current clinical practice is to assess the calcification index on lateral 2-D x-rays as follows: The calcifications are measured lengthwise for the posterior as well as anterior walls at each vertebral segment of the L1 - L4 region, using the midpoint of the intervertebral space above and below the vertbrae as boundaries. The lesions are graded as follows [1] :

0 : No aortic calcific deposits
1 : Small scattered calcific deposits less than 1/3 of the longitudinal wall of the aorta
2 : 1/3 or more, but less than 2/3 of the longitudinal wall are calcified
3 : 2/3 or more of the longitudinal wall are calcified

Individual level-specific severity scores are summarized to yield three different composite scores for aortic calcifications:

(0 - 4) : Affected segments score
         number of individual aortic segments which show calcification are calculated
(0 - 8) : Anterior and posterior affected score
         number of individual aortic segments (both anterior and posterior) which show aortic calcification are summed
(0 - 24) : Anterior - posterior severity score
         the scores of individual aortic segments both for the posterior as well as for the anterior wall are summed

Fig. 1 visualizes this indexing system. The 24-score (or anterior - posterior severity score) is the most expressive score and is used as the comparative measure in this paper.

2   Method

2.1   Overview

The dataset contains 80 hand-annotated x-rays of the lumbar region with pixel intensities ranging from 0 - 2048; 77 of them display various degrees of calcification and 3

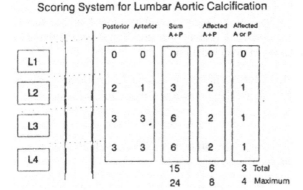

Fig. 1. Semi-quantitative grading

images are not calcified. The idea behind our approach is to simulate how a calcified image would have looked like non-calcified, by inpainting all the calcified areas. The difference between the calcified and the non-calcified image then yields the new calcification index. This way, not only the longitudinal extend but also the density of the calcifications can be expressed.

2.2 Inpainting

Inpainting is from a mathematical point of view, an interpolation problem:
Given a rectangular image u_0 known outside a hole Ω, we want to find an image u - an *inpainting* of u_0 - that matches u_0 outside the hole and which has "meaningful" content inside the hole Ω. From the many different inpainting algorithms TV inpainting [8,9] and Harmonic inpainting [9] were choosen for this work. TV inpainting was chosen for its ability to preserve structures (edges) to some extent, whereas Harmonic inpainting was chosen due to the fact that it provides much smoother solutions. The general Bayes' formulation of inpainting can be expressed as:

$$p(u|u_0) = \frac{p(u_0|u)p(u)}{p(u_0)} \propto p(u_0|u)p(u) \quad \text{since } u_0 \text{ is known.} \tag{1}$$

The *model* term $p(u_0|u)$ models the data formation process. Here we assume that the observed image u_0 is obtained from a clean image u corrupted by additive zero-mean Gaussian noise spatially uncorrelated and stationary, with standard deviation σ outside the hole Ω, and that the data inside Ω has been totally lost. Therefore the model of acquisition-degradation is given by

$$p(u_0|u) = c_1 e^{-\sum_{x \in R \setminus \Omega} \frac{(u(x)-u_0(x))^2}{2\sigma^2}}$$

where c_1 is a normalizing constant. The *prior* term $p(u)$ is usually more difficult to find, since it models the probability that a given array of pixel values represents a meaningful image. In absence of texture, we assume some form of smoothness for images - i.e. the variations of pixel values around a given pixel location should be small. We can, for that purpose, introduce a discrete Gradient operator, $\nabla u(x)$ encoding the local variations of the image around a given pixel location.

TV Inpainting: In order to enforce a reasonable smoothness, we assume a Laplace distribution on these values [10] and we obtain the following prior:

$$p(u) = c_2 e^{-\sum_{x \in R} \frac{|\nabla u(x)|}{\mu}}$$

where c_2 is a normalizing constant and $\mu\sqrt{2}$ the standard deviation. The resulting energy expression can be written as

$$E(u) = \int_R \chi(u - u_0)^2 dx + \lambda \int_R |\nabla u| dx, \tag{2}$$

where χ denotes the function $\chi(x) = 0$ if $x \in \Omega$, $\chi(x) = 1$ otherwise, and $\lambda = \frac{\sigma^2}{\mu}$.

Harmonic Inpainting: For Harmonic inpainting we assume a Gaussian distribution for the prior probability

$$p(u) = c_2 e^{-\sum_{x \in R} \frac{|\nabla u(x)|^2}{2\mu^2}} \tag{3}$$

where c_2 again is a normalizing constant and μ is the standard deviation. The energy term can then be expressed as

$$E(u) = \int_R \chi(u - u_0)^2 dx + \lambda \int_R |\nabla u|^2 dx, \tag{4}$$

where χ denotes the function $\chi(x) = 0$ if $x \in \Omega$, $\chi(x) = 1$ otherwise, and $\lambda = \frac{\sigma^2}{\mu^2}$.

Details regarding the solutions of the respective energy models can be found in the lecture notes of François Lauze [9]

Average Inpainting: This constitutes the simplest form of inpainting, where Ω is filled homogeneously with the value S resulting from averaging over the immediate boundary of Ω according to

$$S = \frac{1}{n} \sum_{i=1}^{n} t_i, \tag{5}$$

where n is the number of boundary pixels and t the respective pixel value.

2.3 Estimating the Noise Level

In order to estimate how well the individual inpainting techniques perfom on the x-ray images, 3000 templates of calcification shape were chosen at random from manual annotations (see Fig. 2). Algorithm 1 describes how each template is placed at a randomly chosen, non-calcified region of a randomly chosen aorta, and how the standard deviations of the pixelwise differences between the inpainted and original areas are calculated. Figure 3 shows regression lines through the calculated standard deviations. The regression lines express the standard deviations in the total pixelwise intensity difference for the three inpainting methods as a function of areasize.

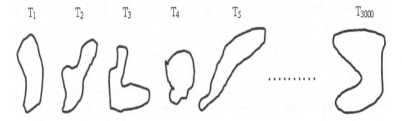

Fig. 2. Background estimation. The 3000 randomly chosen templates used for the respective inpainting schemes.

Algorithm 1. *Background estimation*

---

1. let A = number of pixels in an area circumscribed by a template
2. For $i = 1 \ldots 3000$ do
   - randomly choose an area template
   - randomly choose an image [1:80]
   - randomly choose a non-calcified aorta segment ([1:7],
     4 lumbar segments and 3 intervertebral spaces)
     large enough to center the area template in
   - For $c = 1 \ldots 3$ do
     - inpaint the area circumscribed by the area template
       ([1:3], TV, Harmonic, and Average inpainting)
     - calculate the pixelwise differences between inpainted and original area
     - take the standard deviation of the pixelwise differences and multiply
       by $\sqrt{A}$
3. calculate the regression curves through the sorted standard deviations

---

2.4 Pixelwise Expansion of the Individual Calcifications

Visual inspection of our initial experiments [11] with inpainting of calcified areas made it clear that the inpainting procedures were biased by minute calcific deposits just outside the annotated areas. These calcific rests were missed by the physician and became only apparent when zooming in to pixel-level. Since the inpainting methods rely entirely on boundary information, we had to expand the annotated areas in order to avoid faulty results as much as possible. Thus, the next step was to iterate the inpainting process for each calcified area of an image, so that each area was expanded in order to yield the maximum signal-to-noise ratio (SNR), which was calculated for each pixel along the immediate boundary of the calcified area according to

$$SNR = \frac{I_{inp} - I_{orig}}{std \times area},\tag{6}$$

where I_{inp} denotes the inpainted image, I_{orig} the original image, std the standard deviation of the estimated noise level, and $area$ the number of pixels in Ω. The idea behind the expansion scheme is that all pixels that increase the SNR get included in Ω.

Algorithm 2 illustrates the mechanism in detail and figure 4 shows the results on a test image.

3   Results

Using the iteration scheme described for the noise level estimation, we obtained the results listed in table 1 and visualized in Fig. 3. TV inpainting produces the least error per pixel and Harmonic inpainting follows closely. Average inpainting performs worst. Paired *t-tests* performed on the background data showed significant performance differences for TV vs. Average inpainting ($p < 0.0001$) and Average vs. Harmonic inpainting ($p < 0.0001$). There seems to be, however, no significant difference for TV vs. Harmonic inpainting ($p = 0.3506$).

Having computed a function for the error in background estimation with respect to the area, we tested the mechanics of algorithm 2 on a test image. Figure 4 shows how algorithm 2 detects the majority of the boundary pixels that should be included in the inpainting area of the test image and thus removes the bias from the inpainting procedure.

Having seen that algorithm 2 performs satisfactorily on a test image, we subjected the 77 calcified x-ray images to the algorithm, where in each image all the calcified areas were expanded and finally inpainted using the different inpainting techniques. For each image we summed over the pixelwise differences between the original and inpainted image, which constitutes our new calcium score. In order to assess the quality of our method, we plotted our score against the 24-score of the standard procedure (Fig. 5). From the plots in Figure 5 it is apparent that our method offers more possibilty

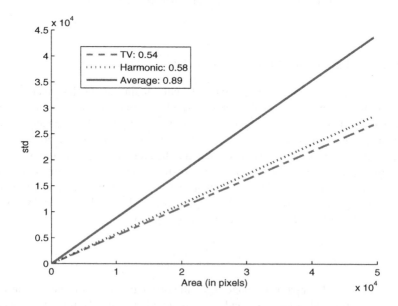

Fig. 3. Background estimation. Regression lines for the 3 different inpainting schemes.

Algorithm 2. *Pixelwise expansion scheme*

1. let N = number of calcified areas in image
2. let B = number of pixels in an isocurve
3. let p denote a pixel

4. For $i = 1 \ldots N$ do
   - inpaint Ω
   - calculate SNR
   - while SNR not max do
     • calculate outer distance map
     • find next isocurve
     • For $j = 1 \ldots B$ do
       * expand Ω by p_j
       * inpaint and calculate SNR
       * if SNR is increased, include p_j
   - inpaint new Ω
   - calculate SNR
5. output SNR

Table 1. The top part of the table displays the p-values resulting from the paired t-tests. The bottom row shows the standard deviations of the pixelwise error for the three inpainting methods.

	TV	Harmonic	Average
TV	1	0.3506	<0.0001
Harmonic	0.3506	1	<0.0001
Average	<0.0001	<0.0001	1
std	0.54	0.58	0.89

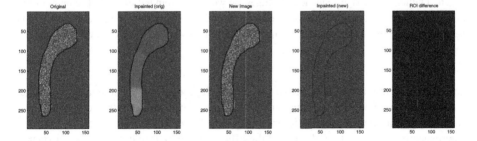

Fig. 4. Algorithm 2 run on a testimage. Left: The original input image with faulty annotation. Second-to-left: The inpainting resulting from the original input image. Middle: The algorithm has detected most of the left-out pixels. Second-to-right: The inpainting resulting from the revised input image. Right: The boundary difference between the original and revised input image.

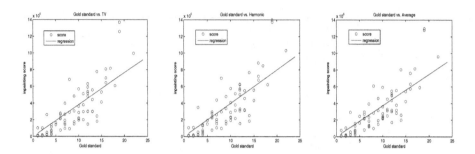

Fig. 5. The scores for the respective inpainting procedures versus the gold standard. Left: The 24-score versus the total differences resulting from TV inpainting. Middle: The 24-score versus the total differences resulting from Harmonic inpainting. Right: The 24-score versus the total differences resulting from Average inpainting.

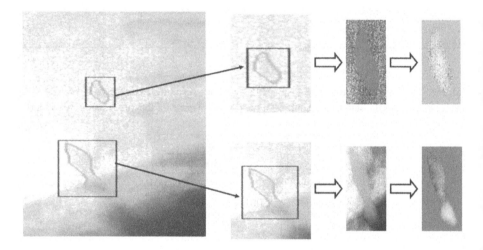

Fig. 6. Outlier. The image sequence illustrates the workflow from left to right. The input image at the start of the sequence contains two calcified areas. The two output images at the end of the sequence, one or each calcified area, contain the differences between the original areas and the inpainted areas.

for discerning the different stages of plaque development than the standard procedure. In many cases where the standard yields the same score for a number of images, our methods find a considerable difference (Fig. 5). The correlation coefficients between the respective inpainting methods and the official 24-score (table 2) show a reasonable correlation, but the new score is able to discern subtle differences, whereas the standard score is not.

The attention gets drawn towards the outliers, that, in spite of a fair general correlation, produce different numbers than expected. In Figure 6, the most extreme outlier of our data set is shown. This particular outlier scores a total of 2978536 (TV) on our

Table 2. The top row of the table shows the correlation coefficients between the inpainting schemes and the 24-score. The bottom row contains the p-values of the respective correlation coefficients.

	TV	Harmonic	Average
cor. coef	0.8284	0.8246	0.8329
p-value	<0.0001	<0.0001	<0.0001

calcification scale even though only two areas of normal size are detected. Looking at the differences between the original and the inpainted subimages however, leads to the conclusion that only plaque density can be the cause of this unexpectedly high score.

4   Conclusions and Discussion

In the present report, we described inpainting-based methods to quantify the degree of atherosclerosis. The findings suggest that this approach could offer better possibilities for the characterization of plaque densisty than the discrete scoring systems that are currently used in epidemiological settings. The statistical tests have shown that TV and Harmonic inpainting are both superior to Average inpainting in terms of their abilities for background estimation. There was however no statistical evidence that points towards preferring TV to Harmonic inpainting, and it remains to be medically evaluated whether or not the considerable extra computational effort involved in TV inpainting as opposed to Harmonic inpainting is justifiable. The preservence of structure, that is characteristic for TV inpainting [9] could prove to be a vital factor, since a considerable amount of structures is introduced by age, variation in body fat distribution, and lifestyle factors of the patient.

Future studies are planned to assess the sensitivity of this method for monitoring changes in aorta calcification compared with currently used semi-quantitative methods and the relation of these measures to the risk profile of the patients. The ability of the method to provide a continuous (not categorical) measure of aorta calcification is expected to provide useful assistance for both epidemiological and pharmacological studies in which monitoring of subtle changes over a period of time is a critical study parameter.

References

1. Leena I. Kauppila et al., "New indices to classify location, severity and progression of calcific lesions in the abdominal aorta: a 25-year follow-up study," *Atherosclerosis* **132**, pp. 245–250, 1997.
2. Wolffe JB and Siegal EI, "X-ray of the abdominal aorta in detection of atherosclerosis," *Clin Med* **69**, pp. 401–406, 1962.
3. Witteman JCM et al., "J-shaped relation between change in diastolic blood pressure and progression of aortic atherosclerosis," *Lancet* **343**, pp. 504–507, 1994.

4. Robert A. ORourke et al., "Expert consensus document on electron-beam computed tomography for the diagnosis and prognosis of coronary artery disease," *Circulation* **102**, pp. 126–140, 2000.

5. D.P.Kiel et al., "Bone loss and the progression of abdominal aortic calcification over a 25 year period: The framingham heart study," *Calcified Tissue International* **68**, pp. 271–276, 2001.

6. Laszlo B. Tanko et al., "Peripheral adiposity exhibits an independant dominant antiatherogenic effect in elderly women," *Circulation* **107**, pp. 1626–1632, 2003.

7. L. Conrad-Hansen et al., "Prediction of the location of the lumbar aorta using the first four lumbar vertebrae as a predictor," in *miip*, M. Sonka and M. Fitzpatrick, eds., **5370**(2), pp. 1271–1290, SPIEpress, 2004.

8. T. Chan and J. Shen, "Mathematical models for local non-texture inpaintings," *SIAM Journal of Applied Mathematics* **62**(3), pp. 1019–1043, 2001.

9. Francois Lauze, "Harmonic and tv inpainting," 2003.

10. Jinggang Huang and David Mumford, "Statistics of natural images and models," *Computer Vision and Pattern Recognition* **1**, 1999.

11. L. Conrad-Hansen et al., "Quantizing calcification in the lumbar aorta on 2-d lateral x-ray images using tv inpainting," in *miip*, M. Sonka and M. Fitzpatrick, eds., SPIEpress,in press, 2005.

Real-Time Simulation of Deformable Soft Tissue Based on Mass-Spring and Medial Representation

Shaoting Zhang[1], Lixu Gu[1,2], Pengfei Huang[1], and Jianfeng Xu[2]

[1] School of Software, Shanghai Jiaotong University, 800, Dongchuan Road,
Shanghai, P.R. China 200240
[2] Computer Science, Shanghai Jiaotong University800 Dongchuan Road,
Shanghai, P.R.China 200240

Abstract. In this paper, we present a novel deformable model for soft tissue simulation in a real-time manner. The innovative model consists of two sub-models: the surface one and the internal one, which are based on Mass-Spring system and Medial Representation respectively. This proposed model is more accurate and efficient than the pure surface Mass-Spring one by taking advantages of Medial Representation to reflect inner attributes of soft tissue. We also optimize the Mass-Spring system in order to refine the appearance of soft tissue movement and reduce its complexity. A real clinical model using a segmented left-kidney is presented as an example in our case study.

1 Introduction

For years, real-time modeling of deformable objects has become increasingly significant in biomedical domain. More and more novices and students practice surgical operations on the virtual objects instead of living animals and cadavers.

Many authors proposed various models in the past decades. Finite Element Method (FEM) [1] and Mass-Spring [2] are considered the most popular methods among them. Meanwhile, M-Rep [3], a sort of model basing on Medial Representation [3], was proposed to represent the global deformation of the objects. However, an ideal soft tissue deforming simulation is still a challenging task due to the complex internal structure and surface appearance of the deformable objects. FEM is the most accurate method for simulating, but it hardly satisfies the real-time requirement because of its high complexity and large numbers of parameter definitions. Surface Mass-Spring System could have acceptable response-time if we limit the number of mass points of the model. Nevertheless, this model contains few internal features of soft tissue [4], which results in low accuracy when to simulate the global deformation. M-rep is applied to simulate the deformation based on medial structure implying the internal information of soft tissue. However, it is limited in the rough appearance of surface and poor efficiency. The novel approach proposed in this paper addresses the problems mentioned above by introducing a hybrid model integrating the advantages of Mass-Spring and Medial Representation.

In order to implement the context mentioned above, the hybrid model is designed as follow. From the medical image data of soft tissue, two types of models are

Y. Liu, T. Jiang, and C. Zhang (Eds.): CVBIA 2005, LNCS 3765, pp. 419–426, 2005.

generated which represent the surface Mass-spring system and the internal model respectively. After that, we will establish a relationship between the two separate models to transfer forces from outside to inside. The strategy is attractive because it reserves both surface information and internal structure. Contrasting to the standard techniques, it can not only simulate the local deformation appropriately, but also reflect the global deformation reasonably.

The paper is organized as follows. In section 2, we provide the methods to obtain the surface Mass-Spring model and the internal model, and then we introduce the hybrid model consisting of them. Some results of the hybrid model are shown in section 3. Finally, we will discuss future work and come to our conclusion in section 4.

2   Soft Tissue Modeling

The complete methodology of soft tissue modeling consists of two core modules: Image Data Processing and Mathematical Modeling, each of which contains two sub-modules. The former includes Balloon Segmentation and Skeleton Extracting, while the latter consists of Surface Modeling and Internal Modeling (Fig. 1).

The whole procedure of the modeling is described here: firstly, Balloon Segmentation is employed to extract the specific soft tissue from medical image dataset; secondly, it establishes the surface model of soft tissue using Mass-Spring System; thirdly, the skeleton of soft tissue is calculated; fourthly, the medial atoms [3] on the skeleton shoot out many spokes implying the boundary information, after which the internal model composed with skeleton and spokes is created; finally, the hybrid model of soft tissue is generated by composing the surface Mass-Spring model and the skeleton structure according to specialized relations. The detail of these steps will be illuminated in the following sections, especially the surface modeling, the internal modeling and the hybrid modeling (Fig. 1).

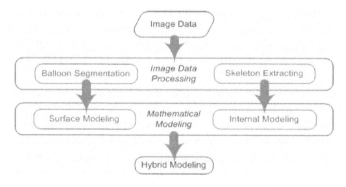

Fig. 1. The flow chart of the whole procedure to model the soft tissue

2.1   Balloon Segmentation for Surface Mesh

Balloon Segmentation is a volumetric Segmentation algorithm based on dynamic deformable meshes [5]. This algorithm is preferred because the data structure of the segmentation's result is appropriate to establish the surface Mass-Spring model as well as its connection with the internal model.

The basis idea of balloon algorithm is to add image-force [5] on an initial mesh object, which could make the object expand or shrink towards the surface of soft tissue. The mesh object will adjust its shape to meet with the boundary of soft tissue as closely as possible after iterating the calculation for specified times, just like a balloon inflated or deflated. Fig. 2 shows the effect while the algorithm is applied on the medical image of a left kidney.

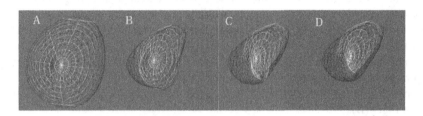

Fig. 2. Balloon Segmentation applied on the medical image of a left kidney. (A) The initial mesh. (B) Iterate for 50 times. (C) Iterate for 100 times. (D) Iterate for 150 times.

2.2 Surface Mass-Spring Modeling

The Mass-Spring system is widely used in simulating the deformation of non-rigid object. The system models an object as a set of masses connected by corresponding springs. The springs' topology used here is based on Balloon Segmentation, which means that each mass connects with its six neighboring points through corresponding springs (Fig. 3(A)).

Spring is a fundamental unit in Mass-Spring model. Fig. 3(B) presents two essential parts of the unit: the elastic equipment and the damper [2]. The former generates elasticity force proportional to the alteration of the springs' length, and the latter engenders damping force proportional to the velocity of mass-points.

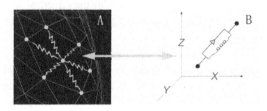

Fig. 3. (A) The springs' layout of the surface model. (B) The basic unit of the spring in the 3D coordinate-system. The triangular module is the damper.

Mass-Spring employs a differential equation to simulate the process of deformation:

$$m_i \ddot{x}_i(t) + c_i \dot{x}_i(t) + \sum_{j \in \sigma(i)} (k_{i,j} * \Delta l_{i,j}) = F_i^{extern} \tag{1}$$

Where x_i, m_i and c_i is the displacement, mass and damping factor of the ith point respectively; $\delta(i)$ represents the neighboring points of the ith point; $k_{i,j}$ is the elastic coefficient of the spring ij; Δl donates the difference between original length and current length of spring ij.

During the implementation, we improve the structure of traditional Mass-Spring system in order to refine the effect of simulation. Firstly, we add a curvature force. Curvature force controls the degree of bending and twisting of soft tissue. We imitate the force by bringing in an assistant spring: angular spring [2]. As shown in Fig. 4(A), P_1, P_2 and P_3 are the surface points of soft tissue. The angular spring links point A with the *mid point* of P_2P_3. Secondly, we induct a concept of fixed position [6] in order to prevent soft tissue from escaping from the original location. Here, we presume that each point has a corresponding fixed spot located in the original position of the point, and the point connects with the spot through springs named return-springs. As a result, soft tissue always has a tendency to go back to the original position. For example, P_1P_1', P_2P_2', P_3P_3' and P_4P_4' are the return-springs whose initial length is zero in Fig. 4(B).

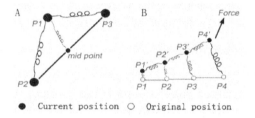

Fig. 4. (A) The angular-spring between *P1* and *mid point*. (B) The return-spring between the original position (*P1, P2, P3, P4*) and the current position (*P1', P2', P3', P4'*).

2.3 Internal Skeleton Modeling

Stephen M. Pizer [3] introduced the "M-Rep" concept, a type of Medial Representation, based on Blum's medial axes. This model uses medial atoms and a particular tuple ($\{x, r, F(\vec{b}, \vec{n}), \theta\}$) [7] [8] to imply the positions of boundary (Fig. 5(A)). Here medial atom represents an interior section of a figure [7]. As a result, M-rep is a sound approach to reflect the internal structure.

In order to establish the internal model, Distance Mapping Method [9] is employed to calculate the skeleton, along which media atoms are selected evenly. Then we simplify M-Rep with the purpose of reducing the model's complexity. We reset the topology of medial atom and implied boundary just like hub and spokes (Fig. 5(B)). Each medial atom (or hub) on the skeleton shoots out several spokes evenly, and the angle between each single spoke and skeleton is a constant value θ. The corresponding tuple is altered to $\{x, r, F(V, \overline{AB}), \theta\}$, where x is the coordinate of the medial atom B; r is the length of the spoke; F is the plane determined by V and $\overline{AB}$; V is the Orientation-Vector of boundary C which links media atom A to boundary C; θ is the angle between skeleton BA and spoke BC.

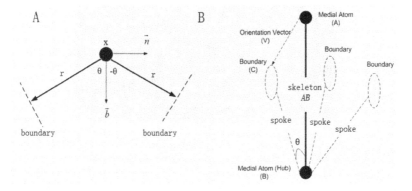

Fig. 5. (A) M-rep in 2D. (B) Simplified Medial Representations in 3D.

The simplified Medial Representations (Fig. 5(B)) are different from M-rep in several ways. Firstly, each tuple in M-rep corresponds with a medial atom, while the one of the simplified corresponds with a spoke. Secondly, the r in M-rep is the radius of corresponding medial atom and the r belonging to the same medial atom should be identical to each other, whereas the one in the simplified model is the length of the relevant spoke and they could be unequal to each other. According to the data of the tuple, we can calculate the position of implied boundary C:

$$\underline{C} = x + R_{v,\overline{AB}}(\theta)\overline{AB} * r_{\overline{BC}} / |\overline{AB}| \tag{2}$$

Where $R_{v,\overline{AB}}(\theta)$ denotes an operator rotating its operand ($\overline{AB}$) by the argument angle in the plane spanned by v and $\overline{AB}$; $|\overline{AB}|$ is the length of the vector $\overline{AB}$.

Other spokes connecting with media atom B are calculated by rotating spoke BC around axis BA and scaling BC to the length of corresponding spoke. All implied boundaries could be obtained by iterating the approach described above.

2.4 The Hybrid Model

The boundaries implied by spokes might not just the points on the surface Mass-Spring model, so the application will relate spokes with surface points by repeating the following step: calculating the coordinate of an implied boundary by formula (2) and finding out its closest point on the surface model. Then, a new spoke, which links the closest surface point and the corresponding medial atom, is established and replaces the old one. The new spoke will be removed if the closest surface point has already related to another spoke. Fig. 6 displays an instance of each model.

The hybrid model is established after the above processes. Then the skeleton and spokes are considered to be springs. Finally, we should set the parameters of the model appropriately in order to simulate soft tissue effectively and efficiently. An automatically recursive approach is employed to set these parameters. Firstly, we

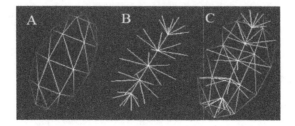

Fig. 6. An example of ellipsoid represented by the three models. (A) Surface Mass-Spring model (B) Internal model with skeleton and spokes (C) The hybrid model.

initialize such parameters as the damping factor (c), the mass (m) of the points and the elastic coefficient (k) of springs on the surface as well as at the inside manually. Here the values of the internal parameters are set much larger than the ones of the surface parameters because the interior of soft tissue is more difficult to deform than the surface. Secondly, a specified force is applied on a surface point. If the displacement of the surface point excesses the maximum threshold determined previously, all of these parameter values on the surface would increase 0.5 times. These values would decrease 0.5 times if the displacement were less than the minimum threshold. The same criterion is also applicable for the internal parameters. After iterating for several times, the program terminates with suitable values for these parameters. By comparing numerous generated parameter values engendered from different initial values and observing the deformation effect using these values, we choose one group of the most appropriate values as the optimum parameters.

3   Experiment Results

The hybrid model application is performed on the computer with an Intel Pentium IV-2.60 GHz CPU and 1.0GMbyte of memory. Visual C++ 7.0 is used as the integrated development environment. There are 458 points on the surface and 24 points on the skeleton. Each atom shoots out 18 spokes ($\theta = 90$ degrees).

The stable state of the left kidney model is showed in Fig. 7(A). The model achieves a reasonable result when deforming on global level (Fig. 7(B)), while the surface Mass-Spring model corrupts under the same large-scale force. The model also gets a refined appearance on local-region deformation (Fig. 7(C) and Fig. 7(D)).

In order to meet the real-time requirement, the deformation should be determined at rates of 15-20 times per second. In our application simulating the left kidney employing the hybrid model, the update rate is 25-40 times per second, which means that the hybrid model satisfies the real-time requirement. Moreover, the surface Mass-Spring model with the same surface structure as the hybrid one is updated at rates of 28-45 times per second, so the hybrid model does not markedly increase its complexity when introducing the internal structure and achieving sound global deformation effect.

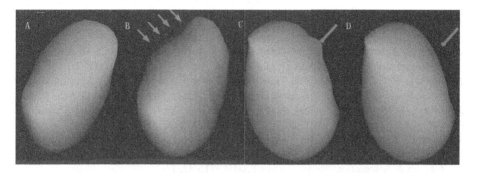

Fig. 7. (A) The left-kidney (B) Global deformation caused by applying large-scale force. (C) Nip the kidney. (D) Release the forceps.

4 Conclusion

In this paper, we present a hybrid model ensuring a sound effect without increasing the computation-time when deformation is applied on either the global level or the local region. We also briefly introduce the Balloon Segmentation appropriate to obtain the mesh structure of soft tissue. Using Balloon algorithm could generate mesh arrangement automatically as well as conveniently. However, it also results in the uneven distribution of springs and points. The density of springs and points near the two acmes is much higher than are others (Fig. 2(D)), which influence the accuracy of simulation. In addition, the method employed to exact the skeleton has some flaws [9]. It could not obtain a precise result when the structure of soft tissue contains some branches.

In future, we endeavor to model a more complex soft tissue, such as heart. We also attempt to improve the accuracy of the current model and reduce the response-time, which is significant in virtual surgery. Moreover, we need to ameliorate the program for generating the mesh structure as well as the algorithm for exacting the skeleton. The recent task is programming on the force feedback mouse, which could make users feel actual about soft tissue.

Acknowledgement

The authors would like to thank Prof. Pizer (University of North Carolina) for bringing the concept of "M-Rep" to Shanghai Jiao Tong University (SJTU) and discussing with us patiently. We also thank Guangxiang Jiang, a member in the Image Based Surgery and Therapy laboratory of SJTU, for contributing his application for extracting the skeleton of the left-kidney recorded in DICOM format, and Feifeng Yang, Xiahai Zhuang for their helpful advices. This work is partially supported by the Shanghai Municipal Research Fund.

References

1. Cover, S. A, Ezquerra, N. F, and O'Brien, J. F.: Interactively Deformable Models for Surgery Simulation. IEEE Computer Graphics & Applications, Vol 13 (1993) 68-75
2. Nedel, L. P., Thalmann, D.: Real Time Muscle Deformations Using Mass-Spring Systems. Proceedings of the Computer Graphics International. Hannover, Germany (1998) 156-166
3. Pizer, S. M., Siddiqi, K., Szekely, G., Damon, J. N.: Multiscale Medial Loci and Their Properties. IJCV Special UNC-MIDAG issue, Vol. 55(2/3) (2002) 155-179
4. Conti, F., Khatib, O., Baur, C.: Interactive rendering of deformable objects based on a filling sphere modeling approach. Proceedings of the 2003 IEEE International Conference on Robotics & Automation. Taipei, Taiwan (2003) 3716-3721
5. Bowden, R. Mitchell, T. A. Sahardi, M.Vision.: Real-time Dynamic Deformable Meshes for Volumetric Segmentation and Visualization. In Proc BMVC, Vol. 1 (1997) 310-319
6. Tanaka, T., Ito, H.: Deformation and Cutting Algorithm of an Organ Model Used for a Laparoscopic Surgery Simulator. Systems and Computers in Japan, Vol. 33 (2002) 1-10
7. Pizer, S. M., Joshi, S., Fletcher, P. T., Styner, M., Tracton, G., Chen, J. Z.: Segmentation of Single-Figure Objects by Deformable M-Reps. Medical Image Computing and Computer-Assisted Intervention (MICCAI 2001), WJ Niessen, MA Viergever, eds. Lecture Notes in Computer Science, Vol. 2208 (2001) 862-871
8. Joshi, S., Pizer, S. M., Fletcher, P. T., Yushkevich, P., Thall, A.: Multiscale Deformable Model Segmentation and Statistical Shape Analysis Using Medial Descriptions. IEEE Transactions on Medical Imaging, Vol. 21 (2002) 538-550
9. Wan, M., Liang, Z., Ke, Q., Hong, L.: Automatic Centerline Extraction for Virtual Colonoscopy. IEEE Transactions on Medical Imaging, Vol. 21 (2002) 1450-1460

Registration of 3D Angiographic and X-Ray Images Using Sequential Monte Carlo Sampling

Charles Florin[2], James Williams[2], Ali Khamene[2], and Nikos Paragios[1]

[1] Ecole Nationale des Ponts et Chaussees,
Champs-sur-Marne, France
nikos.paragios@certis.enpc.fr
[2] Imaging & Visualization Department,
Siemens Corporate Research, Princeton, NJ, USA
{charles.florin, jimwilliams, ali.khamene}@siemens.com

Abstract. Digital subtraction angiography (DSA) reconstructions and 3D Magnetic Resonance Angiography (MRA) are the modalities of choice for diagnosis of vascular diseases. However, when it comes to treatment through an endovascular intervention, only two dimensional lower resolution information such as angiograms or fluoroscopic images are usually available. Overlaying the pre-operative information from high resoluion acquisition onto the images acquired during intervention greatly helps physician in performing the operation. We propose to register pre-operative DSA or MRS with intra-operative images to bring the two data sets into a single coordinate frame. The method uses the vascular structure, which is present and visible from most of DSA, MRA and x-ray angiogram and fluoroscopic images, to determine the registration parameters. A robust multiple hypothesis framework is built to minimize a fitness measure between the 3D volume and the 2D projection. The measure is based on the distance map computed from the vascular segmentation. Particle Filters are used to resample the hypothesis, and direct them toward the feature space's zones of maximum likelihood. Promising experimental results demonstrate the potentials of the method.

1 Introduction

Digital subtraction angiography (DSA), which is based on conventional X-ray, and Magnetic Resonance Angiography (MRA) are the modalities of choice for many diagnostic vascular imaging procedures, as well as for performing and monitoring endovascular interventions. The main advantage is that the DSA and/or MRA data are usually of high resolution and since they are three dimensional in nature, they provide much needed information with regard to the topology of the vessel tree. The drawback is that these acquisitions can not be performed, while the intervention is underway. Mainly because the fact that DSA takes a long time to acquire and requires certain spatial clearance around the patient and MRA scanner are not usually available in the interventional rooms. What is available, and is fast to acquire, is two dimensional conventional projection x-ray images. In order to take advantage of high resolution, three dimensional info from either DSA or MRA, it is desirable to have a registration method, which brings

Y. Liu, T. Jiang, and C. Zhang (Eds.): CVBIA 2005, LNCS 3765, pp. 427–436, 2005.

in the two data sets (i.e., x-ray and 3D DSA or MRA) into a single coordinate frame. The problem at hand is 2D-3D registration problem, which has been investigated in the literature for various applications [4][16][13][25]. Image registration [15] methods can be categorized in two distinct groups: intensity-based and features-based techniques.

Feature-based methods [1,3] are quite popular and rely on a pre-processing often pre-segmentation step where local structures of particular interest like points are determined. Once such structures have been recovered in both images, and correspondence between them have been established registration is obtained through a parametric transformation that aligns the retained local structures. Such methods exhibit low registration complexity once features have been recovered, an important strength. On the other hand their performance heavily depends on the feature extraction that can be viewed as an important limitation.

Global and local similarity measures between the Digitally Reconstructed Radiographs (DRR) and the 2D images are the base of intensity-based methods. Simple criteria like linear correlation [5,12] or correlation ratio [19] were considered to address such a problem. More advanced methods [14,17,22] require the generation of DRRs in an iterative optimization loop. In order to decrease complexity induced by the computation of DRRs in [26] partial DRR were considered, or DRRs have been pre-computated for different starting positions/orientations [20]. The similarity measure is critical for any registration algorithm performance [20]. Mutual information [23] is a prominent approach that was also considered in therapy [18]. Gradient descend methods are the most common approach to recover the registration parameters once the problem has been expressed with an energetic formulation. Nevertheless one can claim that these methods are subject to local minima and have a limited capture range.

To circumvent this limitation, in [21] a technique was proposed that starting from low-order estimates - valid in a limited region - does perform a progressive refinement where the region associated with it is expanded. This method can be qualified as hybrid between a gradient descent and simulated annealing, and showed good results for retinal images. Nevertheless, besides the limitation of having an initial model such a method presents certain limitations: (i) the initial model needs to be close enough to the minimum solution, (ii) the algorithm could not converge when the image features are dispatched into different geometrical clusters. One can address this limitation through a multiple hypothesis assumption that can overcome the case of converging to local minima. Such an approach could be implemented in an efficient fashion if a limited number of features is retained and use similarity measures that exhibit robust scoring of patient position proposals.

To this end, instead of registering the whole volume, we propose to register the vascular structures. To explore different hypothesis without prior models suggests the use of stochastic processes. Recent improvements in computer capabilities dramatically increased the popularity of Monte-Carlo methods, in particular Particle Filters for tracking problem. We propose here to use the Condensation form of sequential Monte Carlo sampling to estimate a cost function gradient, and find the global minimum.

The reminder of this paper is organized as follows: first, the 2D-3D registration problem is presented, along with a function that measures the fitness of any patient position/orientation proposal. Then, the Condensation framework is presented to direct the multiple hypothesis toward the most probable projection hypothesis. Finally, results are presented and compared with standard Nonlinear Least Squares Fitting methods [2].

2   2D-3D Registration

2.1   Problem

2D-3D registration consists in finding the limited number of parameters that define the perspective projection from a given 3D volume to a 2D image (see [FIG. (1)]). A perspective projection from a 3D homogeneous point P to a 2D homogeneous point p is defined with matrix as

$$p = \mathbf{PCT}P, \tag{1}$$

where $\mathbf{T}$ is a 4×4 matrix of the pose relating the pre-operative coordinate frame to the iso-centric coordinate frame of intra-operative imaging device. $\mathbf{C}$ is a 4×4 matrix defining the transformation between the iso-centric coordinate frame and the coordinate frame centered at the x-ray imaging source, which also depends on gantry angles. $\mathbf{P}$ is a 3×4 projection matrix defining the projection cone related to the source-detector geometry. We assume $\mathbf{P}$ and $\mathbf{C}$ are known from a calibration step. $\mathbf{T}$ is the unknown pose that encodes the three translation and three rotation parameters. The problem thus consists of formulating different hypothesis for $\mathbf{T}$, measuring the fitness of each pose hypothesis, and optimizing the best ones.

2.2   Pose Fitness Measure

Intensity based registration approaches require DRR generation, which is then compared with the x-ray or fluoro images at each step of the process. The main bottleneck for intensity based approaches is the speed. In [26], the authors mentioned several minutes for registering the whole intensity volume, most of the time spent on generating the DRR. For this application, we use the vascular structures as features for registration. Vascular structures are easy to segment in most of cases, sparse enough for the

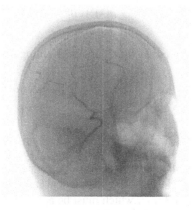

Fig. 1. Contrast enhanced X-ray image of right hemisphere vessels

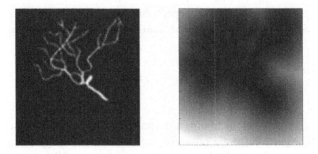

Fig. 2. The projected vascular structure and the distance map associated with it

registration to be faster than intensity-based methods, but yet generally well distributed throughout the organs to capture potential misalignments. One obstacle here is to define a fast and robust measure that characterizes the fitness of the pose. The proposed method uses a prior segmentation of the vessels in the 3D volume of interest and the 2D image. From the 2D segmentation result, a distance map[8] is computed (see [FIG. (2)]). For a given pose matrix $\mathbf{T}$, the measure of fitness is the sum of distances (i.e. D) to the 2D structure for each projected 3D point from the segmented vessel tree:

$$F(\mathbf{T}) = \int_{P \in vessel} D(\mathbf{PCTP}). \tag{2}$$

3 Bayesian Process and Condensation

3.1 Bayesian Process

The Bayesian problem can be simply formulated as the computation of the present state x_t pdf of a system, based on observations from time 1 to time t $z_{1:t}$: $p(x_t|z_{1:t})$. Assuming that one has access to the prior pdf $p(x_{t-1}|z_{1:t-1})$, the posterior pdf $p(x_t|z_{1:t})$ is computed according to the Bayes rule:

$$p(x_t|z_{1:t}) = \frac{p(z_t|x_t)p(x_t|z_{1:t-1})}{p(z_t|z_{1:t-1})}.$$

where the prior pdf is computed via the Chapman-Kolmogorov equation

$$p(x_t|z_{1:t-1}) = \int p(x_t|x_{t-1})p(x_{t-1}|z_{1:t-1})dx_{t-1},$$

and

$$p(z_t|z_{1:t-1}) = \int p(z_t|x_t)p(x_t|z_{1:t-1})dx_t$$

The recursive computation of the prior and the posterior pdf leads to the exact computation of the posterior density. Nevertheless, in practical cases, it is impossible to compute exactly the posterior pdf $p(x_t|z_{1:t})$, which must be approximated. This approximation is performed using Condensation [SEC. (3.2)].

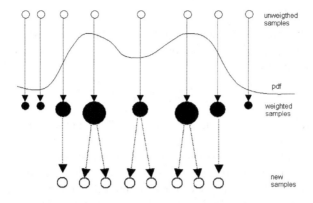

Fig. 3. The resampling process: a random selection chooses the samples with the highest weights where a local perturbation is applied

3.2 Sequential Monte Carlo and Condensation

Condensation [6,11] (Conditional Density Propagation) is a sequential Monte-Carlo technique that is used to estimate the Bayesian posterior probability density function (pdf) with a set of samples [9,24]. A prior set of particles (hypothesis) is used to estimate the probability of different situations (posterior pdf), given the current observation. In terms of a mathematical formulation, such a method approximates the posterior pdf by M random measures $\{x_t^m, m = 1..M\}$ associated to M weights $\{w_t^m, m = 1..M\}$, such that

$$p(x_t|z_{1:t}) \approx \sum_{m=1}^{M} w_t^m \delta(x_t - x_t^m).$$

where each weight w_t^m reflects the importance of the sample x_t^m in the pdf, as shown in [FIG. (3)].

The samples x_t^m are drawn using the principle of *Importance Density* [10], of pdf $q(x_t|x_{1:t}^m, z_t)$, and it is shown that their weights w_t^m are updated according to

$$w_t^m \propto w_{t-1}^m \frac{p(z_t|x_t^m)p(x_t^m|x_{t-1}^m)}{q(x_t^m|x_{t-1}^m, z_t)}. \tag{3}$$

Once a set of samples has been drawn, $p(x_t^m|z_t)$ can be computed out of the observation z_t for each sample, and the estimation of the posteriori pdf can be sequentially updated.

Such a process will remove most of the particles and only the ones that express the data will present significant weights. Consequently the model will lose its ability to track significant changes on the pdf; therefore a resampling procedure has to be executed on a regular basis. Such a process will preserve as many samples as possible with respectful weights. One can find in the literature several resampling techniques. We chose the most prominent one, Sampling Importance Resampling [9], for its simplicity to implement, and because it allows more hypothesis with low probability to survive, compared to more selective techniques such as Stratified Resampling [7].

3.3 Sampling Importance Resampling

The Sampling Importance Resampling (SIR) algorithm [9] consists of choosing the prior density $p(x_t|x_{t-1})$ as importance density $q(x_t|x_{1:t}^m, z_t)$. This leads to the following condition, from [EQ. (3)]

$$w_t^m \propto w_{t-1}^m p(z_t|x_t^m). \tag{4}$$

The samples are updated by selecting $x_t^m \propto p(x_t|x_{t-1}^m)$, and perturbed according to a random noise vector.

The SIR algorithm is the most widely used resampling method because of its simplicity from the implementation point of view. Nevertheless, the SIR uses mostly the prior knowledge $p(x_t|x_{t-1})$, and does not take into account the most recent observations z_t. Such a strategy could lead to an overestimation of outliers. On the other hand, because SIR resampling is performed at each step, fewer samples are required, and thus the computational cost may be reduced with respect to other resampling algorithms.

Since the resampling is based on the prior $p(x_t|x_{t-1})$, and not $p(x_t|x_{t-1}, z_t)$, it does not take into account the most recent observation ; the resampling is suboptimal. Nevertheless, one can notice the process is stationary (the statistics of x_t do not vary with time). Therefore, $p(x_t|x_{t-1})$ can be considered optimal. Further research will investigate the use of Nonlinear Gradient Descent during the resampling step to drive the particles toward the region of interest.

It is important to note that the statistics of x_t (the projection parameters) do not change in time ; the process is stationary. Therefore, if the posterior pdf estimation is put aside, such a Particle Filter is nearly equivalent to some kind of Genetic Algorithm[1]. Nevertheless, if the observation z_t changes in time (e.g. registration of a 3D pre-operative volume with a sequence of fluoro images) and if the registration at one time-step constitutes a prior for the next time step (in other words, if registration for one portal image helps registering the next image), Condensation is exploited to its full extent. This will be explored in further studies.

4 Results and Discussion

4.1 Condensation Performs Better Than Random Search

First, experiments were conducted to compare the method presented in this paper with a purely random search, and the results proved that Condensation used with x particles during z time steps reach a better registration than $x \times z$ random trials (in the experiments, x=64 and z=100).

4.2 Condensation Performs Better Than Levenberg-Marquardt Gradient Descent

Second, experiments were conducted to compare Condensation performance (with respect to the measure presented in [SEC. (2.2)]) with classic nonlinear least square

---

[1] Although Genetic Algorithm cannot be used in this case, since the parameters are dependent.

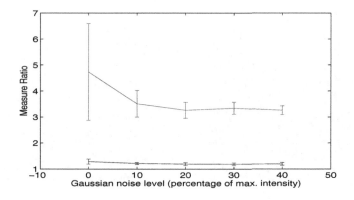

Fig. 4. Comparison of Condensation (blue) and Levenberg-Marquardt (red) performances when gaussian noise is introduced in the portal image

methods to find the minimum of a nonlinear function: Levenberg-Marquardt[2] and Gauss-Newton algorithms. Both Levenberg-Marquardt and Gauss-Newton are highly dependent on initialization, and never led to better results than Condensation (over 100 experiments were made with synthetic portal images from real pre-operative volumes, and random patient poses).

The perspective projection may not be perfect, and for optimal parameters, the subtraction of the two registered images may not be exactly null in real cases. For that matter, white noise has been added to the portal image to test the sensibility of the two algorithms, Condensation and Gradient Descent. The results are presented in [FIG. (4)] and [FIG. (7)].

Tests have been performed about the method sensitivity to segmentation error, and the conclusions are presented in [FIG. (5)]. Whereas the Gradient Descent performances decrease as the segmentation error increases (in Hounsfield units), the Condensation results do not vary. As the error level increases, the global minimum's basin of attraction

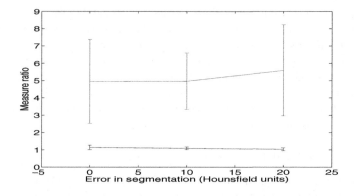

Fig. 5. Comparison of Condensation (blue) and Levenberg-Marquardt (red) performances when segmentation error is introduced

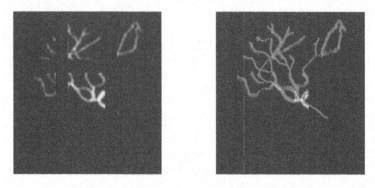

Fig. 6. Condensation converges toward global minimum with missing features

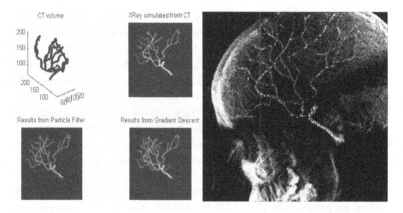

Fig. 7. (L) Comparison between Condensation and Levenberg-Marquardt method performance. (R) Registered vascular structure with 2D projection simulated from original CT data.

(for Gradient Descent) diminishes; consequently, the probability for the Gradient Descent to be correctly initialized diminishes. Since the particles are uniformly initialized in any case, the results are independent of the segmentation error.

For a similar reason, Condensation is independent of the capture range, while any Gauss-Newton / Gradient Descent method inherently depends on the global minimum's basin of attraction width. Furthermore, when features are missing, local minima are created, which are likely to attract the Gradient Descent method. Particle Filters still converge toward the global minimum (see [Fig. (6)]).

4.3   Further Investigation

Condensation can be combined with Gradient Descent, for a more efficient resampling. During the resampling stage, the particles with the most significant weights are selected, and moved along the steepest direction.

Further investigations will also focus on observations that change in time, issues that are naturally handled by Bayesian processes. For a sequence of X-ray images, the Condensation can estimate the parameters pdf at a given time, and use this estimation to actualize the pdf at at the next time step. This application is particularly relevant for features that may or may not be present at time t. Several local minimas can be detected using Particle Filter at time t, and observation at time t+1 may solve the ambiguity.

Last but not least, biplanar acquisition can be exploited to resolve ambiguities and local minimas.

In conclusion, the solution presented in this paper is both computationally light compared to intensity-based methods, and more robust than gradient descent algorithm applied on the same feature-based framework. With a limited number of particles (64 in our experiments), the computational cost (of the order of one minute, using non optimized Matlab code) gives reasonable hopes for real-time applications in the future.

References

1. R. Bansal, L. H. Staib, Z. Chen, A. Rangarajan, J. Knisely, R. Nath, and J. S. Duncan. Entropy-based, multiple -portal-to-3dct registration for prostate radiotherapy using iteratively estimated segmentation. In *MICCAI*, pages 567–578, 1999.
2. D. M. Bates and D. G. Watts. *Nonlinear regression and its applications*. New York, Wiley, 1988.
3. J. Bijhold, M. van Herk, R. Vijlbrief, and J. V. Lebesque. Fast evaluation of patient set-up during radiotherapy by aligning features in portal and simulator images. *Physics in Medicine and Biology*, 36(12):1665–1679, 1991.
4. JV. Byrne, C. Colominas, J. Hipwell, T. Cox, JA. Noble, GP. Penney, and DJ. Hawkes. Assessment of a technique for 2d-3d registration of cerebral intra-arterial angiography. *British Journal of Radiology*, 77:123–128, 2004.
5. L. Dong and A.L. Boyer. An image correlation procedure for digitally reconstructed radiographs and electronic portal images. *International Journal of Radiation Oncology Biology Physics*, 33(5):1053–60, 1995.
6. A. Doucet, J. de Freitas, and N. Gordon. *Sequential Monte Carlo Methods in Practice*. Springer-Verlag, New York, 2001.
7. P. Fearnhead and P. Clifford. Online inference for well-log data. *Journal of the Royal Statistical Society*, 65:887–899, 2003.
8. A. Fitzgibbon. Robust registration of 2d and 3d point sets. In *British Machine Vision Conference*, volume II, pages 411–420, September 2001.
9. N. Gordon. Novel Approach to Nonlinear/Non-Gaussian Bayesian State Estimation. *IEE Proceedings*, 140:107–113, 1993.
10. N. Gordon. On Sequential Monte Carlo Sampling Methods for Bayesian Filtering. *Statistics and Computing*, 10:197–208, 2000.
11. N. Gordon. A Tutorial on Particle Filters for On-line Non-linear/Non-Gaussian Bayesian Tracking. *IEEE Transactions on Signal Processing*, 50:174–188, 2002.
12. D.H. Hristov and B.G. Fallone. A grey-level image alignment algorithm for registration of portal images and digitally reconstructed radiographs. *Medical physics*, 23(1):75–84, 1996.
13. Y. Kita, D. Wilson, and J.A. Noble. Real-time registration of 3d cerebral vessels to x-ray angiograms. In *Proc. Medical Imaging Computing and Computer Assisted Interventions (MICCAI)*, pages 1125–1133, 1998.

14. D. LaRose. *Iterative X-ray/CT Registration Using Accelerated Volume Rendering.* PhD thesis, Robotics Institute, Carnegie Mellon University, Pittsburgh, PA, May 2001.
15. J. Maintz and M. Viergever. A Survey for Medical Image Registration. *Medical Image Analysis*, 2:1–36, 1998.
16. R. A. McLauglin, J. Hipwell, G.P. Penney, K. Rhode, A. Chung, J.A. Noble, and D.J. Hawkes. Intensity-based registration versus feature-based registration for neurointerventions. In *Proc. Medical Image Understanding and Analysis (MIUA)*, pages 69–72, 2001.
17. G. P. Penney, J. Weese, J. A. Little, P. Desmedt, D. L. G. Hill, and D. J. Hawkes. A comparison of similarity measures for use in 2d-3d medical image registration. *IEEE Trans. Med. Imaging*, 17(4):586–595, 1998.
18. D. Plattard, G. Champleboux, P. Vassal, J. Troccaz, and M. Bolla. Epid for patient positioning in radiotherapy: calibration and image matching in the entropid system. In H. Lemke, editor, *Cars*, pages 265–9, 1999.
19. A. Roche, G. Malandain, X. Pennec, and N. Ayache. The correlation ratio as a new similarity measure for multimodal image registration. *Lecture Notes in Computer Science*, 1496, 1998.
20. T. Rohlfing, D. B. Russakoff, M. J. Murphy, and C. R. Maurer, Jr. Intensity-based registration algorithm for probabilistic images and its application for 2-D to 3-D image registration. In Milan Sonka and J. Michael Fitzpatrick, editors, *Medical Imaging: Image Processing*, volume 4684 of *Proceedings of the SPIE*, pages 581–591, February 2002.
21. C. V. Stewart, C-L. Tsai, and B. Roysam. The dual bootstrap iterative closest point algorithm with application to retinal image registration. *IEEE Trans. Med. Imaging*, 22(11):1379–1394, 2003.
22. D. Tomazevic, B. Likar, T. Slivnik, and F. Pernus. 3-d/2-d registration of ct and mr to x-ray images. *IEEE Trans. Med. Imaging*, 22(11):1407–1416, 2003.
23. P. Viola and W. Wells. Aligment by Maximization of Mutual Information. In *ICCV*, pages 16–23, 1995.
24. W. West. Modelling with mixtures. In J. Bernardo, J. Berger, A. Dawid, and A. Smith, editors, *Bayesian Statistics*. Clarendon Press, 1993.
25. D.L. Wilson, D.D. Royston, J. A. Noble, and J.V. Byrne. Automatic determination of optimal x-ray projections for use during endovascular treatments of intracranial aneurysms. *IEEE Transactions on Medical Imaging*, 18(10):973–980, October 1999.
26. L. Zöllei, W. E. L. Grimson, A. Norbash, and W. M. III Wells. 2d-3d rigid registration of x-ray fluoroscopy and ct images using mutual information and sparsely sampled histogram estimators. In *CVPR (2)*, pages 696–703, 2001.

Registration of PET and MR Hand Volumes Using Bayesian Networks

Derek Magee[1], Steven Tanner[1], Michael Waller[2], Dennis McGonagle[2],
and Alan P. Jeavons[1]

[1] School of Computing/Academic Unit of Medical Physics, University of Leeds, UK
[2] Leeds Teaching Hospitals NHS Trust, Leeds, UK
drm@comp.leeds.ac.uk

Abstract. A method for the non-rigid, multi-modal, registration of volumetric scans of human hands is presented. PET and MR scans are aligned by optimising the configuration of a tube based model using a set of Bayesian networks. Efficient optimisation is performed by posing the problem as a multi-scale, local, discrete (quantised) search, and using dynamic programming. The method is to be used within a project to study the use of high-resolution HIDAC PET imagery in investigating bone growth and erosion in arthritis.

1 Introduction

In this paper we present a novel method for the non-rigid registration of high-resolution HIDAC Positron Emission Tomography (PET) and Magnetic Resonance[1] (MR) scan volumes of human hands. To our knowledge we are the first to tackle this particular multi-modal registration problem. This work is part of a wider project to investigate the use of high-resolution list-mode QuadHIDAC^{TM} PET imagery ($\sim 0.5mm^3$ voxel size, Fluorine-18 tracer) for the study of the location of bone growth and erosion in the hands of patients suffering from arthritis. Our method involves fitting a pair of models, based on a set of cylindrical tubes, to the two data sets to be registered and calculating a rigid and a non-rigid (piecewise rigid) transform. The models are fitted by the optimisation of a set of Bayesian networks with respect to annotated volumes. The method is made computationally tractable by posing it as a multi-scale local search problem. Quantisation of the search spaces allows the efficient use of dynamic programming to obtain a globally optimal solution in these spaces.

Lower resolution PET imaging ($\sim 5mm^3$ voxel size) is widely used in brain imaging to extract functional information. However, PET imaging provides little anatomical information. Therefore, it is routinely used in conjunction with MR imaging, which can provide this anatomical information. As PET and MR scans are rarely co-located, data sets must be registered. To quote Myers [1]; "[this has] become a matter of routine in the analysis of brain PET studies". The most popular and successful methods of non-fiducial (physical marker) based registration

---

[1] T2-weighted, fat suppressed, spin-echo coronal images (voxel size $\sim 0.5 \times 0.5 \times 2$mm).

Y. Liu, T. Jiang, and C. Zhang (Eds.): CVBIA 2005, LNCS 3765, pp. 437–448, 2005.

are based around the maximisation of mutual information, or voxel similarity, over a rigid transform (e.g. [2,3,4], see [5] for an overview and evaluation of a number of such techniques). Clearly such rigid transforms are unsuitable in our application domain (figure 5). PET has also been applied to cardiac imaging. Here PET provides metabolism information, which must again be augmented with anatomical information from MR imaging. Akin to our work, Makela *et al.* [6] use a model based technique to perform multi-modal registration. This is based on the fact that the thorax and lung surfaces are clearly visible in both imaging modalities. A deformable template model is fitted to each data set, and the results used to calculate a rigid transformation. Farahani *et al.* [7] describe a prototype system for the spatio-temporally co-located acquisition of PET and MR for brain imaging. There remain some large technical hurdles to be overcome with this approach. If this were widely used (unlikely any time soon due to cost and technical constraints) this will eliminate the need for volume registration. However, multi-modal volume registration is likely to be required for some time to come, especially for high-resolution PET scans (where few uni-modal scanners exist, let alone multi-modal scanners). In our application PET imaging provides information about bone growth and/or erosion. As with previous applications of PET, MR imaging is required to provide anatomical information such as blood vessel and tendon location.

Our approach to the registration problem is partly inspired by the 3D geometric models used in visual tracking. Perhaps the first example of such a model is the WALKER model of Hogg [8] where the body and limbs of a human are modelled as a collection of cylinders. This model is fitted to 2D visual data using edge information. Rehg and Kanade [9] use a similar approach to track the human hand. A simplified 28 D.O.F. cylinder based model is fitted to stereo data using a local optimisation method (Levenburg-Marquart). Stenger *et. al* [10] use a similar model based on a number of 3D quadratics, rather than cylinders, for added realism. Visual tracking has the advantage over medical image analysis applications of having state estimate(s) from previous timesteps to work from. As such, local optimisation over such a large configuration space is possible (although a good initialisation method is required). Felzenswalb and Huttenlocher [11] describe how the effective dimensionality of such optimisation problems may be reduced for certain classes of model using quantisation and dynamic programming. This work is our starting point, and it is described more fully in the following section.

2   Model Fitting as Bayesian Network Optimisation Using Dynamic Programming

Felzenswalb and Huttenlocher [11] pose the problem of fitting a model to sensor data (in the visual tracking domain) as the optimisation of the parameters of a directed graph structured network (a type of Bayesian network). Probabilistic dependencies exist between the data and individual model graph nodes, and between parent and child nodes joined by the directed vertices. In general, finding a globally optimal solution over such a network is an N-P complete problem (and in practice costly approximate methods are often used). However, if the model graph is tree-structured (i.e. there are no loops), and the space of solutions is quantised, a globally optimal solution may be obtained in linear time (w.r.t. the number of nodes in the graph) using dynamic programming (see [11] for full details). The solution in fact has complexity $O(q^2 n)$ (where n is the number of nodes, and q is the number of quantisations of each node parameterisation). Furthermore, the method is made up of two parts; individual node evaluation (complexity $O(qn)$), and belief propagation over the network (complexity $O(q^2 n)$). If the majority of the complexity of the network dependencies is in the former, the solution is approximately linear in both the number of nodes, and the number of quantisations of the individual node parameterisations. The phalanges (rigid finger sections) of a human hand in our PET/MR registration problem may be modelled as tree-structured networks, as illustrated in figure 1.

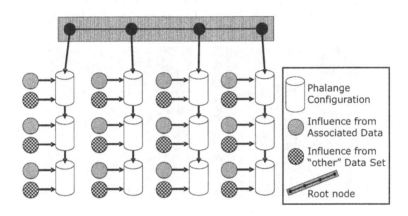

Fig. 1. Hand (four fingers) PET/MR Bayesian Networks Formulation

In our scenario there are two models to be fitted to two data sets (PET and MR). The data sets are linked in that they relate to the same individual. As such, phalange lengths should be similar. The phalanges are parameterised as a tube with 7 parameters (3D start/end and radius). We choose not to constrain the motion of the fingers to a plane (as in [9]), as this is not a useful approximation for our data. However, even with a small number of quantisations per dimension this produces an excessively large number of configurations of each phalange (individual node evaluation has complexity $O(q_d{}^{n_d})$, where q_d is the number of quantisations in each dimension, and n_d is the number of dimensions). The following sections describe an approach that uses two networks per data set, and local quantisation to overcome this computational hurdle.

3   Efficient Model Networks and Their Optimisation

The raw data used in this paper is volumetric and comes from PET and MR scans. Typically volume dimensions are $256 \times 256 \times 16$ for the MR data and $256 \times 256 \times 440$ for the PET data. With this volume of data it is desirable to pre-process the data before evaluating possible model configurations for computational reasons. Another reason for data pre-processing is to identify volumetric areas relating to physical features to assist the model matching/registration process. As there is essentially no common information in the PET and MR scans, other than that an area is within the hand (or not), this is what is used. One common method of identifying regions is volume segmentation. In this process each voxel is labelled as belonging (or not belonging) to a physical structure. For our data this is problematic, as there is much uncertainty over many voxels (especially in the PET data). This task is therefore hard for a skilled human expert, let alone an automated system. This approach also performs little data reduction. We propose a simpler alternative approach to segmentation; point annotation. The principle behind this is that a relatively sparse set of

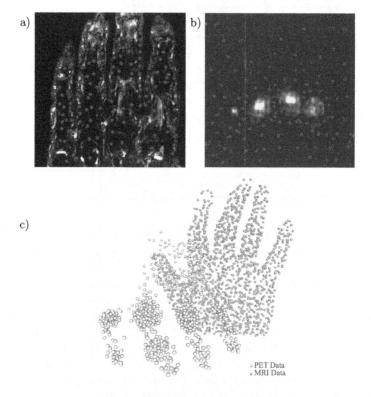

Fig. 2. Examples of Hand Annotation of Data in 2D: a) MR 'hand', b) PET 'not hand', 3D Visualisation of 'hand' PET & MR point clouds

points that are definitely "hand" or "not hand" are identified. This is currently performed in 2D by hand (taking <15 minutes per data set), and is illustrated in figure 2. We believe annotation to be a much simpler process to automate (using region based classifiers) than segmentation for this data, as uncertain points may simply be excluded from the labelling process. It is also a much faster process to carry out by hand. Automation of this process is planned for the near future. The 2D point annotation of multiple volumetric slices is used to form 3D "point clouds" using the slice number to form the third dimension. This is illustrated in figure 2.c. These point clouds allow the definition of probabilistic metrics over the model configuration parameters (see later), and allow quite effective visualisation of the quality of final model configurations.

3.1   Model Initialisation and Local Search

Our approach to reducing the computational complexity of the Bayesian network optimisation is to pose the optimisation as a local search problem. Initial model configurations are specified by hand, and the set of possible configurations investigated are local offsets from this configuration. This allows a rather smaller number of quantisations of each dimension than quantising the complete 7D space of solutions for each phalange. Hand specification of the initial configuration is done by clicking on the approximate start/end points of each phalange in a 2D slice view (as in the annotation in the previous section). The end of a parent phalange and the start a connected child phalange are deemed to be coincident, thus only 16 clicks are required for four fingers (the thumb is ignored only as it is absent in the majority of the data sets used). The radius of each phalange is estimated as $K \times$ phalange length (where K is typically 0.25, which is usually a slight underestimate). Figures 3.a and 3.d show examples of the variable quality of this initial configuration. In particular, the length (and thus radius) of the finger tip phalanges in the MR data is incorrect as they lie partially outside the scan volume. The location of PET data phalanges, especially at the base of the fingers, is up to 10mm from the correct location. Estimated radii in all cases are very approximate, even when the length is near correct.

Two methods are applied to the initial configurations before Bayesian Network optimisation is performed. Firstly a check is made on whether the ends of a phalange lie very close to the edge of the scan volume (i.e. within 5% of the complete range of any dimension from the edge). We term this "phalange validity". If it is the case that one phalange is valid and the other is not the length of the invalid phalange is set to be equal to the valid one. This is done using the valid end of the invalid phalange and its direction vector, as in equation 1.

$$End_{new} = Start_{orig} + Dir_{orig} \times Len_{other} \tag{1}$$

The results of this process are illustrated in figures 3.b and 3.e (which are data sets imaged from the same individual, and only the MR data has invalid phalanges). Once the lengths are corrected, a "greedy" algorithm is used to obtain a better initial estimate of the radius. This works by assigning annotated

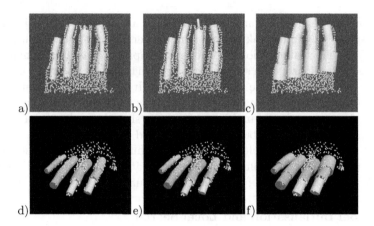

Fig. 3. Example of model Initialisation (MR Data): a) Initial guess, b) Corrected Tube lengths, c) Output of 'Greedy' algorithm, (PET Data): d) Initial guess, e) Corrected Tube lengths, f) Output of 'Greedy' algorithm

hand points to phalanges that contain them[2]. The radii of each tube is increased by increasing factors (typically 1:1.5 in 0.01 steps). The minimum radii that contains a larger number of unassigned annotated hand points than the initial estimate, without containing points assigned to another phalange, is selected. If increasing the radius by one step increases the number of "not hand" annotated points contained within the phalange tube, without increasing the number of "hand" annotated points, expansion of that phalange is halted. This process is repeated until convergence. The results of this process are illustrated in figures 3.c and 3.f.

3.2   Model Fitting Using Multi-scale Optimisation of Two Networks

If each dimension of the 7D configuration space of each phalange tube is divided into 9 evenly spaced quantisations[3] (centred around the initial configuration) the total number of quantisations (q) of each tube is $9^7 = 4,782,969$. As the complexity of the belief propagation is $O(q^2n)$ evaluation of such a network takes of the order of an hour or more on current standard hardware (PIV 3GHz). As we wish to perform this optimisation at multiple scales this would make the registration process rather time consuming. As a computationally efficient alternative, we divide the model into two networks; one relating to the start/end point configuration of the phalange tubes (6D) and one relating to the Radius (1D). Optimisation of a pair of the former is performed in around 30 seconds, and the later is optimised in interactive time. Tables 1-4 describe the various probabilistic factors that are used to form the model networks. These fall into two categories; i) Simple probabilities, calculated as a data proportion (or similar), and ii) Normalised Gaussian probabilities, calculated from some distance d, as in

---

[2] If a point is inside two tubes it is assigned to the tube it is furthest inside.

[3] This is approaching the minimum sensible before solutions are lost between steps.

Table 1. Probabilistic influence factors on individual tube configurations (position/length)

Variable	Description	Form	Notes
P_{cgl_start}, P_{cgl_end}	Distance of start/end from 'curve gradient line' start/end	Norm. Gaussian	S.D. = 0.5×length [1 if 'invalid']
P_{assign}	Proportion of 'assigned' data enclosed	Simple prob.	If <0.95 set to 0.01
$P_{n\_unassign}$	Proportion of nearby (within search range) 'unassigned' data enclosed	Simple prob.	Clipped at 0.9 and scaled [0,1]
P_{len_p}	Difference of length from mean of PET & MR original lengths of this tube	Norm. Gaussian	S.D. = 0.5×length, =PET/MR orig if the other 'invalid', 1 if both 'invalid'
P_{len_sim}	Difference in length from same tube in other data set (current guess)	Norm. Gaussian	S.D. = 0.25×length

N.B. Where length is specified in the notes, this is the initial estimate for that data set

equation 2. Normalised Gaussians are used as $P = 1$ for $d = 0$ (i.e. no influence is had).

$$P = e^{\frac{-d^2}{2\sigma^2}} \tag{2}$$

The Curve gradient line (CGL), used to calculate P_{cgl_start} in table 1), is calculated for each phalange from the mean of the points initially associated with that phalange. For each finger (trio of phalanges), a quadratic is fitted to the points in the 2D plane defined by these points. The gradient (direction) of this quadratic at each mean point defines the CGL (a straight line which passes through the mean). The extent (start/end) of these lines are found by projecting each of the associated points onto the line and calculating the maximum distance in each direction from the mean point. Validity of these lines is calculated in exactly the same way as described in section 3.1. Independence of each factor is assumed, and individual phalange tube configuration influences are combined as a product (equation 3).

$$P_{tube_n} = P_{cgl\_start_n} \times P_{cgl\_end_n} \times P_{assign_n} \times P_{n\_unassign_n} \times P_{len\_p_n} \times P_{len\_sim_n} \tag{3}$$

Independence of topological factors is also assumed, and configuration influences are combined as a product (equation 4).

$$P_{topol_{n,m}} = P_{near_{n,m}} \times P_{straight_{n,m}} \tag{4}$$

Table 2. Probabilistic influence topological factors between parent/child configurations (position/length)

Variable	Description	Form	Notes
P_{near}	Distance between parent end and child start	Norm. Gaussian	S.D. = 0.025×parent length
$P_{straight}$	Dot product of unit direction vectors of parent/child	Simple prob.	Enforces finger straightness

Table 3. Probabilistic influence factors on individual tube configurations (radius)

Variable	Description	Form	Notes
P_{assign}	Proportion of 'assigned' data enclosed	Simple prob.	If <0.95 set to 0.01
$P_{unassign}$	Proportion of 'unassigned' data enclosed	Simple prob.	Clipped at 0.9 and scaled [0,1]
P_{not}	1 - (No. 'not hand' points / No. 'associated' hand points)	Simple prob.	Lower clip at 0.01
P_{enc_other}	If no. assigned to another tube enclosed > no. assigned to this tube × 0.05, P_{enc_other}=0.01, else 1	Simple Prob.	
$P_{rad_{m}atch}$	Difference between radius and initial other model radius	Norm. Gaussian	S.D. = 0.25 × tube radius

Table 4. Probabilistic influence topological factors between parent/child configurations (radius)

Variable	Description	Form	Notes
$P_{dradius}$	Difference in radius between parent and child	Norm. Gaussian	S.D. = 0.25 × parent radius

Radius model network influences are combined as a product in exactly the same way as the start/end model. Belief propagation through each finger (trio of phalange tubes) of the network also assumes independence of factors and is performed separately for each finger (equation 5).

$$P_{finger} = P_{root} \times P_{tube_1} \times P_{topol_{1,2}} \times P_{tube_2} \times P_{topol_{2,3}} \times P_{tube_3} \qquad (5)$$

The globally optimal (maximum) value of P_{finger} for each finger (within the quantised space) is found using dynamic programming. Efficiency savings may be made in this process by bearing in mind all probabilities in equation 5 are < 1 by design. Thus a partial solution that has lower probability than the best solution so far need not be evaluated further in the forward part of the algorithm (in practice saving many evaluations of $P_{topol_{n,m}}$).

P_{root} relates to the probabilistic influence from the root node (figure 1). This is calculated as a normalised Gaussian (equation 2) based on the distance (in the 2D plane defined by the root node, and tube directions) of the start of the base phalange from its "root node projection" (σ is 0.5 × the tube radius). The root node configuration is defined as a straight line in 3D space. This line is calculated by calculating a least squares rigid registration (translation and rotation) between the corresponding start and end points of the PET and MR models (pre-optimisation), using the method of Horn [12]. A straight line is fitted to the 8 registered base phalange start points, again using a least squares error minimisation approach. The pairs of start points (one for each data set) are projected onto this line, and the mean taken as the "root node projection" for that finger. These points are projected back into the original space for the transformed data set (choice of which set to transform makes little difference to the root node projections calculated). It should be noted that the root node configuration is pre-calculated from the initial configuration rather than optimised within the dynamic programming stage as it is the same for both PET and MR networks (which are currently optimised separately). This gives consistency of the starting points of the phalange tubes, which would be expected for data taken from the same patient. The networks are optimised at increasingly finer quantisations / smaller search ranges using the previous optimal as a starting point, as illustrated in figure 4.

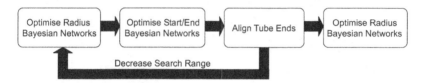

Fig. 4. Multi-scale Network optimisation flowchart

Parent/child end/start points are aligned after each application of the Start-End network optimiser. The iteration detailed in figure 4 is performed 4 times (with the start/end search range halved at each iteration). The total model fitting process (including initialisation) takes just a few minutes to fit models to both data sets.

3.3   Non-rigid Transform Calculation

Once the tube based model has been fitted to corresponding PET and MR datasets, it is a reasonably simple process to calculate a non-rigid (piecewise rigid) transform between the two data sets. This transform may be used to warp one of the data sets (we warp the PET data) into correspondence with the other. First, a global rigid (translation and rotation) transform is calculated from the corresponding start and end points of the phalange tubes in the two models. The closed form least-squares error minimisation method of Horn is used [12]. Calculating local rigid transformations for each (globally aligned) tube pair is performed using the same method. However, at least three points are required for this method, and only two are available (the start & end of the tube). A third point is generated by using principal components analysis (PCA) to calculate the eigenvector of the globally aligned annotated hand points (both sets) with the smallest eigenvalue. This 'minor axis vector' (V_{ma}) defines a plane with the tube direction (T_{dir}) in which the third point lies. This third point is calculated as in equation 6.

$$P_3 = T_{start} + T_{length} \times D_3 \tag{6}$$

Where D_3 is the vector in the plane defined by V_{ma} and T_{dir} perpendicular to T_{dir}, where the dot product of D_3 and V_{ma} is positive. Transformation of any point or voxel within a single tube is simply a matter of performing the global transform, followed by the appropriate tube transform (or the inverse operations in the opposite order for the reverse transform). Points outside the tubes may simply be transformed using the global transform only. In fact we interpolate the transform near the edges and when a point is in more than one tube. Details are omitted for brevity. Figure 5 shows some results of these transforms applied to annotated point and voxel data.

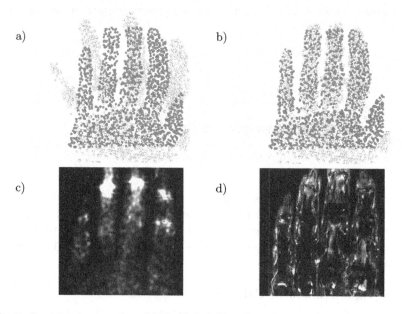

Fig. 5. Registration results; a)&b) Global (Rigid) and Local (Non-rigid) registration applied to annotated hand points, c) Warped PET slice, d) Corresponding MR slice

4   Evaluation

Our method was evaluated by application to a number of data sets. The principal behind the evaluation is that the closest annotated point in the 'other' data set to a registered/transformed 'hand' point should be a hand point. Our chosen evaluation metric is to count the proportion of these 'correct points' for the transforms in either direction. It should be noted that the absolute values presented are fairly meaningless as PET and MR data sets don't image exactly the same part of the hand (parts may be missing in one set or another). However, relative values for a data set demonstrate improvement in registration quality. Results are presented in table 5. Results show a statistically significant improvement (at 5% confidence) in the local and global registrations (especially local) over all data sets after application of our method. Also, local registration always outperforms global registration. Our chosen metric says nothing about the magnitude of registration errors, although by inspection maximum error appears well under

Table 5. Nearest Neighbour Correct Evaluation Results

Data Set	PET→MR Nearest Correct Prop.	MR→PET Nearest Correct Prop.
A	[0.844/0.866]→[0.920/0.970] (0.026)	[0.774/0.821]→[0.816/0.919] (0.325)
B	[*0.834*/0.887]→[*0.829*/0.910] (0.018)	[0.766/0.835]→[0.769/0.909] (0.302)
C	[0.525/0.714]→[0.586/0.906] (0.132))	[0.552/0.762]→[0.651/0.931] (0.374)
D	[0.930/0.931]→[0.951/0.953] (0)	[0.712/0.732]→[0.757/0.841] (0)
E	[0.518/0.520]→[0.704/0.764] (0.054)	[0.689/0.680]→[0.908/0.941] (0.306)
F	[0.880/0.892]→[0.956/0.977] (0.553)	[0.758/0.788]→[0.890/0.914] (0.119)
Mean inc.	[0.069/0.111]	[0.090/0.139]

Results show initial [Global Trans./Local Trans.] → final [Global Trans./Local Trans.] (Raw, for reference)

Italics imply registration fit decrease (for data set GJ PET→MR Global registration only)

5mm. Ground truth would be required to verify this. We plan experiments with imaging phantoms and pseudo-synthetic data to do this verification.

5 Discussion, Future Work and Acknowledgements

We have posed a problem of non-rigid multi-modal volume registration as one of model fitting by optimisation of a set of Bayesian networks. Quantisation, and local search, allow the efficient use of dynamic programming to find a globally optimal solution (within a locally quantised space). Applying this approach iteratively at multiple, decreasing, scales gives robust model fits within a few minutes. We have applied this approach to the registration of PET and MR volumes of hands, for the study of bone growth/erosion in arthritis. The networks we have proposed include no learned (or measured) prior terms. Such terms could easily be included if sufficiently accurate (and useful) models were available. However, it is debatable whether such models would add anything for the application presented as patients with arthritis often have rather unusual hand poses. In the near future we intend to automate the process of hand/not hand point annotation of volumetric data sets. We intend to further evaluate the exact accuracy of registrations using imaging phantoms with easily identifiable localisation points. Evaluation using pseudo-synthetic data is also planned.

D. McGonagle has been funded by the UK Medical Research Council to carry out the high-resolution imaging studies of arthritis used in this paper.

References

1. Myers, R.: The application of PET-MR image registration in the brain. The British Journal of Radiology **75** (2002) 31–35
2. Woods, R., Grafton, S., Holmes, C., Cherry, S., Mazziotta, J.: Automated image registration I. Journal of Computer Assisted Tomography **22(1)** (1998) 139–152
3. Wells, W., Viola, P., Atsumi, H., Nakajima, S., Kikinis, R.: Multi-modal volume registration by maximisation of mutual information. Medical Image Analysis **1(1)** (1996) 35–51

 4. Studholme, C., Hill, D., Hawkes, D.: Automated 3D registration of magnetic resonance and positron emssion tomography brain images by multi-resolution optimization of voxel similarity measures. Medical Physics **24(1)** (1997) 25–35
 5. West, J., Fitzpatrick, M., Wang, M., et al.: Comparison and evaluation of retrospective intermodality brain image registration techniques. Journal of Computer Assisted Tomography **21(4)** (1997) 554–566
 6. Makela, T., Pham, Q., Clarysse, P., Neonen, J., Lotjonen, J., Sipila, O., Hanninen, H., Lauerma, K., Knuuti, J., Katila, T., Magnin, I.: A 3D model-based registration approach for the PET, MR and MCG cardiac data fusion. Medical Image Analysis **7(3)** (2003) 377–389
 7. Farahani, K., Slates, R., Shao, Y., Silverman, R., Cherry, S.: Contemporaneous positron emission tomography and MR imaging at 1.5T. Journal of Magnetic Resonance Imaging **9** (1999) 497–500
 8. Hogg, D.: Model-based vision: A program to see a walking person. Image and Vision Computing **1** (1983) 5–20
 9. Rehg, J., Kanade, T.: Visual tracking of high DOF atriculated structures: An application to human hand tracking. In: Proc. European Conference on Computer Vision. (1994) 35–46
10. Stenger, B., Mendonca, P., Cipolla, R.: Model-based hand tracking using an unscented kalman filter. In: Proc. British Machine Vision Conference. (2001) 53–72
11. Felzenswalb, P., Huttenlocher, D.: Efficient matching of pictorial structures. In: Proc. IEEE Conf. on Computer Vision and Pattern Recognition. (2000)
12. Horn, B.: Closed-form solution of absolute orientation using unit quaternions. Journal of the Optical Society of America **4(4)** (1987) 629–642

Segmentation and Volume Representation Based on Spheres for Non-rigid Registration

Jorge Rivera-Rovelo and Eduardo Bayro-Corrochano

CINVESTAV del IPN, Unidad Guadalajara,
Av. López Mateos 590. Zapopan, México, C.P.45232

Abstract. This paper presents three different tasks: segmentation of medical images, volume representation and non-rigid registration. The first task is a necessary step before volume representation ant it is done with a simple but effective strategy using tomographic images, combining texture and boundary information in a region growing strategy, obtaining good results. For the second task, we present a new approach to model 2D surfaces and 3D volumetric data based on marching cubes idea using however spheres (modeling the surface of an object using spheres allows us to reduce the number of primitives representing it and to benefit -from such reduction- the registration process of two objects). We compare our approach based on marching cubes idea with other one using Delaunay tetrahedrization, and the results show that our proposed approach reduces considerably the number of spheres. Finally, we show how to do non-rigid registration of two volumetric data represented as sets of spheres using 5-dimensional vectors in conformal geometric algebra.

1   Introduction

Image segmentation is a common task in image processing applications and it has a great importance in medical applications. When dealing with tumor segmentation in brain images, one way to solve the problem is by using Magnetic Resonance (MR) images because in such images we have different types of them (for example T1, T2, T1-weighted, T2-weighted, etc); some of them highlight tumor and other structures. Thus, by combining and differentiating them, the task become more easy and an automatic approach for segmentation become possible (see [1]). Other methods use a probabilistic digital brain atlas to search abnormalities (outliers) between the patient data and the atlas (see [2,3]). The use of Computer Tomographic (CT) images is less used because they have not such modalities and the development of an automatic algorithm for segmentation is more complicated; however semi-automatic approaches have been proposed (see [4,5]) using seed points (defined by user) as initialization and growing the region by some method. In this work we use a simple but effective algorithm to segment the tumor: a set of 5 *texture descriptors* is used to characterize each pixel of the image by means of 5×1 template or a 5D-vector; then each vector is compared with the typical vector describing a tumor in order to establish an initialization of the tumor in the image (seed points for tumor tissue). Finally, a

Y. Liu, T. Jiang, and C. Zhang (Eds.): CVBIA 2005, LNCS 3765, pp. 449–458, 2005.
© Springer-Verlag Berlin Heidelberg 2005

region growing strategy is used, combined with boundary information to obtain the final shape of the tumor (this method is explained in Sect. 2).

On the other hand, representation of volumetric objects using primitives like points, lines or planes is a common task. The Union of Spheres proposed in [6] is another possible representation for volumetric data, but the representation is obtained using the Delaunay tetrahedrization and its complexity is $O(n^2)$ in both, time and number of primitives, while our highest number of spheres using our proposed method based on marching cubes is less than $2n$ in the worst case, and some times it is less. We use computer tomography (CT) images to do the experiments, and one of the the surfaces to be modeled is the segmented tumor; n is the number of boundary points in a total of m CT images (slides).

In surgical procedures we have a big problem when surgeon opens the head because of the loss of cerebrospinal liquid, which causes (non-linear) deformation of the internal structures. In this work (see Sect. 4.2) we present a new approach which uses models based on spheres for using such spheres as the entities to be aligned. This is embedded in the Conformal Geometric Algebra (CGA) framework using the TPS-RPM algorithm but in a 5-dimensional space.

2   Segmentation

According to [8,9] segmentation techniques can be categorized in three classes: a) thresholding, b) region-based and c) boundary-based. Due to the advantages and disadvantages of each technique, many segmentation methods are based on the integration of information obtained by two techniques: the region and boundary information. Some of them embed the integration in the region detection (integration through definition of new parameters or decision criterion for the segmentation), while others integrate the information after both processes are completed (integration is performed after both techniques -boundary and region based- have been used to process the image). Within each category for integration of the information, we have a great variety of methods; some of them works better in some cases, some need user initialization, some are more sensitive to noise, etc. This fact make not feasible to determine the best approach to segmentation that integrates boundary and region information because we have not a generally accepted and clear methodology for evaluating the algorithms; additionally, the properties and objectives that the algorithms try to satisfy and the image domain in which they work are different. Interested reader can consult a detailed review of different approaches in [8]. Due to the fact that we are dealing with medical images, we need also to take into account an important characteristic: the texture. Textural properties of the image can be extracted using *texture descriptors* which describe the texture in an area of the image. So, if we use a *texture descriptor* over the whole image, we obtain a new "texture feature image". In most cases, a single operator does not provide enough information about texture, and a set of operators need to be used. This results in a set of "texture feature images" that jointly describe the texture around each pixel. Main methods for texture segmentation are Laws's texture energy filters, Co-occurrence matrices, Random fields, frequency domain methods and Perceptive texture features (see [10] for more details).

When segmenting tomographic images, simple segmentation techniques such as region growing, split and merge or boundary segmentation can not be used alone because such images contain textures of different tissues, similar gray-levels between healthy and non-healthy tissues, and sometimes the boundaries are not well defined. For this reason, we decide to combine not only boundary and region information (as typically it is done), but also to integrate information obtained from texture descriptors and embed that in a region growing strategy. A block diagram of our proposed approach is shown in figure 1.a.

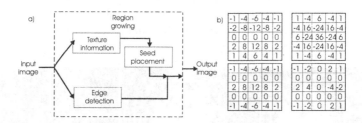

Fig. 1. a) Block diagram of the approach to segment tumors in CT images (region growing strategy combining texture and boundary information); b) Texture descriptors used to obtain the texture information (4 Laws energy masks)

The first step is to characterize each pixel on images, so we use the texture information provided by some of the Laws's masks to characterize them with a five-dimensional vector (named *texture vector*, V_{ij}, for pixel in coordinates (i, j)). Then, to place automatically the seed points for the region growing strategy, we choose only the pixels having a texture vector for the tissue of interest (in this case we are interested in tumor) and use them as initialization (or seeds) for the region growing strategy; boundary information is used to stop the growing of the region. The construction of V_{ij} is explained as follows: the first element, $V_{ij}[0]$, is only to identify if the pixels corresponds to the background ($V_{ij}[0] = 0$) or to the patient's head ($V_{ij}[0] = 1$) - patient's head could be skin, bone, brain, etc.; in order to obtain the texture information, we use a set of four masks of the so called Laws Masks (L5E5,R5R5,L5S5,E5S5-figure 1.b); then we fix the value in a position of V_{ij} with 1's or 0's, depending on if the value is greater than zero or zero, respectively. As a result, each structure (tissue, bone, skin, background) on the medical images used, has the same vector V_{ij} in a high number of its belonging pixels, but not in all of them because of variations in values of neighboring pixels. So we can use the pixels having the texture vector of the object we want to extract to establish them as seed points in a region-growing scheme.

Region growing criterions we use are as follows: we compute the mean μ_{seeds} and standard deviation σ_{seeds} of the pixels fixed as seeds; then, for each neighboring pixel being examined to determine if added or not to the region:

If $I(x, y) = \pm 2\sigma_{seeds}$ and $V_{xy} \neq V_{seed}$ at most in 1 element,then $I(x, y) \in R_t$;

where R_t is the region of the tumor. The stopping criterion takes into account the boundaries of the object. Such boundaries are found processing the image with the Canny filter (having in this form, one more image of information for the processing). So, the growing of the region is in all directions, but when a boundary pixel is found in the *canny image*, the growing in such direction is stopped.

Figure 2 shows results of the process explained before: figure 2.a shows one original CT-image; figure 2.b shows the seed points fixed, which have the texture vector of the tumor; figure 2.c shows the final result after the overall process has ended (the tumor extracted). The overall process takes only few seconds per image and it could be used to segment any of the objects; but in our case, we focus our attention on the extraction of the tumor. After that, the next step is

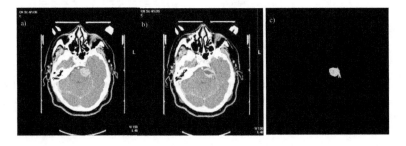

Fig. 2. Results for the segmentation. a) One of the original CT-images; b) Seed points fixed; c) Result for the image of (a) after the whole process (the tumor extracted).

to model the volumetric data by some method. Due to the fact that tumor can be deformed because of the lost of cefalic liquid once the head of the patient is opened, we need a 3D representation of the tumor which allows us to update the shape of the tumor. Next sections present how the spheres are represented in conformal geometric algebra (CGA); then we will show how to build 3D models and register two of them using such entities with TPS-RPM method.

3   Representation of Spheres in CGA

Due to that our objective is not to provide a detailed description of the geometric algebra (GA) and its advantages, we only give a brief introduction and explain how to represent spheres in conformal geometric algebra (CGA) as points in a space of 5 dimensions (because such representation will be used in the non-rigid registration process).

Geometric algebra is a coordinate-free approach to geometry based on the algebras of Grassmann and Clifford. The algebra is defined on a space whose elements are called *multivectors*; a multivector is a linear combination of objects of different grade, e.g. scalars, vectors and k-vectors. It has an associative and fully invertible product called the *geometric* or Clifford product, represented as ab for two vectors a and b, and defined as:

$$ab = a \cdot b + a \wedge b . \tag{1}$$

where $a \cdot b$ represents the *dot* or *inner* product and $a \wedge b$ represents the *wedge* or *exterior* product. The geometric algebra $G_{p,q,r}$ is a linear space of dimension 2^n, where $n = p + q + r$ and p, q, r indicate the number of basis vectors which squares to $1, -1, 0$, respectively. This algebra is constructed by the application of geometric product between each two basis vectors e_i, e_j from the base of the vector space $\Re^{p,q,r}$. Thus $G_{p,q,r}$ has elements of grade 0 (scalars), grade 1 (vectors), grade 2 (bivectors), and so on. The CGA $G_{4,1,0}$ is adequate for representing entities like spheres because there is no direct way to describe them as compact entities in $G_{3,0,0}$ (the geometric algebra of the 3D space); the only possibility to define them is given by formulating a constraint equation. However, in CGA the spheres are the basis entities from which the other entities are derived. These basic entities, the spheres $\underline{s}$ with center p and radius ρ are defined by

$$\underline{s} = p + \frac{1}{2} \left(p^2 - \rho^2 \right) e + e_0 . \tag{2}$$

where $p \in \Re^3$, ρ is a scalar and e, e_0 are defined as in eq. 3 (they are called null vectors), and they are formed with two basis vectors e_-, e_+ additional to the three basis vectors of the 3D-Euclidean space (which have the properties that $e_-^2 = -1; e_+^2 = +1; e_- \cdot e_+ = 0$).

$$e = e_- + e_+; \quad e_0 = \frac{1}{2}(e_- - e_+) \tag{3}$$

In fact, we can think in a conformal point $\underline{x}$ as a degenerate sphere of radius $\rho = 0$. More details on GA and the construction of other entities in CGA can be consulted in [12,13]. We can see eq. 2 as a linear combination: $\underline{s} = \alpha e_1 + \beta e_2 + \gamma e_3 + \delta e_+ + \epsilon e_-$, or represent it as a 5D-vector $\underline{s} = [\alpha \ \beta \ \gamma \ \delta \ \epsilon]^T$. Note that such representation in CGA encodes the center of $\underline{s}$ in α, β, γ, and the radius in encoded in δ, ϵ. Thus, the sphere in CGA is represented with a 5-dimensional vector, which is an adequate representation to make two sets of 5-vectors, one representing the object and the other the deformed object. These sets are obtained by the method explained in next section. Once we have these sets, we will be able to apply the TPS-RPM algorithm in order to do the registration process (see Sect. 4.2).

4   Volume Representation and Non-rigid Registration

In medical image analysis, the availability of 3D-models is of great interest to medicians because it allows them to have a better understanding of the situation, and such models are relatively easy to build. However, in special situations (as surgical procedures), some structures (as brain or tumor) suffer a (non-rigid) transformation and the initial model must be corrected to reflect the actual shape of the object. For this reason, it is important to have a representation suitable to be deformed, with the minor quantity of primitives involved in such representation as possible to make faster the process. In literature we can find the Union of Spheres algorithm (see [6]), which uses the spheres to build 3D-models of objects and to align or transform it over time. Nevertheless, we use the marching cubes algorithm's ideas to develop an alternative method to build 3D models by using spheres, which has the advantage of reducing the number of primitives needed. For space reasons we do not provide an explanation of the Union of Spheres nor the Marching Cubes algorithms, but it can be found in [6,11].

4.1   3D Models Using Spheres

To build a 3D model of the object of interest using spheres, we are based in the marching cubes algorithm (MCA). The principle of our proposal is the same as in MCA: given a set of m slides (CT images), divide the space in logical cubes (each cube contains eight vertexes, four of slide k and four of slide $k+1$) and determine which vertexes of each cube are inside (or on) and outside the surface. Then define the number of spheres of each cube according to figure 3 and eq. 4 (where i is the ith sphere of the case indicated by j), taking the indexes of the cube's corners as the first cube of such figure indicates. Note that we use the same 15 basic cases of the marching cubes algorithm because the total of 256 cases can be obtained from this basis. Also note that instead of triangles we define spheres and that our goal is not to have a good render algorithm (as intended for Marching cubes algorithm), but have a representation of the volumetric data based on spheres which, as we said before, could be useful in the process of object registration.

$$s_{p_i}^j = c_{p_i} + \frac{1}{2}(c_{p_i}^2 - \rho_{p_i}^2)e + e_0$$

$$s_{m_i}^j = c_{m_i} + \frac{1}{2}(c_{m_i}^2 - \rho_{m_i}^2)e + e_0$$

$$s_{g_i}^j = c_{g_i} + \frac{1}{2}(c_{g_i}^2 - \rho_{g_i}^2)e + e_0 \tag{4}$$

Figure 4.a-d shows the results obtained for a set of 36 images of a real patient with a tumor visible in 16 of them (see in figure 4.d the 3D model of the tumor of the real patient). Table 1 is a comparison between the results of the Union of Spheres and our approach for the case of a brain model. The first row shows the worst case with both approaches; second row shows the number of spheres with improvements in both algorithms (reduction of spheres in DT is done by grouping spheres in a single one which contents the others, while such reduction is done using a bigger displacement, $d = 3$, in our approach). The number of boundary points was $n = 3370$ in both cases. It is obvious the reduction in

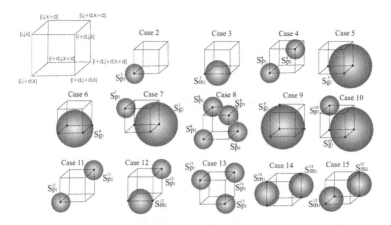

Fig. 3. The basic 15 cases of surface intersecting cubes (defining a different number of spheres with different centers and radius)

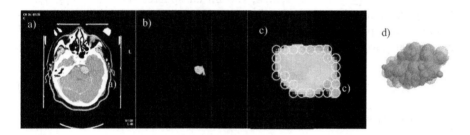

Fig. 4. Real patient: a) Original of one CT slide; b) Segmented object (the tumor); c) Zoom of the approximation by circles according the steps described in section; d) Approximation by spheres of the tumor extracted

the number of primitives obtained with our approach, while maintaining clear enough the representation (even in the worst case).

4.2   Registration of Two Models

Registration problem is frequently founded in computer vision and medical image processing. Suppose you have two points sets and one of them results from the transformation of the other but you do not know the transformation nor the correspondences between the points. In such situation you need an algorithm that find these two unknowns the best as possible. If in addition the transformation is non rigid, the complexity increases enormously. In the variety of registration algorithms existing today, we find some that assume the knowledge of one of this unknowns and solve for the other one; but there are two examples of algorithms that solve for both: Iterated Closest Point (ICP) and Thin plate spline-Robust Point Matching (TPS-RPM). Details of each one of this algorithms can be found

Table 1. Comparison between number of spheres using approach based on Delaunay tetrahedrization and our approach based on marching cubes algorithm; n is the number of boundary points; d is the distance in pixels between vertexes in logical cubes of second approach

n/d	Num of spheres with each approach	
	DT approach	Our approach
3370 / 1	13480	11866
3370 / 3	8642	2602

in [7]; here we assume, for space reasons, the reader knows them. In a past work we presented a comparison between these algorithms for non-rigid registration and we concluded TPS-RPM gives better results. However, we had used only sets of 2D and 3D points. Now we have spheres as points in a 5D-space modeling the object, and these spheres have not only different centers, but also different radius.

Let be $U_I = \{\underline{s}_j^I\}, j = 1, 2, ..., k$, the initial spheres set; $U_F = \{\underline{s}_i^F\}, i = 1, 2, ..., n$, the final spheres set. For the non-rigid registration we follow the simulated annealing process of TPS-RPM explained in [7]. To update the matrix M of correspondence for spheres $\underline{s}_j^I$ y $\underline{s}_i^F$, modify m_{ji} as

$$m_{ji} = \frac{1}{T}e^{-\frac{(\underline{s}_i^F - f(\underline{s}_j^I))^\top (\underline{s}_i^F - f(\underline{s}_j^I))}{T}}. \qquad (5)$$

for outlier entries $j = k + 1$ and $i = 1, 2, ..., n$:

$$m_{k+1,i} = \frac{1}{T_0}e^{-\frac{(\underline{s}_i^F - f(\underline{s}_{k+1}^I))^\top (\underline{s}_i^F - f(\underline{s}_{k+1}^I))}{T_0}}. \qquad (6)$$

and for outliers entries $j = 1, 2, ..., k$ and $i = n + 1$:

$$m_{j,n+1} = \frac{1}{T_0}e^{-\frac{(\underline{s}_{n+1}^F - f(\underline{s}_j^I))^\top (\underline{s}_{n+1}^F - f(\underline{s}_j^I))}{T_0}}. \qquad (7)$$

where T is the parameter of temperature which is reduced in each stage of the optimization process beginning at a value T_0 (remember that TPS-RPM use the simulated annealing process). Then, to update transformation we use the QR-decomposition of M to solve eq. 8 (following the same process explained in [7] and omitted here for space reasons).

$$E_{tps}(d, w) = \|Y - Vd - \Phi w\|^2 + \lambda_1 (w^T \Phi w) + \lambda_2 [d - I]^T [d - I] . \qquad (8)$$

Figure 5.a shows the 3D models as sets of spheres representing the object (the tumor mentioned in figure 4) -one is the initial set (or representation at time t_1); the other is the deformed or expected set (or representation at time t_2)- which must be registered. Figure 5.b shows the results of registration process using TPS-RPM algorithm with the spheres as 5D-vectors in CGA (it shows the

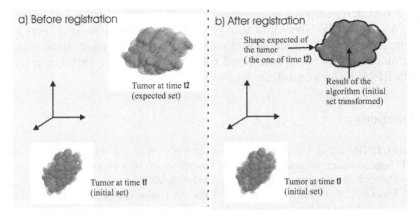

a) Before registration

b) After registration

Shape expected of
the tumor
(the one of time t2)

Tumor at time t2
(expected set)

Result of the
algorithm (initial
set transformed)

Tumor at time t1
(initial set)

Tumor at time t1
(initial set)

Fig. 5. a) Initial and expected sets (the expected set is obtained by a non-rigid transformation of the initial one); b) Initial and result of applying TPS-RPM to align the sets of spheres, represented as 5D-vectors in CGA. Note that the resulting set has been aligned an looks like the initial one.

shape of the expected set for visual comparison). Note that usually, researchers use TPS-RPM with 2D or 3D vectors because they can not go beyond such dimension; in contrast, using CGA we have an homogeneous representation which preserves isometries and uses the sphere as the basic entity. A right comparison must use an algorithm which deals with non-rigid registration without a priori information about correspondences nor transformation as the ICP mentioned above; but in past work we have shown that TPS-RPM solve the problem better than ICP, so we suppress it here for this reason. It is important to highlight that the algorithm adjusted the radius as expected because the CGA 5-vector representing the sphere $\underline{s}$ encodes the information about its center and radius, so both are adjusted at each iteration step of the TPS-RPM algorithm by updating the values of $\alpha, \beta, \gamma, \delta, \epsilon$.

5   Conclusions

We have shown three different but related tasks: 1) A simple but effective approach for image segmentation which combines texture and boundary information and embed it into a region-growing scheme, having the advantage of integrating all the information in a simple process. The algorithm showed be useful despite the limitations of the CT images used (limitations compared with the facilities given by MRI images, commonly used in similar works) and is not the contribution of this work, but a necessary step before the others two tasks. 2) We show how to obtain a representation of volumetric data using spheres. Our approach is based on the ideas exposed in marching cubes algorithm but it is not intended for rendering purposes or displaying in real time, but for reduce the number of primitives modeling the volumetric data and with this saving, make a better registration process; better in the sense of using less primitives in the process. 3) We show how to represent these primitives as spheres in the CGA by means of 5-dimensional vectors which encode the information about the center and radius of the spheres, and using them naturally with the principles of TPS-RPM. Experimental results seem to be promising.

References

1. S. Ho, E. Bullitt, G. Gerig, "Level-set evolution with region competition: automatic 3-D segmentation of brain tumors", *Proceedings of 16th International Conference on Pattern Recognition*, Volume 1, pp. 532-535, 2002.
2. M. Prastawa, E. Bullit, S. Ho and G. Gerig, "A Brain Tumor Segmentation Framework Based on Outlier Detection," *Medical Image Analysis Journal*, 8(3), pp. 275-83, September 2004.
3. N. Moon, E. Bullit, K. van Leemput and G. Gerig, "Model Based Brain and Tumor Segmentation," in *Proceedings of the 16th International Conference on Pattern Recognition*, August 11 - 15, 2002, Quebec City, QC, Canada pp. 528- 531.
4. M.C. Andrade, "An interactive algorithm for image smoothing and segmentation," *Electronic Letters on Computer Vision and Image Analysis*, **4-1**, pp. 32-48, 2004.
5. P. Lin, C. Zheng, Y. Yang and J. Gu, "Medical Image Segmentation by Level Set Method Incorporating Region and Boundary Statistical Information," *9th Iberoamerican Congress on Pattern Recognition*, National Institute of Astrophysics, Optics and Electronics (INAOE), Puebla, Mexico, pp. 654-660, October 2004.
6. V. Ranjan and A. Fournier, "Union of spheres (UoS) model for volumetric data,", in *Proceedings of the Eleventh Annual Symposium on Computational Geometry*, Vancouver, Canada, 1995, C2-C3, pp. 402-403.
7. H. Chui, A. Rangarajan, "A new point matching algorithm for non-rigid registration". *IEEE Conf. on Computer Vision and Pattern Recognition (CVPR)*, Volume 2, pp. 44-51, 2000.
8. X. Muñoz, "Image segmentation integrating color, texture and boundary information," *Ph.D. Thesis in Computer engineering*, Girona, December 2002.
9. K.S. Fu and J.K. Mui, "A survey on image segmentation," *Pattern Recognition*, 12:395-403, 1980.
10. M.J. Chantler, "The effect of variation in illuminant direction on texture classification", *Ph.D. thesis, Dept. Computing and Electrical Engineering*, Heriot-Watt University, August 1994, pp. 67-89.
11. W. Lorensen and H. Cline, "Marching cubes: a high resolution 3D surface construction algorithm," *Computer Graphics*. **21-4**, 163–169, July 1987.
12. E. Bayro-Corrochano and G. Sobczyk, *Geometric algebra with applications in science and engineering*, Birkhuser, 2001.
13. B. Rosenhahn and G. Sommer, "Pose Estimation in Conformal Geometric Algebra," Technical report 0206, Christian-Albrechts-University of Kiel, November 2002, pp. 13-36.

Segmentation of 3D CT Volume Images Using a Single 2D Atlas*

Feng Ding[1], Wee Kheng Leow[1], and Shih-Chang Wang[2]

[1] Dept. of Computer Science, National University of Singapore,
3 Science Drive 2, Singapore 117543
{dingfeng, leowwk}@comp.nus.edu.sg
[2] Dept. of Diagnostic Radiology, National University of Singapore,
5 Lower Kent Ridge Road, Singapore 119074
dnrwsc@nus.edu.sg

Abstract. Segmentation of medical images is an important first step in the analysis of medical images. A lot of research has been performed on the segmentation of complex CT/MR images using the atlas-based approach. Most existing methods use 3D atlases which are more complex and difficult to control than 2D atlases. They have been applied mostly for the segmentation of brain images. This paper presents a method that can segment multiple slices of an abdominal CT volume using a single 2D atlas. Segmentation of human body images is considerably more difficult and challenging than brain image segmentation. Test results show that our method can handle large variations in shape and intensity between the atlas and the target CT images.

1 Introduction

Segmentation of medical images is an important first step in the analysis of medical images. For example, in liver transplant, CT images of the donor are taken. Then, the image regions corresponding to the liver are segmented to compute the liver's volume. Moreover, 3D model of the liver and the blood vessels are reconstructed to help the surgeons plan the surgical procedure.

A lot of research has been performed on the segmentation of CT and MR images. In particular, the atlas-based approach is most suited to segmenting complex medical images because it can make use of spatial and structured knowledge in the segmentation process. Typically, 3D atlases are used to segment the surfaces of the anatomical structures in 3D CT/MR images [1,2,3,4,5,6,7]. However, 3D atlases are more complex and difficult to construct than 2D atlases. There are much more parameters to control in 3D atlases. Thus, 3D atlas-based algorithms tend to be developed for segmenting specific anatomical structures. It is not easy to adapt the algorithms to the segmentation of other anatomical structures by simply changing the atlas.

An alternative is to use multiple 2D atlases to segment a CT/MR volume. In this case, it is necessary to understand how many 2D atlases will be needed to

---

* This research is supported by NUS ARF R-252-000-210-112.

Y. Liu, T. Jiang, and C. Zhang (Eds.): CVBIA 2005, LNCS 3765, pp. 459–468, 2005.

segment all the slices in a volume. The worst case scenario of one atlas per image would defeat the idea of using 2D atlases because the stack of 2D atlases would contain the same amount of complexity as a 3D atlas. It also makes practical application difficult because there are many slices in a typical CT/MR volume. For example, in the case of liver transplant, more than 200 abdominal CT images are taken.

Interestingly, most work on atlas-based segmentation has been focused on brain MR images [1,2,3,8,6] or heart MR images [4,7]. Less work is done on the segmentation of abdominal CT images [5], which is considerably more difficult and challenging than segmentation of brain images.

This paper describes an atlas-based method for segmenting multiple anatomical structures in multiple slices of an abdominal CT volume using a single 2D atlas. The research objective is to investigate how well can a single 2D atlas perform on segmenting various slices in a CT volume of a particular patient. This research can lead to an understanding of the number and types of atlas required to segment various CT images encountered in normal clinical practices.

Test results show that our algorithm can successfully and accurately segment 34 abdominal CT slices of 1mm thickness using a single 2D atlas. Since the 2D atlas differs significantly in shape and intensity from the test CT images, successful test results suggest that the algorithm should work well in segmenting CT images of other patients. Our research work thus contributes to solving the difficult and challenging problem of segmenting human body CT/MR images.

2   Related Work

Atlas-based segmentation is performed using atlas-based registration technique. The registered atlas contours (2D case) and surfaces (3D case) are taken as the boundaries of the segmented anatomical structures. Fully automatic atlas-based segmentation problems map to atlas-based registration problems with unknown correspondence. Solutions to these problems have to solve both the registration and the correspondence problems at the same time. These problems are therefore much more difficult to solve than semi-automatic registration and segmentation, which require some user inputs such as landmark points [9].

An atlas-based segmentation algorithm typically comprises two complementary stages: (1) global transformation of the atlas to roughly align it to the target image, and (2) local transformation or deformation of the atlas to accurately register it to the corresponding image features. Global transformation often serves to provide a good initialization for local deformation. Without a good initialization, local deformation may deform the atlas out of control and extract wrong object boundaries (see Section 3.3 for an example).

In the global transformation stage, spatial information (i.e., relative positions) of various parts of an atlas is used to determine how the atlas should be transformed. Both similarity [2,3,5] and affine [4,6,7] transformations have been used. An iterative optimization algorithm is applied to compute the optimal transformation parameters. In each iteration, the possible correspondence between the atlas and the target is usually determined based on the closest point criterion in the same way as the Iterative Closest Point algorithm [10].

In the local deformation stage, several main approaches have been adopted. The method in [11] applies iterative optimization to determine optimal local affine or 2nd-order polynomial transformations that deform the various parts of the atlas to best match the target. The methods in [4,5] also apply optimization techniques but they represent the 3D atlas surface using B-splines and thin-plate spline constraint. These methods ensure that the extracted surfaces are smooth but they require a large number of parameters to represent complex convoluted surfaces of the brain.

A popular method is to apply the so-called *demons algorithm* [2,3,6,12]. It regards the atlas and the target as images at consecutive time steps, and applies the optical flow algorithm to determine the correspondence between them. As for any optical flow algorithm, it suffers from the so-called *aperture problem* and may not be able to handle large displacements between corresponding points. It is also easily affected by noise and extraneous image features.

Among the existing methods discussed in this section, [5,7] use probabilistic atlases whereas the other methods use non-probabilistic atlases. Although probabilistic atlas contains more information about the variations, it requires sufficient training samples to accurately model the probability distributions.

In addition to applying atlas-based registration technique, [5,7] included a final classification stage that classifies each pixel to a most likely anatomical category. This stage is required because the registration algorithms are not precise enough in aligning the atlas boundaries to the object boundaries in target images. Classification approach can improve the accuracy of the segmentation result. However, it may not be able to handle segmentation of regions which are nonuniform in intensity and texture. For example, the air pocket in the stomach appears to have the same intensity as the background (Section 4, Fig. 3a, 5). Classification algorithms will be easily confused by such nonuniform regions.

Some existing papers have presented quantitative performance measures of their methods. In particular, [2,3] measure similarity index that is proportional to the area of intersection between segmented regions and the ground truth, [12,5] measure the amounts of false positives and false negatives, and [6] measures the mean squared error of corresponding points between the extracted boundaries and ground truth.

3   Automatic Atlas-Based Segmentation

Our method uses a 2D deformable atlas to segment the major components in abdominal CT images. The atlas consists of a set of closed contours of the entire human body, liver, stomach, and spleen, which are manually segmented from a reference CT image given in [13]. As shown in Fig. 1, the reference image is significantly different from the target image in terms of shapes and intensities of the body parts. Such differences are common in practical applications.

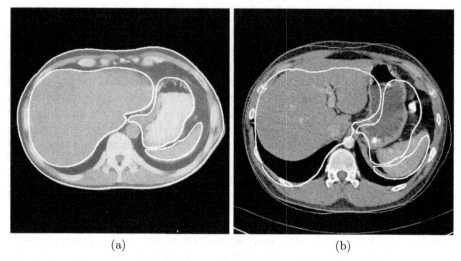

(a)   (b)

Fig. 1. (a) Atlas contours (white curves) superimposed on the reference CT image taken from [13]. (b) Atlas registered onto an target image after global transformation.

Our fully automatic segmentation algorithm consists of three stages:

1. Global transformation of the entire atlas.
2. Iterative local transformation of individual parts in the atlas.
3. Atlas contour refinement using active contour algorithm.

3.1   Global Transformation

This stage performs registration of the atlas to the target input image with *unknown correspondence*. First, the outer body contour of the target image (target contour) is extracted by straightforward contour tracing. Next, the outer body contour of the atlas (reference contour) is registered under affine transformation to the target contour using Iterative Closest Point algorithm [10]. After registration, the correspondence between the reference and target contour points is known. Then, the affine transformation matrix between the reference and target contours is easily computed from the known correspondence by solving a system of over-constrained linear equations. This transformation matrix is then applied to the atlas to map the contours of the inner body parts to the target image.

After global transformation, the centers of the reference contours fall within the corresponding body parts in the target image (Fig. 1b). The reference contours need to be refined to move to the correct boundaries of the body parts.

3.2   Iterative Local Transformation

This stage iteratively applies local transformations to the individual body parts to bring their reference contours closer to the target contours. The idea is to search the local neighborhoods of reference contour points to find possible corresponding target contour points. To achieve this goal, it is necessary to use features that are invariant to image intensity because the reference and target images can have different intensities (as shown in Fig. 1).

Let $N(p)$ denote the normal to the reference contour at point p, and $L(p)$ denote an ordered list of points $\{p_i\}$, $i = -n, \ldots, 0, \ldots, n$, lying on $N(p)$, with $p_0 = p$. Let $I(p_i)$ denote the intensity of point p_i. Then, the ordered list $D(p) = \{I(p_i) - I(p_{i+1})\}$, $i = -n, \ldots, n-1$, is the *intensity difference distribution* (IDD) at p along $N(p)$. IDD depends only on the local intensity difference, which does not differ as much as intensity across images. Thus, IDD is better than intensity for determining corresponding points between the images. In the same way, we can compute the IDD $D'(p')$ of an image point p' along a normal $N(p)$ of the reference contour and with respect to the target image intensities $I'(p_i')$. In the current implementation, $n = 5$, i.e., the length of IDD is 10.

The local search for possible corresponding points is performed as follows, after coarse registration of the atlas and the reference image to the target image by global transformation. For each reference contour point p, a search is performed within a small neighborhood $U(p)$ centered at p and along the normal $N(p)$ for a target image point p' whose IDD $D'(p')$ is most similar to $D(p)$. The difference between $D(p)$ and $D'(p')$ is measured in terms of the Euclidean distance between them. The neighborhood $U(p)$ decreases quadratically over time so that the search process will converge. In the current implementation, the width of the search neighborhood is 100 at the first iteration.

After finding the best matching target image point p' of a reference contour point p, a verification procedure is performed. Shoot a ray from the centroid of the closed reference contour of p to p'. If the number of number of "white" pixels or "black" pixels along the ray in the target image exceeds a predefined threshold, then the point p' is discarded because the intensity of the desired body parts are gray. Otherwise, p' is regarded as a corresponding point of p.

Given the reference contour points p_i whose corresponding points p_i' are found, compute the affine transformation matrix M that maps p_i to p_i'. Then, the matrix M is applied to all reference contour points, including those whose corresponding points are not found.

The above local transformation is repeated iteratively for each closed contour of the body parts individually until the reference contours converge. Therefore, the reference contours of different body parts can be mapped to the corresponding target image contours through different affine transformation matrices that are appropriate for them.

The iterative local transformation algorithm described above is analogous to the Iterative Closest Point (ICP) algorithm [10] in that it iteratively determines the possible correspondence between the reference and the target, and computes the transformation that maps the reference to the target. However, it differs from ICP in that possible correspondence is determined based on most similar IDD, which is a local image feature, instead of nearest position as in ICP. Therefore, it

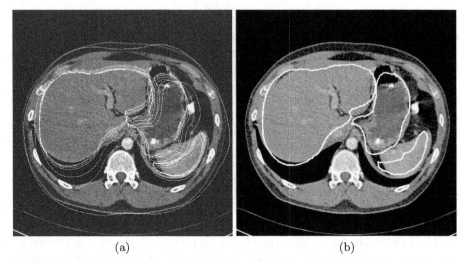

Fig. 2. Iterative local transformation. (a) The white reference contours are iteratively transformed. (b) The result of iterative local transformation after convergence.

can determine the correct correspondence more accurately than ICP. This algorithm can thus be called an *Iterative Corresponding Point* algorithm. Sample results of iterative local transformation are shown in Fig. 2.

3.3   Atlas Contour Refinement

The last stage performs refinement of the atlas contour using active contour, i.e., snake algorithm [14] with Gradient Vector Flow (GVF) [15]. The original snake algorithm has the shortcoming of not being able to move into concave parts of the objects to be segmented. This is because there is no image forces outside the concave parts to attract the snake. GVF diffuses the gradient vectors of the edges outward, and uses the gradient vectors as the image forces to attract the snake into concave parts.

Figure 3(a) illustrates the result of applying snake with GVF on the atlas to refine the contours obtained from iterative local transformation. The final atlas contours now coincide accurately with the actual boundaries of the body parts in the target image.

Note that after global transformation, the discrepancies between the reference contours and the target contours are still quite large (Fig. 1b). If the snake algorithm is applied immediately after global transformation without iterative local transformation, the reference contour is easily attracted to the boundary edges of other body parts (Fig. 3b). This shows that generic deformable models such as active contour (i.e., snake), active shape, and level set can be easily attracted to incorrect boundary edges. Our method resolves this problem by using iterative local transformation to bring the atlas contours closer to the desired object boundaries before applying the snake algorithm.

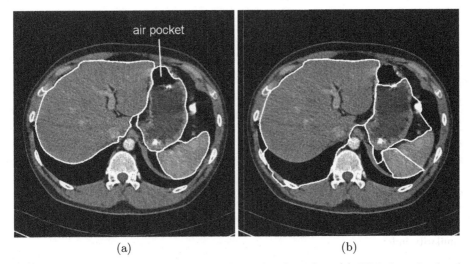

(a) (b)

Fig. 3. Results after contour refinement by snake algorithm. (a) With iterative local transformation (slice 72). (b) Without iterative local transformation.

3.4 Comparisons with Existing Work

Most existing atlas-based approaches adopt a two-stage approach consisting of global transformation followed by local deformation. On the other hand, our method consists of three stages, namely (1) global affine transformation, (2) iterative local affine transformation, and (3) snake deformation. The first two stages are similar to those in [1], but the method in [1] is developed for registering an atlas to a brain surface that is already segmented.

[5] also presented a method for segmenting abdominal CT images. However, their atlas registration algorithm is not accurate enough, and a final classification stage is applied to classify the image pixels into various anatomical categories. In contrast, by adopting a three-stage approach, our atlas registration algorithm is accurately enough to segment the various anatomical parts. Compare to the test results reported in [5,8], our method can handle much more variations between the atlas and the target images.

4   Experiments and Discussion

40 abdominal CT images (from slice 41 to 80) of 1mm thickness of a patient were used in the test. The accuracy of the segmentation result was measured in terms of the area of intersection between the target body part (that was obtained manually) and the segmented regions. This performance measure, called *similarity index S*, was proposed by Zijdenbos et al. [16]:

$$S = 2\frac{|A \cap B|}{|A| + |B|} \tag{1}$$

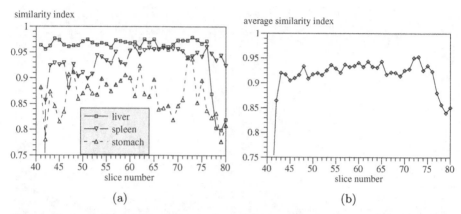

(a)   (b)

Fig. 4. Test results. (a) Similarity indices of liver, spleen, and stomach. (b) Average similarity index.

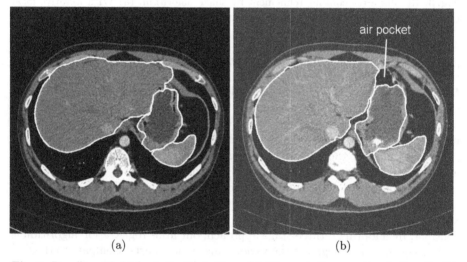

(a)   (b)

Fig. 5. Results with high similarity indices. (a) Segmentation results of slice 48. (b) Segmentation results of slice 60.

where A is the set of pixels of the body part in the target image and B that of the segmented region. When the segmented region coincide exactly with the target body part, $S = 1$.

Detailed segmentation performance of the algorithm is shown in Fig. 4. The liver is well segmented and the algorithm's performance on liver is very stable (Fig. 4a). The similarity indices are greater than 0.95 for slices 41 to 76 (Fig. 3a, 5). From slice 77 onward, the liver is split into two lobes, which is greatly different from that in the atlas image (Fig. 6b).

The algorithm's performance on segmenting the spleen shows a bit variation (Fig. 4a). But the similarity indices are still higher than 0.9 for slices 43 to 80

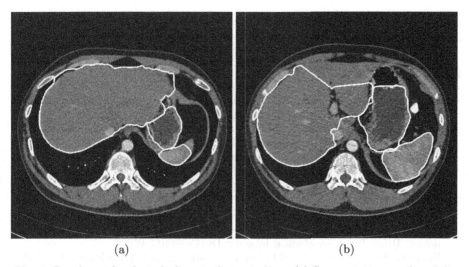

(a)   (b)

Fig. 6. Results with relatively low similarity indices. (a) Segmentation results of slice 42. (b) Segmentation results of slice 77.

(Fig. 3a, 5). For slice 42, the spleen becomes so small that it differs significantly from that in the atlas (Fig. 6a). Thus, the algorithm is not expected to perform well for this case.

The stomach is less well segmented, with the similarity index ranging from 0.8 to 0.95. It is due to the existence of air pocket, which appears as a black region with a very thin wall (Fig. 3a, 5b). When the air pocket is correctly included in the segmentation result (Fig. 3a), or when there is no air pocket (Fig. 5a), then the similarity index is high. The shape of stomach is quite complex. So, sometimes the snake algorithm is attracted to nearby edges that actually belong to the liver and the spleen.

Figure 4(b) illustrates the average performance of the algorithm on segmenting the liver, spleen, and stomach. The similarity index is above 0.9 for slices 43 to 76 (Fig. 3a, 5). That is, with a single 2D atlas, the algorithm can successfully and accurately segment 34 slices of the abdominal CT volume.

5   Conclusions

This paper presented an atlas-based method for segmenting abdominal CT images. It applies three complementary stages, namely global transformation, iterative local transformation, and snake algorithm, to iteratively deform the atlas to register with the target image. Experimental tests show that the algorithm can successfully and accurately segment 34 slices of a CT volume of 1mm thickness using a single 2D atlas. As the reference image that is used to derive the atlas differs significantly in shape and intensity from the target CT images, the successful test results suggest that the algorithm should work well on segmenting CT images of different patients. This research work thus contributes to solving the difficult and challenging problem of segmenting human body images.

References

1. Thurfjell, L., Bohm, C., Greitz, T., Eriksson, L.: Transformations and algorithms in a computerized brain atlas. IEEE Tran. on Nuclear Science **40** (1993) 1187–1191
2. Dawant, B.M., Hartmann, S.L., Thirion, J.P., Maes, F., Vandermeulen, D., Demaerel, P.: Automatic 3-D segmentation of internal structures of head in MR images using a combination of similarity and free-form transformations: Part I, methodology and validation on normal subjects. IEEE Trans. on Medical Imaging **18** (1999) 909–916
3. Hartmann, S.L., Parks, M.H., Martin, P.R., Dawant, B.M.: Automatic 3-D segmentation of internal structures of head in MR images using a combination of similarity and free-form transformations: Part II, validation on severely atrophied brains. IEEE Trans. on Medical Imaging **18** (1999) 917–926
4. Rueckert, D., Sanchez-Ortiz, G.I., Lorenzo-Valdés, M., Chandrashekara, R., Mohiaddin, R.: Non-rigid registration of cardiac MR: Application to motion modelling and atlas-based segmentation. In: IEEE Int. Symp. on Biomedical Imaging. (2002)
5. Park, H., Bland, P.H., Meyer, C.R.: Construction of an abdominal probabilistic atlas and its application in segmentation. IEEE Trans. on Medical Imaging **22** (2003) 483–492
6. Cuadra, M., Pollo, C., Bardera, A., Cuisenaire, O., Villemure, J.G., Thiran, J.P.: Atlas-based segmentation of pathological MR brain images using a model of lesion growth. IEEE Trans. on Medical Imaging **23** (2004) 1301–1314
7. Lorenzo-Valdés, M., Sanchez-Ortiz, G.I., Elkington, A.G., Mohiaddin, R.H., Rueckert, D.: Segmentation of 4D cardiac MR images using a probabilistic atlas and the EM algorithm. Medical Image Analysis **8** (2004) 255–265
8. Aboutanos, G.B., Nikanne, J., Watkins, N., Dawant, B.M.: Model creation and deformation for the automatic segmentation of the brain in MR images. IEEE Trans. on Biomedical Engineering **46** (1999) 1346–1356
9. Lancaster, J.L., Glass, T.G., R., B., Downs, L.H., Mayberg, H., Fox, P.T.: A modality-independent approach to spatial normalization. Human Brain Mapping **3** (1995) 209–223
10. Besl, P.J., McKay, N.D.: A method for registration of 3-D shapes. IEEE Trans. on Pattern Analysis and Machine Intelligence **14** (1992) 239–256
11. Cuisenaire, O., Thiran, J., Macq, B., Michel, C., Volder, A.D., Marques, F.: Automatic registration of 3D MR images with a computerized brain atlas. SPIE Medical Imaging **1719** (1996) 438–449
12. Aboutanos, G.B., Nikanne, J., Watkins, N., Dawant, B.M.: Model creation and deformation for the automatic segmentation of the brain in MR images. IEEE Trans. on Biomedical Engineering **46** (1999) 1346–1356
13. Fleckenstein, P., Jensen, J.T.: Anatomy in Diagnostic Imaging. Munksgaard (1993)
14. Kass, M., Witkin, A., Terzopoulos, D.: Snakes: active contour models. Int. J. of Computer Vision **1** (1987) 321–331
15. Xu, C., Prince, J.L.: Gradient vector flow: A new external force for snakes. In: Proc. IEEE Conf. on Computer Vision and Pattern Recognition. (1997)
16. Zijdenbos, A.P., Dawant, B.M., Margolin, R.A., Palmer, A.C.: Morphometric analysis of white matter lesions in MR images: Method and validation. IEEE Trans. on Medical Imaging **13** (1994) 716–724

Segmenting Brain Tumors with Conditional Random Fields and Support Vector Machines

Chi-Hoon Lee[1], Mark Schmidt[1], Albert Murtha[2], Aalo Bistritz[3],
Jöerg Sander[1], and Russell Greiner[1]

[1] Department of Computing Science,
University of Alberta
[2] Division of Radiation Oncology
[3] Division of Diagnostic Imaging, Department of Oncology,
Cross Cancer Institute, Edmonton AB, Canada

Abstract. Markov Random Fields (MRFs) are a popular and well-motivated model for many medical image processing tasks such as segmentation. Discriminative Random Fields (DRFs), a discriminative alternative to the traditionally generative MRFs, allow tractable computation with less restrictive simplifying assumptions, and achieve better performance in many tasks. In this paper, we investigate the tumor segmentation performance of a recent variant of DRF models that takes advantage of the powerful Support Vector Machine (SVM) classification method. Combined with a powerful Magnetic Resonance (MR) preprocessing pipeline and a set of 'alignment-based' features, we evaluate the use of SVMs, MRFs, and two types of DRFs as classifiers for three segmentation tasks related to radiation therapy target planning for brain tumors, two of which do not rely on 'contrast agent' enhancement. Our results indicate that the SVM-based DRFs offer a significant advantage over the other approaches.

1 Introduction

Support Vector Machines (SVMs) are a popular tool for classification tasks due to their appealing generalization properties; this has led several groups to propose using SVMs for brain tumor segmentation [1,2,3]. However, SVMs assume that data (here, individual voxels) is independently and identically distributed (iid), which is not appropriate for tasks such as segmenting medical images. In particular, SVMs can not consider dependencies in the labels of adjacent pixels/voxels. Markov Random Fields (MRFs), a popular classification technique that models such dependencies, have been used in many medical image segmentation tasks [4,5,6], and have also been used in systems for brain tumor segmentation [5,6,7]. However, *generative* MRFs often do not have the discriminative power of *discriminative* techniques such as SVMs. Conditional Random Fields (CRFs [8]) and their multi-dimensional extension, Discriminative Random Fields (DRFs), are *discriminative* alternatives to MRFs, which have outperformed MRFs for several tasks [9,10]. In the remainder of this section, we

Y. Liu, T. Jiang, and C. Zhang (Eds.): CVBIA 2005, LNCS 3765, pp. 469–478, 2005.
© Springer-Verlag Berlin Heidelberg 2005

review MRFs (Sect. 1.1), CRFs and DRFs (Section 1.2), and SVMs (Section 1.3). Section 2 then describes our recently proposed Support Vector Random Field (SVRF) model, which combines the advantages of both SVMs and CRFs [11]. Section 3 presents an evaluation of these techniques within a system for brain tumor segmentation that uses an extensive MR preprocessing pipeline and a set of multi-scale image-based and 'alignment-based' features.

1.1   Markov Random Fields (MRFs)

Markov Random Fields (MRFs) are widely used in medical image processing applications [4,5,6]. They are ideal for many tasks, and are particularly relevant to segmentation tasks as they allow the classification of one element to depend on the labels of neighboring elements of the observation (image, volume, or sequence). By contrast, traditional classification techniques assume the data is iid, and therefore do not model dependencies in the labels of neighboring elements. MRFs typically use a generative approach, modeling the joint probability of the features of the set of voxels $\mathbf{x} = \{x_1, \ldots, x_n\}$ and their corresponding labels $\mathbf{y}$: $p(\mathbf{x}, \mathbf{y}) = p(\mathbf{x}|\mathbf{y}) \, p(\mathbf{y})$. However, these systems often make simplifying assumptions to make the calculation of the joint probability tractable. This usually involves assuming that the likelihoods have a simple factorized form, such as $p(\mathbf{x}|\mathbf{y}) = \prod_i p(x_i|y_i)$, which involves restrictive independence assumptions, and does not allow the modeling of complex dependencies between the features and the labels. For the MRF in our experiments, we used a Gaussian assumption to factor $p(\mathbf{x}|\mathbf{y})$ (as opposed to a non-parametric alternative such as Parzen Windowing [4]), and used the Hammersley-Clifford method [12] to factor $p(\mathbf{y})$, producing the following model for the posterior, given a set of labeled training data $S = \{\langle x_i, y_i \rangle\}_i$.

$$p(\mathbf{y}|\mathbf{x}) \quad = \quad \frac{1}{Z} \exp \left[\sum_{i \in S} \log(p(x_i|y_i)) \ + \ \sum_{c \in C} V_c(\mathbf{y}_c) \right] \qquad (1)$$

where C is a set of cliques in the neighborhood (here defined as the set of 8 planar neighbors), $V_c(\mathbf{y})$ is a clique potential function of labels for the clique $c \in C$, and Z normalizes over all possible labelings. The Gaussian assumption allows us to use Maximum Likelihood (ML) parameter estimation.

1.2   Conditional and Discriminative Random Fields (CRF, DRF)

Conditional Random Fields (CRFs) are a *discriminative* alternative to the traditionally *generative* MRFs [8]. Rather than modelling the joint likelihood of the features and labels $p(\mathbf{x}, \mathbf{y})$, *discriminative* models directly model the posterior probability of the labels given the features $p(\mathbf{y}|\mathbf{x})$. This subtle difference alleviates the need to model the distribution over the observations. This is important in medical imaging applications, since anatomic structures can have complex shapes that are not easy to model and may not be appropriately modelled by a factorized form of $p(\mathbf{x}|\mathbf{y})$. Since CRFs directly model the posterior, they can relax many of the major simplifying assumptions often made in MRFs. This allows the (tractable) modelling of complex dependencies (a) *between the features of an element and its label*, (b) *between the labels of adjacent elements*, and (c) *between the labels of adjacent elements and their features*, or even other features of the observation.

Discriminative Random Fields (DRFs) are a multi-dimensional extension of 1-dimensional CRFs for lattice-structured data [9]. This extension, combined with the popularity of MRFs in medical imaging applications and the major advantages that CRFs can have in certain situations over MRFs, suggests that DRFs could have a major impact on a number of medical imaging tasks. In our experiments, we used the following DRF model:

$$p(\mathbf{y}|\mathbf{x}) = \frac{1}{Z} \exp\left(\sum_{i \in S} A_i(y_i, \mathbf{x}) + \sum_{i \in S} \sum_{j \in N_i} I_{ij}(y_i, y_j, \mathbf{x})\right) \qquad (2)$$

where A_i is the 'Association' (Observation-Matching) potential for modelling dependencies between the i-th class label y_i and the set of all observations $\mathbf{x}$. The DRF method uses a Generalized Linear Model (GLM) based on Logistic Regression for this potential [9]. The 'Interaction' (Local-Consistency) potential for modelling dependencies between the labels of neighboring elements, I_i, is also a GLM. Non-linear models for both potentials can be induced through a change of basis. Simultaneously determining the optimal parameters of the Association potential and the Interaction potential can be done numerically as a convex optimization problem. The performance of the GLM in DRFs compared to the probability distribution in the first term of MRFs will depend on the application. However, note the important difference between the clique potentials in MRFs and the Interaction potential in DRFs. MRFs indiscriminately smooth over neighboring cliques while DRFs consider the features when taking into account interactions in the labels $\sum_{i \in S} \sum_{j \in N_i} I_{ij}(y_i, y_j, \mathbf{x})$. This is a subtle but important point, since it means a DRF can learn how to optimally use image (and image gradient) information when modeling label dependencies.

DRFs are a powerful method for modeling dependencies in spatial data. There are, however, several problems associated with this method: it is hard to find a good initial labeling during inference, and due to the simultaneous learning of parameters, it tends to overestimate the Interaction potential parameters which can degrade edges during inference (unless regularization is used very carefully). Furthermore, the GLM may not estimate appropriate parameters in data with a high-dimensional feature space or where features may be correlated (as with textural features or multi-modality data) [13]. Because of these factors, in some tasks DRFs will not be advantageous compared to models such as Support Vector Machines.

1.3 Support Vector Machines (SVMs)

Support Vector Machines (SVMs) are a popular tool for classification of data that is independent and identically distributed. SVMs are less sensitive to class imbalance than GLMs, and due to the properties of error bounds, SVMs tend to outperform GLMs, especially in cases where the classes overlap (often the case in medical imaging applications) [14]. SVMs try to maximize the margin between classes (here using the simple linear feature space $x_i \cdot x_j$), by finding the optimal α_i values in the following Quadratic Programming problem (represented in dual Lagrangian form where C is a constant that bounds the misclassification error) [14]:

$$\max \sum_{i=1}^{N} \alpha_i \; - \; \frac{1}{2} \sum_{i=1}^{N} \sum_{j=1}^{N} \alpha_i \, \alpha_j \, y_i \, y_j \, (x_i \cdot x_j)$$

$$\text{subject to} \tag{3}$$

$$0 \le \alpha_i \le C \quad \text{and} \quad \sum_{i=1}^{N} \alpha_i y_i = 0$$

Unlabelled instances are classified using the learned parameters α_i and bias b, by taking the sign of the following decision function [14]:

$$f(x) = \sum_{i=1}^{N} \alpha_i y_i (x \cdot x_i) + b$$

2   Support Vector Random Fields (SVRFs)

An SVM is an iid classifier, which does not consider interactions in the labels of adjacent data points. Conversely, DRFs and MRFs consider these interactions, but do not have the same appealing generalization properties as SVMs. This section will review our Support Vector Random Field (SVRF) model, an extension of SVMs that uses a DRF framework to model interactions in the labels of adjacent data points [11]:

$$p(\mathbf{y}|\mathbf{x}) \;\; = \;\; \frac{1}{Z} \exp \left\{ \sum_{i \in S} \log(O(y_i, \varUpsilon_i(\mathbf{x}))) \; + \; \sum_{i \in S} \sum_{j \in N_i} V(y_i, y_j, \mathbf{x}) \right\} \tag{4}$$

where $\varUpsilon_i(\mathbf{x})$ computes features from the observations $\mathbf{x}$ for location i, $O(y_i, \varUpsilon_i(\mathbf{x}))$ is an SVM-based Observation-Matching potential, and $V(y_i, y_j, \mathbf{x})$ is the Local-Consistency potential over a pair-wise neighborhood structure, where N_i are the 8 neighbors around location i.

2.1   Observation-Matching

The Observation-Matching function maps from the observations (features) to class labels. We would like to use SVMs for this potential. However, the decision function in SVMs produces a distance value, not a posterior probability suitable for the DRFs' framework. To convert the output of the decision function to a posterior probability, we used a modified version of the method in [15]. This efficient method minimizes the risk of overfitting and is formulated as follows:

$$O(y_i = 1, \varUpsilon_i(\mathbf{x})) \;\; = \;\; \frac{1}{1 + \exp(A \times f(\varUpsilon_i(\mathbf{x})) + B)} \tag{5}$$

The parameters A and B are estimated from training data represented as pairs $\langle f(\Upsilon_i(\mathbf{x})), t_i \rangle$, where $f(\Upsilon_i(\mathbf{x}))$ is the real-valued SVM response (here, distance to the separator), and t_i denotes a related probability that $y_i = 1$, represented as the relaxed probabilities: $t_i = \frac{N_+ + 1}{N_+ + 2}$ if $y_i = 1$, and $t_i = \frac{1}{N_- + 2}$ if $y_i = -1$, where N_+ and N_- are the number of positive and negative class instances. Using these training instances, we can solve the following optimization problem to estimate parameters A and B:

$$\min - \sum_{i=1}^{l} [t_i \log O(t_i, \Upsilon_i(\mathbf{x})) + (1 - t_i) \log(1 - O(t_i, \Upsilon_i(\mathbf{x})))] \tag{6}$$

Platt [15] used a Levenberg-Marquardt approach that tried to set B to guarantee that the Hessian approximation was invertible. However, dealing with the constant directly can cause problems, especially for unconstrained optimization problems [13]. Hence, we employed Newton's method with backtracking line search for simple and robust estimation. To avoid overflows and underflows of exp and log, we reformulated (6) as

$$\min \sum_{i=1}^{l} [t_i(A \times f(\Upsilon_i(\mathbf{x})) + B) + \log(1 + \exp(-A \times f(\Upsilon_i(\mathbf{x})) - B))] \tag{7}$$

2.2   Local-Consistency

We use a DRF model for Local-Consistency, since we do not want to make the (traditional MRF) assumption that the label interactions are independent of the features. We adopted the following pairwise Local-Consistency potential:

$$V(y_i, y_j, \mathbf{x}) = y_i y_j (\nu \cdot \Phi_{ij}(\mathbf{x})) \tag{8}$$

where ν is the vector of Local-Consistency parameters to be learned, while $\Phi_{ij}(\mathbf{x})$ calculates features for sites i and j. DRFs use a Φ_{ij} that penalizes for high absolute differences in the features. As we are additionally interested in encouraging label continuity, we used the following function that encourages continuity while discouraging discontinuity: $(\max(\Upsilon(\mathbf{x}))$ denotes the vector of max values of the features):

$$\Phi_{ij}(\mathbf{x}) = \frac{\max(\Upsilon(\mathbf{x})) - |\Upsilon_i(\mathbf{x}) - \Upsilon_j(\mathbf{x})|}{\max(\Upsilon(\mathbf{x}))} \tag{9}$$

Observe that this function is large when neighboring elements have very similar features, and small when there is a wide gap between their values.

2.3   Learning: Parameter Estimation

SVRFs use a sequential learning approach to parameter estimation. This involves first solving the SVM Quadratic Programming problem (3). The resulting decision function is then converted to a posterior probability using the training data and estimated relaxed probabilities. The Local-Consistency parameters are then estimated from the m training pixels from each of the K training images using pseudolikelihood [12]:

$$\widehat{\nu} \quad = \quad \arg\max_{\nu} \prod_{k=1}^{K} \prod_{i=1}^{m} p(y_i^k | y_{N_i}^k, \mathbf{x}^k, \nu) \tag{10}$$

We ensure that the log-likelihood is convex by assuming a Gaussian prior over ν: that is, $p(\nu|\tau)$ is a Gaussain distribution with 0 means and $\tau^2 I$ variance (see [9]). Thus, the local-consistency parameters are estimated using its log likelihood:

$$\widehat{\nu} = \arg\max_{\nu} \sum_{k=1}^{K} \sum_{i=1}^{m} \left\{ O_i^n + \sum_{j \in N_i} V(y_i^k, y_j^k, \mathbf{x}^k) - \log(z_i^k) \right\} - \frac{1}{2\tau} \nu^T \nu \tag{11}$$

where z_i^k is a partition function for each site i in image k, and τ is a regularizing constant that ensures the Hessian is not singular. Keeping the Observation-Matching $(O_i^k = O(y_i, \Upsilon_i(\mathbf{x})))$ constant, the optimal Local-Consistency parameters can be found by gradient descent.

We close by noting that the $M^3 N$ [10] framework resembles SVRFs, as it also incorporates label dependencies and uses a max-margin approach. However, the $M^3 N$ approach uses a margin that magnifies the difference between the target labels and the best runner-up, while we use the 'traditional' 2-class SVM approach of maximizing the distance from the classes to a separating hyperplane. An efficient approach for training and inference in a special case of $M^3 N$s was presented in [16]. However, the simultaneous learning and the inference strategy used still make computations with this model expensive compared to SVRFs.

3   Brain Tumor Segmentation

Segmenting brain tumors is an important medical imaging problem, currently done manually by expert radiation oncologists for radiation therapy target planning. Markov Random Fields [5,6,7] and SVMs [1,2,3,17] have been used in systems to perform this task. We have recently evaluated DRFs and SVRFs for the relatively easy case of segmenting "enhancing tumor areas" [11]. We extend this by providing improved results for this easy case (due to using better preprocessing and features), and results for two much harder segmentation cases. This section will present (i) our experimental data and design, (ii) a summary of the MR preprocessing pipeline and the multi-scale image-based and 'alignment-based' features that afford a significant improvement over those previous results and allow us to address more challenging tasks, and (iii) experimental results comparing SVMs, MRFs, DRFs, and SVRFs within this context for three different segmentation tasks.

Our experimental data set consisted of T1, T1c (T1 after injecting contrast agent), and T2 images (each 258 by 258 pixels) from 7 patients (Fig. 1), each

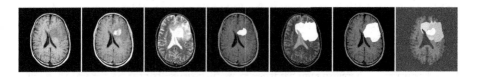

Fig. 1. Left to right: T1 image, T1 image with contrast agent, T2 image, enhancing area label, edema label, gross tumor label, full brain segmentation

having either a grade 2 astrocytoma, an anaplastic astrocytoma, or a glioblastoma multiforme. The data was preprocessed with an extensive MR preprocessing pipeline (described in [3], and making use of [18,19]) to reduce the effects of noise, inter-slice intensity variations, and intensity inhomogeneity. In addition, this pipeline robustly aligns the different modalities with each other, and with a template image in a standard coordinate system (allowing the use of alignment-based features, mentioned below).

We used the most effective feature set from the comparative study in [17]. This multi-scale feature set contains traditional image-based features in addition to three types of 'alignment-based' features: spatial probabilities for the 3 normal tissue types (white matter, gray matter and cerebrospinal fluid), spatial expected intensity maps, and a characterization of left-to-right symmetry (all measured at multiple scales). As with many of the related works on brain tumor segmentation (such as [1,2,6,20]), we employed a patient-specific training scenario, where training data for the classifier is obtained from the patient to be segmented. In order to be fair, all classifiers received the same training and testing pixels, and the testing pixels came from a different area of the volume than the training pixels — here, distant MR slices (this prevents the Random Field models from achieving high scores due to over-fitting.)

In our experiment, we applied 6 classifiers — a Maximum Likelihood classifier (degenerate MRF), a Logistic Regression model (degenerate DRF), an SVM (degenerate SVRF), an MRF, a DRF, and an SVRF — to 13 different volumes, based on various time points from 7 patients.

For each of the Random Field methods, we initialized inference with the corresponding degenerate classifier (ie. Maximum Likelihood, Logistic Regression, or SVM), and used the computationally efficient Iterated Conditional Modes (ICM) algorithm to find a locally optimal label configuration [12].

The 6 classifiers were evaluated over the 13 time points for the following 3 tasks, where the ground truth was defined by an expert radiologist. The first task was the relatively easy task of segmenting the 'enhancing' tumor area — ie. the region that appears hyper-intense after injecting the contrast agent (and including the non-enhancing or necrotic areas contained within the enhancing contour). The second task was the segmentation of the entire edema area associated with the tumor, which is significantly more challenging due to the high degree of similarity between the intensities of edema areas and normal cerebrospinal fluid. The final task was segmenting the Gross Tumor area as defined by the radiologist. This can be a subset of the edema but a superset of the

Table 1. Jaccard Percentage Scores for Enhancing tumor, Edema areas, and Gross Tumor areas (high scores in bold). ML denotes Maximum likelihood and LR denotes Logistic regression.

Study	|| Enhancing Tumor Area						|| Edema Area						|| Gross Tumor Area					
	ML	MRF	LR	DRF	SVM	SVRF	ML	MRF	LR	DRF	SVM	SVRF	ML	MRF	LR	DRF	SVM	SVRF
1-1	23.1	24.6	44.4	46.1	49.7	**52.8**	21.9	21.6	35.7	36.7	57.0	**58.2**	19.3	19.5	39.4	40.9	**40.7**	40.5
2-1	0	0	61.3	61.5	86.4	**87.7**	33.3	34.2	59.2	61.4	88.4	**89.2**	35.4	35.7	65.1	66.1	**78.2**	76.9
3-1	69.2	69.7	61.8	61.8	82.0	**84.8**	34.4	34.4	75.5	77.1	80.7	**82.2**	44.5	46.1	72.9	73.4	77.9	**78.7**
3-2	40.1	40.3	84.8	84.6	84.7	**87.8**	47.6	48.1	73.6	74.1	79.3	**83.1**	51.2	51.3	76.3	76.2	78.1	**80.8**
4-1	26.9	27.3	49.1	50.4	77.8	**81.7**	28.3	29.1	38.6	41.2	53.0	**55.4**	37.4	38.7	39.4	40.1	**41.4**	41.2
4-2	58.9	59.7	68.3	70.2	75.7	**77.9**	43.2	46.8	45.3	46.7	53.7	**57.7**	38.0	40.2	39.7	39.4	62.1	**64.9**
4-3	49.2	50.7	71.3	71.6	87.2	**88.1**	35.4	35.4	69.9	**70.7**	68.2	69.1	66.0	68.5	73.3	**73.5**	64.4	64.5
4-4	65.6	68.2	87.5	87.1	86.0	**89.1**	44.1	43.7	78.6	79.0	76.7	**79.3**	46.7	45.8	83.8	83.5	86.0	**89.0**
5-1	67.0	67.5	52.2	51.4	81.8	**84.3**	47.8	48.6	63.6	65.7	73.8	**76.9**	50.1	50.9	65.3	68.3	82.8	**84.8**
6-1	37.4	37.6	76.4	76.2	78.2	**80.4**	40.3	40.1	79.3	79.7	81.2	**83.7**	46.6	47.6	79.6	79.4	87.6	**88.2**
7-1	63.2	63.0	75.5	76.7	80.0	**81.4**	74.9	77.7	91.2	92.4	93.8	**94.9**	66.4	66.3	71.9	73.2	**74.6**	74.1
7-2	37.7	39.3	75.9	75.8	85.5	**87.3**	39.2	40.4	80.9	82.7	82.1	**82.8**	49.6	52.4	68.3	67.9	72.7	**72.9**
7-3	45.3	45.6	81.8	81.5	87.7	**89.6**	54.1	53.9	79.3	80.7	84.6	**86.5**	43.4	43.7	73.5	72.7	81.6	**83.2**
Ave:	44.9	45.7	68.6	68.8	80.2	**82.5**	41.9	42.6	67.0	68.3	74.8	**76.9**	5.7	46.7	65.3	65.7	71.4	**72.3**

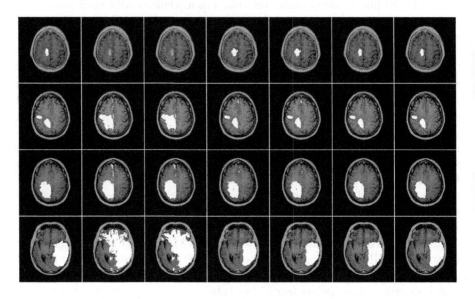

Fig. 2. Classification results for 4 different test slices, where each row shows a different test slice. Top to bottom: 2-1 Enhancing tumor, 7-2 Enhancing tumor, 7-1 Edema, and 4-4 Gross Tumor. Left column to right: Expert Segmentation, ML, MRF, LR, DRF, SVM, SVRF.

enhancing area, and is inherently a very challenging task, even for human experts, given the modalities examined. We used the Jaccard similarity measure to assess the classifications in terms of true positives (tp), false positives (fp), and false negatives (fn): $J = \frac{tp}{tp+fp+fn}$.

Table 1 presents the classification results for the three tasks (example test slice results are shown in Fig 2). For each of the three tasks, SVRFs showed the best performance on average, while SVMs were the second most effective method. The differences in the average scores between all methods across the three tasks were significant at the $p < 0.05$ level based on a paired example t-test. Note that SVRFs were the best in all 13 enhancing tumor cases, 12 of the 13 edema cases, and in the challenging Gross Tumor cases, SVRFs were best 8 times, SVMs best 4 times, and DRFs 1 time. The results from the second patient "2-1", produced an interesting observation: significant overlap between Gaussians in the high dimensional feature space leads ML and subsequently MRFs to misclassify *all* areas as non-tumors. This example shows that inappropriate modeling of $p(\mathbf{x}|\mathbf{y})$ can generates poor performance (see the first row of Fig 2). Although the segmentation tasks for edema and gross tumor areas are very hard, the discriminative approaches, and in particular SVRFs, still produce segmentations that are highly similar to the manual segmentations on average for all 3 tasks.

4   Conclusion

We are currently focusing on methods to allow inter-patient testing scenarios with SVRFs. This necessitates intensity standardization methods as in [17,5], and developing more computationally efficient parameter estimation models. Note that the SVRF results could be improved through the use of non-linear kernels (as in [1,2]), and through more effective inference methods. We are also interested in exploring applications of CRFs in other medical imaging tasks.

This work introduces SVRFs, a method that combines the random field relaxation properties of DRFs (to associate labels of neighboring voxels) with the discriminative properties of SVMs. We then presented experimental results on 3 challenging tasks related to brain tumor segmentation, and found that SVRFs offer a significant performance advantage over 5 other plausible classifiers, including both SVMs and other random field models.

Acknowledgments

R. Greiner is supported by NSERC and the Alberta Ingenuity Centre for Machine Learning (AICML). C.-H. Lee is supported by NSERC, AICML, and iCORE. Our thanks to the Cross Cancer Institute for providing the brain tumor data, Dale Schuurmans for helpful discussions on optimization and parameter estimation, Marianne Morris for help in data acquisition, and other members of the BTGP team.

References

1. Garcia, C., Moreno, J.: Kernel based method for segmentation and modeling of magnetic resonance images. LNCS **3315** (2004) 636–645
2. Zhang, J., Ma, K., Er, M., Chong, V.: Tumor segmentation from magnetic resonance imaging by learning via one-class support vector machine. International Workshop on Advanced Image Technology (2004) 207–211
3. Schmidt, M.: Automatic brain tumor segmentation. Master's thesis, University of Alberta (2005)

4. Held, K., Kops, E., Krause, B., Wells, W., Kikinis, R., Mullter-Gartner, H.: Markov random field segmentation of brain mr images. IEEE TMI **16** (1997) 878–886
5. Gering, D.: Recognizing Deviations from Normalcy for Brain Tumor Segmentation. PhD thesis, MIT (2003)
6. Chen, T., Metaxas, D.N.: Gibbs prior models, marching cubes, and deformable models: A hybrid framework for 3d medical image segmentation. In: MICCAI. (2003) 703–710
7. Capelle, A., Colot, O., Fernandez-Maloigne, C.: Evidential segmentation scheme of multi-echo MR images for the detection of brain tumors using neighborhood information. Information Fusion **5** (2004) 203–216
8. Lafferty, J., Pereira, F., McCallum, A.: Conditional random fields: Probabilistic models for segmenting and labeling sequence data. ICML (2001)
9. Kumar, S., Hebert, M.: Discriminative fields for modeling spatial dependencies in natural images. NIPS (2003)
10. Taskar, B., Guestrin, C., Koller, D.: Max margin markov networks. NIPS (2003)
11. Lee, C., Schmidt, M., Greiner, R.: Support vector random fields for spatial classification. PKDD (2005)
12. Li, S.Z.: Markov Random Field Modeling in Image Analysis. Springer-Verlag, Tokyo (2001)
13. R.Fletcher: Practical Methods of Optimization. John Wiley & Sons (1987)
14. Shawe-Taylor, J., Cristianini, N.: Kernel Methods for Pattern Analysis. Cambridge University Press, Cambridge, UK (2004)
15. Platt, J.: Probabilistic outputs for support vector machines and comparison to regularized likelihood methods. MIT Press, Cambridge, MA (2000)
16. Anguelov, D., Taskar, B., Chatalbashev, V., Koller, D., Gupta, D., Heitz, G., Ng, A.: Discriminative learning of markov random fields for segmentation of 3d scan data. CVPR (2005)
17. Schmidt, M.: Segmenting brain tumors using alignment-based features. Technical report, University of Alberta (2005)
18. McAuliffe, M., Lalonde, F., McGarry, D., Gandler, W., Csaky, K., Trus, B.: Medical image processing, analysis and visualization in clinical research. IEEE CBMS (2001) 381–386
19. Statistical Parametric Mapping: http://www.fil.ion.bpmf.ac.uk/spm/ (Online)
20. Kaus, M., Warfield, S., Nabavi, A., Black, P., Jolesz, F., Kikinis, R.: Automated segmentation of MR images of brain tumors. Radiology **218** (2001) 586–591

Segmenting Cardiopulmonary Images Using Manifold Learning with Level Sets

Qilong Zhang and Robert Pless

Department of Computer Science and Engineering,
Washington University, St. Louis, MO, 63130, USA
{zql, pless}@cse.wustl.edu

Abstract. Cardiopulmonary imaging is a key tool in modern diagnostic and interventional medicine. Automated analysis of MRI or ultrasound video is complicated by limitations on the image quality and complicated deformations of the chest cavity created by patient breathing and heart beating. When these are the primary causes of image variation, the video sequence samples a two-dimensional, nonlinear manifold of images. Nonparametric representations of this image manifold can be created using recently developed manifold learning algorithms. For automated analysis tasks that require segmenting many images, this manifold structure provides strong new cues on the shape and deformation of particular regions of interest. This paper develops the theory and algorithms to incorporate these manifold constraints within a level set based segmentation algorithm. We apply our algorithm, based on manifold constraints to the problem of segmenting the left ventricle, and show the improvement that arises from using the manifold constraints.

1   Introduction

Images of the chest cavity of a particular patient vary due to the imaging geometry, the permeation of contrast agents through different tissues, noise and deformation caused by the patient's breathing and heartbeat. Accounting for the deformation is vital to many image analysis tasks – this is underscored by the many diagnostic protocols that use gated MR-imaging to minimize motion of the heart, and/or held-breath protocols which ask patients to minimize breathing motions.

When many images are taken with the same imaging geometry of the same patient, these images are samples of a manifold with two degrees of freedom in principle: the phase of the heartbeat and the phase of the breathing cycle. When sufficiently many images are available, manifold learning algorithms, (typified by Isomap [1], Locally Linear Embedding (LLE) [2], and Semidefinite Embedding (SDE) [3]), create nonparametric representations of low-dimensional nonlinear manifolds.

The contribution of this paper is to develop an approach that first learns the manifold structure of the images of a particular patient, then exploits this structure to improve segmentation. For segmentation of the left ventricle, for example,

Y. Liu, T. Jiang, and C. Zhang (Eds.): CVBIA 2005, LNCS 3765, pp. 479–488, 2005.

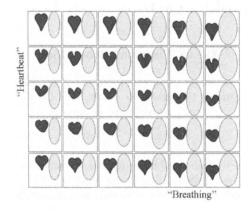

Fig. 1. A cartoon of the manifold structure of a cardiopulmonary video. Manifold learning techniques can automatically parameterize a video sequence by the position of each image on this cardiopulmonary manifold. This manifold structure provides additional cues for segmenting multiple images — for example, motion along the breathing axis simply translates the heart image, while motion along the heartbeat axis deforms the heart shape (with minimal global translational motion). These constraints are more specific and therefore stronger than temporal smoothness constraints. This paper develops methods to enforce these manifold based constraints.

the manifold structure gives strong cues about the shape changes between manifold neighbors. Figure 1 depicts the constraints in the cardiopulmonary manifold. In particular, variations in the breathing phase lead to an approximately uniform translation of the heart, corresponding to a rigid translation of the (2D) shape segments. Alternatively, changes in the heartbeat phase lead to variations in the shape of the heart, but, largely, not its position. These more specific constraints provide stronger cues than those available from just the temporal order of the original video, in which consecutive images often exhibit both a translation and a non-rigid deformation.

For segmentation of MR-imagery, several representation tools allow the description of shapes within an image, and support algorithms that automatically fit these shapes to image data. One such tool is level sets [4,5], which represents 2D shapes as the zero-crossing of a surface. The standard evolution equations which drive the adaptation of the surface to the image data have very natural modifications which allow the level set to enforce manifold based-constraints. In preliminary experimental results, we find that these additional constraints that the manifold imposes on the level set evolution allows segmentation of the left ventricle in images that are too low contrast to support single image segmentation.

The following section gives a very brief background in manifold learning and highlights previous work specializing these algorithms for biomedical applications. This is followed by a description of the standard Level Set framework for object segmentation. Section 3 describes a derivation of new level set evolution equations that enforce the manifold-based constraints on shape changes between images. We conclude with experiments on a low-contrast cine-MRI sequences.

2 Background and Previous Work

This work integrates ideas from level set segmentation and manifold learning. To our knowledge, it is novel to combine these approaches. In order to ground our later presentation, we first introduce, very briefly, some recent research in the use of level sets in biomedical image analysis and an overview of manifold learning.

2.1 Manifold Learning

Image data can be naturally represented as points in a high dimensional data space (one dimension for each pixel). When the set of images has lower *intrinsic* dimensionality, the data set can be mapped onto a lower dimensional space. Principle Component Analysis (PCA) [6] and Independent Component Analysis (ICA) [7] are two algorithms that represent data as linear combinations of basis vectors — the coefficients that specify each image define a linear low-dimensional embedding of the data set.

However, often the number of basis images required to a linearly reconstruct a data set is much larger than the degrees of freedom in the process that generates the images. This has led to a number of methods seeking to parameterize low-dimensional, nonlinear manifolds. These methods measure local distances or approximate geodesic distances between points in the original data set, and seek low-dimensional embeddings that preserve these properties. Isomap [1] extends classic multidimensional scaling (MDS) by substituting an estimate of the geodesic distance along the image manifold for the inter-image Euclidean distance. LLE [2] attempts to represent the image manifold locally by reconstructing each image as weighted combination of its neighbors. SDE [3] applies semidefinite programming to learn kernel matrices which can be used to create isometric embeddings. These algorithms, and others [8,9,10] have been used in various applications, including classification, recognition, tracking, and to a limited extent, biomedical image analysis [11].

2.2 Isomap Embedding of Cardiopulmonary Manifolds

The Isomap procedure for dimensionality reduction starts by computing the distance between all pairs of images (using some distance function such as SSD pixel intensities). Then, a graph is defined with each image as a node and undirected edges connecting each image to its k-closest neighbors (usually choosing k between 5 and 10). A complete pair-wise distance matrix is calculated by solving for the all-pairs shortest paths in this sparse graph. Finally, this complete distance matrix is embedded into some low dimension by solving an Eigenvalue problem (Multidimensional Scaling (MDS) [12]). The dimensionality embedding can be chosen as desired, but ideally is the number of degrees of freedom in

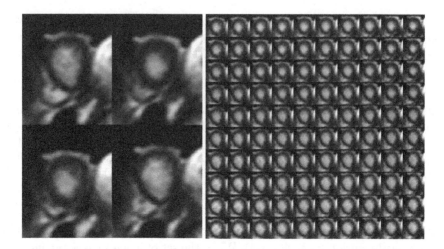

Fig. 2. (left) four images from a 200 image cardiopulmonary cine-MRI sequence of the heart. Note the variation both in the shape of the left ventricle (the white blob roughly centered in the image) and the position of the heart (shifting vertically). (right) A 2D manifold was defined with Isomap, using a Gabor filter-based image distance function. The 2D embedding is interpolated to give a regular sampling of the image manifold, and Section 3 modifies the level set approach to segment images over the entire manifold simultaneously.

the image set, in our case 2 (the two intrinsic dimensions of variability are the heartbeat and breathing).

Previous work that applies manifold learning to biomedical image analysis suggests modifying Isomap to use image distance functions other than pixel intensity differences [13,14]. For data sets with deformable motion, the suggested distance function is computed as the phase difference of local complex Gabor filters:

$$||I_1 - I_2||_{motion} = \sum_{x,y} \Psi(G_{(\omega,V,\sigma)} \otimes I_1, G_{(\omega,V,\sigma)} \otimes I_2) + \Psi(G_{(\omega,H,\sigma)} \otimes I_1, G_{(\omega,H,\sigma)} \otimes I_2)$$

where $G_{(\omega,\{V|H\},\sigma)}$ is defined to be the 2D complex Gabor filter with frequency ω, oriented either vertically or horizontally, with σ as the variance of the modulating Gaussian, and Ψ returns the phase difference of the pair of complex Gabor responses above some threshold τ; we choose τ to be the 50-th percentile filter magnitude. Figure 2 gives 4 example images of the heart, illustrating both the non-rigid and the rigid deformations. The Isomap embedding computes a 2D coordinate for each original image.

An even sampling of this manifold simplifies the numerical implementation of the level set segmentation in the subsequent sections. However, the given image sequence may not be evenly distributed in the manifold space. Ideally, it is desirable to have a continuous image function f to describe all possible cardiopulmonary images. One may interpolate the image function f locally by fitting thin-plate smoothing spline to the given images $\{I_i \mid i = 1 \cdots n\}$ and their associated manifold position $\{(u_i, v_i) \mid i = 1 \cdots n\}$, such that $f(x, y, u, v)$ minimizes the following weighted sum:

$$(1 - p) \sum_{i=1}^{n} |I_i(x, y) - f(x, y, u_i, v_i)|^2 \cdots$$

$$+ p \int \left| \frac{\partial^2 f(x, y)}{\partial u^2} \right|^2 + 2 \left| \frac{\partial^2 f(x, y)}{\partial u \partial v} \right|^2 + \left| \frac{\partial^2 f(x, y)}{\partial v^2} \right|^2 \, du \, dv, \qquad (1)$$

where p is a the smoothing parameter. We use the Matlab toolbox function *tpaps*, which chooses this smoothing parameter "in an ad hoc fashion in dependence on the [data]" [15].

In the next section, we consider how to exploit this manifold structure, in order to assist a level set function to track the left ventricle of a beating heart.

3 Level Set Segmentation

This section refines a standard framework for level set segmentation. The presentation includes background material through Equation 5, after which we extend the approach to segment all images in the data set simultaneously, and enforce additional constraints from the manifold structure.

In n-dimension space Ω, we define the evolving hypersurface C as the boundary $\partial \Omega$ of regions of interest. We call Ω^- the inside of C and Ω^+ the outside of C. For the cases of image segmentation, on approach is to define the contour as an energy minimization problem (the following presentations follows [16]):

$$E(c_1, c_2, C) = \mu \cdot Length(C) + \nu \cdot Area(\Omega^-)$$

$$+ \lambda_1 \int_{\Omega^-} |f(x, y) - c_1|^2 dx \, dy$$

$$+ \lambda_2 \int_{\Omega^+} |f(x, y) - c_2|^2 dx \, dy, \qquad (2)$$

where c_1 and c_2 are constants depending on C and are usually the average of image intensity $f(x, y)$ in the region Ω^- and the outside Ω^+, respectively. All parameter settings, such as λ_1, used in our experiments are listed in Section 4.

In problems of curve evolution, the level set method has been used extensively. Using the level set formulation, the boundary C is represented by the zero level set of a Lipschitz function $\phi : \Omega \to \mathbb{R}$, such that:

$$\begin{cases} C = \partial \Omega = \{(x, y) \in \Omega : \phi(x, y) = 0\} \\ \Omega^- = \{(x, y) \in \Omega : \phi(x, y) < 0\} \\ \Omega^+ = \{(x, y) \in \Omega : \phi(x, y) > 0\} \end{cases}$$

Using the Heaviside and Dirac delta functions with a smoothed approximation of finite width ϵ:

$$H_\epsilon(\phi) = \frac{1}{2} \left[1 + \frac{2}{\pi} \arctan \left(\frac{\phi}{\epsilon} \right) \right], \quad \delta_\epsilon(\phi) = \frac{d}{d\phi} H_\epsilon(\phi) \qquad (3)$$

the energy functional (2) can be written to evaluate the level set function ϕ on the domain Ω:

$$E(c_1, c_2, \phi) = \mu \int_\Omega \delta_\varepsilon(\phi(x,y)) |\nabla \phi(x,y)| dx\ dy + \nu \int_\Omega H_\varepsilon(\phi(x,y)) dx\ dy$$

$$+ \lambda_1 \int_\Omega |f(x,y) - c_1|^2 (1 - H_\varepsilon(\phi(x,y))) dx\ dy$$

$$+ \lambda_1 \int_\Omega |f(x,y) - c_2|^2 H_\varepsilon(\phi(x,y)) dx\ dy \tag{4}$$

Using the calculus of variations, one can recover the following evolution equation which incorporates an artificial time parameter t and converges to minimize $E(c_1, c_2, \phi)$:

$$\frac{\partial \phi}{\partial t} = \delta_\varepsilon(\phi) \left[\mu \nabla \cdot \left(\frac{\nabla \phi}{|\nabla \phi|} \right) - \nu + \lambda_1 (f - c_1)^2 - \lambda_2 (f - c_2)^2 \right] \tag{5}$$

To complete the definition of this evolution, we need to additional define the starting condition, $\phi_0(x,y)$. Section 4 describes the starting conditions used in our experiments. The next section illustrates how to incorporate manifold constraints on the level set solution, including the additions to the energy function E and the solution for the corresponding evolution equation.

3.1   Level Set Segmentation on Image Manifolds

For cardiopulmonary image sequences, the images vary in principle depending on their cardiac phase u and pulmonary phase v — the two degrees of freedom that parameterize the manifold shown in Figure 2. As described in Section 2.2, we use Isomap to automatically parameterize all images, and interpolate the result to generate evenly spaced samples of the image manifold $f(x, y, u, v)$. Accordingly, the contour C that we seek is also a function of u and v, and our goal is to describe C implicitly by the level set function ϕ in 4-dimension space Ω. Thus, a given cardiopulmonary image sequence specifies this contour by extending the energy functional (2) to 4-dimension space:

$$\inf_{c_1, c_2, \phi} E_1(c_1, c_2, \phi), \text{ where } \phi : \mathbb{R}^4 \to \mathbb{R} \tag{6}$$

But the manifold dimensions also correspond to specific kinds of deformation. The breathing of the patient results, approximately, in a translation of the heart. Therefore, we expect the variation of ϕ in the v direction to be a uniform translation. That is, the energy functional change $\frac{\partial \phi}{dv}$ should be consistent with a uniform translation. This induces a level set corollary to the classic optic flow constraint equation [17]:

$$\frac{\partial \phi}{\partial x} \omega_x + \frac{\partial \phi}{\partial y} \omega_y + \frac{\partial \phi}{\partial v} = 0 \tag{7}$$

where $(\omega_x,\ \omega_y)^\top$ is the velocity vector that is constant over any given image, but may vary for different values of u and v.

On the other hand, varying images along the other axis of the image manifold, deformations due to the cardiac cycle lead to image variation with minimal overall translation. For the special case of deformation caused by (non-uniform) heart expansion and contraction, we can express the constraint as:

$$\frac{\partial \phi}{\partial u} = \omega_u \tag{8}$$

where ω_u is constant over the region of the heart for any given u and v. This constraint enforces the condition that moving along the "heartbeat" axis simply adds or subtracts a constant value of the Level Set function ϕ, and therefore enforces that the shape either expands or shrinks.

Enforcing these constraints is natural within the level set framework; both lead naturally to new terms in the evolution of the ϕ function. Computationally, at each time step of the temporal evolution ϕ, we compute three parameters for each sample manifold image (u, v). First, we compute the least-squares estimates of the vector $(\omega_x, \omega_y)^\top$ that corresponds to global motion as we move from one image to another in the u direction on the image manifold. Second, we compute the constant ω_u that defines the change to ϕ the best corresponds to the expansion or contraction of the shape as we move from one image to another on the manifold along the v direction.

That is, for a particular u, v value, we compute first $\omega_x(u, v), \omega_y(u, v)$ by calculating $\frac{\partial \phi}{\partial x}, \frac{\partial \phi}{\partial y}$, and $\frac{\partial \phi}{\partial u}$ over the entire image, and solving the resulting linear system (from Equation (7)). Second, we compute $\omega_u(u, v)$ at a particular point u, v as the mean value (over all x, y) of $\frac{\partial \phi}{\partial u}$.

Once we have computed $\omega_x(u, v), \omega_y(u, v)$, and $\omega_u(u, v)$, we can write the motion constraints as an energy functional:

$$E_2(\phi) = \eta_1 \int_\Omega \left(\frac{\partial \phi}{\partial x}\omega_x + \frac{\partial \phi}{\partial y}\omega_y + \frac{\partial \phi}{\partial v} \right)^2 d\Omega$$

$$+ \eta_2 \int_\Omega \left(\frac{\partial \phi}{\partial u} - \omega_u \right)^2 d\Omega \tag{9}$$

where η_1 and η_2 are blending parameters. The first term enforces rigid changes in shape by penalizing regions of ϕ where the x, y, v derivatives are not consistent with the translation motion, and the second term penalizes the overall mean translational motion of the heart, which is minimal when motion is caused only by the heartbeat.

Solving for the evolution equation such that ϕ minimizes $E_2(\phi)$ gives:

$$\frac{\partial \phi}{\partial t} = 2\eta_1 \left(\frac{\partial^2 \phi}{\partial x^2}\omega_x^2 + \frac{\partial^2 \phi}{\partial y^2}\omega_y^2 + \frac{\partial^2 \phi}{\partial v^2} \right.$$

$$\left. +2\frac{\partial^2 \phi}{\partial x \partial y}\omega_x\omega_y + 2\frac{\partial^2 \phi}{\partial x \partial v}\omega_x + 2\frac{\partial^2 \phi}{\partial y \partial v}\omega_y \right) + 2\eta_2 \left(\frac{\partial^2 \phi}{\partial u^2} - \frac{\partial \omega_u}{\partial u} \right). \tag{10}$$

One can integrate this motion constraint module (9) into the previously defined energy term (6):

$$E(c_1, c_2, \Psi, \phi) = E_1(c_1, c_2, \phi) + E_2(\Psi, \phi). \tag{11}$$

Given an initial level set function ϕ_0, we minimize the above functional (11) by iterating two steps, first using the current estimate of ϕ to estimate c_1, c_2 and solving for $\omega_x(u, v), \omega_y(u, v)$, and $\omega_u(u, v)$, and then evolving ϕ by Equations (5) and (10).

4   Example Application

In cardiovascular imagery, an important application is to measure the dynamic behavior of the human heart, especially the left ventricle [18]. Here we define all

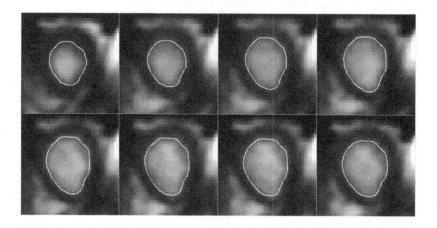

Fig. 3. Segmentation examples of cine-MRI images (from the same data set as shown in Figure 2)

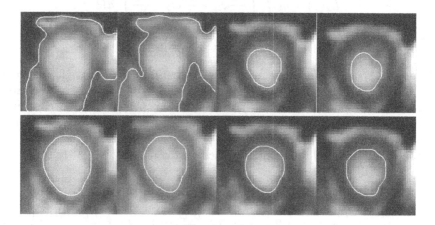

Fig. 4. A comparison of single image based segmentation (top) and the simultaneous solution for all image using the manifold constraints. In the left two images, the single image solution fails because of low contrast, on the right manifold based solution differs and draws a perceptually more reasonable boundary.

the parameters of the algorithm described in the last section and show preliminary results for segmenting a 200 frame cine-MRI sequence (the same data set as shown in Figure 2), using the manifold based constraints.

Our version of the level set algorithm has several parameters. The standard level set parameters λ_1 and λ_2 determine the importance of matching the intensity estimate for the inside and outside of the contour, and are set to $\lambda_1 = \lambda_2 = 1$. The parameter μ penalizes long contour curve lengths, and is set to $\mu = 0.075$. We set the area penalty parameter $\nu = -0.1$, which tends to make the shape grow. We use $\epsilon = 1$ for approximating the Heaviside function H_ϵ and Dirac function δ_ϵ (in Equation (3)).

There are also parameters specific to our modification of the level set function. Our experimental data set has 200 images, and we constructed the image function $f(x, y, u, v)$ of size $40 \times 40 \times 10 \times 10$ to regularly sample the manifold. The blending parameters η_1 and η_2 determine the importance of manifold constraints, and are set to $\eta_1 = \eta_2 = 0.1$. The initial level set $\phi_0(x, y, u, v)$, for each image, is defined by the signed distance function to the circle of radius 6 centered at the image center, with points inside the circle having a negative value. Figure 3 show examples of the segmentation solution for eight consecutive frames using these parameters.

The manifold constraints are most important for images that are especially low contrast or noisy. Figure 4, gives examples of images where the manifold based solution differs significantly from the single image solution. In the first two cases, the manifold constraints show a significant improvement — the single image solutions are wrong because of insufficient contrast. The last two cases show segmented shape boundaries that are different than the single image segmentation, and which may reflect more accurately the correct boundary, although it is difficult to quantify the improvement.

5   Summary and Discussion

This work presents preliminary efforts towards incorporating manifold learning as a tool to provide additional constraints for segmenting cardioplumonary images. This approach can be applied to any application domain for which there is a known manifold structure to the data, and may be extended also to other computational shape representation tools (such as snakes). Furthermore, we believe that many algorithms may be improved through better understanding and exploitation of non-linear image manifold learning algorithms, and tight integration of these with classical analysis tools.

References

1. Tenenbaum, J.B., de Silva, V., Langford, J.C.: A global geometric framework for nonlinear dimensionality reduction. Science **290** (2000) 2319–2323
2. Roweis, S.T., Saul, L.K.: Nonlinear dimensionality reduction by locally linear embedding. Science **290** (2000) 2323–2326

3. Weinberger, K.Q., Saul, L.K.: Unsupervised learning of image manifolds by semidefinite programming. In: Computer Vision and Pattern Recognition. (2004)
4. D.Mumford, Shah, J.: Optimal approximation by piecewise smooth function and associated variational problems. In: Commun. Pure Appl. Math. Volume 4. (1989) 577–685
5. Osher, S., Fedkiw, R.: The Level Set Method and Dynamic Implicit Surfaces. Springer-Verlag, New York (2003)
6. Jolliffe, I.T.: Principal Component Analysis. Springer-Verlag (1986)
7. Hyvärinen, A., Karhunen, J., Oja, E.: Independent Component Analysis. John Wiley and Sons (2001)
8. Donoho, D.L., Grimes, C.: Hessian eigenmaps: Locally linear embedding techniques for high-dimensional data. PNAS **100** (2003) 5591–5596
9. Brand, M.: Charting a manifold. In S. Becker, S.T., Obermayer, K., eds.: Advances in Neural Information Processing Systems 15. MIT Press, Cambridge, MA (2003) 961–968
10. Belkin, M., Niyogi, P.: Laplacian eigenmaps and spectral techniques for embedding and clustering. In: Advances in Neural Information Processing Systems. (2002)
11. Lim, I.S., Ciechomski, P.d.H., Sarni, S., Thalmann, D.: Planar arrangement of high-dimensional biomedical data sets by isomap coordinates. In: Proceedings of the 16th IEEE Symposium on Computer-Based Medical Systems (CBMS 2003). (2003) 50–55
12. Borg, I., Groenen, P.: Modern Multidimensional Scaling: Theory and Applications. Springer-Verlag (1997)
13. Pless, R.: Differential structure in non-linear image embedding functions. In: Articulated and Nonrigid Motion. (2004)
14. Souvenir, R., Pless, R.: Isomap and non-parametric models of image deformation. In: In Proc. IEEE Workshop on Motion and Video Computing, Breckenridge, CO (2005)
15. Matlab version 6.5.0 tpaps documentation. Mathworks Inc. (2002)
16. Chan, T.F., Vese, L.A.: Active contours without edges. IEEE Trans. on Image Processing **10** (2001) 266–277
17. Horn, B.K.P.: Robot Vision. McGraw Hill, New York (1986)
18. Paragios, N.: A variational approach for the segmentation of the left ventricle in cardiac image analysis. International Journal of Computer Vision, (2002) 345–362

Shape Based Segmentation of Anatomical Structures in Magnetic Resonance Images

Kilian M. Pohl[1], John Fisher[1], Ron Kikinis[2],
W. Eric L. Grimson[1], and William M. Wells[2]

[1] Computer Science and Artificial Intelligence Lab,
Massachusetts Institute of Technology, Cambridge, MA, USA
{pohl, fisher, welg}@csail.mit.edu
[2] Surgical Planning Laboratory, Harvard Medical School
and Brigham and Women's Hospital, Boston, MA, USA
{kikinis, sw}@bwh.harvard.edu

Abstract. Standard image based segmentation approaches perform poorly when there is little or no contrast along boundaries of different regions. In such cases, segmentation is largely performed manually using prior knowledge of the shape and relative location of the underlying structures combined with partially discernible boundaries. We present an automated approach guided by covariant shape deformations of neighboring structures, which is an additional source of prior information. Captured by a shape atlas, these deformations are transformed into a statistical model using the logistic function. Structure boundaries, anatomical labels, and image inhomogeneities are estimated simultaneously within an Expectation-Maximization formulation of the maximum a posteriori probability estimation problem. We demonstrate the approach on 20 brain magnetic resonance images showing superior performance, particularly in cases where purely image based methods fail.

1 Introduction

To better understand brain diseases, many neuroscientists analyze medical images for cortical and subcortical structures that seem to be influenced by the disease [1]. The analysis is based on segmentations of the structures of interests, often performed by human experts. However, this manual process is not only expensive, but in addition, it increases risks related to inter- and intra-observer reliability [2]. In this paper, we describe an automatic method, which accurately segments these structures by considering anatomical shape constraints and image artifacts of Magnetic Resonance (MR) images.

The detection of substructures is difficult as many of them are defined by partially discernible boundaries, such as in the case of the boundary between thalamus and white matter [3]. However, the ventricles, the structure above the thalamus, is more easily identified. In order for the ventricles to guide the boundary detection between the thalamus and the white matter, automatic segmentation algorithms use spatial priors [4,5,6]. These spatial priors capture the spatial relationship between structures such as the fact that the ventricles are above the thalamus. This is one example in which neighboring structures are of great utility for segmentation purposes.

Y. Liu, T. Jiang, and C. Zhang (Eds.): CVBIA 2005, LNCS 3765, pp. 489–498, 2005.

These types of priors are often characterized by soft boundaries representing the large spatial variability of a structure within a population. Deformable models offer an alternative as they capture the shape and permissible modes of variation within a population. In contrast to spatial priors on tissue labels, segmentation methods based on deformable models are guided by structure specific boundary conditions such as the length of the boundary in relation to others.

The work of this paper is motived by the class of deformable model-based approaches called active contour methods [7,8,9], in which the shape of an anatomical structure is represented as a level set function in a higher dimensional space. Similarly, our method defines anatomical shape constraints using signed distance maps in combination with the modes of variations of a Principle Component Analysis (PCA) [13]. While active contour methods were originally motivated by physical models [10], many methods are based on a Bayesian framework [11,14,12], which we chose for our algorithm. A Bayesian framework allows us to explicitly model the image inhomogeneities of MR images in order to segment large data sets without manual intervention.

The optimal solution within our framework is defined by a Maximum A posteriori Probability (MAP) estimation problem with incomplete data. From the MAP estimation problem we derive an instance of the Expectation Maximization algorithm (EM). The main contribution of the current work is that while we represent the shape variations through an implicit low-dimensional PCA, we additionally derive from this an explicit space-conditioned probability model by way of the logistic function. When combined with image-coupling and other terms in our Bayesian framework, the mechanism is able to identify shapes that are not restricted to the low-dimensional PCA space.

In contrast to other EM implementations [11,14,15], our method explicitly models the boundary via the shape model. Consequently, we achieve smooth segmentations without underestimating fine structures; a common problem in EM implementations [15]. To demonstrate the capabilities of our approach, we outline 20 sets of MR images into the major tissue classes as well as subcortical structures. The reliability of our approach is determined by the correspondence of the automatic segmentations to expert manual ones.

2   Deriving a Unified Framework for Image Inhomogeneity Correction, Shape Modeling, and Segmentation

The accuracy of outlining structures with indistinct boundaries in MR images significantly depends on properly modeling the boundary of the structure as well as estimating the inhomogeneities in the image. In this section, we develop a unified framework that performs segmentation, shape detection, and inhomogeneity correction simultaneously.

Without additional assumptions, it is difficult to extract the inhomogeneities $\mathcal{B}$ and the shape parameters $\mathcal{S}$ from the MR images I due to their complex dependencies. However, this problem is greatly simplified when formulated as an incomplete data problem via EM. Within this framework, we define the following MAP estimation problem:

$$(\hat{\mathcal{B}}, \hat{\mathcal{S}}) = \arg\max_{\mathcal{B}, \mathcal{S}} \log P(\mathcal{B}, \mathcal{S} | I). \tag{1}$$

In general, this results in a system of equations for which there is no analytical solution. We introduce the labelmap $\mathcal{T}$, which assigns each voxel in the image to an anatomical structure. If $\mathcal{T}$ is known it eases the estimation of $\mathcal{B}$ and $\mathcal{S}$ based on I. In our problem, the labelmap $\mathcal{T}$ is unknown so that the instance of the EM algorithm iteratively determines the solution of [16]. At each iteration, the method improves the estimates $(\mathcal{B}', \mathcal{S}')$ of $(\hat{\mathcal{B}}, \hat{\mathcal{S}})$ through

$$(\mathcal{B}', \mathcal{S}') \leftarrow \arg\max_{\mathcal{B}, \mathcal{S}} E_{\mathcal{T}|I, \mathcal{B}', \mathcal{S}'} (\log P(\mathcal{B}, \mathcal{S}, \mathcal{T}|I)). \tag{2}$$

The expected value is defined as $E_{A|B}(f(C)) \triangleq \sum_A P(A|B)f(C)$.

In our case, Equation (2) is a less complicated MAP problem than Equation (1). However, we would like to further simplify this update rule as it depends on both shape $\mathcal{S}$ and inhomogeneities $\mathcal{B}$. To split Equation (2) into two separate MAP problems, we first rephrase Equation (2) by simply applying Bayes' rule and dropping terms that do not depend on $(\mathcal{B}, \mathcal{S})$:

$$
\begin{aligned}
(\mathcal{B}', \mathcal{S}') &\leftarrow \arg\max_{\mathcal{B}, \mathcal{S}} E_{\mathcal{T}|I, \mathcal{B}', \mathcal{S}'} (\log P(\mathcal{B}, \mathcal{S}|\mathcal{T}, I) + \log P(\mathcal{T}|I)) \\
&= \arg\max_{\mathcal{B}, \mathcal{S}} E_{\mathcal{T}|I, \mathcal{B}', \mathcal{S}'} (\log P(I|\mathcal{T}, \mathcal{B}, \mathcal{S}) + \log P(\mathcal{B}, \mathcal{S}|\mathcal{T}) - \log P(I|\mathcal{T})) \\
&= \arg\max_{\mathcal{B}, \mathcal{S}} E_{\mathcal{T}|I, \mathcal{B}', \mathcal{S}'} (\log P(I|\mathcal{T}, \mathcal{B}, \mathcal{S}) + \log P(\mathcal{S}|\mathcal{T}, \mathcal{B}) + \log P(\mathcal{B}|\mathcal{T}))
\end{aligned} \tag{3}
$$

The optimization procedure decomposes nicely as a consequence of the following independence assumptions: First, we assume independence of I with respect to $\mathcal{S}$ conditioned on $\mathcal{T}$ and $\mathcal{B}$ because our model characterizes each anatomical structure by a stationary intensity distribution [11,14]. Next, we assume independence of $\mathcal{S}$ with respect to $\mathcal{B}$ conditioned on $\mathcal{T}$, as the image inhomogeneities do not influence the shape of a structure. Finally, we assume independence of $\mathcal{B}$ with respect to $\mathcal{T}$ and that the two conditional probabilities $P(I|\mathcal{T}, \mathcal{B})$ and $P(\mathcal{S}|\mathcal{T})$ are defined by the product of the corresponding conditional probabilities over all the voxels in the image space. Thus, Equation (3) simplifies to

$$
\begin{aligned}
(\mathcal{B}', \mathcal{S}') &\leftarrow \arg\max_{\mathcal{B}, \mathcal{S}} E_{\mathcal{T}|I, \mathcal{B}', \mathcal{S}'} (\log P(I|\mathcal{T}, \mathcal{B}) + \log P(\mathcal{S}|\mathcal{T}) + \log P(\mathcal{B})) \\
&= \arg\max_{\mathcal{B}, \mathcal{S}} \sum_x E_{\mathcal{T}_x|I, \mathcal{B}', \mathcal{S}'} [\log P(I|\mathcal{T}_x, \mathcal{B}) + \log P(\mathcal{S}|\mathcal{T}_x)] + \log P(\mathcal{B})
\end{aligned} \tag{4}
$$

The labelmap $\mathcal{T} = (\mathcal{T}_1, \ldots, \mathcal{T}_M)$ is composed of the indicator random vector $\mathcal{T}_x \in \{e_1, \ldots, e_N\}$, where x represents a voxel on the image grid. The vector e_a is zero at every position but a, where its value is one. For example, if $\mathcal{T}_x = e_a$ then voxel x is assigned to the structure a. We now define the E-Step of our EM implementation as

$$\mathcal{W}_x(a) \triangleq E_{\mathcal{T}_x|I, \mathcal{B}', \mathcal{S}'}(\mathcal{T}_x(a)) = 1 \cdot P(\mathcal{T}_x = e_a|I_x, \mathcal{B}'_x, \mathcal{S}') + 0 \cdot P(\mathcal{T}_x(a) \neq e_a|I_x, \mathcal{B}'_x, \mathcal{S}').$$

If we assume that $\mathcal{S}$ is independent of $\mathcal{B}$ then

$$\mathcal{W}_x(a) = \frac{P(I_x|\mathcal{T}_x(a)=e_a, \mathcal{B}'_x, \mathcal{S}') \cdot P(\mathcal{T}_x(a)=e_a|\mathcal{B}'_x, \mathcal{S}')}{P(I_x|\mathcal{B}'_x, \mathcal{S}')} = \frac{P(I_x|\mathcal{T}_x(a)=1, \mathcal{B}'_x) \cdot P(\mathcal{T}_x(a)=1|\mathcal{S}')}{P(I_x|\mathcal{B}'_x, \mathcal{S}')} \tag{5}$$

and Equation (4) reduces to

$$(\mathcal{B}', \mathcal{S}') \leftarrow \arg\max_{\mathcal{B}, \mathcal{S}} \sum_x \sum_a \mathcal{W}_x(a) [\log P(I|\mathcal{T}_x = e_a, \mathcal{B}) + \log P(\mathcal{S}|\mathcal{T}_x = e_a)] + \log P(\mathcal{B}).$$

Now, the M-Step solves the following two separate MAP problems

$$S' \leftarrow \arg\max_{S} \sum_{x} \sum_{a} \mathcal{W}_x(a) \log P(\mathcal{T}_x = e_a | S) + \log P(S) \tag{6}$$

$$\mathcal{B}' \leftarrow \arg\max_{\mathcal{B}} \sum_{x} \sum_{a} \mathcal{W}_x(a) \cdot \log P(I | \mathcal{T}_x = e_a, \mathcal{B}) + \log P(\mathcal{B}) \tag{7}$$

A variety of closed-form solutions for Equation (7) have been proposed in the literature such as by [14] and [11]. The remainder of this paper therefore focuses on Equation (6).

In summary, we find a local maxima to the difficult MAP estimation problem of Equation (1) by solving the simpler Equation (2), derived from an EM formulation. Based on independence assumptions, our instance of the EM algorithm iterates between the E-Step, which calculates $\mathcal{W}$ via Equation (5), and the M-Step, which solves the MAP problems of Equation (6) and Equation (7).

3 Logistic Maps for Shape Probabilities

The solution of Equation (6) greatly depends on the shape representation that defines the space of S and the probabilities that define the relationship of the attributes within our model. This section gives an example for a derivation of this equation. Before we do so, we briefly review the shape representation defined by the signed distance map.

Note, while we adopt a PCA representation of shape information, the final estimate is not restricted to the PCA parameterization of shape. This is facilitated by the use of the logistic function as described in Section 3.2. Consequently, our model captures a broader class of shapes than those methods that are restricted to the PCA model.

3.1 Shape Representation

As mentioned, the results of level set methods [7,8,17] using a PCA model on signed distance maps inspired us to introduce shape constraints in an EM framework. We follow the suggestion by Tsai [7], who applies PCA to all structures simultaneously to capture the covariation between structures. We initially model the shapes of all structures of interest by the distance map $\mathcal{D}$. $\mathcal{D}(x)$ is a vector of dimension equal to the number of structures of interests. It defines the distance of voxel x to the boundary of each structure. Positive values are assigned to voxels within the boundary of the object, while negative values indicate voxels outside the object.

We first turn a set of manual segmentations into signed distance maps and then apply PCA to the maps in order to determine the modes of variations of each structure. The resulting shape model is represented by the eigenvector or modes of variation matrix U, eigenvalue matrix Λ, and $\overline{\mathcal{D}} := (\overline{\mathcal{D}}_1^T, \cdots, \overline{\mathcal{D}}_N^T)^T$, where $\overline{\mathcal{D}}_a$ is the mean distance map of the anatomical structure a. To reduce the computational complexity for the EM implementation, U and Λ are only defined by the first K eigenvectors. In our case K represents 99 % of the eigenvalues' energy, which corresponds to the first five eigenvectors.

The shapes in a specific image are described by the expansion coefficients of the eigenvector representation, which are the shape parameters $S = (S_1, \cdots, S_K)$. S relates to the distance maps by $\mathcal{D}_S = \overline{\mathcal{D}} + U \cdot S$, where $\mathcal{D}_S$ captures the distance maps of all structures of interest. We refer to the distance map of a specific structure a defined by shape S as $\mathcal{D}_{S,a} = \overline{\mathcal{D}_a} + U_a \cdot S$, where U_a are the entries in U corresponding to structure a. This type of shape representation is only appropriate for defining local shape deformations as the space defined by signed distance maps is not a linear vector space. Thus, $\mathcal{D}_{S,a}$ is a local approximation to the manifold of distance maps.

We end this brief description of the shape model by defining the prior over the shape parameters as

$$p(S) = \frac{1}{\sqrt{(2\pi)^K |\Lambda|}} \exp\left(-\frac{1}{2} S^T \Lambda^{-1} S\right), \tag{8}$$

which is based on the hidden Gaussian assumption in PCA.

3.2   Estimating the Shape

In this section, we define the relationship of the unknown labelmap $\mathcal{T}$ and the shape parameter S captured by the conditional probability $P(\mathcal{T}_x = e_a | S)$ of Equation (6). The task is not straight-forward because unlike active contour methods, we also model the unknown labelmap $\mathcal{T}$ and the image inhomogeneities $\mathcal{B}$ explicitly. The shape S captures global characteristics of structures, while $\mathcal{T}$ and $\mathcal{B}$ characterize local properties. Motivated by the need to combine global and local information, we describe the use of the logistic function of the distance transform. The logistic function provides an implicit representation of the shape and an explicit space-conditioned probability model.

As mentioned previously, our model captures the relationship between the shape parameters S (which corresponds to a signed distance map) and the labelmap $\mathcal{T}$ through the conditional probability $P(\mathcal{T}_x = e_a | S)$. Since the random variable $\mathcal{T}_x$ is discrete, we define the conditional probability in terms of a generic shape function $\mathcal{A}(\cdot, \cdot)$ as

$$P(\mathcal{T}_x = e_a | S) \equiv \frac{\mathcal{A}(a, \mathcal{D}_{S,a}(x))}{\sum_{a'} \mathcal{A}(a, \mathcal{D}_{S',a}(x))}.$$

Given the motivation above, a natural choice for this formulation is the logistic function

$$\mathcal{A}(a, v) \equiv \frac{1}{1 + e^{-c_a v}},$$

which maps the distance map to the range [0,1]. For example, if $\mathcal{D}_{S,a}(x)$ is positive, then the voxel is inside the object and $\mathcal{A}(a, \mathcal{D}_{S,a}(x)) \in (0.5, 1]$. The variations within $\mathcal{A}(a, \mathcal{D}_{S,a}(\cdot))$ depend on c_a, which captures the certainty of the method with respect to the shape model. Uncertainty about the shape model is represented by relative small c_a. This results in a wide slope of the spatial distribution (see Figure 1), which allows greater mobility of the boundary. Large c_a define spatial priors with steep slopes, which tend to position the boundary of a structure.

The probability of the segmentation conditioned on the shape is now defined as

$$P(\mathcal{T}_x = e_a | S) = \left(\left(1 + e^{-c_a \mathcal{D}_{S,a}(x)}\right) \cdot \left(\sum_{a'} \frac{1}{1 + e^{-c_{a'} \mathcal{D}_{S,a'}(x)}}\right) \right)^{-1}, \tag{9}$$

so that the MAP estimation problem of Equation (6) transforms to

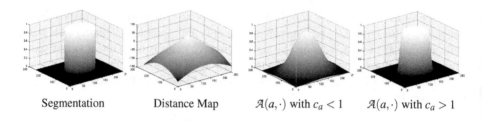

| Segmentation | Distance Map | $\mathcal{A}(a,\cdot)$ with $c_a < 1$ | $\mathcal{A}(a,\cdot)$ with $c_a > 1$ |

Fig. 1. The image to the left is a labelmap of a circle whose corresponding distance map is shown to its right. Based on the distance map, two different logistic functions are plotted. The first logistic function is defined by a large slope ($c_a < 1$) and the second plot represents a logistic function with a steep slope ($c_a > 1$).

$$S' \leftarrow \arg\max_S - \sum_x \sum_a \mathcal{W}_x(a) \left(\log\left(1 + e^{-c_a \mathcal{D}_{S,a}(x)}\right) + \log\left(\sum_{a'} \frac{1}{1 + e^{-c_{a'} \mathcal{D}_{S,a'}(x)}}\right) \right) + \log P(S)$$

$$= \arg\min_S \sum_x \left[\sum_a \mathcal{W}_x(a) \log\left(1 + e^{-c_{a'} \mathcal{D}_{S,a'}(x)}\right) + \log\left(\sum_{a'} \frac{1}{1 + e^{-c_{a'} \mathcal{D}_{S,a'}(x)}}\right) \right] + \frac{1}{2} S^t \Lambda S$$

(10)

Determining a closed form solution to this estimation problem is generally very difficult so that we approximate its solution using Powell's method [18].

In summary, the parameters S are seen within the context of a shape atlas created by PCA on signed distance maps. We relate the shape model to the EM algorithm of the previous section by defining $P(\mathcal{T}_x = e_a | S)$ of Equation (6) as a composition of logistic functions on distance maps. The E-Step of the EM algorithm calculates the $\mathcal{W}$ based on the shape parameters S', intensity I, image inhomogeneities $\mathcal{B}'$, and voxel x.

$$\mathcal{W}_x(a) = \left(\sum_{a'} \frac{P(I_x | \mathcal{T}_x = e_{a'}, \mathcal{B}'_x)}{1 + e^{-c_{a'} \mathcal{D}_{S',a'}(x)}} \right)^{-1} \cdot \frac{P(I_x | \mathcal{T}_x = e_a, \mathcal{B}'_x)}{1 + e^{-c_a \mathcal{D}_{S',a}(x)}}$$

The distribution of $P(I_x | \mathcal{T}_x = e_a, \mathcal{B}'_x)$ depends on the underlying image inhomogeneity model, which is an ongoing discussion [11,14]. We choose the model by Wells et al. [11] that defines $P(I_x | \mathcal{T}_x = e_a, \mathcal{B}'_x)$ by the Gaussian distribution $\mathcal{N}(\mathcal{B}'_x + \mu_a, \Upsilon_a)$. (μ_a, Υ_a) capture the mean and variance of the intensity distribution of the structure a.

The M-Step updates the estimates of the inhomogeneities $\mathcal{B}'$ and shape S' based on the weights $\mathcal{W}_x$. The update rule of $\mathcal{B}'$ (Equation (7)) reduces to a system of linear equations and is solved in closed form [11]. The shape S' is updated according to Equation (10) for which a solution is found via Powell's method [18].

4   Validation

This section compares the accuracy of our new method with (EM-Shape) and without shape modeling (EM-NoShape). Both methods segment 22 test cases into the three brain tissue classes - white matter, grey matter and corticospinal fluid. As in Figure 2, the right (light grey) and left ventricle (light grey) are extracted from the corticospinal fluid, and the grey matter is further parcellated into right (grey) and left (grey) thalamus, and right (black) and left caudate (black). We determine the accuracy of the approaches

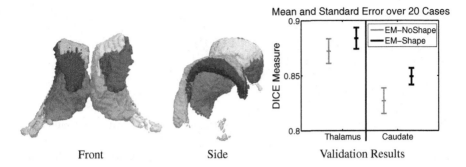

Fig. 2. Different views of a 3D model of the thalamus (grey), the caudate (black), and the ventricles (light grey). The model is based on a segmentation generated by EM-Shape. The graph to the right summarizes the validation results. For both structures EM-Shape performs clearly better than EM-NoShape.

by comparing the automatic segmentations of the thalamus and the caudate to manual ones, which we view as ground-truth.

With respect to EM-Shape, the atlas of Section 3.1 represents the shape of the thalamus, caudate, and the ventricles. The three brain tissue classes are excluded from the dynamic shape model as their spatial distributions are defined by the spatial atlas of [15] and not Equation (9). The model of EM-NoShape represents all anatomical structures by the spatial atlas.

We focus on the thalamus and caudate as they are challenging structures to segment. Purely intensity based segmentation methods, such as EM without spatial priors, cannot outline these structures because part of the boundary is invisible on MR images. Consequently, EM relies heavily on the prior information. In addition, the two structures are characterized by very different shapes (see Figure 2). While the right and left thalamus are shaped like an oval with a hook attached to it, the caudate is defined by long, thin horns wrapped around the ventricles. The segmentation methods also segment the ventricles because they are clearly visible on MR images. This structure further constrains the space of possible solutions for EM-Shape as all structures of interest have to be in proper proportion to each other.

To measure the quality of the automatic generated results, we compare them to the manual segmentations using the volume overlap measure DICE [19]. The graph in Figure 2 shows the average DICE measures and standard error for the two methods with respect to the thalamus and caudate. For the thalamus, EM-Shape achieves a higher average score ($88.4 \pm 1.0\%$; mean DICE score $\pm$ standard error) than EM-NoShape ($87.3 \pm 1.2\%$). The impact of the shape model on the segmentation results is even more apparent in the case of the caudate, where EM-Shape ($84.9 \pm 0.8\%$) is significantly better than EM-NoShape ($82.7 \pm 1.2\%$). The greater accuracy of EM-Shape is attributed to the shape atlas, which better captures the subject specific bending of the horn shaped caudate than the spatial atlas.

The initial DICE score of EM-Shape is generally lower than that of EM-NoShape because the shape model misrepresents the patient specific structures. For example, Figure 3 shows the outcome of EM-Shape after every fifth iteration. Initially, the seg-

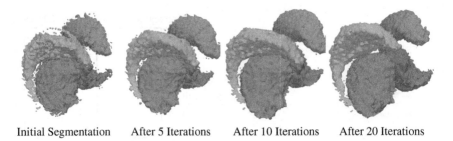

| Initial Segmentation | After 5 Iterations | After 10 Iterations | After 20 Iterations |

Fig. 3. The 3D models are based on the segmentations generated by our new method through 20 iterations. The method is initialized with the mean shape of each structure. The very noisy initial segmentation is an indication of the disagreement between the mean and the patient specific shape. As the algorithm proceeds the shape of the caudate and thalamus adjusts to the patient specific situation. After about 20 iterations the algorithm converges to a smoother segmentation.

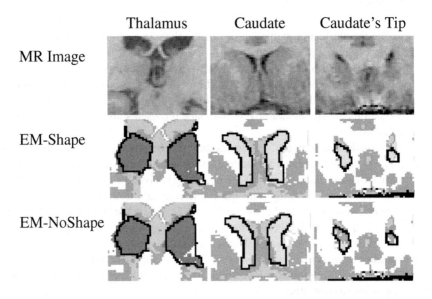

Fig. 4. The figure is a collection of differentsubcortical regions. The black lines in the automatic segmentations are the thalamus or caudate outlined by the human expert. The left column shows a MR image with corresponding segmentations of the oval shaped body of the thalamus with attached hook. The middle column shows part of the caudate which is adjacent to the putamen, another subcortical structure with identical intensity distribution. The right column shows the top of the caudate which is generally is underestimated by EM-NoShape. In all three examples, EM-NoShape performs worse than EM-Shape because the discriminatory power of spatial prior and intensity pattern is too low to determine the boundary of the structure.

mentation is noisy, which indicates discrepancy between the initial shape model defined by the mean shape and the patient specific shape. With each iteration, the arch of the caudate widens and the segmentations get smoother. After 20 iterations the method converges to a solution that generally outperforms EM-NoShape.

As mentioned, it is difficult to determine the exact shape of a structure with weakly visible boundaries. From the MR images, the size of the oval and the position of the hook of the thalamus are often not clearly defined. The top-left image of Figure 4 shows an example of such a scenario. The segmentations are the results of the two automatic segmentation methods where black indicates the outline of the human expert. In this example, EM-NoShape underestimates the hook of the thalamus, which we found to be true throughout this experiment. EM-Shape can better cope with this problem as the shape model adds global constraints to the local analysis of the intensities. An example of a global constraint is the explicit definition of shape dependencies across anatomical structures. This causes the shape of the thalamus to be proportional to one of the easily segmentable ventricles. This impacts the accuracy of EM-Shape as it further constrains the space of possible segmentations.

The other structure of interest in this experiment is the caudate. The structure is adjacent to the putamen, another subcortical structure with an identical intensity distribution. In the MR image of the middle column of Figure 4, the putamen is located on the outside of image. Neither the intensity pattern nor the spatial prior can properly separate these two structures, as indicated by the noisy segmentations of EM-NoShape. The outliers visible in EM-NoShape violate the shape constraints of EM-Shape as the boundary has to satisfy the conditions set by the ventricles and the thalamus.

For both structures, EM-NoShape did not adequately segment the ends of the structure. In the right column of Figure 4, EM-NoShape underestimates the tip of the caudate. The opposite is true for the thalamus where EM-NoShape overestimates the ends. Again, spatial and intensity distributions do not allow discrimination between anatomical structures in this area. In summary, on the 20 test cases our shape based method EM-Shape was performing much better than EM-NoShape, which uses a spatial atlas instead of a shape atlas.

5   Summary and Conclusions

We presented a statistical framework for the segmentation of anatomical structures in MR images. The framework is guided but not restricted to the low-dimensional PCA shape model as the shape representation is turned into space-conditioned probability model using the logistic function. The approach is especially well suited for structures with weakly visible boundaries as it simultaneously estimates the image inhomogeneities, explicitly models the boundaries through a deformable shape model, and segments the MR images into anatomical structures. Our approach was validated by automatically segmenting 20 test cases and comparing the results to a similar EM implementation without shape priors. In general, our new method performs much better. The improvement is primarily due to explicit modelling of the shape constraints along the boundary of anatomical structures.

Acknowledgments. This investigation was supported by the NIH grants K02 MH-01110, R01 MH-50747, R01-NS051826-01, P41 RR-13218, U24 RR021382, and U54-EB-005149. We would also like to thank Bryan Russel and Polina Golland for their helpful comments.

References

1. M. Shenton, R. Kikinis, F. Jolesz, S. Pollak, M. LeMay, C. Wible, H. Hokama, J. Martin, D. Metcalf, M. Coleman, and R. McCarley, "Left temporal lobe abnormalities in schizophrenia and thought disorder: A quantitative MRI study," *New England Journal of Medicine*, vol. 327, pp. 604–612, 1992.
2. R. Kikinis, M. E. Shenton, G. Gering, J. Martin, M. Anderson, D. Metcalf, C. Guttmann, R. W. McCarley, W. Lorensen, H. Line, and F. A. Jolesz, "Routine quantitative analysis of brain and cerebrospinal fluid spaces with MR imaging," *MRI*, vol. 2, no. 6, pp. 619–629, 1992.
3. K. Pohl, J. Fisher, J. Levitt, M. Shenton, R. Kikinis, W. Grimson, and W. Wells, "A unifying approach to registration, segmentation, and intensity correction," in *MICCAI*, 2005.
4. D. Collins, A. Zijdenbos, W. Barre, and A. Evans, "Animal+insect: Improved cortical structure segmentation," *IPMI*, vol. 1613, 1999.
5. M. Leventon, W. Grimson, and O. Faugeras, "Statistical shape influence in geodesic active contours," in *CVPR*, pp. 1316 – 1323, 2000.
6. B. Fischl, A. van der Kouwe, C. Destrieux, E. Halgren, F. Sgonne, D. Salat, E. Busa, L. Seidman, J. Goldstein, D. Kennedy, V. Caviness, N. Makris, B. Rosen, and A. Dale, "Automatically parcellating the human cerebral cortex," *Cerebral Cortex*, vol. 14, pp. 11–22, 2004.
7. A. Tsai, A. Yezzi, W. Wells, C. Tempany, D. Tucker, A. Fan, W. Grimson, and A. Willsky, "A shape-based approach to the segmentation of medical imagery using level sets," *TMI*, vol. 22, no. 2, pp. 137 – 154, 2003.
8. M. E. Leventon, *Statistical Models in Medical Image Analysis*. PhD thesis, Massachusetts Institute of Technology, 2000.
9. J. Yang and J. S. Duncan, "Joint prior models of neighboring objects for 3D image segmentation," in *CVPR*, pp. 314 – 319, 2004.
10. D. Mumford and J. Shah, "Boundary detection by minimizing functionals," in *CVPR*, pp. 22–26, 1985.
11. W. Wells, W. Grimson, R. Kikinis, and F. Jolesz, "Adaptive segmentation of MRI data," *TMI*, vol. 15, pp. 429–442, 1996.
12. P. P. Wyatt and J. A. Noble, "MAP MRF joint segmentation and registration," in *MICCAI*, pp. 580–587, 2002.
13. T. Cootes, A. Hill, C. Taylor, and J. Haslam, "The use of active shape models for locating structures in medical imaging," *Imaging and Vision Computing*, vol. 12, no. 6, pp. 335–366, 1994.
14. K. Van Leemput, F. Maes, D. Vanermeulen, and P. Suetens, "Automated model-based bias field correction of MR images of the brain," *TMI*, vol. 18, no. 10, pp. 885–895, 1999.
15. K. Pohl, S. Bouix, R. Kikinis, and W. Grimson, "Anatomical guided segmentation with non-stationary tissue class distributions in an expectation-maximization framework," in *ISBI*, pp. 81–84, 2004.
16. G. J. McLachlan and T. Krishnan, *The EM Algorithm and Extensions*. John Wiley and Sons, Inc., 1997.
17. J. Yang, L. H. Staib, and J. S. Duncan, "Neighbor-constrained segmentation with level set based 3D deformable models," *TMI*, vol. 23, no. 8, pp. 940–948, 2004.
18. W. Press, B. Flannery, S. Teukolsky, and W. Vetterling, *Numerical Recipes in C : The Art of Scientific Computing*. Cambridge University Press, 2 ed., 1992.
19. L.R.Dice, "Measure of the amount of ecological association between species," *Ecology*, vol. 26, pp. 297–302, 1945.

Simultaneous Segmentation and Motion Recovery in 3D Cardiac Image Analysis

Ling Zhuang[1], Huafeng Liu[1,2], Wei Chen[1], Hujun Bao[1], and Pengcheng Shi[2]

[1] State Key Laboratory of CAD & CG,
Zhejiang University, Hangzhou, China
{zhuangling, chenwei, bao}@cad.zju.edu.cn
eelichf@ust.hk
[2] Department of Electrical and Electronic Engineering,
Hong Kong University of Science and Technology, Clear Water Bay, Hong Kong
eeship@ust.hk

Abstract. Accurate and robust estimation of the three-dimensional left ventricular geometry and deformation has important clinical implications for better diagnosis and understanding of ischemic heart diseases. So far, most image analysis efforts have performed the shape recovery and the motion tracking tasks in separate steps, typically in sequential fashion. In this paper, we present a continuum biomechanics model based framework that performs simultaneous segmentation and motion analysis of the left ventricle from 3D image sequences, achieved through the tracking of the spatiotemporal evolution of a 3D active region model driven by imaging data, statistical priors of the left ventricular boundaries, and cyclic motion models of the myocardial tissue elements. Experiments on 3D canine and human MR image sequences have shown the superiority of the strategy.

1 Introduction

With the rapid development of medical imaging technology, 3D images of the moving heart have become increasingly available from several different imaging modalities such as MR tagging, phase contrast MRI, and cine CT. These images provide the spatiotemporal tomographic insights of the cardiac states of health, and the computer assisted analysis of these images offers quantitative tools for the diagnosis of ischemic cardiomyopathy, the leading fatal disease in the world.

Since ischemic heart diseases often manifest as abnormalities of ventricular geometry, wall kinematics, and myocardial mechanics, there have been many image analysis efforts over the last twenty years devoted to the shape and motion recovery of the heart [1,2,3]. While it has been argued that there are advantages to treat the spatial boundary finding and the spatiotemporal motion tracking as a coherent and unified process to reduce the possibility of error propagation from one step to another, most of the existing efforts do not attempt to tackle the segmentation and motion problems simultaneously, but rather sequentially.

In this paper, we put forward a method of simultaneous segmentation and motion recovery of the left ventricle from 3D image sequences. This variational

Y. Liu, T. Jiang, and C. Zhang (Eds.): CVBIA 2005, LNCS 3765, pp. 499–507, 2005.

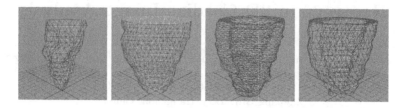

Fig. 1. From left to right: the constructed endocardial and epicardial surface meshes, the dense and coarse volumetric mesh representations of the left ventricle. We use the coarse model here to save computational time.

strategy extends the *active region model* (ARM) [7] to 3D, where each ARM node spatiotemporally evolves under the influences of the internal and external forces towards apparent boundary and structures in the image. Based upon the finite element representation, we adopt the physically meaningful continuum biomechanical model of the myocardium to regularize the intrinsic behavior of the ARM, while node-dependent imaging data, the temporal consistency models of the tissue geometry and kinematics, and the statistical priors of the myocardial tissue distributions are used as driving forces. Experiments on canine and human MR images are used to demonstrate the usefulness of the method.

2   Methodology

The simultaneous segmentation and motion recovery framework is built upon the 3D active region model, which consists of three integral components: a volumetric representation of the left ventricle, a material constitutive law which constrains the intrinsic behavior of the myocardium, and the data- and model-driven external forces which move and deform the left ventricle towards image-defined equilibrium of simultaneous boundary recovery and motion correspondence.

2.1   Finite Element Representation

The left ventricle is represented by a finite element mesh of sampling nodal points, bounded by the endo- and epi-cardial boundaries. To ensure desired computation stability and accuracy, it is very important to have the same resolution in $x-$, $y-$, and $z-$ directions. Thus, for certain images which have coarser inter-plane resolution, the shape based interpolation method is used to create additional between-slice boundary contours from contours of the original slices, rather than interpolating image slices directly [5].[1] After segmentation of the first image frame, we create the Delaunay triangular surface meshes of the endo- and epicardium first, and then construct the volumetric tetrahedra mesh of the left ventricle. Such meshes, as shown in Fig. 1, are reconstructed from canine MR images with original image resolution of $1.64 \times 1.64 \times 5.00$ mm/pixel. After

---

[1] However, when using phase contrast velocity MR images, we do need to interpolate the images for consequent calculations of image forces.

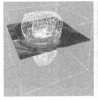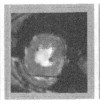

Fig. 2. Segmentation result of the 3D canine MR image sequences at frame #8, left: slice #6, right: slice #10

contour interpolation, the meshes has 1.64mm in-plane resolution and 1.66mm inter-plane resolution (the left volumetric model in Fig. 1), then we got 9540 points and 43200 tetrahedrons, which may spend more than 10 hours to get the motion result using our method. To save computational cost, we have re-sampled the mesh to 4.92mm in-plane and 5.00mm inter-plane resolution (the right volumetric model in Fig. 1), thus we got 1800 points and 7850 tetrahedrons, which only need about 4000s to run.

2.2 3D Active Region Model

For the 3D active region model, we aim to minimize the energy function, measuring the segmentation and motion tracking costs, over the entire LV:

$$E_{total}(\mathbf{u}) = \int_{\Omega} E_{internal}(\mathbf{u}) + E_{external}(\mathbf{u})\mathrm{d}\Omega \qquad (1)$$

where $\mathbf{u}$ is the displacement field defined over the region of interest Ω, such that certain measure on the final configuration of the LV shape and movement reaches steady state of minimum energy. $E_{internal}$ here composes of the internal energy of the LV volume itself, i.e. the elastic energy of the myocardium, while $E_{external}$ consists of data and prior model driven energies discussed later.

Using the finite element method as the numerical framework, we arrive at the following system dynamics equation:

$$KU = F \qquad (2)$$

where K is the stiffness matrix, U is the nodal displacement vector, and F is the generalized external force vector. This equation can be interpreted as that the LV spatiotemporally evolves towards equilibrium state, under the internal spatial constraint of K which provides the relationship between sampling nodes, and the space-time dependent external forces F which enforce segmentation and motion tracking.

By applying the principles from Lagrangian mechanics, we can update the displacement vector with time step τ:

$$(I + \tau K)U^t = (U^{t-1} + \tau F^{t-1}) \qquad (3)$$

where I is an identity matrix and U^t is the displacement at time t. The iteration stops when $\|U^t - U^{t-1}\|$ is below certain threshold.

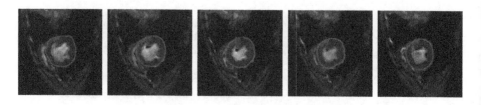

Fig. 3. Segmentation of the 3D canine MR image sequences (mesh intersections with a middle ventricle slice for illustration): frames #1, #3, #5, #7 and #9 (out of 16 frames)

2.3   Continuum Biomechanical Models

We use continuum biomechanical model of the myocardium, instead of the geometrical deformable models, to construct the stiffness matrix K. For computational feasibility, we use linear isotropic material model where the stress (σ) and strain (ϵ) tensors obey the constitutive law:

$$[\sigma] = [C][\epsilon] \tag{4}$$

with:

$$[\epsilon] = \begin{bmatrix} \frac{\partial}{\partial x} & 0 & 0 \\ 0 & \frac{\partial}{\partial y} & 0 \\ 0 & 0 & \frac{\partial}{\partial z} \\ \frac{\partial}{\partial y} & \frac{\partial}{\partial x} & 0 \\ 0 & \frac{\partial}{\partial z} & \frac{\partial}{\partial y} \\ \frac{\partial}{\partial z} & 0 & \frac{\partial}{\partial x} \end{bmatrix} \begin{bmatrix} u \\ v \\ w \end{bmatrix} = [B']\mathbf{u} \tag{5}$$

and the material matrix [C]:

$$[C] = \frac{E}{(1+\nu)(1-2\nu)} \begin{bmatrix} 1-\nu & \nu & \nu & 0 & 0 & 0 \\ \nu & 1-\nu & \nu & 0 & 0 & 0 \\ \nu & \nu & 1-\nu & 0 & 0 & 0 \\ 0 & 0 & 0 & 1-2\nu & 0 & 0 \\ 0 & 0 & 0 & 0 & 1-2\nu & 0 \\ 0 & 0 & 0 & 0 & 0 & 1-2\nu \end{bmatrix} \tag{6}$$

where E and ν are material dependent parameters. The internal energy of the linear isotropic ARM model thus can be expressed as:

$$\begin{aligned} E_{internal} &= \frac{1}{2} \iiint_\Omega [\epsilon]^T[\sigma]\mathrm{d}V \\ &= \frac{1}{2} \iiint_\Omega \mathbf{u}^T[B']^T[C][B']\mathbf{u}\mathrm{d}V \end{aligned} \tag{7}$$

which is a function of strain and stress tensors, and the stiffness matrix is $K = \iiint_\Omega [B']^T[C][B']\,\mathrm{d}V$.

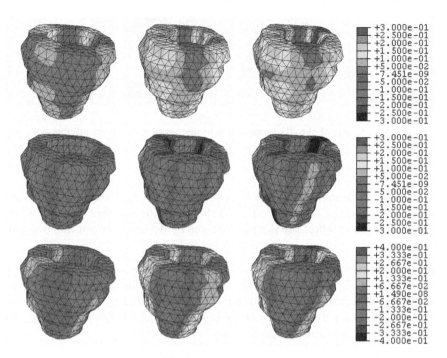

Fig. 4. Estimated strain maps with respect to end-diastole (canine MR images, frames #3, #6, #9 (left to right)): radial strains (top), circumferential strains (middle), and radial-circumferential shear strains (bottom)

2.4   Image/Model Driven External Forces

The external driving force F incorporates both imaging data information and prior modeling constraints that are needed for the simultaneous recovery of the LV shape and motion. It has four primary components: F_{edge} which drags the LV surfaces towards the boundary locations, F_{shape} which preserves the salient feature coherence between image frames, F_{prior} which provides the statistical prior distributions of the myocardial tissue locations, and the spatiotemporal constraints on the myocardial behavior $F_{temporal}(\mathbf{x})$. If $\mathbf{x}$ denotes the nodal position, then the overall external force on a boundary point is the form of:

$$F_{boundary}(\mathbf{x}) = F_{edge}(\mathbf{x})\left[\alpha(\mathbf{x})F_{prior}(\mathbf{x}) + \beta(\mathbf{x})F_{temporal}(\mathbf{x}) + \gamma(\mathbf{x})F_{shape}(\mathbf{x})\right] \quad (8)$$

Here, the algorithm favors locations which are likely edge points while maintains the balance between the prior positional information, the temporal filtering/prediction results, and the salient shape coherence measures between frames.

For all non-boundary nodes, there are no constraints on them being edge points or preserving shape coherence between image frames. Hence, the force term is simplified to:

$$F_{internal}(\mathbf{x}) = \alpha(\mathbf{x})F_{prior}(\mathbf{x}) + \beta(\mathbf{x})F_{temporal}(\mathbf{x}) \quad (9)$$

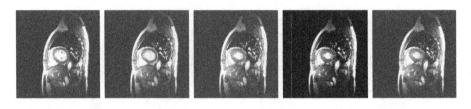

Fig. 5. Segmentation of the 3D human MR image sequences (mesh intersections with a middle ventricle slice for illustration): frames #1, #3, #5, #7 and #9 (out of 20 frames)

All the force components above, $F_{edge}(\mathbf{x})$, $F_{shape}(\mathbf{x})$, $F_{prior}(\mathbf{x})$ and $F_{temporal}(\mathbf{x})$, are normalized to the range of $[0, 1]$, and the weighting constants $\alpha(\mathbf{x})$, $\beta(\mathbf{x})$ and $\gamma(\mathbf{x})$ are selected to reflect the varying data and model conditions at different parts of the heart.

Edginess Measures. For noisy grey level images, it is not appropriate to only use image gradient as the external force since gradient has limited capture range and poor convergence to true boundary concavities. Hence, we have also used the Gradient Vector Flow (GVF) of the image [8], which reaches minimum value at boundary, to construct F_{edge}:

$$F_{edge}(\mathbf{x}) = \frac{|GVF(\mathbf{x})|}{1 + |Grad(\mathbf{x})|} \tag{10}$$

where $|Grad|$ is image gradient and $|GVF|$ is the GVF magnitude.

Prior Measures. In medical image analysis, prior information such as general shape, location, and orientation are often incorporated into the deformable model formulations in order to achieve more robust estimates during shape recovery. In the same spirit, we have used 3D Gaussian distributions $N(\mathbf{x}(k-1), \sigma_1, \sigma_2, \sigma_3)$ as the spatial prior range for any nodes movement between frames, where $\mathbf{x}(k-1)$ is the node's position at the last frame, σ_1, σ_2 and σ_3 are the variances. Then the construction of F_{prior} becomes:

$$F_{prior}(\mathbf{x}) = 1 - N(\mathbf{x}(k-1), \sigma_1, \sigma_2, \sigma_3) \tag{11}$$

In other words, we favor positions which are not far away from the nodal positions at the previous frame.

Shape Coherence Measures. It has been shown in earlier works that shape coherence is a valid criterion in motion recovery of the left ventricular boundary [6]. Thus, we enforce geometrical consistency to establish point correspondence between image frames. Under iso-intensity assumption, we can compute the Gaussian curvature of 3D point directly from image (one frame in the 4D image) [4]:

$$\kappa_x = \frac{1}{\left(f_x^2 + f_y^2 + f_z^2\right)^{3/2}} det \begin{bmatrix} f_{xx} & f_{xy} & f_{xz} \\ f_{xy} & f_{yy} & f_{yz} \\ f_{xz} & f_{yz} & f_{zz} \end{bmatrix} \tag{12}$$

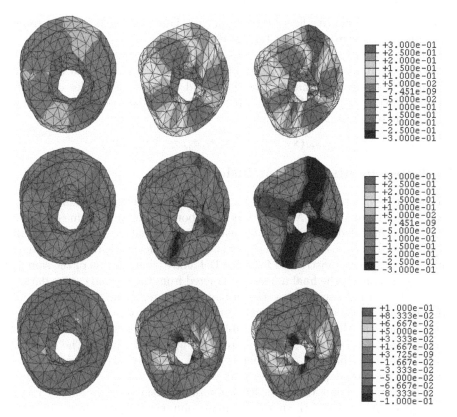

Fig. 6. Estimated strain maps with respect to end-diastole (frame #1) (human MR images, frames #3, #6, #9 (end-systole) (left to right)): radial strains (top), circumferential strains (middle), and longitudinal strains (bottom)

where f_x, f_y, and f_z are the first derivatives of the 3D image intensity, and f_{xx}, f_{xy}, f_{xz}, f_{yy}, f_{yz}, and f_{zz} are the second derivatives. Since the construction of F_{shape} is based on shape coherence, the resulting point should has close curvature to the corresponding point at last frame:

$$F_{shape} = |\kappa_{(x+\delta x)(k+1)} - \kappa_{x(k)}| \tag{13}$$

where $(x + \delta x)$ indicates local search window.

Temporal Measures. Temporal constraints can be put into the model since the heart motion is periodic. A standard Kalman predictor is used to estimate the state vector at frame $k+1$ through: $\hat{z}(k+1|k) = C\hat{z}(k|k)$, where $z = [\bar{\mathbf{x}}, \mathbf{x}, \dot{\mathbf{x}}]$ is the state vector (position, displacement and velocity), $\hat{z}(k+1|k)$ and $\hat{z}(k|k)$ are the estimated state vectors for frame $k+1$ and k respectively, the construction of C is based on the trajectory functions followed by each node, and $\bar{\mathbf{x}}$ should be updated during each estimation. In our experiments, the velocity information adopts the motion fields from the MR phase contrast velocity images or the spatio-temporal intensity flow between images. The phase velocity data should be regularized first to get rid of the noises.

The estimated possible node position $\hat{\mathbf{x}}$ is used to construct a rotated 3D Gaussian distribution $N(\hat{\mathbf{x}}, \sigma_i, \sigma_j, \sigma_k, \theta(\hat{\mathbf{x}}), \phi(\hat{\mathbf{x}}))$, where σ_i, σ_j and σ_k are the variances in the rotated major directions, and θ, ϕ are the angles of the line formed by $\mathbf{x}(k-1)$ and $\hat{\mathbf{x}}(k)$ with respect to the cartesian coordinate. Then we can get the temporal force as follow:

$$F_{temporal}(\mathbf{x}) = 1 - N(\hat{\mathbf{x}}, \sigma_i, \sigma_j, \sigma_k, \theta(\hat{\mathbf{x}}), \phi(\hat{\mathbf{x}})) \tag{14}$$

3   Experiments and Conclusions

We have implemented the algorithm and performed initial experiments on normal canine and human cardiac MRI data sets. For both human and canine cases, myocardium is modeled as an isotropic linear elastic material with Young's modulus 75,000 Pascal and Poisson ratio 0.47 [9]. The left ventricle is represented by linear finite element mesh constructed from the Delaunay triangulation of the sampled points, Fig. 1 shows the final model constructed from the normal canine data.

For the normal canine data, the in-plane and inter-plane image resolutions are 1.64 mm/pixel and 5 mm/pixel respectively, with temporal resolution 40 msec/frame. Visually robust and sensible volumetric segmentation of the endo- and epi-cardial boundaries are presented in Fig. 2 and Fig. 3. The recovered cardiac-specific radial (R), circumferential (C), and R-C shear strain maps of selected frames are depicted in Fig. 4, all with respect to the end-diastolic state.

The normal Human MRI data sets are acquired using breath-hold technique. The image parameters of the normal human volunteer (36 year old male) shown here LV were as following: TR 3.786ms, TE 1.584ms, flip angle 45, 256 × 256 matrix, 8mm slice thickness, pixel spacing 1.5625mm × 1.5625mm. The resulting 3D image set consists of 11 2D image slices per temporal frame, and 20 temporal 3D frames per cardiac cycle. Once again, visually appropriate volumetric segmentation results for this normal human MR data are shown in Fig. 5 for selected frames. The top views of the cardiac-specific strain maps at frames #3, #6, and #9 (end-systole) are shown in Fig. 6, all with respect to end-diastole. As expected for normal heart, the magnitudes of the radial, circumferential, and longitudinal strains increase during the cardiac deformation from ED to ES. The longitudinal strains are relatively small compared with other strains. These indicate that the myocardium is primarily thickened in the radial direction and shortened in the circumferential direction.

These preliminary results demonstrate that the proposed algorithm can be used to perform 3D segmentation and motion field tracking simultaneously. With further experiments and validations, we expect that 3D active region model will find a valuable role for myocardial segmentation and motion analysis.

Acknowledgement

This work is supported in part by the National Natural Science Foundation of China(60403040), by the Hong Kong Research Grant Council under Competitive

Earmarked Research Grant HKUST6031/01E for PCS, by the National Basic Research Program of China (2003CB716104), and by the NSF of China for Innovative Research Groups (60021201).

References

1. A.J. Frangi, W.J. Niessen, and M.A. Viergever. Three-dimensional modeling for functional analysis of cardiac images: A review. *IEEE Transactions on Medical Imaging*, 20(1):2–25, 2001.
2. T. McInerney and D. Terzopolous. Deformable models in medical image analysis: a survey. *Medical Image Analysis*, 1(2):91–108, 1996.
3. J. Montagnat and H. Delingette. 4d deformable models with temporal constraints: application to 4d cardiac image segmentation. *Journal of Medical Image Analysis*, 9:87–100, 2005.
4. Stanley Osher and James A. Sethian. Fronts propagating with curvature dependent speed: Algorithms based on hamilton-jacobi formulations. *Journal of Computational Physics*, 76:12–49, 1988.
5. P. Shi, A. Sinusas, R. T. Constable, and J. Duncan. Volumetric deformation analysis using mechanics-based data fusion: Applications in cardiac motion recovery. *International Journal of Computer Vision*, 35(1):87–107, 1999.
6. P. Shi, A. Sinusas, R. T. Constable, E. Ritman, and J. Duncan. Point-tracked quantitative analysis of left ventricular motion from 3D image sequences. *IEEE Transactions on Medical Imaging*, 19(1):36–50, 2000.
7. L.N. Wong, H. Liu, A. Sinusas, and P. Shi. Spatio-temporal active region model for simultaneous segmentation and motion estimation of the whole heart. In *IEEE Workshop on Variational, Geometric and Level Set Methods in Computer Vision*, pages 193–200, 2003.
8. C. Xu and L. Prince. Snakes, shapes, and gradient vector flow. *IEEE Transactions on Image Processing*, 7(3):359–369, 1998.
9. H. Yamada. *Strength of Biological Material.* The Williams and Wilkins Company, Baltimore, 1970.

Spatial and Temporal Analysis for Optical Imaging Data Using CWT and tICA

Yadong Liu[1], Guohua Zang[1], Fayi Liu[2], Lirong Yan[1], Ming Li[1],
Zongtan Zhou[1], and Dewen Hu[1,3]

[1]College of Mechatronics and Automation, National University of Defense Technology,
Changsha, Hunan, 410073, PRC
[2]Neurophysiology Department, Xiangya Medical college of Center South University,
Changsha, Hunan, 410008, PRC
[3]Key Laboratory of Mental Health, Institute of Psychology, Chinese Academy of Sciences,
Beijing 100101, PRC
dwhu@nudt.edu.cn

Abstract. In this paper a novel temporal-spatial analysis procedure for optical imaging (OI) data of single trail is proposed which exploits the continuous wavelet transform (CWT) to detect the activated voxels of cortex and exploits temporal independent component analysis (tICA) to extract the underlying independent sources whose number is determined by Bayesian information criterion. The neural response signals and the V-signals are picked out by investigating the temporal architecture of the independent sources given by tICA. Simulated data is generated to test the validity of the procedure and then the procedure was applied to two sets of OI data of single trail collected from the rats' HP area. The neural response signals together with the pulse-induced and the 0.1Hz fluctuation signals are extracted from data successfully. The procedure we proposed is a valuable technique for researchers to investigate the temporal and spatial architectures of cortical functional mapping.

1 Introduction

Intrinsic Optical imaging (OI) is relatively a new functional brain imaging technique. It first appeared in 1980's[1] and has been growing rapidly since then. Functional physiological changes, such as increases in the blood volume, hemoglobin oxymetry changes, and light scattering changes, result in intrinsic tissue reflectance changes that are exploited in OI to map functional activities. The technique has high spatial as well as high temporal resolution, and relatively noninvasive. So it is capable to image development and plasticity of neurons in a long duration[1,2]. Assistant with the signal processing methods, OI technique can be exploits to reveal changes of underlying functional chromophores (such as Hb, HbO_2 etc.). These advantages make OI ideal for studying the fine functional organizations of the sensory cortices as well as the physiology of neurovascular couplings at the level of the arterioles, venules, and even capillaries.

One of the leading difficulties of OI technique is how to analyze the signals. The OI data has a poorer signal to noise ratio (0.1%-0.4%) than that of fMRI and EEG.

Y. Liu, T. Jiang, and C. Zhang (Eds.): CVBIA 2005, LNCS 3765, pp. 508–516, 2005.
© Springer-Verlag Berlin Heidelberg 2005

The noises come from illumination, CCD etc., but mainly from physiological factors. The general analysis method of OI data is the first-frame technique which has several serious shortcomings: (1) The different spatial and temporal architectures of neural response signals in different trails can not be revealed. (2) It is difficult to keep the physiological condition of animals homogeneous in a relatively long duration (for example several minutes containing a series of trials) and this may lead to functional pseudo-mapping. (3) Repeating the same stimulus uninterruptedly will make the cortices less sensitive and will finally lead to drift of strength. An improved method is to stimulate the cortices by several different stimuli alternatively which will make the experiment duration too long to keep the physiological condition homogeneous however. (4) The method can not be used to investigate the temporal patterns of functional perfusion and neurovascular physiology. Some researchers have begun to exploit multivariable statistical methods[3] such as PCA and ICA to process the OI data. The neighborhood information is synthesized to obtain the spatial architecture of activated area as well as dynamic response. PCA assumes that the data are made up of a linear sum of signals, which can be decorrelated based on their differences in variance. Functional mapping comes from some one or several principal components which often violates the real situation[3]. The ICA can be classified into sICA and tICA by different assumptions[4,5,6]. It is found in our simulation that the sICA can't get the correct result when the ratio of activated area to total area is larger than about 0.2. The reason may be that the spatial independent assumption doesn't hold [6] in the optical imaging. Usually the tICA is unfeasible because the spatial dimension (which is equal to the number of pixels) of OI data is much higher than temporal dimension[6]. What is more, due to the small magnitude of detectable signals, CCD-induced noises and intrinsic biological heterogeneity, OI data typically has a poor SNR which also make the results of tICA unstable.

In this paper, the continuous wavelet transform (CWT) is exploited to detect the activated voxels in some appropriate resolution levels (subspace) in wavelet coefficients domain. The tICA is then exploited to extract the neural response signal, pulse-induced and 0.1Hz fluctuation signals from OI data of single trial. Because pixels have been per-selected to reduce the spatial dimension and improve SNR, tICA can be successfully applied now.

2   The Introduction of Data Processing Procedure

If a pixel belongs to activated area, its time series will has a sharp variance corresponding to onset of the stimulus. This sharp variance can be detected by wavelet transform and thus detecting the activated voxels is posed as a singularity detection problem[7,8,9].

The physiological factors such as V-signals dominate the noises of OI data and the pulse- and respiration-induced signals are two of the most serious noises. The main difference between the stimulus-induced sharp variance and pulse/respiration-induced signals is not their amplitudes but their durations. In general, if the duration of a stimulus is 2 seconds, the sharp variance needs about 4 seconds to arrive at climax from stimulus onset and about 8-12 seconds to return to baseline. The sharp variance has the comparable amplitude with pulse-induced fluctuation, but has much longer duration than one pulse cycle. In other words, the sharp variance and the pulse/respiration-induced fluctuation have different temporal scales and so can be discerned by wavelet transform. Wavelet transform isolates a deterministic signal into a few large coefficients while the background noises spread across most, if not all, of the wavelet coefficients.

The CWT is applied to decompose the temporal information of each voxel into coefficients associated with both time and scale. The continuous wavelet transform of a function f is defined as

$$Wf(u,s) = \int_{-\infty}^{+\infty} f(t) \frac{1}{\sqrt{s}} \psi^* (\frac{t-u}{s}) dt \; . \tag{1}$$

where ψ is called as the basis function and u and s are integers. If the basis function ψ can be written as $\psi = (-1)^n \theta^{(n)}$ where θ is compactly supported and satisfies $\int_{-\infty}^{+\infty} \theta(t) dt \neq 0$ and then the CWT can be written as

$$Wf(u,s) = s^n \frac{d^n}{du^n} (f * \overline{\theta}_s)(u) \tag{2}$$

where the function f is first filtered by $\theta_s = \theta(t - \bullet / s)$ and then derivated n times. In general, the basis function is intentionally chosen as Gaussian function, that is, f will first be smoothed by a Gaussian function $\psi(s,u)$ and then derivated to generate coefficients of wavelet transform. As is known, the first derivation of a function is called as slope indicating how fast the function varies at some point. If the sharp variance of activation signals survived the smoothness of Gaussian function θ_s, the CTW will generate large coefficient values at the location of sharp variance and its neighborhood. The existence of activation signal can be easily detected by a threshold of coefficient values under some appropriate resolution levels (subspace) in wavelet coefficients domain [7,8].

In this paper, the resolution of images is denoted as $M \times N$ and the time series of the pixel at the location (m,n) in the image is denoted as $\{x_{m,n}(t)\}$ whose length is denoted as L and coefficients of wavelet transform are denoted as $Wx_{m,n}(u,s)$ $u = 1,2 \cdots L, s = 1,2 \cdots S$ where S is the maximum of scales. An indicator function is proposed as formulation (3) to indicate the existence of activation signals.

$$J(m,n) = \sum_{s=s0}^{s1} \frac{\sum_{u=t0}^{t1} Wx_{m,n}^2(u,s)}{\sum_{u=1}^{t0} Wx_{m,n}^2(u,s)} \; . \tag{3}$$

where t_0 and t_1 denote the beginning time point and climax point of the sharp variance separately and $s_0, s_1 (s_0 < s_1)$ denote boundary of the scale subspace. In some step of the procedure, the priori knowledge about the trends in the OI signal and the neural activity is used to select the most appropriate resolution levels (subspace) in wavelet coefficients domain.

The procedure is described in the following by an example of simulated data processing. Firstly conservative initial values are chosen for parameter set $\{t_0, t_1, s_0, s_1\}$ (for example, $t_1 = t_0 + 4$, $s_0 = 21$, $s_1 = 25$). Although these initial values are not the best choices, it is almost always able to detect several activated voxels with them. With a proper scale s under which physiological noises can be efficiently eliminated by θ_s while the singular features of sharp variance survived. The pixel $x(m,n)$ whose corresponding $J(m,n)$ is bigger than some properly set threshold can be considered activated. The average stimulus-induced signal response $\{\bar{x}(t)\}$ $t = 1, 2, \cdots L$ is obtained by adding up the time series of the pixels picked out. The parameter set $\{t_0, t_1, s_0, s_1\}$ is finally confirmed by investigating the temporal architecture of $\{\bar{x}(t)\}$.

The time series of the pixel whose corresponding $J(m,n)$ over the threshold is denoted as x_l. A matrix X_{active} with the dimension $P \times L$ can be formed by x_l used as rows. Except for the neural response signal, the activated area is also influenced by some other factors such as pulse- and respiration-induced fluctuations, 0.1Hz signal and scanner-induced noises which are usually supposed to be independent to each other. So the matrix X_{active} can be considered as the mixing signal matrix [4,5] and the tICA can be exploited on it to extract the neural response signal together with other independent sources in the temporal domain.

The tICA procedure is based on maximizing the nonentropy when the function $G(Y) = 1/\alpha \log \cos \alpha Y$ ($\alpha = 1$) is chosen as the nonlinearity[4,5,6]. The number of the underlying independent components is determined by the Bayesian information criterion (BIC). The stimulus-induced and some other physiological signal responses can be picked out by investigating the temporal architectures of the independent components.

3 Simulation

Simulated data is generated to test the validity of the proposed procedure. A 450-frames image sequence is captured at 15 Hz from the cortex of a SD rat in the absence of any stimulation. A 60×60 child window is further applied to the data set to pick out hindpaw (HP) area. The function

$$f(t) = \begin{cases} 0 & 1 \leq t < 100 \\ \dfrac{\lg e}{\sqrt{2\pi}} e^{-\frac{1}{2}(\frac{\lg(t-10)-\mu}{\delta})^2} & 101 \leq t \leq 450 \end{cases} \quad (4)$$

with parameters ($\delta = 2, \mu = 5$) was exploited to stimulate the neural response signal. Because this function has a sharp ascendant trend and a relatively slow descendant trend alike the stimulus-induced intrinsic OI signal response. This simulated neural response signal is added to the white area as shown in Fig.2-a. All the parameters are evaluated according to the intrinsic optical signals.

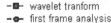

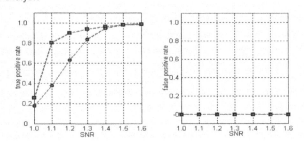

Fig. 1. The true and the false positive rates under different SNR

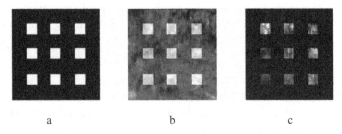

a   b   c

Fig. 2. The Fig. 2-a is the simulated activity map and the Fig.2-b and 2-c are the activation map given by first frame analysis and our procedure separately

The parameter set { t_0, t_1, s_0, s_1 } is evaluated to be {200, 350, 10, 15} by the presented method. In this paper, the SNR is defined as the ratio between standard deviation of the neural response signal to the pixels' mean standard deviation. The SNR varies from 1.0 to 1.6 with a step length of 0.1. Z-score statistics is used to map the $\{J(m,n)\}$ and the threshold is denoted as 4. The true and false positive rates under different SNR are shown in Fig.1. As can be seen, the procedure we proposed has improved true positive rate significantly without raising the false positive rate. The $\{J(m,n)\}$ whose corresponding SNR is 1.0 is given as an example in Fig.2-c. The simulated activated area is remarkably distinct from the background. The activation map given by the first-frame analysis under the same SNR is shown in Fig.2-b. The underlying independent sources given by tICA are shown in Fig.3. The first one is the simulated neural response signal, the second and the third one is the 0.1Hz and pulse-induced signal separately.

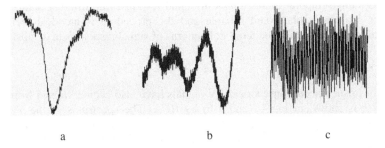

a   b   c

Fig. 3. The underlying independent sources given by tICA: the first one is the simulated neural response signal. The second one and the third one is the 0.1Hz signal and the pulse-induced signal respectively.

4 Intrinsic OI Data Processing

4.1 Animal Preparation and Data Collection

A dental drill is used to thin the skull over the interested cortical area uniformly until the arterioles and veins could be visualized in the field of the view of the detector. Silicon oil is applied to the skull in order to increase the translucency of the skull in the duration of the imaging period. Optical imaging series are collected by a slow-scan digital CCD working at 15Hz scanning frequency. The CCD has a 12-bit analog-to-digital converter. The duration of one trail is 30 seconds and altogether 450 frames of images are collected. Five LCDs with narrow range of wavelength 560 ± 10nm powered by a high-quality regulated voltage-stabilized power supply is used for illumination. The stimulus appeared at the 5th and 15th second respectively in the two trails. The durations of the stimulus are all 2 seconds.

4.2 Spatial and Temporal Architectures of Neural Response Signal

The proposed procedure is applied to two OI data sets and the results are illuminated in Fig. 4. The activation map obtained from the first data set is shown in Fig. 4-a. The average time course of pixels in the red areas (the pixels whose $J(m,n)$ is larger than 3) is shown in Fig.4-b. As can be seen, the response reaches the maximum in the 5th second from the onset of the stimulus and returns to the baseline in the following 2 seconds. The red area is highly task-related and its signal response extracted by tICA is shown in Fig.4-c. The activation map obtained from the second data set is shown in Fig.4-d and the corresponding stimulus-induced signal response of the red area is shown in Fig.4-e. In this trial, the response reaches the maximum in about 2.5 seconds (which is as half as that of first data set) from the onset of the stimulus and returns to the baseline in the following 10 seconds (which is as four times as that of first data set). As can be seen, the neural response signals have different temporal and spatial architectures in different trials even if the data sets are collected from the same animal and so the pseudo-mapping would unavoidably pollute the result if the same model assumptions and parameter set were used for different data sets. The procedure we proposed needs not model assumptions and the parameter set is evaluated by investigating temporal architectures of signal responses in different data set.. So the results are more robust and reliable and the procedure is an ideal technique for investigating the spatial and temporal patterns of signal responses in details.

4.3 V-Signals

Except for neural response signals, V-signals have also been extracted from two data sets (as is shown in Fig.4-f and 4-h) by tICA. The spectrums of the V-signal are shown in Fig.4-g and 4-i and it can be seen that V-signals from the two trials all contain two periodic components at the frequency of about 0.1Hz and 1.7Hz. Because the 1.7Hz V-signal has about the same frequency as the respiration, it is assumed that this V-signal was induced by respiration. It should be pointed that the same V-signals can also been extracted from the time series of pixels in the blue area.

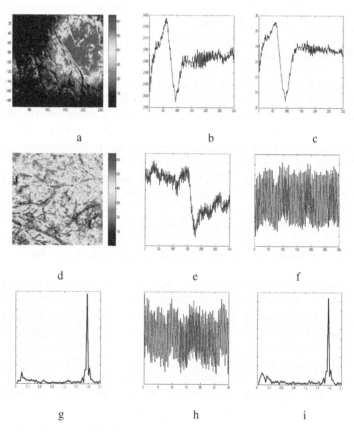

Fig.4. The activation map of the first and second data sets are illuminated in Fig.4-a and 4-d respectively. The neural response signals extracted by tICA from time series of pixels in the red areas shown in Fig.4-a and 4-d are illuminated in Fig.4-c and 4-e. The average time series of pixels in the red area in Fig.4-a is illuminated in Fig.4-b. The V-signals extracted from the first and the second data set are illuminated in Fig.4-f and 4-h and the Fourier spectrums of the V-signals are illuminated in Fig.4-g and 4-i.

The 0.1Hz V-signal was first found in the intrinsic OI signal from rodent somatosensory cortex in 1996 by Mayhew and Askew [10] and was intensively investigated in 1998 by Mayhew and Hu [11]. At the same year the two-photon laser scanning microscopy was applied by Kleinfeld[12] to image the motion of the red blood cells in the individual capillaries that lie as far as 600um below the pia mater of primary somatosensory cortex in the rat, this depth encompassed the cortical layers with the highest density of neurons and capillaries. Some other researchers have also found the 0.1Hz V-signal in fMRI data from the human's visual cortex[13,14]. The 0.1Hz V-signal is considered to be related with some inherent metabolism mechanism, that is, regional cerebral blood flow vibrates round some baseline to keep the dynamic balance of HbO_2 and Hb in the cortex tissue.

The 0.1Hz V-signal, as a physiological noise source, limits the sensitivity of optical and MRI techniques and so many researchers have tried to remove it from the signals. Mayhew and Hu[11] have applied the general linear model technique to extract this kind of V-signal by simulating the V-signal by sine wave with different frequency and phase. Actually one can not precisely forecast the frequency and phase of V-signal which may drift from baseline during the data collection. These weaknesses limit the application of the general linear model. TICA is a data-driven technique which needs not model the signal response, frequency and phase beforehand and hence is a valuable method to investigate the V-signals.

5 Conclusion

The procedure proposed in the paper can be exploited to investigate the spatial and temporal architectures of neural response signals as well as the V-signals of intrinsic OI signals. It can help the researchers to synthesize spatial and temporal information of the data to research the information processing mechanism of cortex. The procedure can also be applied to fMRI and EEG data.

Acknowledgement

This work is supported by National Natural Science Fund of China (30370416), Distinguished Young Scholars Fund of China (60225015), Ministry of Education of China (TRAPOYT Project) and Ministry of Science and Technology of China (Grant 2001 CCA04100),.

Reference

[1]   Grinvald, A., Frostig, R.D. et al.: Optical Imaging of Neural Activity. Physiol Rev., 68 (1988) 1285–1365

[2]   Bonhoeffer, T., Grinvald, A. et al.: The Layout of Iso-orientation Domains in Area 18 of Cat Visual Cortex: Optical Imaging Reveals a Pinwheel-like Organization. J. Neurosci., 13 (1993) 4157–4180

[3]   Stetter, M., Schiebl, I. et al.: Principal Component Analysis and Blind Separation of Sources for Optical Imaging of Intrinsic Signals. NeuroImage, 11 (2000) 482 –490

[4]   McKeown, M.J., Sejnowski, T.J. et al.: Independent Component Analysis of fMRI Data: Examining the Assumptions. Human Brain Mapping, 6 (1998) 368–372

[5]   McKeown, M.J., Makeig, L. et al.: Analysis of fMRI Data by Blind Separation into Independent Spatial Components. Human Brain Mapping, 6 (1998) 160–188

[6]   Calhoun, V.: Spatial and Temporal Independent Component Analysis of Functional MRI Data Containing a Pair of Task-related Waveforms. Human Brain Mapping, 13 (2001) 43–53

[7]   Stone, J.V., Porrill, J. et al.: Spatial, Temporal and Spatiotemporal Independent Component Analysis of fMRI Data. Proc. Leeds Statistical Research Workshop, Leeds, England (1999)

[8]   Desco, M., Hernabdez, J.A. et al.: Multiresolution Analysis in fMRI: Sensitivity and Specificity in the Detection of Brain Activation. Human Brain Mapping, 14 (2001) 16 – 27

[9]   Brammer, M.J.: Multidimensional Wavelet Analysis of Functional Magnetic Resonance Images. Human Brain Mapping, 6 (1998) 378–382

[10]   Ruttimann, U.E., Unser, M. et al.: Statistical Analysis of Functional MRI Data in the Wavelet Domain. IEEE Transactions on Medical Imaging, 17(2) (1998) 142 –154

[11]   Mayhew, J., Hu, D.W. et al.: An Evaluation of Linear Model Analysis Techniques for Processing Images of Microcirculation Activity. NeuroImage, 7 (1998) 49–71

[12]   Mayhew, J., Askew, S. et al.: Cerebral Vasomotion:0.1-Hz Oscillation in Reflected Light Imaging of Neural Activity. NeuroImage, 4 (1996) 183–193

[13]   Kleinfeld, D., Mitra, P. et al.: Fluctuations and Stimulus-induced Changes in Blood Flow Observed in Individual Capillaries in Layers 2 through 4 of Rat Neocortex. Proc. Natl. Acad. Sci. USA, 95 (1998) 15741–15746

[14]   Kiviniemi, V., Jauhiainen, J. et al.: Slow Vasomotor Fluctuation in fMRI of Anesthetized Child Brain. Magnetic Resonance in Medicine, 44 (2000) 373–378

[15]   Kiviniemi, V., Heikki, J. et al.: Independent Component Analysis of Nondeterministic fMRI Signal Sources. NeuroImage, 19 (2003) 253–260

Stereo Matching and 3-D Reconstruction for Optic Disk Images

Kai Zhang[1], Xu Xi[2], Zhang Li[3], and Wang Guoping[1]

[1] School of Electronics Engineering and Computer Science,
Peking University, 100871, China
zk@graphics.pku.edu.cn
[2] Department of Clinical Medicine,
The First Military Medical University, 510515, China
[3] Ophthalmology Center, The Fifth People's Hospital of Foshan,
528000, China

Abstract. 3-D visualization of optic disk surface is very useful in diagnosis and observation of some eye diseases. It helps physicians in understanding and interpreting the stereo disc photographs(SDPs) which is widely used in clinical situations. This paper proposed a segment-based stereo matching algorithm, which represents the fundus structure as a Bayesian network and applies belief propagation(BP) to solve the maximum a posterior(MAX) estimation. Only ground control pixels(GCPs) of the BP results are retrieved and the dense disparity map is obtained by cubic interpolation and Gaussian blurring to ensure smoothness. The resulted 3-D retinal surface shows our approach is promising.

1 Introduction

Retinal diseases such as diabetic retinopathy and glaucoma can damage the optic nerve, resulting in visual loss and blindness. Because the loss of vision is irrevocable, timely diagnosis and treatment are particularly significant. Now stereo disc photograph(SDP) is one of widely used techniques in clinical situations to record the objective status of the optic nerve head (ONH). However, the diagnostic information and the interpretation of those images are dependent on the expertise of the clinician. In such cases the 3-D visualization of the retina is especially useful. Subtle details such as size, shape, and color of pathological features can be easily detected and evaluated in the 3-D graphics, which makes diagnosis more easier.

However, relatively less work has been done on the computer generated 3-D visualization of retinal surface. E. Corona et al. [1] introduced power cepstrum and cross correlation techniques for image correspondence and surface reconstruction. The disparity map obtained was on pixel level and large window cubic B-spline operation was used for smoothing, which made the final 3-D surface less accurate. K. Deguchi et al. [2] assumed the fundus formed part of sphere and created a sphere equation. This method is not practical because the recovered shape of the fundus was fixed to a sphere which would not allow some abnormal

Y. Liu, T. Jiang, and C. Zhang (Eds.): CVBIA 2005, LNCS 3765, pp. 517–525, 2005.
© Springer-Verlag Berlin Heidelberg 2005

features to be accurately displayed. Xu et al. [3] and Kong et al. [4] generated 3-D surface of the retina by two stereo optic images using feature-based matching methods. As far as we known, due to the need for dense depth maps for a variety of applications and also due to improvements in efficient and robust intensity-based matching methods, interest in feature-based methods has declined in the last decade.

On the other hand there exists a considerable body of work on the dense stereo correspondence problem in computer vision field, and computational stereo for extraction of 3-D scene structure has been an intense area of research for decades. [5,6] have provided an exhaustive comparison of dense stereo correspondence algorithms. Graph cut [7] and belief propagation [8,9] have been shown to be among the best performers. Segment-based stereo algorithms arise recently [7,10], which are based on the assumption that there are no large disparity discontinuities inside homogeneous color segments. Usually the segmentation technique is integrated within other frameworks and achieves strong performance.

We take advantages of both the color segmentation technique and the Bayesian belief propagation method, and propose a new intensity-based matching algorithm. Image segmentation representation is used to reduce the high solution space and enforce disparity smoothness in homogeneous color regions. Bayesian method models the fundus structure as a Bayesian network, encapsulates data cost and smooth cost into the message transfer mechanism, and applies the belief propagation to solve the maximum a posterior(MAP) estimation. When belief propagation finished for both images the pixels satisfying the consistency constraint are termed as ground control points(GCPs) [5,10]. Smooth dense disparity map was obtained using cubic interpolation and Gaussian blurring based on the recognized GCPs. While the depth is inversely proportional to the disparity between two matching points, 3-D reconstruction is trivial if we assume the internal and external parameters of the stereo cameras are all known.

The rest of the paper is organized as follows: The proposed algorithm is presented in detail mainly focus on how to define cost function and how to apply belief propagation to obtain disparity map in section 2. Then we provide experimental results in section 3 to demonstrate the algorithm's strong performance. Finally, we make conclusions in Section 4.

2   Stereo Matching and 3-D Reconstruction

The algorithm proposed in this paper consists of various steps mainly including image segmentation, stereo matching and 3-D reconstruction. One of the most challenging step is to detect corresponding pixels between two images, and we discuss this issue in detail from 2.3 to 2.5. Fig. 1 gives out the block diagram of proposed algorithm.

2.1   Definitions

Here we introduce some denotations. We use a pair of horizontally rectified stereo images to ease the description of the algorithm through out the paper.

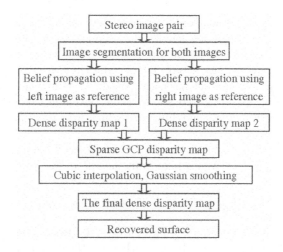

Fig. 1. The flowchart of our proposed stereo matching and 3-D reconstruction algorithm

Let I_L denote the left image and I_R denote the right image. Let $I_L(p)$ denote the intensity of the left image pixel p and $I_R(q)$ the intensity of the right image pixel q. Let $D(p)$ denote the disparity of pixel p. A pair $(p, D(p))$ is termed as a match, which could be considered as a 3-D point. S and T are used to denote image segment, and $D(S)$, $D(T)$ are their disparities respectively.

2.2 Image Segmentation

Our approach is built upon the assumption that large disparity discontinuities only occur on the boundaries of homogeneous color segments. Therefore any image segmentation algorithm that decomposes an image into homogeneous image segments will work for us. In our current implementation, mean-shift image segmentation algorithm [11] is used. We assume that pixels inside the same segment have the same disparity and our algorithm actually assigns each segment a disparity. This assumption makes our method very simple and efficient. Also we noticed the fundus is a smooth surface and there is no occlusion in it, so over-segmentation technique is adopted for more accurate approximation.

2.3 Cost Function

There are two kinds of cost functions. Smooth cost function enforces smoothness by penalizing discontinuities, i.e., imposing penalties if different disparities are assigned to neighboring segments. The smooth cost is easy calculated in proposed algorithm:

$$Cost_{smooth}(S, T, D(S), D(T)) = \varepsilon \times \frac{Peri(S,T)}{Peri(S) + Peri(T)} \times \Lambda(S,T) \quad (1)$$

where S and T are neighboring segments, $Peri(S)$ and $Peri(T)$ are the border length of S and T, $Peri(S,T)$ is the common border length between segment S

and T, and ε is a user-defined const to adjust the cost value. $\Lambda(S,T)$ has value 0 if S and T's disparity difference is less than or equal to one, otherwise 1. $\Lambda(S,T)$ is inspired by the fact that the fundus is a smooth surface so the neighboring segments' disparity difference should be no more than one.

Data cost function is pixel intensity based. The data cost function of the proposed algorithm contains two levels: pixel matching cost which eliminates sampling errors and segment matching cost which measures the disagreement of segments.

The simplest pixel cost function is as the absolute difference of intensity between the two pixels. Given a pixel p in the left image and a possible match $(p, D(p))$:

$$Cost^{\beta}_{Data}(p, D(p)) = |I_L(p) - I_R(p - D(p))| \tag{2}$$

However, this measure is inadequate for discrete images, because image sampling can cause this difference to be large wherever the disparity is not an integral number of pixels and in this case every 3-D point's intensity is distributed over several pixels. Typically, the sampling problem is alleviated by using some linearly interpolated intensity functions in a method that are insensitive to sampling (Birchfield and Tomasi, [12]).

In practice, we found Birchfield and Tomasi's method just alleviated sampling error on one side, but failed when sampling error occurred on both sides especially in textureless regions. We improved their method and achieved better effects. Consider three pixels q_l, q, q_r in right image: $q_l = p - (D(p) + 1)$, $q = p - D(p)$, $q_r = p - (D(p) - 1)$. We believe that sampling error occurs if and only if the dissimilarity between p and q_l, q, q_r is not greater than a predefined threshold λ:

$$Cost_{Data}(p, D(p)) = \frac{1}{|\{q_i\}|} \sum_{q_i \in \{q_i\}} Cost^{\beta}_{Data}(p, p - q_i) \tag{3}$$

where $\{q_i\} = \{q_i | q_i \in \{p - (D(p) + 1), p - D(p), p - (D(p) - 1)\} \wedge Cost^{\beta}_{Data}(p, p - q_i) \leq \lambda\}$, and $|\{q_i\}|$ denotes the element count of $\{q_i\}$.

Segment cost is defined as an average of all pixels' cost. Consider segment S and let $|S|$ denote the pixel count in S, so we can write:

$$Cost_{Data}(S, D(S)) = \frac{1}{|S|} \sum_{p \in S} Cost_{Data}(p, D(S)) \tag{4}$$

Just as window-based cost functions, (4) is also a kind of local constraint. However, window-based measurements usually make large errors in the disparity discontinuous boundaries because of intensity break [5,6]. On the contrary in image segment since pixel intensities are all similar, the disparity break is prohibited, and as mentioned in section 2.2, there are no occlusion in fundus image, so (4) is accurate and is much more robust than previous window-based cost functions.

2.4   Loopy Belief Propagation

In the literature of probabilistic graph models [8,9], a Bayesian network is an undirected graph as shown in Fig. 2. Nodes $\{u_i\}$ are hidden variables and nodes $\{vi\}$ are observed variables. The posterior $P(\{u_i\}|\{v_i\})$ can be factorized as:

$$P(\{u_i\}|\{v_i\}) \propto \prod_{u_s \in \{u_i\}} \Phi(u_s, v_s) \prod_{u_s \in \{u_i\}} \prod_{u_t \in N(u_s)} \Psi(u_s, u_t) \qquad (5)$$

Where $\Phi(u_s, v_s)$ is called the local evidence for node u_s, $\Psi(u_s, u_t)$ is called the compatibility matrix between nodes u_s and u_t, and $N(u_s)$ is the neighbors of u_s. If the number of discrete states of u_s is C, $\Psi(u_s, u_t)$ is an $C \times C$ matrix and $\Phi(u_s, v_s)$ is a vector with C elements.

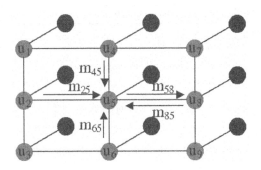

Fig. 2. A regular Bayesian network and message passing flow. Red nodes are hidden variables and blue nodes are observable variables. The message passing through u_s to u_t is denoted as m_{st}. The message sent from node u_5 to u_8 is updated as: $m_{58} = \beta max_{u_5} \Psi(u_5, u_8) \Phi(u_5, v_5) m_{25} m_{45} m_{65}$. The belief at node u_5 is computed as: $b_5 = \beta \Phi(u_5, v_5) m_{25} m_{45} m_{65} m_{85}$.

In the stereo correspondence case, we use the left image as reference view, denote the segments in the left image and corresponding pixel set in the right image as hidden and observed nodes respectively, and link neighboring segments by edges, then we get an irregular Bayesian network. Assuming that the segments in reference image follow an independent identical distribution, we can define the function $\Phi(u_s, v_s)$ and $\Psi(u_s, u_t)$ as:

$$\Phi(u_s, v_s) = exp(-Cost_{Data}(u_s, D(u_s))) \qquad (6)$$

$$\Psi(u_s, u_t) = exp(-Cost_{Smooth}(u_s, u_t, D(u_s), D(u_t))) \qquad (7)$$

It is obviously that the MAP estimation of $P(\{u_i\}|\{v_i\})$ in (5) is equal to the scene disparity map, i.e., the maximum probability is corresponding to the minimum cost. For the Bayesian network, exact inference is usually intractable due to the large state space of nodes [8,9]. Among several approximation methods loopy belief propagation [13] is promising, which has a linear time complexity proportional to the number of hidden nodes and has been applied successfully to stereo vision problems [9]. Belief propagation is an iterative inference algorithm that propagates messages in the network. Let m_{st} be the message that node u_s sends to u_t, and b_s be the belief at node u_s. Note that m_{st} and b_s are both vectors with C elements. Usually the belief propagation using a "max-product" message update rule. For example, in Fig. 2, the message sent from node u_5 to u_8 is updated as: $m_{58} = \beta max_{u_5} \Psi(u_5, u_8) \Phi(u_5, v_5) m_{25} m_{45} m_{65}$. The belief at node u_5 is computed as: $b_5 = \beta \Phi(u_5, v_5) m_{25} m_{45} m_{65} m_{85}$. β is the normalization constant, which can be ignored safely. The belief propagation algorithm we used is given in Algorithm.1, and the disparities of nodes u_s and u_t in (6) and (7) are those values which achieve the maximum belief currently.

Algorithm 1. Belief propagation algorithm

Input: A Baysian network
Output: The maximum a posterior estimation

1 Initialize $\Psi(u_s, u_t)$, $\Phi(u_s, v_s)$ and all messages m_{st}
2 Using "max-product" update rule:

$$m_{st}^{k+1} = max_{u_s} \Psi(u_s, u_t) \Phi(u_s, v_s) \prod_{u_r \in N(u_s)/u_t} m_{rs}^k \qquad (8)$$

where k is iterative step, and $N(u_s)/u_t$ are the neighboring nodes of u_s except u_t
3 Compute beliefs:

$$b_s = \Phi(u_s, v_s) \prod_{u_r \in N(u_s)} m_{rs}, u_s^{MAP} = argmax(b_s) \qquad (9)$$

2.5   Dense Disparity Map Retrieval

To get more smooth disparity map of fundus, we use the output of belief propagation algorithm just for the retrieval of GCPs. Here we define GCP as the pixel which satisfying the consistency constraint, i.e., pixel p in the left image is GCP if and only if $D(p) = D(p - D(p))$, where $p - D(p)$ is a right image pixel. By denoting left image and right image as reference view respectively, we can get two different dense disparity maps of left image, then consistency constraint is applied to get sparse GCP map. As done in [3] and [4], cubic interpolation and Gaussian blurring are used to get the final smoothing dense map.

2.6   3-D Reconstruction

The 3-D reconstruction from dense disparity map is trivial if we have known the cameras' internal and external parameters. Refer to Fig. 3, which is a sketch map of a typical stereo equipment. We define the baseline T of the stereo pair to be the line segment joining the optical centers O_L and O_R. Both camera coordinates axes are aligned and the baseline is parallel to the camera x coordinate axis. The depth of a point in space P imaged by the two cameras is defined by intersecting the rays from the optical centers through their respective images of P, p and p'. Given the baseline T and the focal length f of the cameras, depth at P may be computed by similar triangles as:

$$Z = f\frac{T}{d} \qquad (10)$$

where d is the disparity of P, $d = x - x'$ (see Fig. 3).

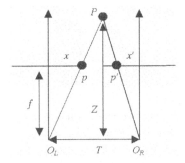

Fig. 3. The geometry of stereo equipment. Depth at a space point P can be computed by similar triangles.

Once dense disparity map is computed, the final 3-D retinal representation can be reconstructed using (10).

3   Experimental Results

Two stereo fundus pairs and the corresponding final disparity maps are shown in Fig. 4. The resulted 3-D retinal surfaces are rendered in OpenGL environment, using the original images as textures. From the 3-D contour images, we can see that the optic cups and retinal vessels clearly and intuitively, helping physicians in understanding and interpreting the SDPs.

4   Conclusions

A novel stereo matching and 3-D reconstruction approach has been proposed in this paper. Image segmentation technique uses the image segment as matching unit other than individual pixel, and this make our algorithm much simple and efficient. Two level data cost functions eliminate the image noise and sampling error effectively. The fundus structure was modeled as a Bayesian network, and belief propagation was applied to get the MAP estimation. The resulted 3-D retinal surfaces are smooth and clearly typical, which show our approach is promising.

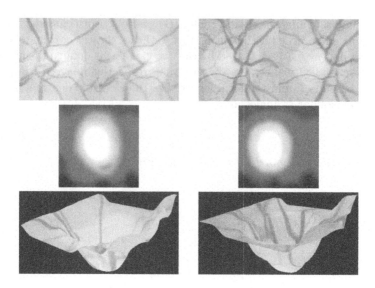

Fig. 4. The top row: the original two stereo fundus images. the middle row: the corresponding smooth dense disparity maps. The bottom row: the corresponding 3-D surfaces rendered in OpenGL environment and observed from the same view point, using the original left images as texture source. Experience shows that the recovered surfaces correspond to the real 3-D surfaces of the eyes very well.

Acknowledgements

This work is supported by the National Basic Research Program of China(973 Program) under Grant No.2004CB719403 and the National High Technology Research and Development Program of China under Grant No.2004AA115120.

References

1. E. Corona, S. Mitra, M. Wilson, T. Krile, Y. H. Kwon, and P. Soliz. Digital Stereo Image Analyzer for Generating Automated 3-D Measures of Optic Disc Deformation in Glaucoma.IEEE Transactions on Medical Imaging, 2002,vol.21(no.10):1244-1253.
2. K. Deguchi, D. Kawamata, K. Mizutani, H. Hontani and K. wakabayashi. 3D Fundus Shape Reconstruction An Display from Stereo Fundus Images. IEICE Trans. INF. & SYST., 2000,vol.E83-D(no.7).
3. J. Xu and O. Chutatape. 3-D Optic Disk Reconstruction from Low-Resolution Stereo Images Based on Combined Registrations and Sub-pixel Matching.Proceedings of the 26th Annual International Conference of the IEEE EMBS.
4. H. J. Kong, S. K. Kiml, J.M. Seo, K. H. Park, H. Chung, K. S. Park and H. C. Kim.Three Dimensional Reconstruction of Conventional Stereo Optic Disc Image.Proceedings of the 26th Annual International Conference of the IEEE EMBS.

5. D. Scharstein and R. Szeliski. A Taxonomy and Evaluation of Dense Two-Frame Stereo Correspondence Algorithms. International Journal of Computer Vision, 2002, vol.47 (no.1): 7-42.

6. M. Z. Brown, D. Burschka, and G. D. Hager. Advances in computational stereo. IEEE Transactions on Pattern Analysis and Machine Intelligence, August 2003, vol.25(no.8): 993-1008.

7. Li Hong and George Chen. Segment-based Stereo Matching using Graph Cuts. In IEEE Computer Vision and Pattern Recognition: 2004. 74-81.

8. J. Yedidia,W. T. Freeman, and Y. Weiss. Understanding Belief Propagation and Its Generalizations. In International Joint Conference on Artificial Intelligence, Distinguished Papers Track: 2001.

9. Jian Sun, Nan-Ning Zheng, and Heung-Yeung Shum. Stereo Matching using Belief Propagation. IEEE Transactions on Pattern Analysis and Machine Intelligence, 2003, vol.25(no.7): 787-800.

10. Yichen Wei and Long Quan. Region-Based Progressive Stereo Matching. In IEEE Computer Vision and Pattern Recognition: 2004. 106-113.

11. D. Comaniciu and P. Meer. Mean shift: A robust approach toward feature space analysis. IEEE Transactions on Pattern Analysis and Machine Intelligence, 2002, vol.24(no.5): 603-619.

12. S. Birchfield and C. Tomasi. Depth Discontinuities by Pixel-to-Pixel Stereo. International Journal of Computer Vision, 1999, vol.35 (no.3): 269-299.

13. J. Pearl. Probabilistic Reasoning in Intelligent Systems: Networks of Plausible Inference. San Mateo, Calif.: Morgan Kaufmann Publishers, 1988.

Total Variation Based Iterative Image Reconstruction

Guoqiang Yu[1], Liang Li[2], Jianwei Gu[2], and Li Zhang[2]

[1] Department of Application Science,
Nuctech Company Limited, Beijing, P.R. China 100084
[2] Department of Engineering Physics, Tsinghua University,
Beijing, P.R. China 100084

Abstract. Image reconstruction is an active research field and plays an important role in many applications . In this paper, we propose a new approach. Firstly, we introduce the minimum total variation (TV) criterion in the optimization process of image reconstruction; secondly, we introduce the level set method to obtain the solution. The TV principle has been studied intensively in the community of image processing and computer vision. The TV constrained minimization problem is convex and has a unique solution. The standard level set method provides the way to get the solution. We validated the proposed model on both toy data and real data. The experimental results show that the TV principle has the advantages of reducing noise and artifacts and preserving edges. The experiments also indicate that the proposed method is suitable and applicable to practical applications.

1 Introduction

Image reconstruction has been extensively reasearched and is important in many applications[3]. Taking the computed tomography (CT) reconstruction as an example, the problem can be stated as following. Suppose we have collected a set of measurements. Each measurement represents the summation or line integral of the attenuation coefficients of an object along a particular ray path. The measurements are taken from different views as shown in Fig.1. Then, how do we reconstruct the original image of attenuation coefficients from these measurements?

Many reconstruction algorithms are proposed, including two main classes [3], filtered back projection (FBP) algorithms and iterative algorithms. FBP algorithms have the advantages of fast speed and less memory needs. However, they suffer from the noise and require complete data. Further more, the prior knowledge about the original image is hardly incorporated in the model. Iterative approaches have been important because of their superior performance in the above context. With the rapid development of computer technology, iterative algorithms receive increasingly more attention. Iterative algorithms may be categorized according to their optimization criteria and the ways of updating an intermediate image with observed data. In fact, image reconstruction is

Y. Liu, T. Jiang, and C. Zhang (Eds.): CVBIA 2005, LNCS 3765, pp. 526–534, 2005.
© Springer-Verlag Berlin Heidelberg 2005

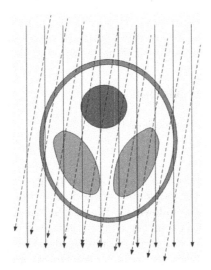

Fig. 1. A sketch map of computed tomography. The real-line and dot-line denote the different views.

an inverse problem and it is an ill-posed problem in CT due to the noise and the incomplete data. A common remedy to such inverse problems is to apply additional constraints. Different constraints correspond to different criterions, such as least square error criterion, maximum smoothness criterion, maximum entropy criterion and Bayesian criterion. Due to the huge data dimension, the implementation is also very important. The algebraic reconstruction techniques (ART), simultaneous iterative reconstruction techniques (SIRT) and expectation maximization (EM) algorithm are the primary implementation algorithms widely used in the community [6].

Our proposed algorithm is an iterative algorithm. As mentioned above, iterative algorithms can be categorized according to their criteria and their implementation. This paper contributes in these two aspects. Firstly, we introduce the total variation (TV) criterion [5] to optimize the objective function. Then, a numerical implementation scheme is presented in the level set formula [9].

The total variation principle is widely applied in the community of image processing and computer vision. The total variation is based on the bounded variation functional space [1]. It can reduce the noise level while preserving edges [10]. Moreover, the objective function from minimizing the total variation is convex, thus the solution to the minimization problem exists and is unique [2], which means that, wherever we start from, it converges and arrives at a global minimum. A time dependent partial differential equation (PDE) can be derived from the minimization model through the calculus of variation method. This PDE can be efficiently implemented with standard level set tools [7]. The implementation is robust, stable, convergent and fairly fast [8,4].

The organization of this paper is as follows. After this introduction, section 2 formulates the proposed model for image reconstruction problem and some properties of this model are also discussed. The numerical implementation is presented in section 3. Experimental results are shown in section 4, including a toy illustration and a real data test. Finally, we conclude this paper in section 5.

2   Reconstruction Model

The imaging system can be modelled as,

$$p = Ru + n \tag{1}$$

where p is the measured data, R stands for the projection matrix, n is the noise in the measurement or the randomness inherited in the system, u is the image to be reconstructed. In the following, without confusing, we will call n as noise. The projection matrix R is from the imaging physics. For example, for an X-ray CT, the matrix R is a linear operator and describes the line integral procedure. Due to its randomness, the noise n is not known exactly. However, we can get some knowledge of the noise such as its mean and standard deviation. In this paper, we assume the noise is Gaussian with zero mean and its stand deviation being δ. Then, the problem is to reconstruct the image u from the observed data p, given the knowledge of R and some statistical knowledge of n.

Due to the existence of the noise, we can't expect that the projection of the true image equals to the observed data. Instead, we expect that the mean square of their difference equals the mean square deviation of the noise.

Denote $\hat{u}$ as the estimation of the true image, we expect that

$$\int_{\Omega} |p - R\hat{u}|^2 = \delta^2 \tag{2}$$

However, there are many solutions satisfying the equation 2. We need to find a reasonable one. The total variation principle states that the solution with the minimum total variation is the best estimation. Then, the reconstruction problem is to solve the following constrained optimization problem

$$\text{Minimize } \int_{\Omega} |\nabla u|$$

$$\text{Subject to } \int_{\Omega} |p - Ru|^2 = \delta^2 \tag{3}$$

This problem is naturally linked to the following unconstrained problem

$$\text{Minimize/Find a critical point of } \int_{\Omega} |\nabla u| + \frac{\lambda}{2} |p - Ru|^2 \tag{4}$$

for a given positive Lagrange multiplier λ. Chambolle and Lions have proved that these two energy functionals have the same solution [2]. In the following, when we say the optimization problem without particular notion we refer this unconstrained case.

The space of functions with bounded variation (BV) is an ideal choice for a total variation based optimization problem since BV provides regularity but also allows sharp discontinuities (edges) [10]. That is why the total variation based model can preserve the edges. The existence and uniqueness of the solution for a total variation based optimization problem has been established in the BV space. For a noisy image, the TV model has larger energy, so this model tends to reduce the noise while preserving the edges without blurring or rings. These properties make the TV model suitable to the image reconstruction where there are sharp discontinuities and noise needs to be reduced. In addition, the uniqueness of the solution release the burden of finding a good initialization.

3   Numerical Implementation

Through the calculus of variation the Euler-Lagrange equation of the equation 4 can be easily obtained as

$$0 = -\nabla \cdot \left(\frac{\nabla u}{|\nabla u|} \right) + \lambda R^T (Ru - p) \tag{5}$$

where R^T denotes the transpose of the projection matrix R. The solution image should satisfy this equation. Since the uniqueness of the solution, if we find some u satisfying this equation, we can say that it is just the best estimation of the true image under the total variation criterion. Finding the u satisfying the equation 5 is not an easy task. Usually a time dependent PDE can be established as

$$u_t = \nabla \cdot \left(\frac{\nabla u}{|\nabla u|} \right) - \lambda R^T (Ru - p) \tag{6}$$

When the PDE reaches its steady state, $u_t = 0$. Then, the equation 5 is satisfied.

Direct numerical approximation to the equation 6 is unstable. So Osher etc. [7] proposed to multiply the whole Euler-Lagrange equation 5 bywith the magnitude of the gradient and the new time evolution model reads as follows

$$u_t = |\nabla u| \nabla \cdot \left(\frac{\nabla u}{|\nabla u|} \right) - |\nabla u| \lambda R^T (Ru - p) \tag{7}$$

Notice here that $|\nabla u| \geq 0$, so the treatment doesn't change the solution of the equation 5.

The equation 7 is in the Hamilton-Jacobi [8] form. More exactly, it is the mean curvature flow with external force. The standard level set method can be applied to obtain an robust and stable numerical solution to the equation 7. The equation 7 has both parabolic and hyperbolic terms, $|\nabla u| \nabla \cdot \left(\frac{\nabla u}{|\nabla u|} \right)$ and $-|\nabla u| \lambda R^T (Ru - p)$. These two terms should be discretized differently.

Let u_{ij}^n be the approximation to the value $u(x_i, y_j, t_n)$, where $x_i = i\Delta x$, $y_j = k\Delta y$, and $t_n = n\Delta t$, with Δx, Δy, Δt being the spatial step sizes and the time step size, respectively. We define the quantity $w_{ij}^n = \lambda R^T (Ru_{ij}^n - p)$. Then the numerical scheme for the equation 7 reads as the following

$$\frac{u_{ij}^{n+1} - u_{ij}^n}{\Delta t} = s_{ij}^n - G_{ij}^n w_{ij}^n \tag{8}$$

where

$$s_{ij}^n = \frac{g_{ij}^{xx}({g_{ij}^y}^2 + \varepsilon) - 2g_{ij}^{xy} g_{ij}^x g_{ij}^y + g_{ij}^{yy}({g_{ij}^x}^2 + \varepsilon)}{{g_{ij}^x}^2 + {g_{ij}^y}^2 + \varepsilon} \tag{9}$$

$$g_{ij}^x = \frac{u_{i+1,j}^n - u_{i-1,j}^n}{2\Delta x} \tag{10}$$

$$g_{ij}^y = \frac{u_{i,j+1}^n - u_{i,j-1}^n}{2\Delta y} \tag{11}$$

$$g_{ij}^{xx} = \frac{u_{i+1,j}^n - 2u_{ij}^n + u_{i-1,j}^n}{\Delta x^2} \tag{12}$$

$$g_{ij}^{yy} = \frac{u_{i,j+1}^n - 2u_{ij}^n + u_{i,j-1}^n}{\Delta x^2} \tag{13}$$

$$g_{ij}^{xy} = \frac{u_{i+1,j+1}^n - u_{i-1,j+1}^n - u_{i+1,j-1}^n + u_{i-1,j-1}^n}{2\Delta x \Delta y} \tag{14}$$

$$G_{ij}^n = \begin{cases} \sqrt{\max((a+)^2, (b-)^2) + \max((c+)^2, (d-)^2)}, & \text{if } w_{ij}^n > 0 \\ \sqrt{\max((a-)^2, (b+)^2) + \max((c-)^2, (d+)^2)}, & \text{if } w_{ij}^n < 0 \\ 0, \text{otherwise}, \end{cases} \tag{15}$$

where $a+ = \max(a, 0)$, $a- = \min(a, 0)$, and so on,

$$a = \frac{u_{i,j}^n - u_{i-1,j}^n}{\Delta x} \tag{16}$$

$$b = \frac{u_{i+1,j}^n - u_{i,j}^n}{\Delta x} \tag{17}$$

$$c = \frac{u_{i,j}^n - u_{i,j-1}^n}{\Delta y} \tag{18}$$

$$d = \frac{u_{i,j+1}^n - u_{i,j}^n}{\Delta y} \tag{19}$$

Here, we introduce a regularization term ε to avoid the occurrence of zero denominator. The Courant-Friedriches-Lewy (CFL) condition for this scheme is $\Delta t \leq c\Delta x^2$, where c is independent of the ∇u and depends on the maximum absolute value of w_{ij}^n. In general, the smaller the absolute value of w_{ij}^n is, the larger Δt is.

4   Experiments

In this section, we present two experimental results, one for synthesized toy data and the other for real data. We will show that the total variation based recon-

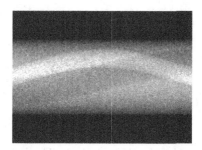

Fig. 2. The noisy projection data for the toy example

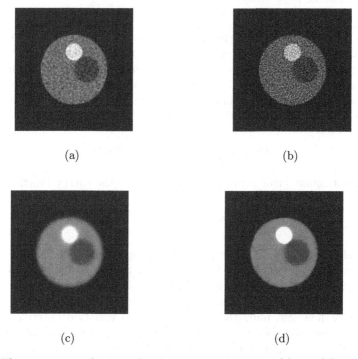

Fig. 3. The reconstructed images for the toy data. Subfigure (a) and (b) are based on FBP method and least square error, respectively. Notice that both these two approaches result in noisy reconstructions. Subfigure (c) shows the reconstructed image from the maximum smoothness method. The noise is reduced greatly. However, the edges are blurred. Subfigure (d) is the result of our proposed method. The image is smooth while the edges are preserved.

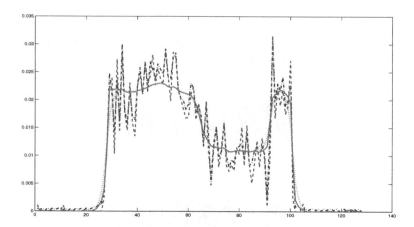

Fig. 4. Profiles of reconstructions for the central row. The dash-dot, dash, dot, and solid lines stand for the reconstructions from FBP, least square error, maximum smoothness and total variation, respectively.

struction can reduce noise while preserving edges. This method is not sensitive to the initialization conditions. In all experiments, we initialize randomly. The experiments indicate that the algorithm is stable and convergent. To demonstrate the advantages of our proposed algorithm, we compare to other three classical algorithms: FBP, maximum smooth reconstruction and least square error reconstruction. The maximum smooth reconstruction minimizes the following energy functional

$$E(u) = \int_{\Omega} |\nabla u|^2 + \frac{\lambda}{2} |p - Ru|^2 \tag{20}$$

and the least square error reconstruction minimizes the energy functional

$$E(u) = \int_{\Omega} |p - Ru|^2 \tag{21}$$

Fig.2 shows the case of noisy projection data for the toy example. The reconstructed images based on the four algorithms are illustrated in Fig.3. All the reconstructed images are of 128 × 128. Both FBP and least square error criterion suffer from heavy noise. The maximum smoothness criterion reduces the noise greatly, however, blurs the edges. The total variation criterion not only reduces noise but also preserves the edges. The profiles at the central rows of the reconstructions demonstrate their performance more clearly as shown in Fig.4.

The real data of a closestool with a metal nail in the hole is collected from an X-ray CT. The projection data is shown in Fig.5. The reconstructed image is 256 × 256. The reconstructed image with FBP is demonstrated in Fig.6(a). We can see the metal artifacts and the image is noisy. Fig.6(b) shows the result by minimizing total variation. The TV based reconstruction gets a fairly smooth image with sharp edges and suppresses the metal artifacts greatly. These prop-

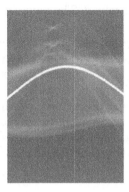

Fig. 5. The projection data for the case of real data

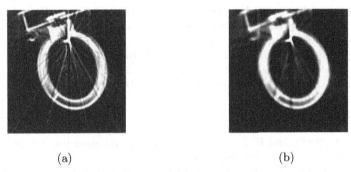

(a)   (b)

Fig. 6. The reconstructed images from the real data. Subfigure (a) is with FBP. The image is corrupted by noise and metal artifacts. Subfigure (b) is the result from our proposed method. The noise and the artifacts are suppressed greatly while the edges are preserved.

erties can enhance the human perception and simplify the post processing such as segmentation and object recognition.

5   Conclusion

In this paper, we proposed a novel iterative reconstruction approach based on the total variation principle, which tends to reduce noises and preserve edges. The reconstruction is modelled as a constrained optimization problem and the energy functional is stated. Through the calculus of variation, the necessary condition of the minimum is obtained. We construct a time dependent PDE from this condition. When the PDE arrives at its steady state, we say the condition is met. Since the proposed energy functional is convex, the PDE's steady state is the solution of the minimization problem. To numerically approximated the PDE, we adopt the level set method. The numerical scheme is presented. Our adopted scheme is stable and robust. The numerical and practical experiments confirm this point.

We demonstrated two experiments, one on the toy data and the other on the real data. Both these two experiments show the advantages of the proposed approach. Notice that the reconstructed images are not of small size. The proposed approach can be applied in real applications.

There is also something requiring further investigation. One is that the space resolution is lost to some extent although the proposed method can get smooth results with edges preserving. Another is the speed. Since the propose energy is convex, some numerical schemes with faster speed may exist. Both are our further research interests.

References

1. G. Aubert and P. Kornprobst. *Mathematical Problems in Image Processing: Partial Differential Equations and the Calculus of Variations*, volume 147 of *Applied Mathematical Sciences*. Springer-Verlag, 2002.
2. Chambolle and P-L. Lions. Image recovery via total variation minimization and related problems. *Numer. Math*, 76(2):167–188, 1997.
3. Jiang Hsieh. *Computed Tomography: Principles, Design, Artifacts and Recent Advances*. SPIE Press, 2003.
4. J.A.Sethian. *Level Set Methods and Fast Marching Methods*. Cambridge University Press, second edition, 1999.
5. S. Osher L. Rudin and E. Fatemi. Nonlinear total variation based noise removal algorithms. *Phys. D*, 60:259–268, 1992.
6. Jiang M. and Wang G. Development of iterative algorithms for image reconstruction. *Journal of X-Ray Science and Technology*, 10:77–86, 2002.
7. Antonio Marquina and Stanley Osher. Explicit algorithms for a new time dependent model based on level set motion for nonlinear deblurring and noise removal. *SIAM Journal on Scientific Computing*, 22(2):387–405, 2001.
8. Stanley Osher and Ronald Fedkiw. *Level Set Methods and Dynamic Implicit Surfaces*. Springer-Verlag, 2003.
9. Stanley Osher and James A Sethian. Fronts propagating with curvature-dependent speed: Algorithms based on Hamilton-Jacobi formulations. *Journal of Computational Physics*, 79:12–49, 1988.
10. F. Park T. Chan, S. Esedoglu and A. Yip. *Mathematical Models in Computer Vision: The Handbook*, chapter Total Variation Image Restoration: Overview and Recent Developments. Springer, 2005.

Voronoi-Based Segmentation of Cells on Image Manifolds

Thouis R. Jones[1], Anne Carpenter[2], and Polina Golland

[1] MIT CSAIL, Cambridge, MA, USA
[2] Whitehead Institute for Biomedical Research, Cambridge, MA, USA

Abstract. We present a method for finding the boundaries between adjacent regions in an image, where "seed" areas have already been identified in the individual regions to be segmented. This method was motivated by the problem of finding the borders of cells in microscopy images, given a labelling of the nuclei in the images. The method finds the Voronoi region of each seed on a manifold with a metric controlled by local image properties. We discuss similarities to other methods based on image-controlled metrics, such as Geodesic Active Contours, and give a fast algorithm for computing the Voronoi regions. We validate our method against hand-traced boundaries for cell images.

1 Introduction

Image cytometry, the measurement of cell properties from microscopy images, has become an important tool for biological research. In particular, high-throughput experiments rely on automatic processing of images to deal with the large amount of data they produce [3]. A fundamental operation in cell-image analysis is identifying individual cell boundaries. This is often difficult because there are many different staining protocols, leading to dramatically different appearances for cells. Moreover, the difference between cell interior and cell border may not be very pronounced (see Figures 1 and 2). Identification of individual cells allows much more powerful analysis of the resulting data than methods that provide only mean measurements for cell populations. For example, expression data from a protein interaction chip cannot differentiate a bimodal population and a unimodal population if they have the same mean expression levels. Measurements of individual cells prevents conflation of subpopulations.

It is almost always the case that the nuclei of cells are more easily identifiable, because they have a more uniform appearance and shape, are brighter relative to the background when stained, and do not abut one another, as cells do. They are also usually interior to the cells. This leads us to phrase the problem of segmenting cells as one of identifying boundaries between regions given "seeds" in individual regions from which to start the segmentation. Current methods for identifying cells for image cytometry sometimes use a fixed offset around the nuclei. However, this fixed offset requires tuning to different cell types, and does not provide information about phenotypes that cause changes in cell size or shape [2].

Y. Liu, T. Jiang, and C. Zhang (Eds.): CVBIA 2005, LNCS 3765, pp. 535–543, 2005.

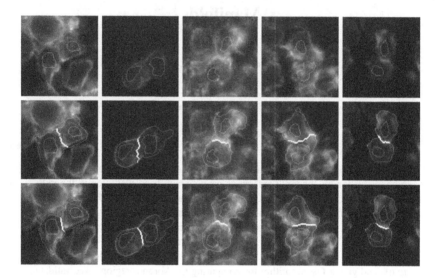

Fig. 1. Typical results from our algorithm. Internal shapes are seed regions, taken from manual segmentation of nuclei, and are the same in both rows. Bold lines show cell/cell boundaries that are compared. Top row: Cell images, with nuclei outlined. Middle row: Automatic segmentation with our method. Bottom row: Manual segmentation.

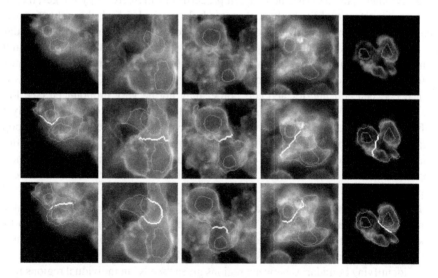

Fig. 2. Five worst outliers from evaluation set, as measured by distance between manual and automatic segmentation boundaries. Internal shapes are seed regions, taken from manual segmentation of nuclei, and are the same in both rows. Bold lines show cell/cell boundaries that are compared. Top row: Cell images, with nuclei outlined. Middle row: Automatic segmentation with our method. Bottom row: Manual segmentation.

Another common approach is to use watershed segmentation to identify cell boundaries [1,8], however, this is often fragile. Watershed segmentation treats the image as a height field, and segments pixels according to which minimum a drop of water would flow to if placed on that pixel in the height field. Morphological operations are used to impose a limited set of minima, equivalent to our seed regions. Watershed is quite unstable, because a single noisy pixel can allow large groups of pixels to change segmentation, by creating a gap leading to a different minimum. We avoid this fragility in two ways: first, by comparing neighborhoods of pixels rather than individual pixels, and second, by including a regularization factor to provide reasonable behavior when the image data does not contain a strong enough edge between two seed regions. In the limit, our regularization approaches a 2D Voronoi segmentation, i.e., pixels are assigned to the nearest seed region measured in the image plane, without reference to image features.

Our approach is to define a metric in the image plane and to calculate distances from seed regions according to this metric. Pixels are then assigned to cells according to their distance from the corresponding nucleus under that metric. The metric uses information about image edges, both their strength and their orientation, as well as a regularization term corresponding to inter-pixel distance within the image.

2 Method

Our method operates by computing a discretized approximation of the Voronoi regions of each seed on a manifold with a metric controlled by local image features. The metric defines the incremental distance in a particular direction in the image/manifold. Its behavior is such that adjacent pixels with similar surrounds are close to one another, while pixels whose surrounds differ are treated as farther apart.

We introduce a Riemannian metric defined in terms of the image $\mathcal{I}$ and a regularization parameter λ, as

$$\mathbf{G} = \frac{\nabla \mathbf{g}(\mathcal{I}) \nabla \mathbf{g}^T(\mathcal{I}) + \lambda \mathbf{I}}{1 + \lambda}, \tag{1}$$

where $\mathbf{I}$ is the 2×2 identity matrix. The function $\mathbf{g}$ maps images to images, and in our application is generally a small-radius blur. The effect of this blur is to combine a weighted neighborhood in the gradient computation, to avoid relying too much on single (noisy) pixel values. Infinitesimal distances under $\mathbf{G}$ are measured by

$$||d\mathbf{x}||_{\mathbf{G}}^2 \equiv d\mathbf{x}^T \mathbf{G} d\mathbf{x} = \frac{(d\mathbf{x}^T \nabla \mathbf{g}(\mathcal{I}))^2 + \lambda(d\mathbf{x}^T d\mathbf{x})^2}{\lambda + 1}. \tag{2}$$

The first term in the numerator of (2), $||d\mathbf{x}^T \nabla \mathbf{g}(\mathcal{I})||^2$, increases distances measured parallel to large gradients in $\mathbf{g}(\mathcal{I})$. The regularization effect of λ can be seen by

$$\lim_{\lambda \to \infty} ||d\mathbf{x}||_{\mathbf{G}}^2 = d\mathbf{x}^T d\mathbf{x} = ||d\mathbf{x}||_2^2, \tag{3}$$

i.e., $\mathbf{G}$ becomes more Euclidean as λ increases.

Given (2), we can compute the distance between any two points in an image as the shortest path between those points. We use a discretized approximation, i.e., a chamfer distance, applied to an 8-connected neighborhood. This approximation to the distance is generally no worse than 10% of the correct value [7], which for our application is generally not more than a single pixel.

Pixels overlapping seed regions are initialized to be distance 0 from their seed, and the distances of the remaining pixels are computed by Dijkstra's algorithm [6]. Each pixel is labelled with the seed it is closest to, i.e., the Voronoi region of that seed in the manifold defined by (2). Computing the seed-to-pixel distances in this manner also makes it trivial to limit the segmentation to a predetermined foreground region (for example, the result from a global thresholding step).

The computation of Voronoi regions places the boundary between two adjacent regions at pixels that are equidistant from each seed, as measured on the manifold from (2). The inter-pixel distance is larger where the image is changing more according to $\nabla \mathbf{g}(\mathcal{I})$, so boundaries tend to align with image differences. The regularizing parameter λ allows the user to make the manifold more "flat" according to prior knowledge about region shapes, and the choice of $\mathbf{g}$ (e.g., the radius of smoothing) controls how sensitive distances are to small features. In this work, we use a narrow (3- or 5-pixel radius) Gaussian blur for $\mathbf{g}$.

2.1 Connection to Geodesic Active Contours

Our algorithm is related to Geodesic Active Contours [5]. The full details of that work are not given here, but we discuss the connection briefly.

Active contours can be seen as finding a shortest path in a Riemannian space, where distances between pixels are defined by an edge stopping function $g : \mathbb{R}^+ \to \mathbb{R}^+$.[1] Examining equation (8) from Caselles *et al.* [5] helps establish the similarity:

$$\text{Min} \int_0^1 g(|\nabla \mathcal{I}(\mathcal{C}(q))|)|\mathcal{C}'(q)|dq \qquad (4)$$

where $\mathcal{I}$ is the image, $\mathcal{C}(q)$ is the curve on image that we are minimizing over, and q is the parameter along the curve. The edge stopping function g is strictly decreasing and positive, with $g(\infty) = 0$. The effect of g's interaction with $\nabla \mathcal{I}$ is such that the minimum curve follows larger gradients in the image.

The minimization can also be written as (equation (12) of [5])

$$\text{Min} \int_0^{\mathcal{L}(\mathcal{C})} g(|\nabla \mathcal{I}(\mathcal{C}(s)|)ds \qquad (5)$$

where s is the arclength parameter for $\mathcal{C}$, and $\mathcal{L}(\mathcal{C})$ is the length of $\mathcal{C}$. Therefore, active contours can be seen as seeking a minimum length curve where the length depends on image characteristics [5].

Our goal is different from active contours, since we hope to find boundaries between regions corresponding to different seeds. However, we do seek shortest paths with a distance metric controlled by image characteristics. We do not wish to follow boundaries, as in active contours, but rather to avoid them (equivalent to making boundaries "far"

---

[1] In this subsection, g is an edge stopping function, not the same as $\mathbf{g}$ in the previous subsection.

from the seed regions in our formulation). However, just as Voronoi regions can be defined in terms of shortest paths, our segmentation algorithm can be defined in terms of shortest paths defined by equation (1) and image properties. The metrics in the two approaches differ, specifically in their treatment of edges in the image: edges in the active contour setting have a metric that makes points along the edge closer, while our metric makes the points across the edge more separated. Moreover, active contours use a directionally uniform metric, while ours is not, since it is larger across edges rather than along them. However, the goal is the same: allow the computation of inter-pixel distances that simplify the problem at hand and map it to a simpler framework. In both cases, the problem reduces to that of finding shortest paths (though this is simply a jumping-off point for active contours to more powerful and efficient methods such as level-sets).

3   Experiments and Evaluation

In order to provide insight into the behavior of the metric defined in (1), we experiment with synthetic data and adjust λ, trading off the effect of image features on the region segmentation versus the Euclidean distance from the seed. As can be seen in Figures 3 and 4, the segmentation approaches the Voronoi diagram of the seed regions (i.e., ignoring image features) as λ increases. Also, note that in the noisy example less regularization (i.e., a lower value for λ) is needed to achieve similar segmentations because the noise makes the edges in the image less pronounced than in the noise-free example. In effect, increasing noise provides a form of regularization.

Our algorithm is currently part of an automatic image cytometry program [4], and has been used in a variety of experiments with several cell types of varying morphologies. To evaluate our algorithm on real world data, we compare it to the manual segmentation of cell images. Sixteen images taken from Drosophila cells stained for DNA (to label nuclei) and Actin (a cytoskeletal protein, to show the cell body) were outlined. First, nuclei were outlined by hand. The nuclear outlines were overlaid on the cell images, and one cell per nucleus was outlined. Our algorithm was then applied to the same cell images and nuclear-outlines data, and the results compared by computing the signed distance between boundary pixels. It effectively computes the distance for each pixel in the automatic segmentation boundary to the corresponding manual segmentation boundary. Hand-outlined nuclei were used, rather than automatically segmented nuclei, since our algorithm does not address nuclei segmentation, and we want the comparison to be as meaningful as possible. In general, automatic segmentation of nuclei is fairly simple (See section 1.)

Our algorithm does not compute a foreground/background separation, but instead relies on a such a label for each pixel to be given as input. For comparing our algorithm to the manual segmentation, we compute the foreground pixels as the union of cells identified in the manual segmentation. Methods exist for automatically choosing a foreground/background labelling, but distinguishing foreground from background is not part of our algorithm.

For the purposes of this comparison, we also use seed regions from hand-outlined nuclei. In general, nuclei are more compact, separated, and brightly stained than cells,

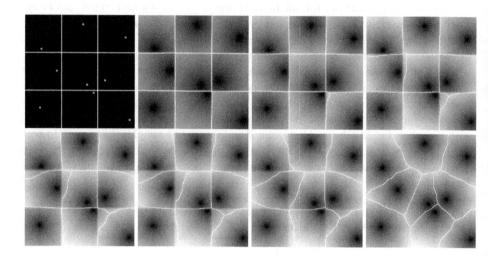

Fig. 3. Synthetic example. The input image is in the upper left, with seed sites marked with dots. From left to right across the two rows, the resulting distances calculated with our metric are shown, with the resulting segmentation overlaid white lines, for λ equal to 0.2, 0.3, 0.4, 0.5, 0.6, 0.8, and 3.0. The segmentation lines follow the ridges in the distances function. As can be seen, as λ increases, the segmentation approaches the Voronoi diagram of the seed regions.

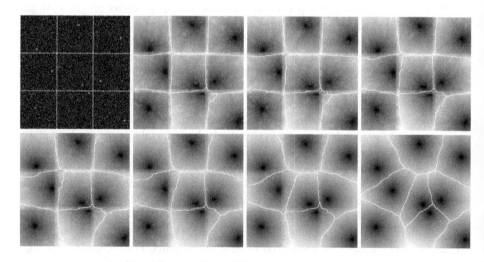

Fig. 4. Synthetic example with noise. The same input as in Figure 3 is used, with zero-mean Gaussian noise with standard deviation 0.5 added to each pixel. Edges were 1.0 and background was 0.0 before noise was added. The layout is the same as in Figure 3, but with λ equal to 0.025, 0.05, 0.075, 0.1, 0.125, 0.2, and 0.75.

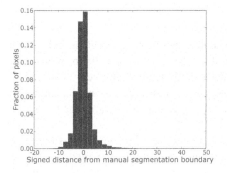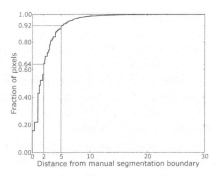

Fig. 5. Combined histogram for the signed distances and cumulative distribution of absolute distances from automatic segmentation to manual segmentation for the sixteen images in our test set

and so are usually easily segmented by simple thresholding. We chose to use the nuclei from manual segmentation in order to keep the conditions for manual segmentation and our algorithm as similar as possible.

Under these conditions, our algorithm is only responsible for computing cell-cell boundaries, rather than cell-background boundaries, which are fixed. We therefore only consider the distance between boundary pixels in the two images that have a common cell-label on either border. When evaluating the algorithm, we use the one-sided signed distance (negative inside cells) from the automatic segmentation to the manual segmentation. We set λ in (1) to 0.05 times the distance between the average foreground and background pixel intensities on a per-image basis. This value for λ was found to be close to optimal in our experiments, with fairly stable behavior for a reasonably large range (within a factor of two). Our test set includes a wide variety of cell types, with different sizes and morphologies. In general, most applications would have more homogeneous data, to which λ should be tuned.

Sixteen images made up the test set. Each image was roughly 512x512 pixels on a side, with cells roughly 25 pixels in diameter, and 80 cells per image on average. Across the entire set, there were 21.6k pixels on a cell-cell boundary in the automatic segmentation. A histogram of their signed distances with respect to the manual segmentation is shown in Figure 5. Sixty-four percent (14.0k) of the boundary pixels in the automatic segmentation are within 2 pixels in distance from the corresponding manual boundary. Ninety-two percent (19.8k) of the pixels are within 5 pixels. The accuracy of the hand-labelling is around 3 pixels, based on the width of the marker used to outline the cells.

Typical results on the test set are shown in Figure 1. We show the top 5 worst outliers from the data set, based on maximum boundary distance, in Figure 2. In some cases, the automatic method has "chosen" a different edge in the image to use as the cell-cell boundary. In others, the close proximity of the nucleus to a cell boundary has caused the automatic segmentation to move past the boundary chosen in the manual segmentation, causing large deviations between the two.

4   Discussion

In some segmentation tasks seed regions for segmentation are easily identified. Nuclei act as such seed regions in our application, the segmentation of cells in microscopy images. The more difficult task is finding the boundaries between cells that share a common border. Cell appearance in the images is not uniform, varying depending on the type of cells and the protocol used to stain them, and simplistic approaches are not sufficiently accurate or robust.

We have demonstrated an algorithm for segmentation of image regions based on seed areas that respects image boundaries as defined by a difference operator. The algorithm computes an approximation of the Voronoi region of a seed on a manifold, implicitly defined by a difference operator that operates on image neighborhoods. The only assumption that the algorithm relies on is that images change more near the borders of regions. This is similar to the behavior of Geodesic Active Contours, with an inversion in the behavior of the metrics near edges. We approximate distances using a chamfer-like difference operator, and use Dijkstra's algorithm for computing individual regions quickly.

Our algorithm is currently implemented in an automatic image cytometry package [4], and has been used successfully in several experiments with a variety of cell types and morphologies. We have compared our algorithm to manual segmentation by an expert of microscopy cell images. Our algorithm performs well. There are a few failure cases, perhaps due to the fairly simple prior on cell shape and size that our metric implies. A more complex prior could incorporate measures of, e.g., cell roundness or cell area. Although our method is more accurate for segmenting cells than others, such as using fixed offsets from nuclei or the watershed transform, the true test of its usefulness is in whether it produces more accurate measurements of cellular phenotypes. In order to understand how segmentation accuracy affects measurement accuracy, we plan to validate against data from flow cytometry or another method not based on image processing.

In the future, we would like to explore other choices for g in (1). It might also be possible to use the distance defined by our metric to compute foreground/background labellings and to detect poorly-segmented cells.

Acknowledgements

The authors would like to thank In-Han Kang for his work on validation of the algorithm, and Chris Gang for the hand-outlined nucleus and cell images.

References

1. S. Beucher "The Watershed Transformation Applied to Image Segmentation," *Scanning Microscopy International*, Vol. 6, pp.299–314, 1992.
2. Boutros M., A. Kiger, S. Armknecht, K. Kerr, M. Hild, B. Koch, S. Haas, Heidelberg Fly Array Consortium, R. Paro and N. Perrimon "Genome-wide RNAi Analysis of Cell Growth and Viability in Drosophila," *Science*, Vol. 303, pp. 832–835, 2004.

3. A.E. Carpenter and D.M. Sabatini "Systematic Genome-wide Screens of Gene Function," *Nature Reviews Genetics*, Vol. 5, pp. 11–22, 2004.
4. "CellProfiler: versatile software for high throughput image analysis," A.E. Carpenter, T.R. Jones, D.B. Wheeler, D.A. Guertin, I.H. Kang, P. Golland, and D.M. Sabatini, *in preparation.*
5. V. Caselles, R. Kimmel, and G. Sapiro "Geodesic Active Contours," *Int. J. Comput. Vision*, Vol. 22, pp. 61–79, 1997.
6. E. W. Dijkstra "A Note on Two Problems in Connection with Graphs," *Numerische Math.*, Vol. 1, pp. 269–271, 1959.
7. U. Montanari "A Method for Obtaining Skeletons Using a Quasi-Euclidean Distance," *Journal of the ACM*, Vol. 15, pp. 600-624, 1968.
8. C. Wählby "Algorithms for Applied Digital Image Cytometry," PhD Thesis, 2003

Parcellating the Intra-splenium Based on the Traced Fiber from Tractography

Gaolang Gong[1], Tianzi Jiang [1], Sheng Xie [2], and Fuchun Lin[1]

[1] National Laboratory of Pattern Recognition, Institute of Automation,
Chinese Academy of Sciences, Beijing 100080, P. R. China
{glgong, jiangtz}@nlpr.ia.ac.cn
[2] Department of Radiology, Peking University First Hospital,
Beijing 100034, P. R. China

Abstract. In this paper, we presented an indirect approach which automatically separates the splenium of corpus callosum on mid-sagittal slice of diffusion tensor image (DTI). The callosal fibers were first extracted to decide the corresponding location in the 2D splenium. Using some specific features determined from their geometric properties, the fibers crossing the splenium were clustered into three bundles, which interconnect bilateral temporal, parietal and occipital lobes, respectively. The sub-regions of the splenium were then demarcated by mapping the clusters to the splenium. Similar distribution pattern of these three sub-regions were obtained by applying our method to two real data sets, which indicated the potential applicability of this approach for the further studies of the splenium.

1 Introduction

For years, large numbers of neuroimaging studies concerned with the corpus callosum were carried out, in which some rigid partition schemes were employed to partition the callosum into several sub-regions directly on the mid-sagittal slice [1,2]. The splenium was accordingly defined as the posterior fifth part of the corpus callosum along its anterior–posterior dimension [2]. Pathological effects on the splenium have been reported in a range of neurological disorders such as Alzheimer's Disease [3]. However, the splenium does not carry homogeneous fibers connecting single functional cortical area, but contains several fiber groups connecting the bilateral temporal, parietal and occipital lobes, respectively [1]. The sub-regions of the splenium in terms of the cortical connectivity may provide more specific information of splenium, and these sub-regions can be used as ROI definition and further taken as separated factors in related studies, which would help to understand the underlying meaning of their changes.

The geometric characteristics of fiber groups connecting distinct cortical areas were supposed to be different, which can be used to distinguish different fiber groups. Previous anatomical studies employed some tracers to separate different fiber groups, but these methods were time-consuming and limited to the animal and postmortem study. Recently, the advent of diffusion tensor imaging (DTI) made it possible to study different white matter tracts in human brain, non-invasively [4].

Y. Liu, T. Jiang, and C. Zhang (Eds.): CVBIA 2005, LNCS 3765, pp. 544 – 550, 2005.
© Springer-Verlag Berlin Heidelberg 2005

As a relatively new MRI technique, diffusion tensor imaging can provide information about the diffusion of water molecules in the brain tissue [4], and it has become the preferred modality for the white matter studies. Tracking algorithms based on DTI have been widely developed to reconstruct the white matter tracts, called tractography [5,6,7]. Very recently, some research works have been dedicated to further application of the traced fiber from DTI tractography. For example, some investigations clustering the traced fibers to bundles are emerging [8,9,10]. On the other hand, the property analysis of white matter tracts has also been extensively studied in the assessment of a wide variety of degenerative, neurological, psychiatric and developmental disorders using DTI [11]. These existing researches were mainly based on the manual ROI-drawing. In contrast, some groups have proposed some fiber-based methods analyzing the white matter property along the traced fiber [12,13].

In this paper, we attempt to use the information of 3D tract from DTI to parcellate intra-splenium structures. The fibers crossing the splenium are first reconstructed from tractography. Then some relative simple features are determined from the traced fiber, which are the positions of start-point, end-point and centroid point. Based on these specific features, k-means clustering is employed to ascertain the clusters of fibers. The clusters are then mapped to the 2D mid-sagittal slice to obtain the sub-regions of the splenium.

2 Materials and Method

In our experiment, 3D diffusion-weighted data was acquired with single-shot echo planar imaging (EPI) sequence from a 1.5-Tesla MR scanner (GE signa 1.5T Twin-speed). The diffusion sensitizing gradients were applied along 13 non-collinear directions with b-value=1000 s/mm^2, together with an acquisition without diffusion weighting (b-value = 0). The acquisition parameters were as follows: Time of Repetition (TR)=10s; Time of Echo (TE)=85ms; matrix=128×128; FOV=22×22cm; Number of excitation (NEX)=4; slice thickness=3mm without gap. The data was interpolated to 1×1×1 mm for further process.

2.1 Reconstruction of Fiber Crossing Splenium from Tractography

The diffusion tensor field was calculated from the diffusion-weighted image according to the Stejskal and Tanner Equation [14]. The eigenvector corresponding to the largest eigenvalue was assumed to represent the orientation of local white matter tract (i.e. principal direction). Here, the tracking algorithm proposed by Lazar *et al.* [15] was applied to reconstruct the fibers crossing splenium. It can be briefly summarized as follows: First, corpus callosum was drawn out manually on the color-map [16] of the mid-sagittal slice from DTI dataset. Then splenium was determined. And seed points distributed regularly were defined in each pixel of the splenium. The tracking algorithm moved a fixed distance (in this case 0.2mm) along the principal direction from each seed point. With diffusion tensor deflection, new diffusion orientation was estimated from the continuous tensor field at this new position, the algorithm then moved the distance towards the new orientation. The movement continued until the FA was below some threshold (in this case, 0.2). The algorithm parameters were:

deflection operator $n = 2$, $\alpha_1 = 1, \alpha_2 = \alpha_3 = 0.5$ (Eq.(3)of the Lazar *et al.*); $f = 0.5$, $g = 0.5$ (Eq.(4) of the Lazar *et al.*). A traced fiber f_i was represented by a set of ordered 3D points p_k^i with total number N_i and intuitively parameterized by arc-length, the fiber set Ω crossing splenium for each subject was as follows:

$$\Omega = \{ f_i \, ; i = 1, \cdots, M \} \quad where \, f_i = \{ p_k^i \, ; k = 1, \cdots, N_i \}$$

2.2 Determining the Features Specific to the Traced Fiber Crossing Splenium

Although most of callosal fibers interconnect homologous hemispheric cortical areas, there exist a substantial number of heterotopic connections, ending in asymmetrical cortical areas [17]. Therefore, only unilateral splenium fibers were extracted to determine the features. Here, we chose the traced fibers traveling in the right hemisphere.

Feature 1: Start-Point of the Fiber
The start-point (i.e. *seed point*) position and end-point position were important properties for a traced fiber. The start-point indicates the location of one fiber on the mid-sagittal slice of splenium. Naturally, the start-points are supposed to be close to each other in the splenium when the fibers connect homologous cortical area and are assigned to the same cluster. The Euclidean distance D_s between the start-points of a pair of fibers (f_i, f_j) was hereby defined to measure the location closeness of these fibers in the 2D splenium:

$$D_s(f_i, f_j) = \left\| p_1^i - p_1^j \right\|, \, \| \cdot \| \text{ is the Euclidean norm}$$

Feature 2: End-Point of the Fiber
The end-point is the direct indicator of the cortical areas connected by this fiber, which is the essential information of connectivity for the fiber clusters. The Euclidean distance D_e between end-points was consequently assigned to measure the homogeneousness of cortical areas connected by a pair of fibers (f_i, f_j). Actually, the callosal fibers travel coherently near the mid-sagittal slice, and become increasingly dispersed when the fibers extend toward to the cortex. Therefore, significant difference between the different fiber bundles would be diminished when using the end-point near the cortex. For this reason, the segment beyond a fixed length (in this case 60mm, i.e. *300 steps with length of 0.2mm*) of the traced fibers was removed to obtain the resulted end-point. The remained part of each fiber would keep the significant difference between different fiber bundles if using its end-point position.

$$D_e(f_i, f_j) = \left\| p_{N_i}^i - p_{N_j}^j \right\| \quad \text{with} \quad N_i = \begin{cases} 300 & N_i \geq 300 \\ N_i & N_i < 300 \end{cases}$$

Feature 3: Centroid of the Fiber
Apart from the features above, the shape of the traced fiber should also be considered. However, the shape description for a 3D curve is a very difficult issue. Here, a crude

measure for the shape description, the position of centroid for a 3D curve, was adopted. The shape distance D_c was defined as the Euclidean distance of the paired centroids between a pair of fiber (f_i, f_j). Actually, the reconstructed fibers were variable in length. In this case, the Euclidean distance of centroids between two fibers was absolutely increased by the difference of the fibers length. To overcome this problem, the corresponding segment of the longer fiber was determined by searching the equal length to the shorter fiber. Then Euclidean distance of centroids between the shorter fiber and corresponding segment of the longer fiber was calculated as the shape difference of the two fibers:

$$D_c(f_i, f_j) = \left\| C^i - C^j \right\|$$

with
$$\begin{cases} C^i = mean(f_i') \ with \ f_i' = \{ p_k^i \ ; k = 1, \cdots, N_j \} \\ C^j = mean(f_j) \end{cases} \quad when \ N_i \geq N_j$$

$$\begin{cases} C^i = mean(f_i) \\ C^j = mean(f_j') \ with \ f_j' = \{ p_k^j \ ; k = 1, \cdots, N_i \} \end{cases} \quad when \ N_i \geq N_j$$

Distance Between a Pair of Fibers Crossing Splenium

Two fibers were defined to be similar if they had similar geometric shape and their start-points (and end-points as well) were located very close. Based on the above selected feature, the distance D of two fibers was defined as the sum of those distances with a weighted factor respectively:

$$D = \alpha_s * D_s + \alpha_e * D_e + \alpha_c * D_c$$

2.3   Clustering the Traced Fiber

Based on the distance defined above, the classical K-means method was used to cluster the fibers [18]. The splenium anatomically carries the fibers connecting three different (*i.e.* parietal, occipital and temporal) lobes; the number of clusters was hence

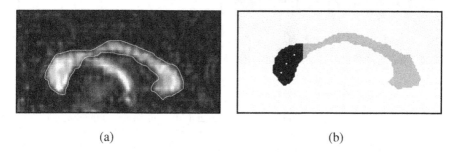

(a)   (b)

Fig. 1. (a): the FA-map of mid-sagittal slice from DTI dataset. (b) The illustration for the initial fiber location: Three white landmarks denoted the three initial fibers while the splenium was marked by black.

defined as three. Another problem in the K-means method is the determination of the initial centers whose location would affect the results. In this study, we chose the three initial fibers distributed uniformly along the superior-inferior and anterior-posterior dimension of splenium (**Fig.1**.b). The clusters of the fibers were then mapped to the 2D splenium in terms of their seed-points.

3 Results

The method was tested on two DTI data sets acquired from two subjects. All algorithms were implemented in Matlab. The results, including sub-regions and their. corresponding unilateral fibers, were demonstrated in **Fig. 2** Three clusters, corresponding to parietal, occipital and temporal lobe, were illustrated by black, white and gray, respectively.

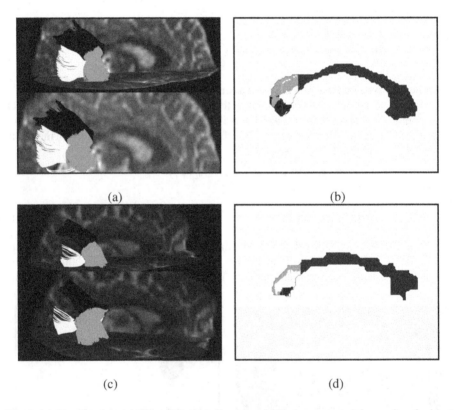

Fig. 2. (a): Top (*i.e.* (a) and (b)) and Bottom (*i.e.* (c) and (d)) demonstrated the results of subject 1 and subject 2, respectively. Left (*i.e.* (a) and (c)): the reconstructed fibers crossing the splenium using tracking algorithm, and the fibers were illustrated with 2 different viewing angles (up and down) for each subject. The fibers in the same cluster were displayed with the same intensity. Right (*i.e.* (b) and (d)): the sub-regions of splenium. The sub-regions were also marked with the same intensity corresponding to their fibers.

4 Discussions and Conclusion

This study proposed an indirect framework parcellating the intra-splenium based on the hypothesis that fiber groups crossing the splenium connecting distinct cortical areas can be distinguished with their geometric and spatial information. Under consideration of the special structure of unilateral fibers initiated from the 2D splenium, the start-point, end-point and centroid were chosen as the features when searching the distance between fibers. The fibers were assigned to the same cluster when these features were close to each other. The clusters were then mapped to the splenium and sub-regions were extracted.

Previous anatomical study demonstrated that the splenium carries fibers connecting temporal, parietal and occipital lobes, which help to determine the fiber cluster number clearly. In fact, the parcellating framework in this paper can be directly extrapolated to the subdivision of the total corpus callosum. However, the issue has not been carried out here because determining the sub-regions number of the total corpus callosum is another crucial research task and beyond the scope of this research.

The real DTI data sets of two subjects were tested with our approach. The results demonstrated similar distribution pattern of the three sub-regions in the two datasets, which would validate our method to some extent. The sub-region associated with parietal, occipital and temporal lobe (marked by black, white and gray, respectively in **Fig.2**) was located in the dorsal, posterior-ventral and anterior-ventral splenium, respectively. The fibers connecting bilateral parietal lobes travel like a forceps with superior-posterior orientation, while the fibers connecting bilateral occipital lobe orient posteriorly. The fibers connecting bilateral temporal lobe are called tapetum anatomically, which travel along the inferior orientation and form the roof of part of the lateral ventricle of the brain.

The results also showed that there were some outliers for each cluster, which might attribute to noise (*i.e.* false fiber reconstructed by the tracking algorithm). Noted that our method was highly dependent on the tracking algorithm, whose validation is still a challenge in the DTI field. Moreover, since the existing tracking algorithm cannot settle down the bifurcation problem [6], bifurcation of fibers near the boundary of different sub-regions of splenium would produce errors. The errors might be the factor resulting in the ratio difference of three sub-regions observed between the two subjects. Improvement of tracking algorithm and image quality would improve the robustness of our method.

In conclusion, the novel framework was presented to parcellate the intra-structure of spenium and our preliminary experiment demonstrated the validity of this method. The extracted sub-regions would provide more detailed information of the splenium and can be further applied to explore the functions of distinct parts of splenium. Furthermore, analysis based on different fiber groups crossing splenium can be performed.

Acknowledgements

The authors would like to thank Xiaobo Li for her carefully proof-read the final version of the manuscript and to Yong He, Chaozhe Zhu and Fang Qian for their comments and support for this work. This work was partially supported by the Natural

Science Foundation of China, Grant Nos. 30425004 and 60121302, and the National Key Basic Research and Development Program (973), Grant No. 2004CB318107.

References

1. Thompson PM, Narr KL, Blanton RE, Toga AW: Mapping structural alterations of the corpus callosum during brain development and degeneration. In: Zaidel E, Iacoboni M, editors. The parallel brain: the cognitive neuroscience of the corpus callosum. Cambridge, MA: MIT Press. 93–130 (2002)
2. Witelson SF: Hand and sex differences in the isthmus and genu of the human corpus callosum. A postmortem morphological study. Brain 112 (1989) 799–835
3. Lyoo IK, Satlin A, Lee CK, Renshaw PF: Regional atrophy of the corpus callosum in subjects with Alzheimer's disease and multi-infarct dementia. Psychiatry Res 74 (1997) 63–72
4. Basser P and Pierpaoli C: Microstructural and physiological features of tissues elucidated by quantitative-diffusion-tensor MRI. J Magn Reson, B 111 (1996) 209–219
5. Conturo TE, Lori NF, Cull TS, Akbudak E, Snyder AZ, Shimony JS, Mckinstry RC, Burton H and Raichle ME: Tracking neuronal fiber pathways in the living human brain. Proc Natl Acad Sci USA, 96 (1999) 10422–7
6. Mori S, Fiber tracking: principles and strategies – a technical review. NMR in Biomedicine 15 (2002) 468–480
7. Xu D, Mori S, Solaiyappan M, van Zijl PCM, and Davatzikos C: An framework for callosal fiber distribution analysis. Neuroimage 17 (2002) 1131–1143
8. Ding Z, Gore JC, and Anderson AW: Classification and quantification of neuronal fiber pathways using diffusion tensor MRI. Mag Reson Med. 49 (2003) 716–721
9. Brun A, Knutsson H, Park HJ, Shenton ME, Westin CF: Clustering Fiber Traces Using Normalized Cuts. In: Medical Image Computing and Computer-Assisted Inter-vention (MICCAI 2004) 368–375
10. Corouge I, Gouttard S, Gerig G: A Statistical Shape Model of Individual Fiber Tracts Extracted from Diffusion Tensor MRI. In: Medical Image Computing and Computer-Assisted Inter-vention (MICCAI 2004) 671–679
11. Kubicki M, Westin CF, Maier SE, Mamata H, Frumin M, Ersner-Hershfield H, Kikinis R, Jolesz FA, McCarley R and Shenton ME: Diffusion Tensor Imaging and Its Application to Neuropsychiatric Disorders. Harvard Rev Psychiatry November/December (2002) 324–336
12. Fillard P, Gilmore J, Piven J, Lin WL and Gerig G (2003): Quantitative Analysis of White Matter Fiber Properties along Geodesic Paths. In: Medical Image Computing and Computer-Assisted Inter-vention (MICCAI2003) 16–23
13. Gong GL, Jiang TZ, Zhu CZ, Zang YF, Wang F, Xie S, JX Xiao and XM Guo: Asymmetry analysis of cingulum based on scale-invariant parameterization by diffusion tensor imaging. Human Brain Mapping 24 (2005) 92–98
14. Stejskal EO, Tanner JE: Spin diffusion measurements: spin echoes in the presence of a time-dependent field gradient. J Chem Phys 42 (1965) 288–292
15. Lazar M, Weinstein DM, Tsuruda JS, Hasan KM, Arfanakis K, Meyerand ME, Badie B, Rowley HA, Haughton V, Field A, Alexander AL: White Matter Tractography Using Diffusion Tensor Deflection. Human Brain Mapping 18 (2003) 306 –321
16. Pajevic S, Pierpaoli C: Color schemes to represent the orientation of anisotropic tissues from diffusion tensor data: application to white matter. Magn Reson Med 42(1999) 526–540
17. Nolte J: The human Brain: An introduction to its Functional Anatomy, Mosby (1999)
18. Duda RO, Hart PE, Stork DG: Pattern classification. 2nd Edition, John Wiley & Sons (2000)

Motion Compensation and Plane Tracking for Kinematic MR-Imaging

Daniel Bystrov, Vladimir Pekar, Kirsten Meetz, Heinrich Schulz,
and Thomas Netsch

Philips Research, Röntgenstr. 24-26, D-22335 Hamburg, Germany

Abstract. The acquisition of time series of 3D MR images is becoming feasible nowadays, which enables the assessment of bone and soft tissue in normal and abnormal joint motion. Fast two-dimensional (2D) scanning of moving joints may also provide high temporal resolution but is limited to a single, predefined slice. Acquiring 3D time series has the advantage that after the acquisition image processing and visualization techniques can be used to reformat the images to any orientation and to reduce the through-plane motion and undesired gross motion superimposed on the relevant joint movement. In this publication, we first review such post-processing techniques for retrospective tracking of viewing planes according to a single moving rigid body (e.g. bone). Then, we present new numerical schemes for optimally tracking viewing planes according to the movement of multiple structures to compensate for their through-as well as in-plane motion. These structures can be specified in an interactive viewing program, and the motion compensated movies can be updated and displayed in real-time. The post-processing algorithms require a 4D motion-field estimation which also can be utilized to interpolate intermediate images to present the final movies in smooth cine-loops and to significantly improve the visual perceptibility of complex joint movement.

1   Introduction

Starting in the late eighties, MRI has been used for imaging of moving joints [11,16]. Most approaches were based on fast 2D imaging, which limited the studies to a single predefined view of a few anatomical structures. In addition, in order to keep the anatomy of interest stable within the imaging plane, devices are needed to restrain a part of the joint [7], thereby limiting the freedom of movements. As a result, pathological behaviour in the kinematics of the investigatated structures may be reduced or completely suppressed. For better diagnostic value of kinematic MR studies, unrestricted patient motion inside the scanner is preferable.

In contrast to relatively tight cylindrical scanners, the new generation of open MRI-systems facilitate kinematic orthopedic studies, since the motion of a patient is much less limited by the design of the magnet. Also the aquisition and reconstruction time is constantly improving; currently the time for aquiring a high resolution 3D volume (e.g. $256^2 \times 100$) is between 10 and 60 seconds. For the acquisition of real-time joint motions active markers can be used, which can be located

Y. Liu, T. Jiang, and C. Zhang (Eds.): CVBIA 2005, LNCS 3765, pp. 551–560, 2005.

inside the aquisition loop of the MRI-system, see e.g. [1,4]. Because such markers are attached from outside to the patient's skin, this results in fat and skin sliding artifacts, see [6,10]. Therefore, the markers only give an orientation for the exact position of the inspected joint and small in- and through plane motion occur. Thus, in either case a post-processing of kinematic 3D datasets is essential for the acceptance and benefit of kinematic time series of moving joints in the clinical routine. Simply presenting the original slice data in a cine-loop will still be compromised by through-plane displacements of the anatomy and "jerks" between frames, both of which hamper the visual analysis of the movement.

In this publication, the retrospective tracking of a viewing plane and selection of the coordinate system inside the viewing plane in order to compensate the in- and though plane motion of one or more anatomical structures through time-series of 3D MR datasets is presented. The method does not require the segmentation of these anatomical structures but is based on an estimation of a continous motion field obtained by elastic image registration of the sequence of volumes. The result of this registration can also be utilized for the interpolation of intermediate frames in order to present the motion compensated movies in smooth cine-loops. The registration of a sequence of volumes is a computationally expensive task and should be done in a separate, offline step. After that, the motion compensation algorithms and also the frame interpolation technique can be computed in real-time while presenting the result in a viewing interface. The user can then interactively specify the anatomical structures whose motion should be compensated; see [9,15].

For the development and presentation of the viewing and motion compensation functionality, time series of 3D-volumes were used, which were simulated by acquiring sequences of stepwise moved resting joints. Surely, for the clinical applications of the presented functionalities the real-time acquisition of active joints is required, see e.g. [3].

The paper is organized as follows: in section 2, the post-processing algorithms for kinematic 4D MRI data sets are described. First, elastic image registration is used for the estimation of the motion. Afterwards, the resulting motion fields are used for the smooth interpolation of intermediate frames and for the compensation of motion for a single rigid body. Then the motion field is utilized to separately compensate through- and in-plane motion in the presence of multiple non-rigidly moving structures (e.g. multiple bones). In section 3, the quality of the motion estimation is analyzed as well as the motion compensation using several kinematic datasets. Finally, the integration of the presented algorithms in a prototype for an interactive viewing software for kinematic 4D data is described.

2   Post-processing of 4D Time Series

2.1   Motion Field Estimation with Image Registration

The registration of two images is defined as finding a correspondence mapping for each point of a reference image on an anatomically corresponding point in a target image. The registration task for sequences of kinematic images of joints and soft tissue is motivated by the conservation of intensity: It is assumed, that a grey value of a particle is constant along its trajectory.

For a sequence of time steps $t_0 < t_1 < \ldots < t_N$ and gray scale images $I_i := I(t_i) : \Omega \mapsto \mathbf{R}$ of a field of view $\Omega \subset \mathbf{R}^3$, we are looking for spatial transformations $T_i := T(t_i) : \Omega \mapsto \mathbf{R}^3$, which minimize the distance between I_i and I_{i+1}. A suitable distance function for subsequent images of a kinematic study is the sum of squared differences:

$$dist_{\text{SSD}}(\Omega, I, J) := \frac{1}{|\Omega|} \int\limits_{p \in \Omega} |I(p) - J(p)|^2 dp. \tag{1}$$

Then, for a given transformation space $\mathcal{T}$ the minimizing transformation yields the required correspondence mapping

$$T_i := \operatorname*{argmin}_{T \in \mathcal{T}} dist_{\text{SSD}}(\Omega, I_i \circ T, I_{i+1}). \tag{2}$$

Since the field of view Ω is a bounded domain, parts of the anatomy can leave or enter it. In such cases boundary conditions in (1) are very important for the global registration result. One possibility to compensate for missing image information at the boundaries could be a model of the anatomy or the image beyond the boundary: e.g. the extent of the image I_i with a black surrounding. Another solution for the boundary value problem is, to exclude the boundary from the computation in (1):

$$T_i := \operatorname*{argmin}_{T \in \mathcal{T}} dist_{\text{SSD}}(T(\Omega) \cap \Omega, I_i \circ T, I_{i+1}). \tag{3}$$

The range of the transformation space $\mathcal{T}$ needs to be limited, in order to prevent that the domain $T(\Omega) \cap \Omega$ gets too small. This is equivalent to a limit of the maximal expected velocity of the observed objects.

For the motion estimation in kinematic studies, two different types of transformation spaces were tested: Firstly, a B-spline registration approach as described in [8,14]. The algorithm uses a dual multiscale method: the image is downsampled in a hierarchy of images and also the B-spline transformation space is organized hierarchically. Secondly, elastic deformation fields were used, which model the transformations as the effect from a set of localized Gaussian forces with adaptable location, strength and elastic properties applied to an infinite elastic medium [12].

The numerical minimization of (3) can be done efficiently with a local optimization technique, which is applicable, if the images are sufficiently "close" and the motion between two frames is limited. For the examples shown here, the Levenberg-Marquard optimization [13] was used.

2.2   Generating Additional Frames Using Motion Interpolation

For the improvement of the visual quality of the motion, the registration field as described in the previous section can be used to interpolate intermediate frames

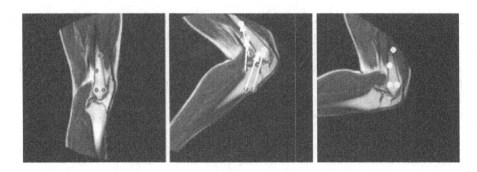

Fig. 1. Sequence of moving knee (femur, patella, tibia) 1) Landmarks are placed in the first frame (femur). 2) Motion of landmarks is estimated. 3) Viewing plane is adapted to avoid motion of landmarks.

between acquired images, analogous to B-frames in MPEG-streams, which are basically a linear interpolation of the gray values along the estimated trajectories [5]. For two consecutive frames $I_i = I(t_i)$ and $I_{i+1} = I(t_{i+1})$ an intermediate frame

$$I(t) := (1 - t) \cdot I_i \circ T'(t) + t \cdot I_{i+1} \circ T''(t) \qquad (4)$$

at time $t \in [t_i,\ t_{i+1}[$ can be estimated using two intermediate motion fields $T'(t),\ T''(t) : \Omega \mapsto \mathbf{R}^3$ with

$$T''(t) \circ T_i = T'(t) := \mathsf{id} + t \cdot (T_i - \mathsf{id}). \qquad (5)$$

The transformation $T''(t)$ can be approximated linearly with a first order inversion of the motion field estimation T_i of the elastic image registration

$$T''(t) \approx \mathsf{id} - (1 - t) \cdot (T_i - \mathsf{id}). \qquad (6)$$

Together with (4) and (5) this yields an approximation for the intermediate frame, depending only on the acquired volumes and the estimation of the motion field T_i between these volumes:

$$\begin{aligned} I(t) \approx \quad & (1 - t) \cdot I_i \circ (\mathsf{id} + t \cdot (T_i - \mathsf{id})) \\ & + t \cdot I_{i+1} \circ (\mathsf{id} - (1 - t) \cdot (T_i - \mathsf{id})). \end{aligned} \qquad (7)$$

If the motion field T_i is properly estimated, (7) will not only crossfade between the images, but also transports edges along piecewise linear trajectories, smoothing the frame transitions, which enhances the visual quality of the resulting videos.

2.3   Homogeneous Motion Compensation for Previously Selected Landmarks

The display of joint movements in the original acquisition slice orientation is compromised by through- as well as in-plane motion and provides a confusing impression for the viewer. It is therefore desirable to automatically adjust the viewing plane according to the motion of previously selected anatomical structures. This virtually fixes those structures in the resulting video. The structures of interest are specified by a set of landmarks, and their motion is compensated by tracking these landmarks using the estimated motion field as described in section 2.1. This approach can easily be integrated in a user interface enabling the interactive selection and variation of structures of interest whose motion should be compensated.

The motion compensation algorithm is applied iteratively to derive coordinate systems for all frames starting from an initial frame. The method is illustrated for selecting a coordinate system in the second frame, starting from the first frame. A right-handed Euclidean coordinate system (c, N) is defined by a center $c \in \mathbf{R}^3$ and an orthogonal matrix $N \in \mathbf{R}^{3 \times 3}$ with $N^t N = I$ and $\det(N) = 1$. Given a coordinate system (c, N), a finite set $P \subset \mathbf{R}^3$ of landmarks in the first frame, and the location $T(P) \subset \mathbf{R}^3$ of these landmarks in the subsequent frame, we are looking for an Euclidean coordinate system (c', N'), so that the following expression is minimized:

$$\underset{(N', c')}{\operatorname{argmin}} \sum_{p \in P} \| N' \cdot (T(p) - c') - N \cdot (p - c) \|_2^2 \tag{8}$$

In [2] an explicit solution for the minimization of (8) using a singular-value decomposition is given. Since the cost for the minimization of (8) is marginal (for a moderate number of points), the coordinate systems can be computed while reformatting the 3D-volumes and displaying the movie.

2.4   Separating In-Plane from Through-Plane Motion

Using the method for selecting viewing coordinate systems as descibed in the previous section, the motion of rigid bodies can be compensated by locating three or more points on these structures; e.g. the femur in a study of the human knee. In more complex scenes with elastic structures or independently moving rigid bodies, e.g. a kinematic study of the shoulder, one may want to suppress the through-plane motion of the humerus without compensating the rotational in-plane motion of the upper arm; see figure 4. In order to achieve this, one needs to differently compensate the two motion components. With a small modification of the minimization term (8), one can formulate an adequate minimization problem. In contrast to minimizing the global motion of the landmarks P, only the motion perpendicular to the current viewing plane is compensated. We are then looking for a Hessian-representation of the viewing plane $N'_{.,3} \cdot p - d'_z = 0$, $p \in P$, of the subsequent frame, which minimizes:

$$\sum_{p \in P} (N'_{.,3} \cdot T(p) - d'_3 - N_{.,3} \cdot (p - c))^2. \tag{9}$$

After the computation of the viewing plane (with parameters $d'_3 \in \mathbf{R}$, $N'_{.,3} \in \mathbf{R}^3$ with $\| N'_{.,3} \|_2 = 1$) the 2D-coordinate system inside the viewing plane can be adjusted, so that the in-plane motion of a second finite list $Q \subset \mathbf{R}^3$ of landmarks is compensated by minimizing:

$$\sum_{q \in Q} (N'_{.,1} \cdot T(q) - d'_1 - N_{.,1} \cdot (q - c))^2$$
$$+ (N'_{.,2} \cdot T(q) - d'_2 - N_{.,2} \cdot (q - c))^2. \tag{10}$$

Because of the orthogonality conditions $N'^t N' = I$, this can be solved with a 2D version of a rigid pointset-registration technique as described in [2]. Then, the center c' of the coordinate system is $c' = N' \cdot d'$.

If the points in P are colinear, the solution of (9) is not unique. Furthermore, the direction of $N'_{.,3}$ is not unique, if the points in P or $T(P)$ are coplanar. For a small number of landmarks P and Q these singularities will lead to confusing and "uncontrollable" flipping of the coordinate axis. It is therefore easier to combine the optimization tasks (9) and (10) in a single minimization by a weighted sum:

$$\operatorname*{argmin}_{(c',N')} \sum_{p \in P} \|D_p \cdot ((N' \cdot (T(p) - c') - N \cdot (p - c))\|_2^2. \tag{11}$$

D_p are diagonal matrices $D_p = \operatorname{diag}(\omega_p^{\mathsf{in}}, \omega_p^{\mathsf{in}}, \omega_p^{\mathsf{out}})$, with nonnegative weights $\omega_p^{\mathsf{in}}, \omega_p^{\mathsf{out}} \geq 0$, which separately penalize in-plane- and through-plane motion of the points $p \in P$.

An explicit formula for the minimizing center c', in dependance on the coordinates N', can be found by setting the derivative of (11) to zero and using $I = N' \cdot N'^t$:

$$c' = N'^t \cdot D^{-1} \sum_{p \in P} D_p^t D_p (N'T(p) - N(p - c)) \quad \text{with} \quad D = \sum_{p \in P} D_p^2. \tag{12}$$

The orthognal matrix N' can be expressed in terms of three angles and thus (11) has three optimization parameters. The minimum of (11) can be approximated using a gradient based optimization algorithm, e.g. the Levenberg-Marquard method as described in [13], which converges rapidly for a moderate numbers of points (less then 0.1 sec on a 1.8 GHz Pentium for 10 landmarks).

3   Results

The approach has been tested for different 4D kinematic MR data sets of the knee and the shoulder (acquired with a Philips Intera 1.5 T and Philips Panorama 1 T scanner). The MR datasets were obtained using T1-weighted 3D gradient echo sequences for seven different positions of the studied joint. The spatial resolution of the knee images were $1.6^2 \times 5 \, \mathrm{mm}^3$ ($256^2 \times 36$ voxels) and the shoulder images $1^2 \times 1.8 \, \mathrm{mm}^3$ ($256^2 \times 100$ voxels).

3.1   Image Registration

For the image registration with B-splines the knee sequences were downsampled into three and the shoulder sequences into four hierarchical levels. The same

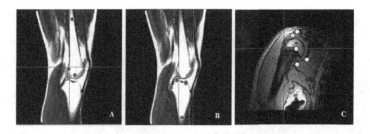

Fig. 2. Sets of reference points of A) femur, B) tibia and C) shoulder

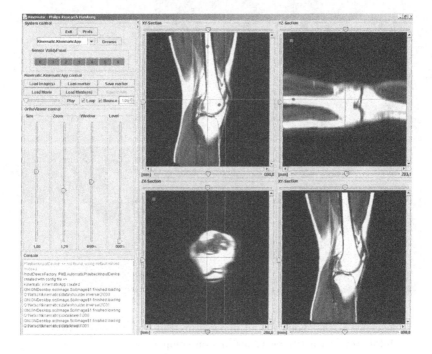

Fig. 3. User interface of the kinematic viewing station

number of levels was used for the multiscale pyramid for the transformation space. The highest level for the knee images consisted of 8^3 B-spline nodes and 16^3 for the shoulder images. The image registration method with localized Gaussian forces was applied in both cases with $3^2 \times 2$ control points for the forces initially starting with an equidistant grid. The qualitative results as well as the computational costs with this transformation space are comparable with the B-spline registration approach.

The quality of the motion field estimation has been analyzed in detail in [9,15]. Here, two aspects of the resulting motion fields were tested: first, the sequence of images was registered in the positive time direction, then the sequence was reversed and again registered. Then, several landmarks were manually

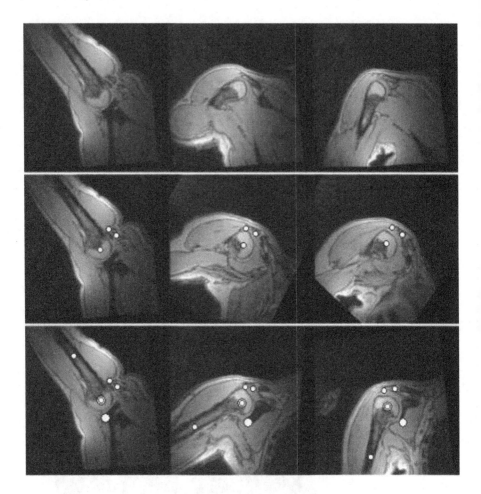

Fig. 4. Sequence of the shoulder and upper arm. Top row: without motion compensation. Middle row: with homogeneous motion compensation as described in section 2.3; the humerus leaves the plane and the chest rotates. Bottom row: Humerus stays in plane as well as the selected acromion; the smaller points ($\omega_p^{in} = 0$, $\omega_p^{out} = 1$) specify anatomical structures which should stay inside the viewing plane; the bigger points ($\omega_p^{in} = 1$, $\omega_p^{out} = 0$) in the chest and at the cap of the humerus prevent the motion of the chest within the viewing plane.

located in the first frame of the sequences as shown in figure 2. These landmarks were transported first in positive time direction, and afterwards backwards using the registrations of the reversed image sequence. Finally, the distances of the resulting positions were compared to the original set. Using seven images for a time sequence the mean Euclidean error for the 12 registration steps is about 0.5 mm and the maximum error is about 1 mm per landmark per registration. Thus, the error for the specified landmarks is in the order of the image resolution.

The second evaluation was a test for the rigidity of the elastic registration fields at the bones. For that purpose several sets of landmarks were located in the first frame of the knee, as well as in the ligaments of the shoulder sequence. The landmarks were transported with the elastic deformation field and afterwards the rigid component of the motion was computed as explained in section 2.3. The mean error of this correction step was about 0.5 mm and for the shoulder ligaments about 1.2 mm per landmark, which was also in the order of the image resolution.

3.2   Interactive Motion Compensated Viewing Software

As depicted in figure 3, the motion compensation and interpolation algorithms were integrated in a program for interactively inspecting 4D kinematic data sets. A detailed description of this software and the integration of the motion compensation algorithm for a single rigid body (as described in section 2.3) can be found in [9,15]. The program consists of three windows, with the common orthoviewer functionality, allowing to navigate through a 3D volume. In a forth window at the lower right a movie of the kinematic sequence is displayed. In the orthoviewer windows the set P of landmarks can interactively be placed in 3D. If the set P of landmarks is changed or the viewing parameters of the upper left window is changed the movie is immediately updated without visible delay. The weights for penalizing in- and through plane motion can be adjusted interactively for each landmark separately: In- and through-plane motion for a landmark can be ajusted in the range of ω_p^{in}, $\omega_p^{out} \in [0, 1]$ and the resulting movies change continously and controllably with moderate changes of these weights.

The usability of the tools has been validated by clinical experts, who have reported that the tool enables a good immobilization of all interesting anatomical structures and that the interactive viewing program allows unprecedented insights into a joint's kinematic behaviour.

4   Conclusion

In conclusion, elastic image registration has successfully been utilized for estimating a motion field in time series of 4D kinematic data sets. The motion field is used to compensate the motion of user selected landmarks, and to dynamically adjust the viewing plane according to the motion of the landmarks. Furthermore the motion field is employed to cross-fade between acquired volumes and to present the final movies in smooth cine-loops. The algorithms which are based on the motion field estimation, are computationally efficient and have been integrated in a viewing workstation that facilitates viewing of 4D kinematic data sets. It allows to observe any user defined anatomical structure from any view point in real-time. Unrestricted from any pre-defined view point, the clinical expert is able to examine and to fixate any anatomical structure during the movement of the joint.

References

1. Ackerman, J.L., et al.: Rapid 3D tracking of small RT coils. In: Proc. 5th Annual Meeting SMRM, (1986) 1131
2. Arun, K.S., et al.:   Least-Squares Fitting of Two 3-D Point Sets.   IEEE Trans. Pat. Anal. Mach. Intell. **9** (1987) 698–700
3. Brossmann, J., et al.: Patellar tracking patterns during active and passive knee extension: evaluation with motion-triggered cine mr imaging. Radiology **187** (1993) 205–212
4. Dumoulin, C.L., et al.: Real-time position monitoring of invasive devices using magnetic resonance. Magnetic Resonance in Medicine **29** (1993) 411–415
5. Le Gall, D.: MPEG: A video compression standard for multimedia applications. Commun. ACM **34** (1991) 46–58
6. Gilles, B., et al.: Bone motion analysis from dynamic MRI: acquisition and tracking. Proc. Int. Conf. on Medical Image Computing and Computer Assisted Intervention (MICCAI) (2004) 942–949
7. Hodge, D.K., et al.: Dynamic MR imaging and testing in glenohumeral instability. J. Magn. Reson. Imaging. **13** (2001) 748–756
8. Kabus, S., et al.: B-spline registration of 3D images with Levenberg-Marquardt optimization. Proc. SPIE Medical Imaging (2004) 304–313
9. Meetz, K., et al.: Viewing workstation for 4D kinematic MR joint studies. Proc. Comp. Assisted Radiology and Surgery (CARS) (2005) 68–73
10. Magnenat-Thalmann, N., et al.: Hip joint reconstruction and motion visualization using MRI and optical motion capture. Proc. of the Austrian, German and Swiss Society for Biomedical Technology Congress (EMB) (2003) 20–23
11. Melchert, U.H., et al.: Motion-triggered cine MR imaging of active joint movement. Magn. Reson. Imaging **10** (1992) 457–460
12. Pekar, V., Gladilin, E.: Deformable image registration by adaptive gaussian forces. Proc. ECCV 2004 Workshop CVAMIA and MMBIA (2004) 317–328
13. Gill, P.E., et al.: Practical Optimization. Academic Press (1981)
14. Rueckert, D., et al.: Nonrigid registration using free-form deformations: Application to breast MR. IEEE Trans. Med. Imaging **18** (1999) 712–721
15. Schulz, H., et al.: Real-time interactive viewing of 4D kinematic MR joint studies. Medical Image Computing and Computer-Assisted Intervention (MICCAI) (2005)
16. Shellock, F.G., et al.: Kinematic MR imaging of patella-femoral joint: comparison of passive positioning and active movement techniques. Radiology **184** (1992) 574–577

Author Index

Angelopoulou, Anastassia 210
Astley, O. 178
Audette, M.A. 178
Axel, Leon 93
Ayache, Nicholas 1
Ayvacı, Alper 388

Bao, Hujun 499
Bayro-Corrochano, Eduardo 449
Bellardine, Carissa 367
Betke, Margrit 367
Bhandarkar, S.M. 146
Bistritz, Aalo 469
Bond, Sarah L. 399
Bourgeat, Pierrick 51
Brady, J. Michael 261, 399
Bystrov, Daniel 551

Carpenter, Anne 535
Celi, Juan Carlos 251
Chen, Terrence 114
Chen, Wei 499
Chen, Ying 200
Cheng, Lishui 61, 160
Chinzei, K. 178
Chowdhury, A.S. 146
Christiansen, Claus 230
Chung, Albert C.S. 281, 314
Cohen, Laurent D. 335
Comaniciu, Dorin 388
Conrad-Hansen, Lars A. 409
Crozier, Stuart 51
Cunningham, Michael L. 302

Dam, Erik 230
de Bruijne, Marleen 170, 409
Delingette, H. 178
Diallo, Mamadou 251
Ding, Feng 459

Echigo, Tomio 271
Ee, Xianhe 200

Fan, Xian 61, 160
Ferris, Daron 240
Fischl, Bruce 135

Fisher, John 489
Florin, Charles 427
Folkesson, Jenny 230
Fripp, Jurgen 51
Fuchs, A. 178

Gan, Rui 281
Geurts, Pierre 220
Golland, Polina 3, 535
Gong, Gaolong 13, 544
Greiner, Russell 469
Grimson, Eric 3, 135, 261, 489
Gu, Jia 240
Gu, Jianwei 526
Gu, Lixu 419
Guoping, Wang 517

Hakansson, Johan 240
Hansson, Ulf 240
He, Yong 13
Hing, Anne V. 302
Howe, Tet Sen 200
Hu, Dewen 508
Huang, Ke 103
Huang, Pengfei 419
Huang, Rui 82
Huang, Thomas S. 114

Jeavons, Alan P. 437
Jiang, Tianzi 13, 544
Jones, Thouis R. 535

Kanade, Takeo 24
Khamene, Ali 251, 427
Kikinis, Ron 489
Krolik, Jeffrey 346
Kubota, Toshiro 324

Lange, Holger 240
Lauze, François 409
Law, W.K. 314
Learned-Miller, Erik 291
Lee, Chi-Hoon 469
Leow, Wee Kheng 200, 459
Li, Fuchun 13
Li, Hua 335, 356

Li, Kang   24
Li, Liang   526
Li, Ming   508
Li, Shuyu   13
Li, Wenjing   240
Li, Xiaobo   13
Liang, Meng   13
Liao, Rui   346
Lin, Fuchun   544
Lin, H. Jill   302
Liu, Fayi   508
Liu, Huafeng   499
Liu, Yadong   508
Luan, Hongxia   378
Lutchen, Kenneth   367

Magee, Derek   437
Marée, Raphaël   220
McGonagle, Dennis   437
McKeown, Martin   346
Meetz, Kirsten   551
Metaxas, Dimitris N.   82, 93
Mewes, Andrea J.U.   51
Mullally, William   367
Murtha, Albert   469

Netsch, Thomas   551
Nielsen, Mads   409
Noble, J. Alison   25

Okada, Kazunori   324
Olsen, Ole Fogh   230
Ourselin, Sébastien   51

Paragios, Nikos   427
Pavlovic, Vladimir   82
Pekar, Vladimir   551
Peng, Zhigang   189
Pettersen, Paola   230
Piater, Justus   220
Pless, Robert   479
Pohl, Kilian M.   489
Pongnumkul, Suchit   271
Pons, Jean-Philippe   135
Prince, Jerry L.   72
Psarrou, Alexandra   210

Qian, Zhen   93
Qi, Feihu   378

Revett, Kenneth   210
Ritter, E.   146
Rivera-Rovelo, Jorge   449
Rocha, Kelvin R.   72
Rodríguez, José García   210
Rousson, Mikael   251
Ruiz-Correa, Salvador   302

Sagawa, Ryusuke   271
Sander, Jöerg   469
Sauer, Frank   251
Schmidt, Mark   469
Schulz, Heinrich   551
Ségonne, Florent   135
Shapiro, Linda G.   302
Shen, Dinggang   378
Shen, Hong   189
Shi, Pengcheng   499
Shi, Yonggang   189
Speltz, Matthew L.   302
Stewart, Charles V.   31
Sze, Raymond W.   302

Tang, Songyuan   13
Tanko, Laszlo B.   409
Tanner, Steven   437
Tek, Hüseyin   388
Tian, Lixia   13
Tollner, E.W.   146

Van Raad, Viara   125, 240

Wai, Lionel C.C.   261
Waller, Michael   437
Wang, Shih-Chang   459
Warfield, Simon K.   51
Wehenkel, Louis   220
Wells, William M.   291, 489
Williams, James   427

Xiang, Yang   314
Xie, Sheng   544
Xu, Jianfeng   419
Xu, Xi   517

Yagi, Yasushi   271
Yan, Lirong   508
Yan, Michelle   103
Yang, Jie   61, 160
Ye, Jian   314
Yezzi, Anthony   72, 335, 356
Yin, Wotao   114

Yu, Guoqiang   526
Yu, J.C.   146

Zang, Guohua   508
Zang, Yufeng   13
Zhang, G.   146
Zhang, Kai   517
Zhang, Li   517
Zhang, Li   526

Zhang, Qilong   479
Zhang, Shaoting   419
Zheng, Yuanjie   160
Zhou, Xiang Sean   114
Zhou, Zongtan   508
Zhu, Chaozhe   13
Zhu, Yun   61, 160
Zhuang, Ling   499
Zöllei, Lilla   291

Lecture Notes in Computer Science

For information about Vols. 1–3655

please contact your bookseller or Springer

Vol. 3765: Y. Liu, T. Jiang, C. Zhang (Eds.), Computer Vision for Biomedical Image Applications. X, 563 pages. 2005.

Vol. 3752: N. Paragios, O. Faugeras, T. Chan, C. Schnoerr (Eds.), Variational, Geometric, and Level Set Methods in Computer Vision. XI, 369 pages. 2005.

Vol. 3751: T. Magedanz, E.R. M. Madeira, P. Dini (Eds.), Operations and Management in IP-Based Networks. X, 213 pages. 2005.

Vol. 3750: J.S. Duncan, G. Gerig (Eds.), Medical Image Computing and Computer-Assisted Intervention – MICCAI 2005, Part II. XL, 1018 pages. 2005.

Vol. 3749: J.S. Duncan, G. Gerig (Eds.), Medical Image Computing and Computer-Assisted Intervention – MICCAI 2005, Part I. XXXIX, 942 pages. 2005.

Vol. 3744: T. Magedanz, A. Karmouch, S. Pierre, I. Venieris (Eds.), Mobility Aware Technologies and Applications. XIV, 418 pages. 2005.

Vol. 3739: W. Fan, Z. Wu, J. Yang (Eds.), Advances in Web-Age Information Management. XXIV, 930 pages. 2005.

Vol. 3738: V.R. Syrotiuk, E. Chávez (Eds.), Ad-Hoc, Mobile, and Wireless Networks. XI, 360 pages. 2005.

Vol. 3735: A. Hoffmann, H. Motoda, T. Scheffer (Eds.), Discovery Science. XVI, 400 pages. 2005. (Subseries LNAI).

Vol. 3734: S. Jain, H.U. Simon, E. Tomita (Eds.), Algorithmic Learning Theory. XII, 490 pages. 2005. (Subseries LNAI).

Vol. 3733: P. Yolum, T. Güngör, F. Gürgen, C. Özturan (Eds.), Computer and Information Sciences - ISCIS 2005. XXI, 973 pages. 2005.

Vol. 3731: F. Wang (Ed.), Formal Techniques for Networked and Distributed Systems - FORTE 2005. XII, 558 pages. 2005.

Vol. 3728: V. Paliouras, J. Vounckx, D. Verkest (Eds.), Integrated Circuit and System Design. XV, 753 pages. 2005.

Vol. 3726: L.T. Yang, O.F. Rana, B. Di Martino, J. Dongarra (Eds.), High Performance Computing and Communcations. XXVI, 1116 pages. 2005.

Vol. 3725: D. Borrione, W. Paul (Eds.), Correct Hardware Design and Verification Methods. XII, 412 pages. 2005.

Vol. 3724: P. Fraigniaud (Ed.), Distributed Computing. XIV, 520 pages. 2005.

Vol. 3723: W. Zhao, S. Gong, X. Tang (Eds.), Analysis and Modelling of Faces and Gestures. XI, 4234 pages. 2005.

Vol. 3722: D. Van Hung, M. Wirsing (Eds.), Theoretical Aspects of Computing – ICTAC 2005. XIV, 614 pages. 2005.

Vol. 3721: A. Jorge, L. Torgo, P. Brazdil, R. Camacho, J. Gama (Eds.), Knowledge Discovery in Databases: PKDD 2005. XXIII, 719 pages. 2005. (Subseries LNAI).

Vol. 3720: J. Gama, R. Camacho, P. Brazdil, A. Jorge, L. Torgo (Eds.), Machine Learning: ECML 2005. XXIII, 769 pages. 2005. (Subseries LNAI).

Vol. 3719: M. Hobbs, A.M. Goscinski, W. Zhou (Eds.), Distributed and Parallel Computing. XI, 448 pages. 2005.

Vol. 3718: V.G. Ganzha, E.W. Mayr, E.V. Vorozhtsov (Eds.), Computer Algebra in Scientific Computing. XII, 502 pages. 2005.

Vol. 3717: B. Gramlich (Ed.), Frontiers of Combining Systems. X, 321 pages. 2005. (Subseries LNAI).

Vol. 3715: E. Dawson, S. Vaudenay (Eds.), Progress in Cryptology – Mycrypt 2005. XI, 329 pages. 2005.

Vol. 3714: H. Obbink, K. Pohl (Eds.), Software Product Lines. XIII, 235 pages. 2005.

Vol. 3713: L. Briand, C. Williams (Eds.), Model Driven Engineering Languages and Systems. XV, 722 pages. 2005.

Vol. 3712: R. Reussner, J. Mayer, J.A. Stafford, S. Overhage, S. Becker, P.J. Schroeder (Eds.), Quality of Software Architectures and Software Quality. XIII, 289 pages. 2005.

Vol. 3711: F. Kishino, Y. Kitamura, H. Kato, N. Nagata (Eds.), Entertainment Computing - ICEC 2005. XXIV, 540 pages. 2005.

Vol. 3710: M. Barni, I. Cox, T. Kalker, H.J. Kim (Eds.), Digital Watermarking. XII, 485 pages. 2005.

Vol. 3709: P. van Beek (Ed.), Principles and Practice of Constraint Programming - CP 2005. XX, 887 pages. 2005.

Vol. 3708: J. Blanc-Talon, W. Philips, D. Popescu, P. Scheunders (Eds.), Advanced Concepts for Intelligent Vision Systems. XXII, 725 pages. 2005.

Vol. 3707: D.A. Peled, Y.-K. Tsay (Eds.), Automated Technology for Verification and Analysis. XII, 506 pages. 2005.

Vol. 3706: H. Fuks, S. Lukosch, A.C. Salgado (Eds.), Groupware: Design, Implementation, and Use. XII, 378 pages. 2005.

Vol. 3704: M. De Gregorio, V. Di Maio, M. Frucci, C. Musio (Eds.), Brain, Vision, and Artificial Intelligence. XV, 556 pages. 2005.

Vol. 3703: F. Fages, S. Soliman (Eds.), Principles and Practice of Semantic Web Reasoning. VIII, 163 pages. 2005.

Vol. 3702: B. Beckert (Ed.), Automated Reasoning with Analytic Tableaux and Related Methods. XIII, 343 pages. 2005. (Subseries LNAI).

Vol. 3701: M. Coppo, E. Lodi, G. M. Pinna (Eds.), Theoretical Computer Science. XI, 411 pages. 2005.

Vol. 3699: C.S. Calude, M.J. Dinneen, G. Păun, M. J. Pérez-Jiménez, G. Rozenberg (Eds.), Unconventional Computation. XI, 267 pages. 2005.

Vol. 3698: U. Furbach (Ed.), KI 2005: Advances in Artificial Intelligence. XIII, 409 pages. 2005. (Subseries LNAI).

Vol. 3697: W. Duch, J. Kacprzyk, E. Oja, S. Zadrożny (Eds.), Artificial Neural Networks: Formal Models and Their Applications – ICANN 2005, Part II. XXXII, 1045 pages. 2005.

Vol. 3696: W. Duch, J. Kacprzyk, E. Oja, S. Zadrożny (Eds.), Artificial Neural Networks: Biological Inspirations – ICANN 2005, Part I. XXXI, 703 pages. 2005.

Vol. 3695: M.R. Berthold, R. Glen, K. Diederichs, O. Kohlbacher, I. Fischer (Eds.), Computational Life Sciences. XI, 277 pages. 2005. (Subseries LNBI).

Vol. 3694: M. Malek, E. Nett, N. Suri (Eds.), Service Availability. VIII, 213 pages. 2005.

Vol. 3693: A.G. Cohn, D.M. Mark (Eds.), Spatial Information Theory. XII, 493 pages. 2005.

Vol. 3692: R. Casadio, G. Myers (Eds.), Algorithms in Bioinformatics. X, 436 pages. 2005. (Subseries LNBI).

Vol. 3691: A. Gagalowicz, W. Philips (Eds.), Computer Analysis of Images and Patterns. XIX, 865 pages. 2005.

Vol. 3690: M. Pěchouček, P. Petta, L.Z. Varga (Eds.), Multi-Agent Systems and Applications IV. XVII, 667 pages. 2005. (Subseries LNAI).

Vol. 3689: G.G. Lee, A. Yamada, H. Meng, S.H. Myaeng (Eds.), Information Retrieval Technology. XVII, 735 pages. 2005.

Vol. 3688: R. Winther, B.A. Gran, G. Dahll (Eds.), Computer Safety, Reliability, and Security. XI, 405 pages. 2005.

Vol. 3687: S. Singh, M. Singh, C. Apte, P. Perner (Eds.), Pattern Recognition and Image Analysis, Part II. XXV, 809 pages. 2005.

Vol. 3686: S. Singh, M. Singh, C. Apte, P. Perner (Eds.), Pattern Recognition and Data Mining, Part I. XXVI, 689 pages. 2005.

Vol. 3685: V. Gorodetsky, I. Kotenko, V. Skormin (Eds.), Computer Network Security. XIV, 480 pages. 2005.

Vol. 3684: R. Khosla, R.J. Howlett, L.C. Jain (Eds.), Knowledge-Based Intelligent Information and Engineering Systems, Part IV. LXXIX, 933 pages. 2005. (Subseries LNAI).

Vol. 3683: R. Khosla, R.J. Howlett, L.C. Jain (Eds.), Knowledge-Based Intelligent Information and Engineering Systems, Part III. LXXX, 1397 pages. 2005. (Subseries LNAI).

Vol. 3682: R. Khosla, R.J. Howlett, L.C. Jain (Eds.), Knowledge-Based Intelligent Information and Engineering Systems, Part II. LXXIX, 1371 pages. 2005. (Subseries LNAI).

Vol. 3681: R. Khosla, R.J. Howlett, L.C. Jain (Eds.), Knowledge-Based Intelligent Information and Engineering Systems, Part I. LXXX, 1319 pages. 2005. (Subseries LNAI).

Vol. 3679: S.d.C. di Vimercati, P. Syverson, D. Gollmann (Eds.), Computer Security – ESORICS 2005. XI, 509 pages. 2005.

Vol. 3678: A. McLysaght, D.H. Huson (Eds.), Comparative Genomics. VIII, 167 pages. 2005. (Subseries LNBI).

Vol. 3677: J. Dittmann, S. Katzenbeisser, A. Uhl (Eds.), Communications and Multimedia Security. XIII, 360 pages. 2005.

Vol. 3676: R. Glück, M. Lowry (Eds.), Generative Programming and Component Engineering. XI, 448 pages. 2005.

Vol. 3675: Y. Luo (Ed.), Cooperative Design, Visualization, and Engineering. XI, 264 pages. 2005.

Vol. 3674: W. Jonker, M. Petković (Eds.), Secure Data Management. X, 241 pages. 2005.

Vol. 3673: S. Bandini, S. Manzoni (Eds.), AI*IA 2005: Advances in Artificial Intelligence. XIV, 614 pages. 2005. (Subseries LNAI).

Vol. 3672: C. Hankin, I. Siveroni (Eds.), Static Analysis. X, 369 pages. 2005.

Vol. 3671: S. Bressan, S. Ceri, E. Hunt, Z.G. Ives, Z. Bellahsène, M. Rys, R. Unland (Eds.), Database and XML Technologies. X, 239 pages. 2005.

Vol. 3670: M. Bravetti, L. Kloul, G. Zavattaro (Eds.), Formal Techniques for Computer Systems and Business Processes. XIII, 349 pages. 2005.

Vol. 3669: G.S. Brodal, S. Leonardi (Eds.), Algorithms – ESA 2005. XVIII, 901 pages. 2005.

Vol. 3668: M. Gabbrielli, G. Gupta (Eds.), Logic Programming. XIV, 454 pages. 2005.

Vol. 3666: B.D. Martino, D. Kranzlmüller, J. Dongarra (Eds.), Recent Advances in Parallel Virtual Machine and Message Passing Interface. XVII, 546 pages. 2005.

Vol. 3665: K. S. Candan, A. Celentano (Eds.), Advances in Multimedia Information Systems. X, 221 pages. 2005.

Vol. 3664: C. Türker, M. Agosti, H.-J. Schek (Eds.), Peer-to-Peer, Grid, and Service-Orientation in Digital Library Architectures. X, 261 pages. 2005.

Vol. 3663: W.G. Kropatsch, R. Sablatnig, A. Hanbury (Eds.), Pattern Recognition. XIV, 512 pages. 2005.

Vol. 3662: C. Baral, G. Greco, N. Leone, G. Terracina (Eds.), Logic Programming and Nonmonotonic Reasoning. XIII, 454 pages. 2005. (Subseries LNAI).

Vol. 3661: T. Panayiotopoulos, J. Gratch, R. Aylett, D. Ballin, P. Olivier, T. Rist (Eds.), Intelligent Virtual Agents. XIII, 506 pages. 2005. (Subseries LNAI).

Vol. 3660: M. Beigl, S. Intille, J. Rekimoto, H. Tokuda (Eds.), UbiComp 2005: Ubiquitous Computing. XVII, 394 pages. 2005.

Vol. 3659: J.R. Rao, B. Sunar (Eds.), Cryptographic Hardware and Embedded Systems – CHES 2005. XIV, 458 pages. 2005.

Vol. 3658: V. Matoušek, P. Mautner, T. Pavelka (Eds.), Text, Speech and Dialogue. XV, 460 pages. 2005. (Subseries LNAI).

Vol. 3657: F.S. de Boer, M.M. Bonsangue, S. Graf, W.-P. de Roever (Eds.), Formal Methods for Components and Objects. VIII, 325 pages. 2005.

Vol. 3656: M. Kamel, A. Campilho (Eds.), Image Analysis and Recognition. XXIV, 1279 pages. 2005.